Order no 17095   £45. C

D1423484

P001915

The Upper Limb and Hand

The Upper Limb and Hand

Nicholas Barton

Emeritus Consultant Hand Surgeon, Nottingham University Hospital

and

Patrick Mulligan

Consultant Hand Surgeon, Royal Orthopaedic Hospital, Birmingham

W.B. Saunders Company Limited London
London Edinburgh New York Philadelphia Sydney Toronto

WB SAUNDERS
An imprint of Harcourt Publishers Limited

First published 1999

ISBN 0 7020 2236 5

British Library Cataloguing in Publication Data
A catalogue record for this book is available from the British Library

Library of Congress Cataloging in Publication Data
A catalog record for this book is available from the Library of Congress

Note
Medical knowledge is constantly changing. As new information becomes
available, changes in treatment, procedures, equipment and the use of drugs
become necessary. The editors/authors/contributors and the publishers
have, as far as it is possible, taken care to ensure that the information given
in this text is accurate and up-to-date. However, readers are strongly
advised to confirm that the information, especially with regard to drug
usage, complies with the latest legislation and standards of practice.

The
publisher's
policy is to use
**paper manufactured
from sustainable forests**

Typeset by PTU Edinburgh
Printed in Hong Kong

Contents

Contributors

Nicholas Barton, FRCS Eng
Emeritus Consultant Orthopaedic Hand Surgeon,
Nottingham University Hospital,
Queen's Medical Centre, Nottingham

Tim Bunker, FRCS Eng, MCh Orth
Consultant Orthopaedic Surgeon,
Princess Elizabeth Orthopaedic Centre,
Royal Devon and Exeter Hospital, Exeter

Michael Craigen, FRCS Ed, FRCS Orth
Consultant Orthopaedic and Hand Surgeon,
Royal Orthopaedic Hospital, Birmingham

James Crossan, FRCSG
Consultant Hand Surgeon,
Western Infirmary, Glasgow

Tim Davis, ChM, FRCS Eng
Consultant Orthopaedic Hand Surgeon,
Nottingham University Hospital,
Queen's Medical Centre, Nottingham

Colin Dent, FRCS Eng, FRCS Orth
Senior Lecturer and Honorary Consultant
Orthopaedic Surgeon, University of Wales
College of Medicine, Cardiff

Peter G Lunn, FRCS Eng, FRCS Ed
Consultant Orthopaedic and Hand Surgeon,
Pulvertaft Hand Centre,
Derbyshire Royal Infirmary, Derby

Patrick Mulligan, FRCS Eng, FRCSG
Consultant Hand and Orthopaedic Surgeon,
Royal Orthopaedic Hospital, Birmingham

Ian A Trail, MD, FRCS Ed
Consultant Upper Limb Surgeon,
Wrightington Hospital, near Wigan, Lancashire

Michael Waldram, FRCS Ed (Orth)
Consultant Orthopaedic and Hand Surgeon,
Royal Orthopaedic Hospital,
Birmingham

Preface

When we became orthopaedic surgeons, there was only one examination in Britain devoted exclusively to the practice of orthopaedic surgery: that was the M. Ch. Orth. of the University of Liverpool. In order to take this, one had to work in or around Liverpool. All the other English-speaking nations had recently developed examinations in the specialty. In contrast, the Royal Colleges of Surgery examined us in many subjects but not the one in which we were going to practice for the rest of our lives. The F.R.C.S. had long ceased to mark the end of training and had become a licence to start Higher Surgical Training. Another important factor was that we had no postgraduate specialist surgical qualification which was recognised in any other country. This was plainly ridiculous and we added our support to those campaigning to introduce an examination in orthopaedic surgery.

The Royal College of Surgeons of Edinburgh led the way. Under the stimulus of J.I.P. James, who was Professor of Orthopaedic Surgery in Edinburgh at that time, a Speciality Fellowship was introduced in 1979. There was one in orthopaedic surgery and one in neurosurgery; cardio-thoracic surgery followed in 1982. This went on for eleven years. The examination remained optional but soon established an acceptance of quality. The benefits were quickly apparent to both candidates and examiners. It was an entirely clinical and *viva voce* format. The standard was high and the pass-rate variable. It was not an easy exam and was said to compare favourably with the examination in the Royal Australasian College of Surgeons. It was even accepted as an equivalent qualification there.

One of the obstacles to the development of such an examination was the fact that there are four Royal Colleges concerned: those of England, Edinburgh, Glasgow and Ireland. It was and still is, difficult to get agreement between the four Colleges about any change. In due course, however, the advantages of the Edinburgh examination were seen and all of the Colleges agreed to collaborate. It was now accepted that a recognition of the standard of Higher Surgical Training by assessment in the form of an examination was essential in all the surgical specialities.

A new Intercollegiate Examination, building on the experience gained in Edinburgh, was introduced in 1990 and takes place twice a year in each of the Colleges in turn. The examiners are drawn from Fellows of all four Royal Colleges. At first, this too was voluntary but in 1991 it became a requirement for accreditation, together with a completed training in one of the Training Programmes which had been inspected and approved by the Specialist Advisory Committee. The format of the examination and adjudication is constantly under review by the Intercollegiate Board.

What used to be the final F.R.C.S. had a pass rate of about 20% and was a formidable hurdle, many failing at the first attempt. The F.R.C.S. (Orth.) examination can only be taken by those who have completed four years of orthopaedic training and, therefore, one would expect most of them to pass. This is, in fact, what happens and the pass-rate is over 80%. Those who have undertaken good clinical work, read the appropriate literature and, most of all, have a sound instructional course will probably pass so there is no need to regard it as a frightful ordeal. If one is a member of the small number who do not pass, it is frequently because of nervousness which prevents a candidate from giving his best and this experience should make it easier to pass the next time around. Sometimes failure is related to inadequacies in the Training Programme provided but a curriculum should help to prevent this. The "clinicals" – long cases and short cases – are crucial because if this aspect is failed, doing well in the other parts of the examination does not allow redemption. Where a sub-standard (but not dreadful) performance in one of the vivas can be compensated for by an above-average performance in other vivas, failure in the clinicals can make it impossible to pass. The clinical exam is held in a hospital ward, clinic or hall, in circumstances very different from normal practice, but it is best approached as though you were presenting the case to the consultant with whom you work or meeting the patient for the first time in a clinic.

The examiners are not there to trip up the candidates. On the contrary, they want to give you an opportunity to show what you know. If the examiner seems to be trying to point you in a particular direction, it is wise to follow this advice. He may, out of habit, use the opportunity to teach you something. On some subjects, opinions differ and most examiners accept this, but it is unwise to argue with the examiner. It may be that you actually know more about a particular subject than the examiner, but try not to make this too obvious. Many examiners like to ask about classifications as these give a quick reference to knowledge of a particular subject. You will have to know the accepted classifications of various diseases and treatments. We distinguish between stages and types. If a disease progresses through different stages, then you must know these and that necessarily involves knowing the order in which the stages occur. It is reasonable to expect you to know them as Stage I, Stage 2, etc. However, where a condition is divided for the purpose of classification into different types, what you need to know are the types and not necessarily the numbers or letters which have been arbitrarily assigned to each.

Finally, remember that it is also a hard day for the examiner. Asking questions about the same subject throughout the day is tiring. For variety the examiner may ask you about an eponym ("Who was Colles?") It does not matter if you do not know the answer; this is to be regarded as light relief. The examiner will welcome any variation and, if you bring up a subject or diagnosis, he is likely to seize upon it for diversion, so don't mention anything you are not willing to pursue. This is usually the explanation when the candidate comes out and says "The bastard grilled me about hydatid cysts" or some other rarity; in most cases the candidate brought it up himself!

This book is one of a series primarily intended to prepare you for the F.R.C.S. Orth, though it should also be of use to orthopeadic and hand surgeons in other countries, to plastic surgeons wishing to learn more about the hand, and to hand therapists. There is to be another volume devoted to trauma. We felt that injuries to tendons and nerves are such an important part of hand surgery that they should be included in this Upper Limb volume. We decided also to cover here other soft-tissue injuries, in particular dislocations and subsequent instability, but fractures of the upper limb will be dealt with in a future WB Saunders publication.

We hope you will find this book interesting and readable. We are grateful to the contributors, who have put a lot of study, thought and work into preparing their chapters. Three of them are or have been examiners, two have master's degrees in orthopaedics and four have taken and passed either the Intercollegiate F.R.C.S. Orth. or its Edinburgh predecessor; one had to take it twice and considers himself especially well qualified to contribute to this book! It should prepare you for the examination and, in some cases, may contain more detail than you will be asked. It is an *aide memoire*.

Good luck, but it shouldn't really be needed!

Nicholas Barton
Patrick Mulligan

1

The Shoulder

Tim Bunker

The shoulder specialist is in a most fortunate and privileged position. In every clinic he will encounter such a rich parade of shoulder pathology. He will see patients with impingement, small cuff tears, large cuff tears, cuff arthropathy, anterior dislocations, posterior dislocations, multidirectional and volitional dislocations, frozen shoulders, rheumatoid shoulders, osteoarthritic shoulders and a weird and wonderful panoply of secondary arthritides. The icing on the cake are the neurological conditions which attend the shoulder clinic: the winging scapulae, the thoracic outlet syndromes, neuralgic amyotrophy and a variety of nerve palsies. On top of this come the curios: the Sprengels, the obstetric plexus palsies, glenoid dysplasias, the muscular dystrophies as well as disorders of the acromioclavicular and sternoclavicular joints.

However, fortune and privilege come with obligations. Diagnosis is difficult and the surgeon is obliged to spend time, to expend effort and to be diligent in observing the patient. The majority of shoulder disorders affect ligament, tendon, muscle and nerve rather than bone or joint and therefore do not show on radiographs. Diagnosis thus depends on clinical skills, taking a detailed history, making a thorough examination and then applying intellectual vigour to come to a correct diagnosis. This is not to ignore the benefit of investigation, for plain radiographs, magnetic resonance imaging (MRI) and arthroscopy are often needed to confirm or refute a diagnosis, but investigations play a far smaller role in diagnosis of shoulder disorders than do radiographs in the hip and arthroscopy in the knee.

The explosion of interest in surgery of the shoulder has come about for two reasons. First, we have come to understand the pathology behind most shoulder conditions, even such enigmas as the frozen shoulder. This has allowed the planning of rational and logical treatment for virtually all shoulder conditions. Second, surgery has become so predictable and reliable that we can effectively treat most conditions around the shoulder. It is incredible to look back just 15 years when all that could be offered to patients with shoulder pain was an injection of steroid, a manipulation or a Putti Platt operation. Now there is acromioplasty for impingement, effective methods of cuff repair using suture anchors, capsular shifts and Bankart's with anchors for dislocations, third-generation unconstrained modular shoulder replacements for arthritis, nerve grafts and muscle transfers for neurological disorders and increasingly effective arthroscopic techniques.

This is not to be complacent, for there are many challenges waiting to be solved. Shoulder surgeons still argue over many aspects of our sub-speciality: the aetiology of shoulder disorders, methods of diagnosis, which investigations to use and when, the indications for surgery and the timing of surgery. On the practical side we have no consistently effective surgical solution for the massive rotator cuff tear, cuff arthropathy and recurrent posterior dislocation. Shoulder replacements are no longer experimental but still have a long way to go before functional results are as good or as consistent as knee or hip replacements. Finally rehabilitation protocols are continuing to evolve and improve.

In summary, if you are creative and energetic and want a career which is both intellectually and practically challenging and which will keep you occupied, intrigued and professionally fulfilled, then you could do worse than specialising in disorders of the shoulder.

FUNCTIONAL ANATOMY OF THE SHOULDER

This book assumes that as an orthopaedic surgeon you have a reasonable grasp of musculoskeletal anatomy. However, in order to master the theory and practice of shoulder surgery there are several aspects of the functional anatomy of the shoulder region which need to be reviewed. Normal shoulder function is dependent on the synchronous and correctly orchestrated motion of the clavicle, scapula and humerus as well as the joints which bind them together.

Bony anatomy

The clavicle

This is a flat bone formed in membrane. The bone is subcutaneous, with only the supraclavicular nerves coursing over it. It is the only bony strut supporting the arm. It acts with the first rib as a nut-cracker in the thoracic outlet syndrome. It is commonly fractured and was the cause of death of both King William III and Sir Robert Peel, the founder of the police force.

The scapula

The scapula is the heart of the shoulder. Its body is formed by intramembranous ossification. The glenoid fossa has two ossification centres. Failure of development of the inferior centre leads to primary glenoid dysplasia. The acromion has two ossification centres. Failure of fusion of the acromion to the scapula occurs fairly commonly, in fact in 7% of people, leading to the os acromiale. The os acromiale is associated with impingement and rotator cuff tears, as it can hinge down on its pseudarthrosis impacting against the rotator cuff.

The coracoid is the key to the anterior surgical approach to the shoulder, the deltopectoral approach. It is an easily palpated landmark and a watershed which has a safe surgical approach on its lateral side and the lurking danger of the brachial plexus and neurovascular bundle on its medial side. Four ligaments attach to the coracoid: the coracohumeral which contracts in frozen shoulder, the coraco-acromial which is responsible for many of the changes of impingement, and the conoid and trapezoid ligaments which tear in acromioclavicular

joint dislocation. Two muscles originate from the coracoid, the short head of biceps and the coracobrachialis, and one inserts into it, pectoralis minor. Release the pectoralis minor from the coracoid and you have instant access to the infraclavicular brachial plexus.

The acromion is highly developed in humans. Of all the primates, only the chimpanzee has an acromion anything like the size of the human acromion. Of course if you have a large acromion it impedes brachiation through the trees, but it does give you a massive platform for a powerful deltoid. The disadvantage of this oversized acromion is that if you work overhead or continue to swing through the trees you are likely to get impingement of the acromion against the rotator cuff; in particular you will abut the anterior edge of the acromion against the insertion of the supraspinatus tendon. Dr Charles Neer noted that certain changes appeared to occur to this anterior edge of the acromion which were associated with shoulder pain and rotator cuff tears. He found a characteristic ridge of proliferative spurs where the coraco-acromial ligament inserts into a crescentic footprint on the undersurface of the anterior acromion. In the later stages of the disease, this area becomes eburnated where it is literally polished by rubbing against the underlying cuff.

Dr Neer's protegé Dr Bigliani found that there were differing morphological shapes to this anterior acromion. By looking at the sagittal cross-section of the acromion, he found that some acromions have a flat undersurface (type I), some are curved (type II), and some are so curved that the anterior acromion actually hooks down towards the rotator cuff (type III). The latter, Bigliani type III hooked acromions, are found in a high proportion of patients with rotator cuff tears, although, as you will find when we come to discuss impingement, this is a topic which is hotly debated.

The glenoid is pear-shaped, 35 mm in height and 25 mm from front to back. It is concave and appears on the skeleton and in radiographs to have a shallower radius of curvature than the humeral head. However, the cartilage surface is highly congruent with the humeral head and this means that the articular hyaline cartilage is thick at the periphery and thin in the centre. This thinning of the cartilage in the centre of the glenoid gives the typical appearance of a 'grey spot' in the centre of the articular surface as seen arthroscopically. The surface of the glenoid is very small compared to the humeral head, a feature which is beneficial in that it allows the shoulder to be the most mobile joint in the body, but also leads to the Achilles' heel of the shoulder: its readiness to dislocate. The articular surface is enlarged by the glenoid labrum which also acts as the anchor for the long head of biceps tendon and the glenohumeral ligaments.

Proximal humerus

The proximal humerus consists of a spherical epiphysis mated to a cylindrical metaphysis. The epiphysis has three centres of ossification, one for the head, one for the greater tuberosity and a third which can really be ignored because the centre for the lesser tuberosity appears in the fifth year and coalesces with the centre for the greater tuberosity in the same year, so blink and you will miss it!

The centre of rotation of the spherical epiphysis does not lie on the line of the centre of the shaft of the humerus. It lies medial to this line (medial offset) and posterior to it (posterior offset). This offset is important in relation to the geometry of shoulder replacement. The head of the humerus is retroverted 21° from both the coronal plane of the body and the transepicondylar plane.

The ligaments of the glenohumeral joint

The glenoid labrum

Although the labrum is not a ligament, it is the anchor for the glenohumeral ligaments and the major site of disruption in traumatic dislocation. The labrum is a complete fibrocartilaginous circle which is wedge-shaped in cross-section, much like the meniscus of the knee. When discussing sectors of the labrum, we use a convention of dividing the face of the glenoid like a clock face. The 12 o'clock position is the superior pole of the glenoid where the long head of biceps arises from the labrum and is contiguous with it. Both long head and labrum are anchored to the supraglenoid tubercle at this 12 o'clock position. By convention 3 o'clock is always the anterior rim of the glenoid. Thus the clockface is clockwise for the right shoulder, but runs anticlockwise for the left shoulder! The labrum is subject to variations between the 2 o'clock and 3 o'clock positions. These are variants of normal

and are not associated with pathology. Thus at the 2 o'clock position the labrum may be detached from the bone. This normal variant leaves a sublabral hole which should not be confused with a Bankart tear. If such a detached but normal labrum is associated with an abnormal middle glenohumeral ligament which is cord-shaped and arises from the long head of biceps tendon then this is called a 'Buford complex' and is again a variant of normal. From 3 o'clock to 9 o'clock, the normal labrum is firmly attached to the glenoid; any detachment at this point is pathological (the Bankart lesion).

The coracohumeral ligament

This is a very strong but oft-neglected ligament with a tensile failure at 360 newtons, making it three-and-a-half times as strong as the superior glenohumeral ligament which accompanies it. The coracohumeral ligament runs from the base of the coracoid to the intertubercular groove of the humerus. If we compare the hip and the shoulder, then the analogue of the coracohumeral ligament is the Y-shaped ligament of Bigelow, said to be the strongest ligament in the body.

The superior glenohumeral ligament

This arises from the glenoid labrum at the 1 o'clock position and runs just anterior to the tendon of long head of biceps. Half-way to its insertion, it starts to blend with the coracohumeral ligament so that the latter forms the cross-bar of a T and the superior glenohumeral ligament, lying perpendicular, makes up the downstroke of the T. As these ligaments merge and course laterally, they wrap around the long head of biceps tendon and make up the internal reflection of the pulley for the long head of biceps as it passes into the sulcus.

The middle glenohumeral ligament

The middle glenohumeral ligament is highly variable in its structure. It courses obliquely from the labrum at 2 o'clock to the lesser tuberosity of the humerus. It may be a thin veil of tissue, or a strong cord-like band. There is an outpouching of the capsule above this ligament which forms the subscapular recess or bursa.

The inferior glenohumeral ligament

This is the most important of the glenohumeral ligaments for it is the main restraint against anterior dislocation when the arm is in the vulnerable position of apprehension. The inferior glenohumeral ligament originates from 4 o'clock to 8 o'clock on the face of the glenoid. It can be likened to a hammock in which lies the head of the humerus. The hammock has guy-ropes at the front and back (the anterior band and the posterior band) and a sheet between the bands which is the thinner capsule of the infraglenoid recess. Selective cutting experiments have shown that it is the primary restraint against anterior dislocation.

Ligaments of the acromioclavicular joint

The superior acromioclavicular ligament

This is the superior capsule of the acromioclavicular joint. Spanning the top of the joint, it suspends the intra-articular disc of the acromioclavicular joint.

Conoid and trapezoid ligaments

The conoid and trapezoid ligaments pass from the coracoid process to the clavicle. As such they are vital to the stability of the acromioclavicular joint and are torn in dislocation of this joint. Like the anterior cruciate in the knee, when they fail they are irreparable and their function has to be replaced with an augment, usually the coraco-acromial ligament.

Coraco-acromial ligament

The coraco-acromial ligament is not a true ligament of the acromioclavicular joint. However, it runs close and is a most important ligament as, together with the acromion and the coracoid, it makes up the coraco-acromial arch which is the secondary joint of the shoulder. This ligament may be triangular, quadrangular or multibanded. If the shoulder movement is dysfunctional for any reason, then the coraco-acromial ligament will come under increasing strain and will react to this. In so doing it will thicken and will show those features over its footprint of insertion to the anterior undersurface of the acromion which are described by that awful term 'enthesopathy'. The ligament insertion thickens, there are reactive changes with spur formation and the insertion gradually becomes disorganised. Because there are very fine tolerances in the movement of this secondary joint, any space-occupying lesion will rub against supraspinatus and lead to impingement and pain. Laboratory studies have shown that the ligament is highly innervated.

Ligaments of the sternoclavicular joint

The capsule of the sternoclavicular joint is thickened as the anterior and posterior sternoclavicular ligaments. The joint contains an intra-articular disc. The medial end of the clavicle is bound to the first rib by the anterior and posterior costoclavicular ligaments. The right and left clavicles are bound together by the inter-clavicular ligament.

The muscles of the rotator cuff

Supraspinatus

This is a bipennate muscle arising from the supra-spinatus fossa and supplied by the suprascapular nerve. It inserts into the greater tuberosity of the humerus. Characteristically impingement lesions and rotator cuff tears originate 7 mm behind the leading edge of this tendon, at the point of its insertion. The insertion is multilayered, the deep portion being weaker and apt to tear first: the 'rim rent' tear of Codman.

Infraspinatus

This is also bipennate, arising from the infraspinous fossa and also supplied by the suprascapular nerve. It is only affected by rotator cuff tears once the whole of the supraspinatus has detached. Teres minor is supplied by the axillary nerve, and thus there is a neural watershed between the two muscles which we use as the surgical approach into the posterior aspect of the shoulder.

Subscapularis

This is a powerful multipennate muscle arising from the front of the scapula and supplied by two nerves directly from the posterior cord of the brachial plexus. Purely muscular in its lower third, it progressively becomes more tendinous as we pass upward to its superior border which is a thick intra-articular tendinous structure, the secondary landmark of shoulder arthroscopy. The insertion blends with the capsule of the joint but can be easily separated for its fibres all run laterally whereas the capsule is much more amorphous. The junction of its middle and lower thirds is marked by the anterior circumflex humeral artery and its two venae commitante and is a key landmark in the deltopectoral approach to the shoulder.

Surgical anatomy of the nerves

Axillary nerve

The axillary nerve is one of the two terminal branches of the posterior cord, the other being the radial nerve. The axillary nerve immediately passes into the quadrilateral space with the posterior circumflex artery and vein. The quadrilateral space is really a conduit passing under the shoulder joint whose roof is the lower margin of subscapularis, then the axillary fold of the capsule of the shoulder joint and finally the lower border of teres minor. The bottom of this conduit is made of the upper margins of the tendons of latissimus dorsi and teres major; the medial wall of the conduit is the long head of triceps and the lateral wall is the metaphysis of the humerus. Tenotomising the superior 7 mm of the tendon of latissimus dorsi where it attaches to the humerus allows the quadrilateral space to be opened and the neurovascular bundle is exposed. On leaving the tunnel, the axillary nerve supplies teres minor and sends off its sensory branch to the skin. The nerve then clings to the deep surface of deltoid, still with its accompanying artery and vein, 5 cm from the acromion in women and 6 cm in men. The nerve is vulnerable to surgical dissection and the placement of sutures in the inferior capsule and is also vulnerable to deltoid-splitting approaches and retraction of the deltoid.

Musculocutaneous nerve

The musculocutaneous nerve is one of the two terminal branches of the lateral cord, the other being the lateral root of the median nerve. In dissection of the infraclavicular brachial plexus, this is the most superficial nerve. It enters the conjoined tendons of short head of biceps and coracobrachialis, 2 cm distal to the coracoid. The nerve supplies both these muscles and is vulnerable to self-retaining retractors placed on the conjoined tendon and to traction during operations which transpose the coracoid process, such as the Bristow operation.

Suprascapular nerve

The suprascapular nerve leaves the upper trunk of the brachial plexus and travels with the suprascapular artery to the scapular notch. Here the artery travels above the transverse ligament and the nerve below. The nerve gives two motor branches to supraspinatus and then passes around the spine of the scapula to supply infraspinatus. The nerve is vulnerable to compression both within the suprascapular notch and at the spinoglenoid notch, and is vulnerable to the surgeon's knife during mobilisation of rotator cuff tears and in posterior approaches to the glenoid.

Thoracic outlet

The thoracic outlet is a triangular pyramid. The triangular base of this pyramid consists of trapezius posteriorly, the first rib medially and the clavicle acts as the hypotenuse. This pyramidal shape is bisected by scalenus anterior passing to the scalene tubercle of the first rib. The subclavian vein passes anterior to scalenus and the artery with the brachial plexus posteriorly.

TAKING A HISTORY FOR SHOULDER DISORDERS

It is sensible to have a coherent framework for taking a history and the scheme devised by the research committee of the American Shoulder and Elbow Surgeons (ASES) is logical, thorough and reproduceable (*Figure 1.1*). The ASES proforma has a patient self-evaluation section which allows the patient to record pain, activity and instability. Patients also complain of stiffness, weakness, crepitus and deformity, but these are best assessed during the examination.

Most patients are referred to an orthopaedic surgeon because of *pain*. It is essential to glean from the patient the site, nature, severity, radiation, onset, duration, exacerbation and easing factors for this pain.

The first question the surgeon has to answer is whether the pain is true shoulder pain or referred pain. True shoulder pain originates around the shoulder and

SHOULDER ASSESSMENT FORM
AMERICAN SHOULDER AND ELBOW SURGEONS

Name:		Date
Age:	Hand dominance R L Ambi	Sex: M F
Diagnosis:		Initial Assess? Y N
Procedure/Date:		Follow-up: M; Y

EXETER SHOULDER SERVICE: Patient assessment form

Welcome to the Exeter Shoulder Clinic. Please answer the patient assessment section of this page to the best of your knowledge. (The first half of the sheet; the surgeon will fill in the lower half once he has seen you). This form allows the surgeon to objectively assess your shoulder pain and your progress towards recovery. Thank you for your help.

PATIENT SELF-EVALUATION

Are you having pain in your shoulder? (circle correct answer)   Yes   No

Mark where your pain is

Do you have pain in your shoulder at night?	Yes	No
Do you take pain medication (aspirin, Advil, Tylenol etc.)?	Yes	No
Do you take narcotic pain medication (codeine or stronger)?	Yes	No
How many pills do you take each day (average)?	pills	

How bad is your pain today (mark line)?

0 |_____| 10
No pain at all   Pain as bad as it can be

Circle the number in the box that indicates your ability to do the following activities:
0 = Unable to do; 1 = Very difficult to do; 2 = Somewhat difficult; 3 = Not difficult

ACTIVITY	RIGHT ARM	LEFT ARM
1. Put on a coat	0 1 2 3	0 1 2 3
2. Sleep on your painful or affected side	0 1 2 3	0 1 2 3
3. Wash back/do up bra in back	0 1 2 3	0 1 2 3
4. Manage toileting	0 1 2 3	0 1 2 3
5. Comb hair	0 1 2 3	0 1 2 3
6. Reach a high shelf	0 1 2 3	0 1 2 3
7. Lift 10 lbs. above shoulder	0 1 2 3	0 1 2 3
8. Throw a ball overhand	0 1 2 3	0 1 2 3
9. Do usual work - List:	0 1 2 3	0 1 2 3
10. Do usual sport - List:	0 1 2 3	0 1 2 3

	Yes	No
Does your shoulder feel unstable (as if it is going to dislocate?)	Yes	No

How unstable is your shoulder (mark line)?

0 |_____| 10
Very stable   Very unstable

PHYSICIAN ASSESSMENT

RANGE OF MOTION	RIGHT		LEFT	
Total shoulder motion Goniometer preferred	Active	Passive	Active	Passive
Forward elevation (Maximum arm-trunk angle)				
External rotation (Arm comfortably at side)				
External rotation (Arm at 90° abduction)				
Internal rotation (Highest posterior anatomy reached with thumb)				
Cross-body adduction (Antecubital fossa to opposite acromion)				

INSTABILITY

0 = none 1 = mild (0 - 1 cm translation)
2 = moderate (1 - 2 cm translation or translation to glenoid rim)
3 = severe (> 2 cm translation or over rim of glenoid)

Anterior translation	0 1 2 3	0 1 2 3
Posterior translation	0 1 2 3	0 1 2 3
Inferior translation (sulcus sign)	0 1 2 3	0 1 2 3
Anterior apprehension	0 1 2 3	0 1 2 3
Reproduces symptoms?	Y N	Y N
Voluntary instability?	Y N	Y N
Relocation test positive?	Y N	Y N
Generalized ligamentous laxity?		Y N
Other physical findings		

Examiner's name _____   Date

SIGNS

0 = none; 1 = mild; 2 = moderate; 3 = severe

SIGN	Right	Left
Supraspinatus/greater tuberosity tenderness	0 1 2 3	0 1 2 3
AC joint tenderness	0 1 2 3	0 1 2 3
Biceps tendon tenderness (or rupture)	0 1 2 3	0 1 2 3
Other tenderness - List:	0 1 2 3	0 1 2 3
Impingement I (Passive forward elevation in slight internal rotation)	Y N	Y N
Impingement II (Passive internal rotation with 90° flexion)	Y N	Y N
Impingement III (90° active abduction - classic painful arc)	Y N	Y N
Subacromial crepitus	Y N	Y N
Scars - location:	Y N	Y N
Atrophy - location:	Y N	Y N
Deformity - describe	Y N	Y N

STRENGTH
(record MRC grade)

0 = no contraction; 1 = flicker; 2 = movement with gravity eliminated
3 = movement against gravity; 4 = movement against some resistance; 5 = normal power.

	Right	Left
Testing affected by pain?	Y N	Y N
Forward elevation	0 1 2 3 4 5	0 1 2 3 4 5
Abduction	0 1 2 3 4 5	0 1 2 3 4 5
External rotation (Arm comfortably at side)	0 1 2 3 4 5	0 1 2 3 4 5
Internal rotation (Arm comfortably at side)	0 1 2 3 4 5	0 1 2 3 4 5

Figure 1.1 The American Elbow and Shoulder Surgeons form. Adapted from Richards et al. (1992), with permission from the *Journal of Shoulder and Elbow Surgeons*.

radiates to the muscles of the arm, around the insertion of deltoid. When severe, this pain will radiate down to the radial border of the forearm and on to the radial border of the wrist; very occasionally it will radiate to the thenar eminence. Trapezius may ache, either due to radiation from the shoulder or because the scapula is being overused to protect the glenohumeral joint.

Beware the patient whose pain radiates into the hand, for this is the pattern of referred pain from the C6 and C7 nerve roots. Similarly beware of the patient whose pain radiates to the ulnar side of the forearm, the axilla or the chest, for this is the radiation from the thoracic outlet, the lower trunks of the brachial plexus (C8, T1), or the C8 and T1 roots. In patients with such radiation, always suspect a neurological cause for their pain and perform a careful and thorough neurological examination.

Referred pain from the viscera (gall-bladder to right shoulder and myocardium to left shoulder) is mentioned in every textbook, but search as I may, I have yet to see one in over 3000 consecutive patients who have been referred to my shoulder clinic.

The onset of the pain is of vital import. An insidious onset is seen in impingement, frozen shoulder and arthritis. A history of mild to moderate injury accompanies a rotator cuff tear and subluxation, and a more violent injury is associated with dislocation and fractures. A sudden crescendo onset of agonising pain can only be acute calcific tendonitis.

Ask which movements make the pain worse. Typically the pain is worse on reaching out in rotator cuff disorders. In recurrent subluxation or dislocation the pain is maximal in the position of apprehension. Acromioclavicular joint pain is maximal on cross-body adduction. In thoracic outlet syndrome the pain is made worse by lifting. Prompt the patient and then listen to the reply. *Night pain* is often a feature of shoulder disorders.

The patient's analgesic consumption should be noted. Enquire as to what treatment has already been given and its effect, for you will not inspire confidence if you recommend a form of treatment which the patient has already tried and which has failed!

The ability to perform a specific function depends on a complex interaction of range of motion, pain and power. The ASES proforma lists the degree of difficulty in performing ten *activities*: putting on a coat, sleeping, washing the back, wiping the bottom, combing the hair, reaching a high shelf, lifting 10 lbs above shoulder-height, throwing a ball, doing usual work and doing usual sport. In fact this is very comprehensive and tests elevation (reach, lift and throw), internal rotation (washing back and wiping bottom), external rotation (putting on a coat and combing hair), power (lifting 10 lbs), speed (throwing) and enquiry into work and sport is very revealing. Beware if the patient is right-handed and complains of pain in the left shoulder; then you have to phrase the combing question differently and ask how the patient washes their hair. Don't ask men how they put on their bra!

Instability is a difficult symptom to quantify. Patients usually complain of the shoulder coming out, or not feeling predictable or feeling vulnerable.

The ASES proforma can be used for research purposes and, if needed, a score can be used by using the formula $((10 - VAS) \times 5) + (5/3 \times \text{cumulative ADL score})$ giving the score out of 100.

If the radiation of pain sounds like a referred pattern, then ask about any neurological symptoms such as pins-and-needles, clumsiness, weakness and sympathetic-induced changes such as skin discoloration, mottling, cold sensitivity and absence or excessive sweating.

At this point it is important to enquire after any relevant previous medical or surgical history. Diabetes is associated with frozen shoulder, sickle-cell disease with avascular necrosis of the humerus and Erhlers–Danlos syndrome with multidirectional dislocation of the shoulder, but do not jump to conclusions. Also ask after what medications the patient is taking and what allergies they have.

By this stage you should have a good idea of what the diagnosis is and can go forward to the examination.

EXAMINATION OF THE SHOULDER

Examination starts as the patient enters the room. Even the introductory handshake can be most revealing, from the shoulder shrug of the massive rotator cuff tear to the engulfing hand of the acromegalic arthropathy. Observe the patient carefully whilst taking the history, for sometimes these observations will run counter to those seen during the formal examination. The patient with referred pain from the neck may move the neck fully and rapidly whilst a history is being taken, but with exaggerated sloth during the formal examination.

The human frame has two upper limbs for the sole purpose of giving a control side for the surgeon to compare with the symptomatic side. Examination should always start with the assumed normal side. The patient should be undressed from the waist upward, ladies retaining their brassière. Observe the patient as he takes off his shirt for this is a complex movement and allows the surgeon to assess range, rotation, speed, power and pain. The surgeon stands behind the upstanding patient. Firstly, observe the posture of the patient; look for any wasting of infraspinatus and deltoid, for deformity such as winging of the scapula or swelling of the acromioclavicular joint and finally for evidence of scars.

Tenderness is not as useful a sign at the shoulder as it is in the hand or around the elbow, for the majority of the shoulder is hidden by the bony acromion. However, the sternoclavicular joint, the acromio-clavicular joint and the impingement area can all be palpated for tenderness. The impingement area is the insertion of supraspinatus into the greater tuberosity which is palpable just in front of the acromion; feel in particular for a sulcus and eminence, indicating a rotator cuff tear.

At this point the surgeon can test for *shoulder joint movement*. A hand should be placed on the scapula as the patient actively elevates the arm. The reason for this is twofold: firstly to assess the contribution of scapulo-thoracic and glenohumeral motion and secondly to feel for crepitus during motion. *Subacromial crepitus* varies from the soft abrasive rumble of impingement, to the clicking and crunching of the edges of a full-thickness tear catching on the acromion, to the 'stiction-friction' of sclerotic bone on sclerotic bone with arthritis. These again are different from the labral clicking and grinding of subluxation, the clunking of dislocation, the crunching of the worn acromioclavicular joint and the washerboard clacking of snapping scapula and osteochondromata. Again the good shoulder is tested against the bad.

During elevation the surgeon looks to see if pain is reproduced through the painful arc, the so-called *impingement sign*. This is assessed in forward elevation, abduction and on internal rotation with the arm forward flexed 90°.

If active movement is restricted then *passive elevation* should be assessed. This is done by asking the patient to stoop down and observing whether a greater arc of elevation can be achieved. *External rotation* is now tested comparing good to bad side and active to passive movement, using the forearm as a goniometer with the elbow to the side. *Internal rotation* is measured as a composite movement of the highest vertebral level which can be reached by the thumb. The normal internal rotation reach is to the lower pole of the scapula (T7).

Power should be tested next using the MRC grade (0–5) for forward elevation, abduction, external rotation and internal rotation.

Although most textbooks mention Yergason's test for biceps this is very unreliable and is best forgotten.

The next phase of the examination is to test for *instability*. This is time-consuming and is only needed on those patients in whom instability lies in the differential diagnosis of their pain. The degree of *anterior and posterior translation* is assessed with the patient lying supine on the couch. The surgeon holds the patient's wrist comfortably in his axilla, places his non-dominant hand on the scapula and with his dominant arm grasps the proximal humerus. The patient's arm is tested at 90°, 110° and 120° of abduction. In each position, the surgeon forcibly pulls and pushes the head forwards and backwards on the glenoid. The degree of movement of the head on the glenoid is graded from 0 (normal), 1 (excessive movement but not to rim), 2 (head moves to edge of glenoid), 3 (severe: head dislocates over rim of glenoid). This test, the anterior and posterior drawer, is incorrectly described in most textbooks and is only of use if tested with the patient lying and the arm abducted.

Next the patient is tested for the *sulcus sign*. This is inferior displacement of the head on the glenoid as the arm is forcibly distracted down. If positive, a sulcus appears between the acromion and the humeral head. This is a sign of multidirectional instability.

The patient is then brought up into the position of apprehension (90° abduction and full external rotation). If the patient winces and protects the shoulder, this is a positive *apprehension test*. Pressure is then applied to the humeral head, pushing it backwards on the glenoid. If this manoeuvre leads to relief of the patient's pain, this is termed a positive *relocation test*.

The *posterior jerk test* is the test for recurrent posterior subluxation or dislocation. Once again, this test is poorly described in the standard texts. With the patient standing and the surgeon standing behind the affected shoulder, the surgeon places his left hand (for the right shoulder; right hand for the left shoulder) on the posterior aspect of the patient's scapula, with his thumb placed over the back of the humeral head, 2 cm below the posterior edge of the acromion. The surgeon then takes the forearm of the patient in his right hand (for the right shoulder; left for the left) and twists the arm into full internal rotation. The arm is then elevated with some 10° of adduction. As the arm elevates to 30°, the head can be felt to displace posteriorly and then to slip right out of joint. When the arm has been elevated to 70°, this elevation is maintained and the arm is taken from the plane of elevation to the plane of abduction and, in doing so, the head will relocate with an almighty thud.

Finally the patient should be tested for *generalised joint laxity*. The patient scores one point for laxity of each wrist in flexion, each little finger in extension, recurvatum of each elbow and recurvatum of each knee and finally the ability to bend right forwards and place the palm of both hands flat on the floor. This gives a maximum score of 9.

If the surgeon believes that the pain is referred, then a full *neurological examination* should be performed. Neck tenderness and movement are tested. Power should be tested in biceps (C5/6), ECRB/L (C6), triceps (C7), FDP (C8) and the intrinsics (T1). Sensibility should be tested through the dermatomes of C4 to T1. The biceps, triceps and supinator reflexes should be tested. Peripheral perfusion, skin colour and sweating should be assessed as well as examination for Horner's syndrome.

Roos' overhead exercise test should be performed for thoracic outlet syndrome. In this test the patient holds both hands above shoulder level and repeatedly squeezes and releases the hands. If positive this brings on the patient's pain within three minutes. Adson's vascular test and the military bracing test are not as sensitive as Roos' test.

INVESTIGATION OF SHOULDER DISORDERS

Plain radiographs

By the time the history has been accurately taken and the patient fully examined, the application of a few moment's intellectual vigour should give an accurate diagnosis in 95% of patients. These few moments of intellectual vigour are gained by telling the patient that you are now going to inspect their radiograph (*Figure 1.2*). Whatever the radiologist says, any patient whose pain is severe enough to warrant referral to an orthopaedic surgeon should at the minimum have a true anteroposterior (AP) radiograph of the shoulder joint. The first time that you make a diagnosis of frozen shoulder in a 60-year-old lady with a stiff painful shoulder and then have to modify your diagnosis when you spot the secondary tumour of the proximal humerus on the radiograph will persuade you to expend one radiograph on each patient referred to you.

The true AP radiograph is very useful in the orthopaedic patient referred with shoulder pain, but remember that every injured patient should have a trauma series for the shoulder which includes mandatory AP and lateral scapular views and an axillary if possible.

The *true AP radiograph* is taken with the arm in neutral; the beam is centred on the joint line and angled at 30° to the sagittal plane to line up parallel to the surface of the glenoid. The film is examined for joint space narrowing, cysts, sclerosis and osteophytes. The inferior osteophyte on the humeral head is the earliest sign of glenohumeral arthritis. Remember to look at the acromioclavicular joint for signs of degenerative change, especially downward-pointing osteophytes which could cause impingement. The early

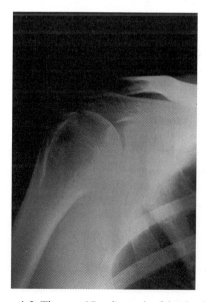

Figure 1.2 The true AP radiograph of the shoulder.

signs of impingement are sclerosis on the undersurface of the acromion, the so-called 'sourcil' (French for eyebrow) sign. Later in the disease, a spike of bone may be seen within the insertion of the coracoacromial ligament. Watch out for the irregularity of the acromial apophysis which can be difficult to spot on the true AP radiograph. In rotator cuff tears, the greater tuberosity shows irregularity, small cysts and sclerotic circles and small enthesopathic osteophytes. The humeral head subluxes superiorly, causing a break or step in Shenton's line of the shoulder (the usual smooth arc between the medial border of the scapula and the medial border of the proximal humerus). Reduction of the acromiohumeral interval should be interpreted with caution, because if the film is not centred properly the interval may appear narrowed when it is in fact normal. Look for calcific deposits in the rotator cuff. By definition the radiograph must be normal in frozen shoulder.

The *axillary radiograph* is of less benefit in the un-injured patient, but abnormalities of the coracoid and acromial apophyses are more easily recognised on this view. Do not try to gauge glenoid version from this view, as the same glenoid will appear to have different version according to the scapular rotation relative to the X-ray beam.

The *lateral scapular view* is useful in patients with pseudo-winging from scapulothoracic space-occupying lesions such as osteochondromas, but these are exceedingly rare.

Some surgeons advocate the *Neer outlet view* in patients with impingement. This is a lateral scapular view centred on supraspinatus and angled 10° caudally. This may show morphological abnormalities of the anterior acromion, or impingement by bone spurs in the coraco-acromial ligament or on the acromio-clavicular joint.

The *Stryker notch* view is best used to demonstrate the Hill–Sachs lesion of recurrent anterior dislocation.

Special views are needed for *acromioclavicular joint* disease. These are an AP radiograph in the plane of the thorax centred on the acromioclavicular joint and coned down, a 10° cephalic tilt of the acromio-clavicular joint and an axillary radiograph. Views needed for *sternoclavicular* disease are an anteroposterior view of both clavicles with 40° cephalic tilt (serendipity view). Often tomograms or CT are needed for the sternoclavicular joint.

Injection studies

Now that you have taken a history, examined the patient and seen the plain radiograph, it is time to consider confirming your diagnosis with injection studies. Three studies are useful.

The impingement test is used to confirm your suspicion that rotator cuff disease is the cause of your patient's shoulder pain. For this test 2 ml of 2% lignocaine are injected into the subacromial space. Using a 23G needle 1.25 inches long, the subacromial space is entered from the anterolateral approach. As the coraco-acromial ligament is traversed, a gritty obstruction is felt and then a sudden release as the needle tip passes into the subacromial space. At this point the needle should be in up to its hub. The space is aspirated. If synovial fluid is withdrawn, this confirms a full-thickness rotator cuff tear. The lignocaine is then inserted and allowed to fix for 5 min. The three impingement signs are then repeated and the response to the anaesthetic noted. The patient's pain should be virtually abolished in impingement and reduced by 50% in cuff tears. A therapeutic dose of corticosteroid can be mixed with the lignocaine if the surgeon wishes both a diagnostic and therapeutic effect from this injection.

If the *acromioclavicular joint* is suspected as the seat of the pain, 1 ml of 2% lignocaine can be injected directly into it. This is a small joint and, when worn, difficult to inject. Look at the radiographs first, as the obliquity of the joint varies. Palpate the osteophytes and push the clavicle to get differential movement between the bone at each side of the joint. Confirmation of entry is shown by lignocaine going into and then being withdrawn with ease. Again the patient's response is judged after 5 min and the injection can be combined with 25 mg hydrocortisone acetate.

The *glenohumeral joint* can also be infiltrated with lignocaine: 5 ml of 2% lignocaine is used from the posterior arthroscopy portal. A slightly longer 18G needle may be needed, or in very muscular or obese patients, a 20G spinal needle. Confirmation of entry is made by injection and aspiration.

Injection studies are extremely useful; indeed mandatory before a patient is booked for acromioplasty.

Arthrography

Arthrography may be considered archaic by some, but it is simple, cost-effective and still (apart from arthroscopy) the only way to detect partial-thickness deep surface tears. However, its role has been taken over by MRI for the detection and quantification of full-thickness tears. Arthrography can still confirm a frozen shoulder which has a typical arthrographic appearance of a small-volume contracted joint with obliteration of the subscapularis bursa and, as yet, there is no specific MRI appearance for this condition. Some surgeons still use double-contrast arthro-tomography to look for Bankart lesions in suspected anterior instability, but again this has been superseded by double-contrast CT scanning and gadolinium-enhanced MRI. Arthrography is uncomfortable for the patient, and demanding of expensive radiologist's hands-on time.

Ultrasonography

Ultrasonography went through a period of favour for examining the insertion of supraspinatus. It is simple to use and devoid of radiation exposure, but requires expert interpretation. Like ultrasonographic examina-tion of other regions, a lot of information is gleaned during the procedure as the shoulder is moved under the small-parts probe. This dynamic information can not be conveyed in the snap-shot films, so the surgeon either has to do the test himself or place great faith in his ultrasonographer.

CT arthrography

CT arthrography is favoured by many surgeons for looking at Bankart lesions. However, interpretation may be difficult, particularly in differentiating between a normal sublabral hole in the 2 o'clock position and a Bankart tear in the 3 o'clock position. Many surgeons would therefore favour EUA (Examination Under Anaesthetic) arthroscopy as the gold-standard investiga-tion for suspected dislocation. Even with 2 mm slices, coronal reconstruction of CT scans is so crude that it has no value in interpreting cuff tears. Essentially this is a method of investigation which can only give accurate data in the axial plane. CT arthrography is uncomfortable for the patient and expensive in terms of radiologist's time; it is invasive, lacks sagittal and coronal reconstruction, and has a high radiation dose for the patient. However, it gives better views of bony contours than MRI and is useful in fracture work.

3D CT scanning

This is very useful in interpreting difficult fracture patterns, especially three- and four-part fractures of the proximal humerus and glenoid fractures.

MRI

Magnetic resonance imaging (MRI) is rapidly becoming the imaging modality of choice for the shoulder. However, although there is no ionising radiation, MRI is still not patient-friendly. The patient has to be loaded head first into the core of the machine, which is extremely claustrophobic, and this is made worse by the terrific noise made by pres-ent-generation machines. Any movement leads to artefacts. The procedure usually takes 20 min. Special shoulder coils have to be used as the shoulder is off-centre from the core of the machine. Orthogonal reconstruction has to be computed to generate scans in the coronal oblique and sagittal oblique direction of scapula and glenoid. Esoteric MRI effects such as the 'angle phenomenon' may make interpretation dif-ficult.

Despite these potential disadvantages and its cost, MRI has led to a revolution in shoulder imaging. In full-thickness tears this is the investigation of choice (*Figure 1.3*). It shows not only that there is a tear, but where the tear is, its size, the degree of retraction, the consistency of the tear edges and, most importantly,

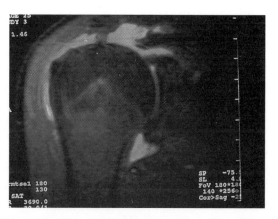

Figure 1.3 MRI of a full thickness rotator cuff tear: the area of discontinuity in supraspinatus tendon can clearly be seen, as can the elevation of the humeral head in relation to the glenoid.

the quality of the residual supraspinatus muscle in terms of atrophy and fatty degeneration.

However, MRI is still very misleading in impingement and partial-thickness tears. In a recent study, 20 asymptomatic patients were scanned and all were reported by an experienced MRI radiologist as having an abnormal cuff and 30% as having a partial tear. How often must the lesson be learned that investigations should be interpreted in the light of clinical findings and never before?

Diagnostic arthroscopy

Diagnostic arthroscopy remains the gold-standard for investigating the shoulder. The disadvantage is that the patient needs admission to hospital (even as a day case) and general anaesthesia. There has been a vogue for arthroscopy under scalene block in the USA with the patient in the beach-chair position, which has not transferred across the Atlantic. The apparatus needed for shoulder arthroscopy is standard knee equipment: a normal arthroscope with video-facility, conventional probes, hand instruments and power shaver. The shoulder arthroscopist will also need a distraction system, shoulder cannulae and some method for pressure infusion of fluid.

Arthroscopy should always be preceded by examination under anaesthetic. The shoulder should be put through a full range of movement to exclude passive restriction of movement. The shoulder should then be tested for instability. First, *the load and shift test* is performed. The surgeon places one hand on the scapula to stabilise it and holds the patient's flexed elbow in his other hand. The arm is brought into the position of apprehension (90° of abduction and full external rotation) and then the humeral head is forced forwards in order to translate or dislocate it anteriorly. This is the shoulder equivalent of the Barlow's test for DDH (Developmental Dysplasia of the Hip). Compressive load is then applied to the elbow to load the head against the glenoid, like the valgus-internal rotation stress in the pivot shift test of the knee. With the load applied, force is used to relocate the humeral head, the equivalent of the Ortolani test. The clunk of relocation is a sure sign of recurrent anterior dislocation (Grade III, as for anterior drawer). Lesser degrees of subluxation may be felt, with or without a grating feeling coming from the torn labrum.

Following the load and shift test, the sulcus sign is sought and finally the posterior jerk test.

Now the patient is placed in the lateral decubitus position, under general anaesthetic with endotracheal intubation, and the forequarter is prepared and draped. The posterior portal for shoulder arthroscopy lies 1 cm below and medial to the posterior angle of the acromion. The trochar and cannula are aimed diectly at the coracoid process. The video-arthroscope is swapped for the trochar and entry is confirmed before the fluid irrigation is turned on.

Examination of the joint is performed according to an established pattern so that every part of the shoulder is seen. The long head of biceps tendon is the primary landmark of shoulder arthroscopy (*Figure 1.4*) and, as such, is the starting point and the finish point of every examination. It is first examined at its origin from the labrum, making sure that there is no SLAP tear (Superior Labrum, Anterior to Posterior). The tendon is then traced from its origin across the joint to the bicipital tunnel. Often there is a mesentery or vinculum running from the capsule to the tendon. This may be a single or multiple strand of synovium or a complete

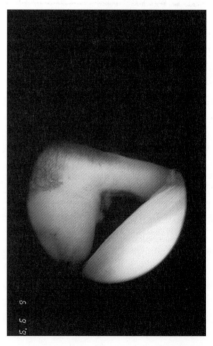

Figure 1.4 Arthroscopic view of the long head of biceps tendon.

sheet. The superior surface of the tendon is inspected for inflammation at the entrance to the tunnel.

Supraspinatus is next surveyed, being very careful to inspect its insertion to the greater tuberosity, as this is where rotator cuff tears start. The arthroscope is then taken underneath biceps to examine the superior triangle of the joint; this is the triangle bounded by the biceps, labrum and top surface of the subscapularis tendon and forms the entrance to the subscapularis recess which is termed the foramen of Weitbrecht. The foramen of Weitbrecht is a favoured hiding place for loose bodies and is the area which contracts in frozen shoulder. The tendon of subscapularis is the secondary landmark of shoulder arthroscopy and is always crossed obliquely by the middle glenohumeral ligament.

The arthroscope must now traverse the tight space between the head and the glenoid on its way to the inferior part of the shoulder: the infraglenoid recess. In the normal shoulder this traverse is so tight that the arthroscope will suddenly flick from the superior part of the joint to the infraglenoid recess. Indeed, if it fails to flick then the shoulder is judged to be over-loose and this is called the *positive drive-thru sign*. If the shoulder is extremely loose, then not only does the arthroscope not flick through from top to bottom but the arthroscopist can take the arthroscope down the back of the joint and see right through to the front of the joint; this is called the *positive see-through sign* and is again a sign of excessive shoulder joint laxity. You will notice the different spelling of these two signs which show from which side of the Atlantic they originate! The experienced arthroscopist will anticipate the flick-through and control and prevent it so that a good view is obtained of the anterior labrum and the origin of the inferior glenohumeral ligament during the traverse of this tight strait. This is the area of the labral detachment which is called the Bankart lesion. Bankart lesions come in all shapes and sizes from a small cleft to the total absence of labrum with cartilage and bone loss on the anterior labrum.

The infraglenoid recess should be quite capacious. It is another favoured site for loose bodies, and is contracted in frozen shoulder. The neck of the humerus leads on to the posterior aspect of the humerus. The synovial reflection has a bare area posteriorly which has small pits and vessels entering the bone; this should not be mistaken for a Hill–Sachs lesion. The posterior surface of the humerus is then observed for a Hill–Sachs lesion and the arthroscope comes back up the synovial reflection of the insertion of infraspinatus to the long head of biceps. At this stage the posterior labrum has not been seen, so the arthroscope is rotated and withdrawn and the posterior labrum traced back down to the infraglenoid recess and back up again to long head of biceps.

As in arthroscopy of the knee, you will now want to introduce a probe to palpate any area of the joint which you suspect is abnormal. The arthroscope is taken through the joint so that the lens rests against the synovium of the rotator interval just above the superior edge of subscapularis. Holding the cannula in place, the lens system is withdrawn and swapped for the sharp cannula, which is thrust forwards to come out through the skin of the front of the shoulder. At this point the patient is impaled on the trochar/cannula which enters posteriorly, travels through the shoulder and emerges anteriorly. Either a cannula can now be railroaded over the trochar/cannula to enter the joint from the front, or the trochar is withdrawn, the hook probe placed a measured distance down the arthroscope cannula so that its tip will be within the joint and then the arthroscope cannula is withdrawn again inside the joint, disengaged from the probe and the video-arthroscope inserted. Now the surgeon has the arthroscope within the joint from the posterior portal and has established an anterior portal with either a cannula or the probe. If a cannula has been placed, the hook-probe is now inserted through it.

Triangulating with the probe, the same routine is followed to re-examine the joint, probing all the structures as they are passed. Finally, if a cannula has been inserted into the anterior portal, the arthroscope can be replaced through this to examine the posterior aspect of the joint and the anterior glenohumeral ligaments from a different perspective. It is quite confusing to the novice to do this for everything is back to front; the surgeon may wish to move to the opposite side of the table to maintain his co-ordination in relation to the picture at this point. This completes the shoulder joint arthroscopy but not the examination, for that is incomplete until the subacromial bursa has been examined.

The shoulder is distracted towards the patient's feet to change the subacromial space from a potential to an actual space. The trochar/cannula is then inserted from the anterolateral approach to the subacromial space.

If in doubt, aim forwards to enter the bursa. If the bursa has been entered then a glorious view will be apparent, but if not then red-out or cobwebs are the usual appearance. Navigation within the subacromial bursa is difficult because the landmarks are not as obvious as within the shoulder. It may be helpful to insert one or two needles into the bursa from each side of the coraco-acromial ligament to aid navigation. Usually the acromion, coraco-acromial ligament, deltoid and supraspinatus tendon can be seen. The rotator cuff is inspected for impingement or rotator cuff tears. Interestingly it is far easier to enter and navigate the bursa if a full-thickness rotator cuff tear is present, for the subacromial bursa will have already been filled from the glenohumeral arthroscopy. The acromion is then inspected for an impingement lesion of the insertion of the coraco-acromial ligament. This completes the investigation.

Haematological examination

This is rarely of benefit in the diagnosis of shoulder disorders. The exceptions to this are investigating avascular necrosis (which may be caused by lymphoma and, in the coloured population, by sickle-cell disease), vitamin B12 estimation in patients with peripheral neuropathies, and factor viii levels in haemophiliac arthropathy. Investigating the arthritides, sepsis and tumours where the CRP (C-Reactive Protein) and ESR (Erythrocyte Sedimentation Rate) are essential markers.

Biochemical tests

Biochemical tests are rarely needed. In chronic renal failure there may be deposition of amyloid in the coraco-acromial ligament leading to impingement. Diabetes is often associated with frozen shoulder. Creatine phosphokinase may be raised in myopathies presenting as winging of the scapula. Electrophoresis will be mandatory in the differential of tumours around the shoulder.

Microbiological testing

This will be necessary in suspected infection. Unusual infections can present at the shoulder, particularly at the sternoclavicular joint. Even osteomyelitis from such rare causes as *Salmonella typhi* may present at the shoulder.

Viral serology may be needed around the shoulder; for instance human parvovirus 19 has recently been linked to neuralgic amyotrophy.

Surgery and biopsy

Surgical exploration and biopsy is, of course, the final investigation. Once again it is rarely needed, due to the battery of less-invasive investigations detailed above. It is the final arbiter of rotator cuff disease and of dislocation and is essential in cases of infection and tumour.

At the end of this exhaustive process the patient should be assured that the diagnosis is not in doubt.

SURGICAL APPROACHES TO THE SHOULDER

In this section the author will assume that the reader has performed the standard approaches to the shoulder and will concentrate on the hints and tricks to gain even better exposure. All approaches must abide by Henry's laws: the exposure should be safe, should follow anatomical watersheds between nerve territories, should allow a good exposure of the tissues to be excised, repaired or replaced, and should be extensile. Inept shoulder surgery appears as a bloody procedure performed with discomfort down a deep dark hole. The shoulder surgeon uses three tricks to obtain exposure: adrenaline in the skin to stop bleeding, extensile exposure and special shoulder retractors. These are the secret weapons of shoulder surgery.

The deltopectoral approach to the shoulder

This is the standard approach for Bankart repair and capsular shift and is extended for shoulder replacement.

Preoperative preparation

The patient should give informed consent. The post-operative physiotherapy rehabilitation should be outlined both by surgeon and physiotherapist. Prophylactic antibiotic should be administered if prosthetic material such as suture anchors or a shoulder replacement are to be implanted. This is routine for all approaches.

Anaesthesia

The patient should be given a general anaesthetic with endotracheal intubation. The anaesthetic circuit should allow the anaesthetist and all his equipment to remain at the foot end of the table. This is necessary for all general anaesthetic procedures on the shoulder. The skin in the line of the incision is infiltrated with 1:200,000 adrenaline solution by the surgeon in the anaesthetic room so that it has time to work before the skin is incised.

Positioning

The patient is placed supine on the operating table and pulled to the edge of the table so that the armpit of the operated side is in line with the edge of the table. This allows the arm to be fully extended. It also allows the patient to fall off the table, a situation which must be guarded against! A small sandbag placed on the medial border of the scapula protracts the shoulder and allows easier access. The author uses the poly-sling in its plastic wrapper instead of a sandbag for it is the correct size and then the surgeon knows it is both in theatre and easily accessible at the end of the operation. A ring is placed under the patient's head and the eyes must be padded and taped to prevent accidental splashing with antiseptic. Finally a theatre hat is placed on the patient to keep hair well away from the operative field.

Draping

The operating department assistant (ODA) holds the patient's hand whilst the forequarter is surgically prepared from the sternum to the table and from the nipple to the earlobe, the arm being prepared to the wrist. An adherent exclusion drape is then placed on the dried skin. The surgeon triple-gloves his dominant hand, and holds the prepared forearm, taking the weight from the ODA. The surgeon then takes the patient's unprepared hand in his triple-gloved hand while the assistant peels the top glove off the surgeon on to the patient and then repeats with the second glove followed by a surgical stocking which is rolled up to the armpit. Using a skin-marker pen, the outline of the clavicle, acromion and coracoid are drawn on the skin. The line of the skin incision is outlined with hash marks for closure and with a final artistic flourish the surgeon draws a mouth and pair of eyes over the patient's head, warning the assistants that retribution will follow should they dare rest anything on the patient's face! The drapes are then tucked under the head-ring and an adhesive op-site seal is placed over the surgical site. Finally the arm is placed on a padded and draped Mayo stand. The surgeon stands in the axilla, the first assistant at the point of the shoulder and the scrub nurse opposite the surgeon and assistant.

The incision

The incision is made in the line of relaxed skin tension. In the male this incision lies along the line of coracoid to armpit crease, 5 cm long in the thin man but longer in the obese or well-muscled. In the young woman, a cosmetic approach can be used which starts in the skin-crease of the armpit but heads back across the axilla instead of upward to the coracoid. The skin is then undermined up as far as the coracoid, allowing the incision to be literally pulled up towards the coracoid by the assistant. The deltopectoral split is then exposed. Often this is marked by the cephalic vein but the vein may not be immediately apparent, in which case it may be found by using the fat stripe which marks the interval. If it still cannot be found, dissect up towards the clavicle where the triangular space will be encountered between deltoid and clavicular head of pectoralis and then work down from there.

The deltopectoral groove is a safe portal of access as it is crossed by only three structures. These are the acromial artery, the cephalic vein and the deltoid artery with its venae comitante. The deltoid artery is a branch of the thoraco-acromial trunk and should be ligated and divided in the standard deltopectoral approach, whereas the cephalic vein should be preserved. The cephalic vein is always left on deltoid, for it has a host of tributaries entering it from deltoid and none or rarely a single tributary from pectoralis major.

The dissection

The whole key to this approach is the ability to place a Kolbel self-retaining shoulder retractor between deltoid and the conjoined tendon (short head of biceps and the coracobrachialis). In order to do this, the arm is abducted to 90° and deltoid is mobilised from the proximal humerus and subacromial bursa. Two structures are at hazard. The first is the anastomosing branch from the posterior circumflex artery which enters the humerus at the level of the top edge of pectoralis major; this must be diathermied and divided or, if large, ligated and divided. This anastomosing branch is the final branch of the posterior circumflex artery which runs with the axillary nerve and the nerve is the second structure at risk. The clavipectoral fascia is now incised along the lateral border of the conjoined tendon, from the level of the pectoralis major tendon to the coraco-acromial ligament. The Kolbel retractor is inserted to give a perfect view of the shoulder.

The key to the successful repair of dislocations is in the separation of the anterior capsule from subscapularis. In order to get a good low repair or a proper capsular shift you will need to get to 6 o'clock on the labrum and to the postero-inferior capsule. To do this, the anterior circumflex humeral artery and its two venae comitante must be ligated and divided; this vessel marks the junction of the tendinous middle third of subscapularis from the lower muscular one-third. Some textbooks suggest that this vessel should be preserved, on the pretext that to operate below it endangers the axillary nerve and that to tie it off jeopardises the blood supply to the head of the humerus. The riposte to such a philosophy is that firstly exposure is inadequate without dividing the lower third of subscapularis, secondly the anterior circumflex is not an end-artery and has a rich anastomosis from its descending branch, and thirdly that no surgeon should operate in this area if he has not been trained to a sufficient standard that he is capable of demonstrating the axillary nerve and protecting it through the operation. Indeed this is the next step in the dissection. The top centimetre of the tendon of latissimus dorsi is tenotomised from the humerus, and teres major is retracted downwards to open up the quadrilateral space thereby exposing the posterior circumflex artery and vein and, behind them, the axillary nerve. Now the nerve has been seen, the surgeon is in a position to avoid it; if he has no clue where it is, avoiding it becomes a matter of luck rather than judgement.

A retractor is now placed in the rotator interval (the thin section of capsule between subscapularis and supraspinatus) to mark the superior aspect of the subscapularis tendon and two stay-sutures are placed in the tendon of subscapularis. The elbow is brought close to the patient's side and the arm held in external rotation, putting subscapularis on the stretch, and a careful vertical tenotomy is performed using cutting diathermy. The tendon fibres of subscapularis run from medial to lateral and spring apart when cut. The tendon is gradually sectioned and, as the cut goes deeper, there comes a time when the last fibres spring apart and then the capsule presents itself. The capsule is not under tension and is amorphous; it is far easier to find at the lower third of subscapularis where the muscular fibres separate easily from the capsule, whereas the capsule blends more with subscapularis towards its superior border. Once the plane of the capsule is defined, it is cleaned with a swab. Now the whole of the capsule is on view; a stay-suture is placed within it, the rotator interval opened and a vertical tenotomy made in the capsule 5 mm medial to the sectioned stump of subscapularis. The joint is now exposed.

The extensions for total shoulder replacement

A more extensile approach is required for preparation of the face of the glenoid in shoulder replacement than in the Bankart exposure, where it is just the anterior margin of the glenoid which needs to be exposed.

A better mobilisation of deltoid is required, which necessitates ligation and division of the cephalic vein and the acromial artery. Deltoid must never be violated as that would compromise the postoperative rehabilitation. The second manoeuvre is the complete pectoralis major tenotomy (Perthes approach). This gives an outstanding exposure for shoulder replacement.

Closure

Subscapularis is closed with interrupted number 1 vicryl. The deltopectoral groove falls back together and requires no sutures. The subcutaneous tissue is reapproximated and the skin closed with a subcuticular suture. Drains are not required for Bankart repair or shift, but should be placed following shoulder replacement. The arm is rested in a sling.

The Matsen 'deltoid on' exposure of the rotator cuff

This is the standard approach for open acromioplasty and rotator cuff repair.

Preoperative preparation

The patient is counselled that during acromioplasty the environment is created to allow healing of the rotator cuff; a process which takes eight weeks. Prior to cuff repair the patient is told that, for the first three months, they will wonder why they had the operation, and warned that there will be a numb patch lateral to the incision due to division of supraclavicular nerve fibres. Hairy men are told that they will awake with an area of their leg which has been shaved for the earthing plate of the diathermy! The patient is advised as to the physiotherapy regime they must undertake.

Anaesthesia

Anaesthesia is as for the deltopectoral approach.

Positioning

Traditionally the patient is positioned as for the deltopectoral approach. However, the author prefers to operate with the patient in the lateral decubitus position, with the patient as far up the table as possible, and with reverse Trendelenburg. This allows the surgeon to stand at the head of the table, and operate straight into the top of the shoulder; whereas, in the traditional approach, the surgeon has to adopt a cock-robin attitude to see into the incision, which is very tiring. The lateral-decubitus position allows exposure of the back of the shoulder, and the supraspinatus fossa. This is essential when repairing large rotator cuff tears.

Draping

This is as for the deltopectoral approach.

Incision

The incision is placed in the line of the skin creases. The landmarks of the incision are the acromioclavicular joint and the coracoid process. The incision extends 7–14 cm cephalad from the coracoid process. The skin is undermined on the plane of deltotrapezius fascia laterally, so that the lateral edge of the acromion can be seen, and 3 cm medial to the acromioclavicular joint. The skin edges are retracted using stay-sutures through the skin.

Dissection

An incision is now made in the deltotrapezius fascia, in line with the muscle fibres of both deltoid and trapezius. This creates two flaps, medial and lateral, which are in continuity, for the trapezius fascia, the periosteum over the acromion and the deltoid fascia are contiguous. Matsen, in his original description, placed the line of this split at the mid-point between the lateral edge of the acromion and the acromioclavicular joint. The problem with siting the incision in the fascia at this point is that it is the very thinnest part of the periosteum and is difficult to repair. This has put some surgeons off this approach. However, by moving this split 5 mm medial, it can be made in the thickest part of the fascial sheet, the superior acromioclavicular ligament, right over the joint itself. Not only does this make closure much more secure, but it allows exposure of the acromioclavicular joint as well. It also allows extensions, either into trapezius or even into a scapular osteotomy.

The two flaps are lifted from the bone using electrocautery, with the needle on the bone itself so that every Sharpey fibre is harvested. As deltoid is split, the clavipectoral fascia comes into view, along with the thickening of the clavipectoral fascia, the coraco-acromial ligament. At this point the acromial artery will be encountered, running just anterior to the acromion in a small cushion of fat, deep to deltoid and superficial to the coraco-acromial ligament. This must be diathermied and divided. The coraco-acromial ligament is now exposed by placing a swab upon it, and pushing the swab down between it and deltoid, until the whole of the ligament is exposed and clean.

The junction between the free edge of the coraco-acromial ligament and the clavipectoral fascia is incised. If fluid is revealed, then a cuff tear is present. The ligament is cut from its insertion into the undersurface of the acromion, and is stored for later use. The rotator cuff is now inspected, prior to performing the acromioplasty.

Extensions

If the acromioclavicular joint is degenerate it is excised (see rotator cuff repair). In massive tears extension into trapezius or a step-cut scapular osteotomy are required.

Closure

The medial flap and the lateral flap are closed using number 1 vicryl. If there is any doubt as to the strength of the attachment of the anterior deltoid to the acromion, extra interosseous sutures are placed to secure it. The subcutaneous tissues are re-approximated and the incision closed with a subcuticular suture.

The posterior approach to the shoulder

This is the routine approach for recurrent posterior instability and fractures of the glenoid.

Preoperative preparation

The patient is counselled that he/she may require a plaster spica postoperatively.

Anaesthesia

This is as for the deltopectoral approach.

Positioning

The patient is placed in the lateral-decubitus position with reverse Trendelenburg.

Draping

This is as for the deltopectoral approach.

Incision

This is placed in Langer's line, from the spine of the scapula, aiming for the axillary skin crease. This gives a far better cosmetic result than the old transverse approach along the spine of the scapula. The skin edges are undermined and retracted on stay-sutures.

Dissection

Deltoid is split in the line of its fibres for 5 cm caudal from the spine of the scapula. To go further is to endanger the axillary nerve. The surgeon next encounters a very thick sheet of fascia which is the deep deltoid fascia; this needs to be split in the line of the incision. A retractor is now placed so that the posterior rotator-cuff muscles can be seen. The problem

for surgeons who rarely undertake this approach is that they know that they should split the muscles between infraspinatus and teres minor, but can't find the gap. Sometimes the split is obvious and sometimes it is not. The way around this is to remember that infraspinatus is a bipennate muscle and its tendon is always very obvious. Measure the amount of muscle above the tendon, and then measure this same distance off below the tendon, and this will always bring you onto the opening. The infraspinatus is retracted superiorly and the teres minor inferiorly, exposing the posterior capsule of the joint.

Extensions

If the exposure is not good enough, deltoid can be lifted from its insertion into the spine of the scapula, to widen the exposure of the rotator-cuff. If the exposure of the capsule is too small, then infraspinatus can be divided on stay-sutures.

Closure

Deltoid is repaired. The subcutaneous tissue repaired, and the skin is closed subcuticularly.

DISLOCATIONS, ACUTE AND RECURRENT

Restraints

The incredible thing about the shoulder is not that it should dislocate (*Figure 1.5*) but that a joint with such minimal constraint should ever remain located! Before considering the mechanisms and types of dislocation, we should consider the restraints which act to keep the shoulder in joint. The shoulder has three overlapping levels of restraint: those which keep the joint located at rest, those which locate it during movement and those which restrain it at the extremes.

Restraints acting at rest

These are the forces which keep the joint located even under anaesthetic.

1. *Bony restraint:* the glenoid fossa is tiny compared to the humeral head so there is very little first-line bony constraint. However, the coraco-acromial arch

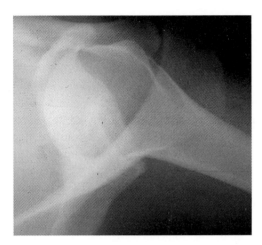

Figure 1.5 Radiograph of an anterior subcoracoid dislocation of the shoulder.

acts as a bony second line of restraint. The coraco-acromial arch subtends an angle of 115° and prevents the shoulder dislocating superiorly or posterosuperiorly. The shoulder may sublux upwards if there is a cuff tear, but can only dislocate if the acromion fractures or if a surgeon has removed part of this arch. This still leaves a vulnerable 245° antero-inferiorly, inferiorly and postero-inferiorly.

2. *The labrum* acts in four ways. It enlarges the glenoid. It also acts as a 'chock-block' to restrain the head, like the chock-blocks which are placed in front of and behind the wheels of aeroplanes. The labrum also acts much like a plumber's plunger (used to clean out drains), or the rubber suction pad of a child's toy arrow, and sticks to the humeral head. Finally the labrum is the anchor for the ligamentous restraints and long head of biceps.

3. *Physical restraints:* the pressure inside the shoulder joint is 4 mmHg below atmospheric. If the capsule of a cadaver shoulder is vented, it will dislocate. Adhesion–cohesion is a physical force which acts between two wetted surfaces and prevents them being pulled apart. The best example of this is the analogy of two wetted glass microscope slides which will slide one on the other but which cannot be pulled apart. The sheer muscular bulk of the muscles prevents dislocation; you can imagine that it would be more difficult to try to dislocate Arnold Schwarzenneger's shoulder than that of an anorexic fashion model!

Restraints acting during movement and under load

1. *The rotator cuff muscles* act in synchrony to control and prevent dislocation. If the cuff muscles are damaged, then subluxation or dislocation will occur. Examples of this are the upward subluxation with rotator cuff tears, and the dislocation seen in paralyses such as poliomyelitis.

2. *Proprioception:* for the cuff to act properly it must have an intact biofeedback loop. The most easily damaged part of this loop is proprioception and there is evidence accumulating which shows that proprioception may be altered in patients with recurrent dislocation.

3. There is evidence that the rotator cuff can *dynamically tension* the ligaments with which it blends close to its insertion.

Restraints acting at the limit

1. *The glenohumeral ligaments:* as the shoulder reaches the limits of movement, the ligaments tighten to prevent dislocation. When the shoulder moves beyond its allowable range, something has to give and that something is the ligamentous restraint. The inferior glenohumeral ligament, and in particular its thick anterior band, is the major restraint to anterior dislocation. Under extreme load the anterior band of the inferior glenohumeral ligament will fail in one of two ways: either it will avulse from the bone, pulling the labrum with it (the Bankart lesion) or it will fail in mid-substance and stretch out. The major restraints to posterior dislocation are the coracohumeral ligament and the posterior capsule.

2. *Long head of biceps* acts both passively and dynamically to restrain the shoulder against dislocation. Under extreme load it will fail and this is usually seen as an avulsion of the biceps anchor, the so-called SLAP tear.

So much for theory, but what happens in reality? Baker arthroscoped 45 patients with acute anterior dislocation of the shoulder and classified the ligamentous injuries into three groups:

Group I (6/45) had a tear of the capsule without any damage to the labrum. The shoulder was stable under anaesthetic. There was haemorrhage between the middle and inferior glenohumeral ligaments and a minimal haemarthrosis.

Group II (11/45) had a partial labral tear. The shoulder subluxed under anaesthetic. There was variable instability and a moderate haemarthrosis.

Group III (28/45) was by far the commonest and also the most severe. There was complete disruption of the anterior labrum with frank dislocation under anaesthesia. A large haemarthrosis was present and 18 had a Hill–Sachs lesion (the osteochondral infarction in the posterior aspect of the humeral head, caused by impaction on the anterior glenoid margin, during the first traumatic dislocation).

Classification

Shoulder instabilities are classified according to degree, direction, recurrence and aetiology. The degree of instability varies from subluxation to locked dislocation. The direction of instability may be anterior, which is by far the commonest, multidirectional or posterior. The first dislocation is an acute event but if the shoulder dislocates a second or further times, then it is classified as recurrent. The aetiology may be trauma (the commonest) or congenital laxity or it may be a combination of both. Extremely rare causes are voluntary dislocation, paralysis and congenital dysplasia.

Acute traumatic anterior dislocation

This is by far the commonest form of dislocation; of all acute dislocations 96% are anterior and 4% posterior. The patient is often a young sportsperson injured on the field. The event is very traumatic for it takes a great force to rip a young shoulder out of joint. Often the event will be a forceful tackle ending in several players falling to the ground. The arm is usually in the position of apprehension (90° abducted and in full external rotation) but it occurs so rapidly and the patient is in such agony that the position is not reported. The patient knows that the shoulder 'is out'. On examination the shoulder is deformed. Sensibility should be tested in the axillary chevron area (that area of skin supplied by the axillary nerve) and for the musculocutaneous nerve (radial side of forearm) and in the hand. A trauma series of radiographs must be taken to confirm dislocation and exclude an associated fracture of the greater

tuberosity or surgical neck. Reduction is a matter of urgency for the longer the shoulder is out the more difficult it will be to reduce.

Reduction should be performed under general anaesthetic, but often this is a counsel of perfection as you can't always find an anaesthetist when you want one; in that case, reduction should be performed under intravenous analgesia and sedation. The Kocher manoeuvre is out of favour because it may cause additional damage during reduction. One of the gentlest and best methods is that of Matsen. The patient lies supine on the couch with a swathe around the chest for counter-traction by an assistant. Traction is applied to the arm by the surgeon who wears a 6 inch crepe bandage wrapped around his waist and forming a loop into which the arm is placed with the elbow bent to a right angle. As the surgeon leans back, he can apply a full 70 kg of traction and gently rock the forearm to unlock the Hill–Sachs impression from the anterior glenoid. This allows the shoulder to be gently reduced. If this fails, then general anaesthetic with muscle relaxant must be used. Neurological status should again be checked after reduction, which is confirmed by further radiographs.

There is controversy over how long the shoulder should be immobilised following a first-time anterior dislocation. Several prospective studies have shown no difference between one week versus three weeks in a sling. The pragmatic view favours three weeks internal rotation in the young athlete but a sling, merely for comfort, over the first week in the older patient in whom stiffness is a more common complication than recurrent dislocation.

Acute posterior dislocation

Acute posterior dislocations are rare and all too often missed, for the signs are subtle on a true AP radiograph. For this reason such a radiograph is a favoured weapon of the examiner in the FRCS Orth. If an examiner shows you an AP radiograph of the shoulder, explain in the nicest possible way that a lateral is mandatory in any trauma case and request that you see it before commenting on the AP film. Posterior acute dislocation may occur after trauma, epileptic siezure or electrocution. The patient is in pain. The clinical deformity is not as gross as that of anterior dislocation. The arm is held in internal rotation and cannot be brought into external rotation. After neurological assessment, a trauma series of radiographs should be taken. Reduction is performed under general anaesthesia or intravenous analgesia with sedation. The reduction manoeuvre is the opposite of that for anterior dislocation: traction and countertraction are applied with the arm in adduction instead of abduction and the head has to be rocked off the posterior glenoid rim. The arm should be rocked into internal rotation first, to disengage it, and then lifted off the posterior rim. Following reduction, the arm should *not* be placed in a sling in internal rotation as this is an unstable position. The arm may either be held at the side in external rotation by using three strips of 4-inch elastoplast wound from the medial side of the arm, around the front of the arm and then taped to the patient's back to keep the arm in external rotation, or the patient should be placed in a plaster-of-Paris spica with the arm in 30° of external rotation.

In irreducible cases or missed *neglected posterior dislocation*, open reduction will be required. Open reduction is performed using the standard deltopectoral approach. The long head of biceps is identified and the lesser tuberosity is osteotomised to enter the joint. The head is then disengaged from the glenoid and reduced. The reason for the locked nature of this dislocation is the massive reversed Hill–Sachs lesion, so this defect is now filled with the bone block of the lesser tuberosity which is screwed into the defect using AO lag screws. This procedure is termed the Neer modification of the McLaughlin procedure. If the defect is greater than 30% of the head, consideration should be given to using an allograft segment from a stored femoral head from the bone bank and, in exceptionally large defects, humeral head replacement. However it should be stressed that the Neer–McLaughlin operation is usually adequate.

Recurrent anterior dislocation

Incidence. A recent well-controlled Scandinavian prospective multicentre study showed that 50% of patients under the age of 40 will have a re-dislocation within three years if they have been treated conservatively. About 70% of patients with a Bankart and Hill–Sach's lesions seen arthroscopically at their initial dislocation will re-dislocate and of those who do not re-dislocate 65% will have severe shoulder symptoms. About 85%

of the first re-dislocations were after minor trauma and the rest atraumatic. Thus it can be seen that re-dislocation is a major cause of shoulder disability in younger patients.

Aetiology. It should be stressed that not all dislocations are the same and nor should they be treated in the same manner. At one end of the spectrum lies the traumatic recurrent dislocator, and at the other end of the spectrum is the atraumatic recurrent dislocator. This can be stated more clearly; patients at one end of the spectrum are 'torn loose' and at the other 'born loose'. Matsen has labelled these ends of the spectrum TUBS and AMBRI. TUBS stands for *T*raumatic, *U*nidirectional, has a *B*ankart lesion, treated by *S*urgery. AMBRI stands for *A*traumatic, *M*ultidirectional, *B*ilateral, treated by *R*ehabilitation; if surgery is needed *I*nferior capsular shift is performed. In reality most dislocations lie somewhere between the two ends of the spectrum and possess elements of both.

Earlier in this century surgeons looked for the Holy Grail of dislocation, the 'Essential Lesion'. However, we now understand that recurrence is caused by slackness in the anterior capsule, which may be from a stretch lesion of the capsule or from avulsion of the capsule either from the glenoid (Bankart lesion, *Figure 1.6*) or much more rarely from the humerus, and more often from a combination of both. These lesions may be associated with a Hill–Sachs impression fracture, loose bodies, chondral or bony damage to the glenoid rim, SLAP tears (avulsion of the origin of biceps and the attached labrum), rents in the rotator interval, tears in subscapularis, tears in the rotator cuff, avulsion fractures of the greater tuberosity, and of course neurological

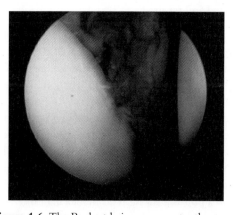

Figure 1.6 The Bankart lesion, as seen at arthroscopy.

lesions. We now understand that there is not one Bankart lesion but a cluster of lesions from a small Bankart cleft to a massive capacious cavern at the front of the glenoid. The pathology of dislocation is complex indeed. Surgery should be aimed at repairing these individual lesions and associated lesions and the surgery should be tailored to the patient.

Indications for surgery. The days of having to earn an operation by seven dislocations are long gone. Surgery for the repair of dislocation is simple, safe and effective. The surgical dissection is mainly blunt dissection, for only two structures have to be cut by the surgeon to get to the capsule: the skin and subscapularis. Anaesthesia in this group of young fit patients is safe. The average length of stay in hospital is under 24 hours for open surgery in the best of hands. The operation is said to have a 97% success rate but some of the papers which purport to equal this success rate of Rowe should be looked upon with some scepticism because the follow-up in many of these studies is of the order of 50%; in reality the recurrence rate is more like 10% than 3%.

The indication for repair is the first re-dislocation within two years in a patient under 40 years. For patients under the age of 25 years some surgeons are moving to shoulder arthroscopy within ten days of reduction and, if this confirms a Baker type III lesion (which has a 70% chance of re-dislocation within three years), offering the patient the chance of immediate repair.

The surgical repair. Surgery is performed through the deltopectoral approach. The type of repair depends on the pathological findings. Each area of pathology is addressed and repaired.

1. Bankart lesion. This is exposed and the front of the glenoid cleaned of soft tissue and decorticated so that the bone is bleeding over the whole area of the defect. Two or three suture-anchors are then placed, using a drill and drill guide to position them precisely on the glenoid rim and making sure that they do not damage the articular surface. There are numerous suture anchors on the market (Mitek, TAG, Revo screw, Harpoon, Corkscrew, FASTak) and the choice is up to the surgeon as they all have a pull-out strength far higher than the breaking strain of the suture material used.

The labrum/capsule complex is then captured by the suture and repaired down onto the anchors in the zone of healing.

2. The capsular stretch lesion. If the capsule itself is lax, it will need to be plicated. Usually the slack will need to be taken out inferiorly as well as laterally and this means performing a Neer capsular shift. A T-capsulotomy is performed, giving two triangular flaps; the bottom flap is taken up and laterally and the top flap is overlapped and taken down and laterally. Finally the flaps are sutured to each other.

3. The rotator interval lesion. The rotator interval is often stretched out and must be sutured closed. This is a vital part of the capsular shift procedure.

4. The SLAP lesion. If there is a SLAP lesion this must be repaired.

5. Loose bodies should be removed.

6. Bony Bankart lesion. If present this should be repaired. If the flake of bone is minute, it can be treated as a soft tissue Bankart and repaired down to a prepared bed with a suture anchor. If it is large enough to take a small fragment screw, then it should be internally fixed.

7. Humeral avulsion of the capsule should be repaired to the humerus with suture anchors.

8. Rotator cuff tears should be repaired.

9. If there is severe chondral or bony damage to the anterior glenoid lip then a bone block procedure such as a Bristow procedure should be considered. (Bristow neither suggested nor performed this operation: it was devised by Arthur Helfet and named by him in honour of Bristow, who before this had no surgical memorial.) The Bristow operation should also be considered for patients who recurrently dislocate following a failed previous repair.

Arthroscopic repair underwent a vogue during the 1980s. However, a high failure rate after arthroscopic staple repair, along with a high complication rate from loosening of the staples led to the demise of this form of repair. Arthroscopic suture repair then came into favour but the capsule could only be repaired to the 2 o'clock and 3 o'clock position, whereas the Bankart defect is at 5 o'clock, so there was a basic concept failure with this form of repair. Suture anchor repair then came into vogue but is so difficult, especially the intra-articular knot-tying, that it has not become popular. Different techniques to get a low anterior portal, such as the Resch slalom approach, show some promise but as yet there is no simple effective method of predictable arthroscopic repair. Moreover arthroscopic capsular plication can only be performed by laser techniques at present. Until arthroscopic repair is as safe and predictable as open repair, it should be regarded as a promising but experimental procedure.

Rehabilitation. The patient is returned to the ward in a sling which is worn for three weeks. During this three weeks the patient is allowed to do elbow extensions, pendulum swings, forearm fist/wrist/twist exercises and shoulder shrugs. After three weeks the patient starts a formal physiotherapy programme to regain movement and then to strengthen the arm. The patient should not be involved in sport for three months, contact sport for six months and overhead sport for one year.

Recurrent posterior dislocation

Recurrent posterior dislocation is one of the challenging areas still facing shoulder surgeons, for we still have no consistently effective method of treating this condition.

Presentation. The patient presents with a story of the shoulder coming out. Often the patient may be able to put the shoulder out. Beware this is not habitual or voluntary dislocation. Genuine recurrent patients do not make a habit of dislocating their shoulders, nor do they seek to gain from it. The problem is that their humerus drops out of the back of the socket with extreme ease whenever the arm is elevated with the arm internally rotated.

Investigation. The patient will often be able to demonstrate the dislocation in the clinic and the resounding clunk of relocation. The surgeon is able to demonstrate a positive jerk test. Plain radiographs are normal. A CT scan may be used to see if there is glenoid retroversion, but this is rarely present.

Treatment. Physiotherapy strengthening exercises to bulk up infraspinatus are unlikely to help in this condition. Teaching the patient to elevate the arm with the palm up (in external rotation) may help for the shoulder only dislocates in internal rotation. The recurrence rate following operation is 30–50%, so it is best to avoid surgery if at all possible and this type of surgery should be performed by a specialist shoulder surgeon.

Surgery may consist of:

1. Posterior capsular shift. This may be enough, but the capsule is very thin and often double-breasting tissue paper only leaves you with two-ply tissue paper.
2. Posterior capsular shift and glenoid osteotomy. This is favoured by some surgeons but the results are similar to plication alone and it is technically more demanding.
3. A Boyd and Sisk transfer of long head of biceps. This is a rather difficult procedure requiring combined anterior and posterior approach to the shoulder.
4. Internal rotation osteotomy of the surgical neck of the humerus. There are only two small series in the world literature. It is theoretically attractive but as yet unproven.
5. Posterior bone block.

Multidirectional instability (MDI)

Presentation. The typical patient presenting with MDI is a thin teenage girl. There is no history of injury. The patient is often hyperlax with recurvatum of fingers, wrist, elbows and knees: she may be balletic or gymnastic or a keen swimmer. She will present with shoulder pain and a feeling of the shoulder coming out. She can always reduce the shoulder herself and it may come out with extreme ease, for instance at night. The dislocations occur without volition and she has nothing to gain from them. Indeed they will often stop her from doing sports which she enjoys and is good at.

Examination. She will have an excess of rotation at the shoulder with 80° to 90° of external rotation of the shoulder joint and internal rotation up to T4 or T5. All the elements of instability will be present on examination. There is excessive anterior and posterior translation, but the key sign is a positive sulcus sign which is pathognomonic of MDI. There is usually an excess of movement and there is also a positive sulcus sign in the asymptomatic shoulder. There may be a family history of MDI.

Investigation. Plain radiographs and CT scans are usually normal. At arthroscopy there is a very capacious capsule with positive drive-thru' sign and positive see-through sign.

Treatment. This is by physiotherapy rehabilitation exercises consisting of a rotator cuff strengthening programme with TheraBand (commercially available elasticated bands), progressing to weights and proprioceptive exercises. Some authors claim an 80% success rate with such a rehabilitation programme. This is not this author's experience.

If rehabilitation fails to work, then a Neer capsular shift should be performed. This is a very successful procedure in the skeletally mature patient but is less successful in the extremely young patient (age 13–14 years).

Voluntary dislocation (wilful dislocation)

It was an ancient Egyptian who wrote in the Edwin Smith Papyrus that some disorders are 'conditions not to be treated'. Voluntary dislocation is probably one of those. However, strict diagnostic criteria must be made before this diagnostic label should be applied. The patient must be dislocating the shoulder for secondary gain. Often this will be to draw attention to bullying at school, or to try to control over-demanding parents.

These patients must be differentiated from those with recurrent posterior dislocation. When asked to demonstrate the dislocation, a patient with recurrent posterior dislocation must internally rotate the arm and then elevate it beyond 30°. In contrast, patients with voluntary dislocation will dislocate the joint without moving the arm; in this conditions the shoulder is pulled from its socket by muscle power, usually latissimus dorsi or pectoralis major. It may be difficult to tell MDI and voluntary dislocation apart. One key factor is, of course, that the patient with voluntary dislocation is mad, but they may not be overtly mad and they are often highly intelligent, scheming and conniving patients. This is where the surgeon should be extremely careful, for surgery is doomed to failure.

Treatment should be aimed along two parallel tracks. First the patient should be assessed by a clinical psychologist to try to get to the key question of secondary gain. Second the patient should be taught which muscles are powering up and pulling the shoulder out and enter a biofeedback programme in order to get this under control. Unfortunately it is often not in the patient's best interest to get better until they have achieved their secondary gains!

It is tempting to try to short-circuit this lengthy psychological battle by defunctioning the offending muscle which they are using to pull the shoulder out of joint. However, our results from using botulinum toxin in these patients has been disappointing for they have rapidly found another unparalysed muscle to use to pull the shoulder out again. Surgical tenotomy is a tempting alternative to the surgeon, but once again this is often only a temporary palliative because the patient will find another muscle with which to pull the shoulder out.

Dislocation from lower motor neurone palsy

Patients with a flaccid paralysis of the shoulder girdle, from polio or from a brachial plexus palsy, may present with symptomatic shoulder dislocation. In the former, this may well be painful, and in the latter may not be painful but may compromise arm function in a C5–6 palsy. Soft tissue procedures will not work in such a patient and they should be considered for shoulder fusion, the ultimate treatment for shoulder dislocation.

Congenital glenoid dysplasia

This is an extremely rare cause of dislocation. The largest series in the world literature consists of 16 patients, only 8 of whom had symptoms of instability. It is a condition best treated by a rehabilitation exercise programme. Surgery is rarely needed.

ROTATOR CUFF DISEASE: IMPINGEMENT TO CUFF TEAR

Rotator cuff disease accounts for more than one-third of all referrals to shoulder clinics. There is a spectrum of rotator cuff disease starting with impingement and progressing to small, moderate, large or massive cuff tears. The final end-point of rotator cuff disease is cuff tear arthropathy. Patients with rotator cuff tears have consistent physical signs which are crying out to be demonstrated in an examination. When we talk about rotator cuff disease we are really talking about the tendon of insertion of supraspinatus: 90% of rotator cuff pathology occurs in the anterior half of the final 3 cm of the tendon of supraspinatus. It therefore pays dividends to get to know this tendon intimately.

Anatomical relationships of the supraspinatus muscle and its tendon

The tendon of supraspinatus arises centrally within the muscle belly for this is a bipennate muscle. As the tendon forms, it migrates towards the anterior edge of supraspinatus and then flattens to form a broad flat tendon of insertion which inserts into a footprint some 2 cm × 1 cm on the greater tuberosity of the humerus. Posteriorly the tendon becomes confluent with the tendon of infraspinatus. Anterior to the tendon is the rotator interval of the capsule which is strengthened by the coracohumeral and superior glenohumeral ligaments.

The deep surface of the tendon merges with the superior capsule of the joint, which in turn is directly in contact with the humeral head. This deep surface of the tendon has a poor blood supply and is therefore slow to heal if injured. The tendon has to pass through a bony tunnel whose floor is the humeral head and whose roof is the coraco-acromial arch. The arch is made of acromion, acromioclavicular joint and coraco-acromial ligament. The subacromial bursa lies between the tendon and the arch and allows gliding of one in relation to the other. Any space-occupying lesion within this tunnel will cause a stenosis, for the tolerances here are minute, and any stenosis will impinge against the tendon and abrade it. This abrasion is the impingement lesion. Arthroscopically the impingement lesion looks like a circular ulcer where the bursa is rubbed through and the underlying cuff is fibrillated.

Pathology of impingement

Neer observed in a series of 100 cadaver scapulae that 11 showed bony changes on the undersurface of the acromion. This change only affected the anterior sector of the inferior surface and consisted of proliferative spurs or eburnation of the bone. He found similar lesions in every patient he operated on for rotator cuff disease and postulated that it was impingement of these bone spurs on the supraspinatus which caused impingement. This led him to champion the anterior acromioplasty as a highly effective operation to relieve pain in impingement. However, the bone is covered by soft tissue and in this case the soft tissue is the footprint of insertion of the coraco-acromial ligament.

Uhtoff examined the histology of the acromion and its attached coraco-acromial ligament in patients with impingement and found four grades of increasing severity of injury to the insertion of the ligament. Grade 1 was a loss of areolar tissue. Grade 2 was localised thickening of the insertion, with or without bone spurs. Grade 3 was break-up of the fibres of insertion of the ligament with irregularity of the undersurface of the acromion and Grade 4 was eburnation of the acromial bone and loss of the coraco-acromial ligament insertion.

There is also a strong association between degenerative changes of the acromioclavicular joint, in particular inferior osteophytes and rotator cuff disease.

Taking the theme of bony changes further, Bigliani (Neer's protegé) showed an association between morphological changes of the anterior acromion and rotator cuff disease. Edelson demonstrated an association between rotator cuff disease and an overdeveloped anterior acromion which projected forwards beyond the clavicle. The human acromion is the largest and most developed in the animal world. It is big enough already and anything which makes it bigger may cause impingement.

Aetiology of rotator cuff disease

We have seen how thickening of the bone and overlying soft tissue of the insertion of the coraco-acromial ligament occur in rotator cuff disease. It is postulated that these changes, along with osteophytes on the acromioclavicular joint, cause a stenosis of the supraspinatus outlet leading to impingement. The question is 'what causes these changes to occur?'

The changes may be related to age. Many studies show a direct relationship between age and the severity of cuff pathology. Perhaps changes in morphology are genetic so some patients are predestined to get cuff pathology. However the big question is 'do the changes to the acromion caused by primary rotator cuff dysfunction lead to a degree of upward subluxation of the head which will cause increased tension in the coraco-acromial ligament, which will then thicken in response and develop enthesopathic changes at its insertion?' This is the classic chicken-and-egg situation.

Ozaki has studied the pathological changes not only of the acromion, nor just the acromion and its ligament insertion, but has examined whole blocks of tissue consisting of humerus, rotator cuff, ligament and acromion. He showed that the first change to be seen is a partial-thickness tear of the deep surface of the supraspinatus insertion. This could be found before changes to the acromion and ligament. However, changes to the ligament and acromion never occurred without a deep surface tear of the cuff insertion. This would tend to imply that the egg came before the chicken!

What of the aetiology of rotator cuff tears? Neer stated categorically that 95% of rotator cuff tears were caused by impingement. Today we recognise that this figure may be too high. There are possibly three causes of rotator cuff tears: impingement, tendon fibre failure and major trauma. Of these, tendon fibre failure is probably the commonest.

Classification

Impingement

This is classified into three grades:

1. Neer stage I: reversible oedema and inflammation of the supraspinatus tendon. This is associated with excessive overhead use in young adults (aged 25–40). Treatment is conservative with a good prognosis for return to normality.
2. Neer stage II: fibrosis of the rotator cuff. These are permanent and irreversible changes to the rotator cuff causing pain on exercise which does not recover with rest. The patient is usually aged around 40 years and may require subacromial decompression.
3. Neer stage III. Although this is termed a stage of impingement, it actually means that there is a partial or full-thickness tear of the rotator cuff. There is bony alteration of the anterior acromion with bone spurs.

Partial thickness tears

These may be classified according to site (articular side or bursal side; deep surface or top surface) and by thickness (grade 1 = less than a quarter thickness; grade 2 = less than half thickness; grade 3 = more than half thickness). However, if you are fascinated by classifying partial thickness tears, you are really taking the examination too seriously and should think about taking a holiday!

Rotator cuff tears

These can be classified by size and by shape. Size is important because the results of surgical repair are directly proportional to the size of the tear: the watershed for a good result from surgery is 4 cm.

1. Small   <1 cm
2. Moderate   1–3 cm
3. Large   >3 cm
4. Massive   >5 cm

The shape is important because the method of repair and placement of sutures depends on the shape. Tears may be a split (very rare), L-shaped (common), reverse L-shaped, crescentic or trapezoid.

Clinical presentation of impingement

A patient aged 40–50 years presents with true shoulder pain which is worse on reaching out and with overhead activities, and also occurs at night. The pain is aggravated by internal rotation. On examination there is mild tenderness over the greater tuberosity. There is minimal wasting of the rotator cuff. On active elevation, the patient winces as the arm goes through the painful arc of movement. This pain is aggravated by internal rotation of the arm when it is held at 90° elevation. There may be soft crepitus when the arm passes through this arc. External rotation is symmetrical. Internal rotation is limited and exhibits end-point pain. Power is normal. The pain is dramatically relieved by injection of local anaesthetic into the subacromial bursa.

One special form of impingement is acute calcific tendonitis. This presents in a spectacular fashion. The patient is admitted to the emergency room with a history of crescendo pain in the shoulder. This starts as an acute toothache-like pain which builds over a period of a few hours into a searing, pacing-the-room, agonising pain which brings tears to the eyes of the strongest of people. Acute calcific tendonitis is one of the few shoulder emergencies. Compassion alone means that the surgeon should immediately flood the subacromial bursa with local anaesthetic and then either needle the calcific deposit, or decompress it arthroscopically or open.

Beware the sportsperson presenting with impingement-type pain, for this may represent impingement secondary to instability or the posterior impingement described by Walch where the posterosuperior glenoid impinges on the deep surface of the cuff in the throwing position.

Clinical presentation of a tear of the rotator cuff

Remember the aphorism 'Grey hair equals cuff tear'. Codman's description of the clinical presentation of a patient with a rotator cuff tear still can not be bettered sixty years after it was written. 'A labourer, aged over forty, with a previously normal shoulder, injures the shoulder and has an immediate but brief pain with severe pain the following night. There is loss of power in elevating the arm but no restriction when stooping, and a faulty scapulohumeral rhythm. There is a tender point, sulcus and eminence at the insertion of supraspinatus which causes a wince and crepitus as the tuberosity disappears under the acromion as the arm is passively elevated and which reappears on descent of the arm. The radiograph is normal.'

The only point of dissent one may have with Codman is in that the radiograph often shows tell-tale signs of a rotator cuff tear by the time the patient presents to the orthopaedic surgeon. The pathological changes to the undersurface of the acromion may be seen on radiographs as a 'sourcil' sign when the sclerosis of the undersurface of the acromion mimics an eyebrow above the shoulder. A spike of bone may show in the insertion of the coraco-acromial ligament and there are often signs of degenerative change in the acromioclavicular joint. All these changes may be seen in impingement and small rotator cuff tears.

Rotator cuff tears which have been present for some time will be accompanied by bony changes on the greater tuberosity in the form of irregularity, small cysts with sclerotic rings (*Figure 1.7*). At a later stage the humeral head will sublux upward with a reduced acromiohumeral interval or a break in 'Shenton's line of the shoulder', which is the elliptical arch formed by the medial border of the scapula and the medial border of the humeral metaphysis.

Further investigation of impingement and rotator cuff tears

Arthrography

Double-contrast arthrography is now an obsolete investigation. It does show deep surface partial-thickness tears and full-thickness tears but its weakness is that it is an invasive investigation which only shows the presence of a tear but gives little information about its extent or shape, nor the quality of the remaining tendon and muscle. It has been superseded by MRI scanning.

Ultrasonography

Ultrasonography may show a full-thickness rotator cuff tear. Its advantage is that it is cheap and does not involve ionising radiation. Against this, it is difficult to interpret and the main extent of any tear is under the acromion and therefore inaccesible to ultrasound. Dynamic ultrasonography gives more information than static ultrasonography.

Magnetic resonance imaging

This is the investigation of choice for full-thickness rotator cuff tears as it will show the presence, position, extent and shape of the tear, the quality of the remaining tendon and the quality of the supraspinatus muscle

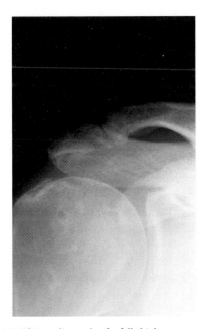

Figure 1.7 Plain radiograph of a full thickness rotator cuff tear. Note the irregularity of the greater tuberosity and the elevation of the humeral head in relation to the glenoid.

in terms of its bulk and whether there is fatty degeneration of the muscle. However, MRI is less specific for impingement, with a high level of false-positive results. MRI is not invasive but is expensive.

Arthroscopy

This is even more expensive than MRI. However, it is more specific for impingement and partial-thickness tears. Partial tears can be inspected from the joint side and from the bursal side. From the bursal side the impingement lesion looks like an ulcer with fibrillation of the bursal side of the tendon. A 'kissing' lesion can also be seen on the deep surface of the acromion. The advantage of arthroscopy is that the surgeon can proceed, in the patient who has given consent, to treat the lesion either by arthroscopic acromioplasty or by open techniques. This makes it cheaper in the long run than MRI.

Conservative treatment of impingement and cuff tears

Impingement lesions often respond to *injection of corticosteroid* into the subacromial bursa. The mode of action is probably to reduce the level of inflammation, thereby reducing the amount of stenosis within the supraspinatus outlet. If the first injection is of marked benefit to the patient, it is allowable to give up to three injections. Recent laboratory studies on the supraspinatus tendon of the rat indicate that more than three injections may lead to permanent damage to the tendon.

Physiotherapy may be useful in impingement. The patient should be taught strengthening exercises to the rotator cuff using TheraBand. This will lead to better centering of the head and reduce the amount of impingement. A recent Scandinavian study compared physiotherapy for impingement using proprioceptive neuromuscular facilitation (PNF) exercises against arthroscopic acromioplasty and placebo; PNF and acromioplasty were effective and placebo was not. The key is that 'hands-on' rehabilitation is effective in impingement: ultrasonography and various other mechanical devices are as useful as a hot water bottle – soothing whilst applied but of no long-term benefit. Both steroid injection and hands-on physiotherapy may also be of benefit in small rotator cuff tears, for the same reasons as they are helpful in impingement.

In irreparable rotator cuff tears in the elderly, assessment by the *occupational therapy* department may be of assistance. Loops sewn into clothing will aid dressing. Angled sponges may help washing, a bracket on the wall to hold a hair drier may allow drying, and a bidet with drier may aid in personal hygiene. All kitchen equipment can be brought to a suitable level. Teapot-tippers and angled knives, lightweight irons and old-fashioned pull-up clothes lines may be of great help.

Indication for surgery

Impingement

Neer's indications still stand. A patient with a normal life expectancy and of general good health, over the age of 40, with a history and clinical features of impingement, must have a positive response to injection of local anaesthetic into the subacromial bursa. The patient must have failed to respond to conservative methods of treatment over a period of six months.

Rotator cuff tear

A patient with a normal life expectancy and of good general health who is aged under 65 years (biologically not chronologically) with a proven symptomatic rotator cuff tear under 4 cm in extent should undergo operative repair as soon as is possible.

Patients over the age of 65 or with tears in excess of 4 cm may be considered for surgery by an expert surgeon depending on the severity of their symptoms.

Surgery for impingement

Arthroscopic subacromial decompression

Certain criteria must be met before considering arthroscopic subacromial decompression. The patient must have proven impingement. The bursa must be un-scarred and highly distensible so that a 'perfect view' is obtained at surgery (*Figure 1.8*). The surgeon must be properly trained in the technique and must be performing the technique regularly with a high success rate. The operating theatre must be adequate in terms of the training of scrub nurses, and have available a correctly functioning power shaver, a pump or other means to distend the bursa, a distraction apparatus, an arthroscopic electrosurgery apparatus to arrest bleeding

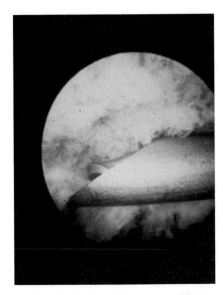

Figure 1.8 Arthroscopic subacromial decompression.

and the ability to turn the procedure to an open technique should problems arise during surgery. An audit of the results of surgery should be kept, for recent studies have shown that in the hands of 'ordinary' surgeons the results are far poorer than the results of the highly skilled pioneers of this technique: (50% success against 80% for open surgery).

The ability to perform this operation depends on a good view within the bursa of the acromion, coraco-acromial ligament and the rotator cuff. In order to get a good view, the arthroscope should be brought in to the bursa from the lateral portal. Pins may be inserted to help orientation within the bursa. The shaver may be introduced either from an anterolateral portal or from the posterior portal. If a special wide-bore inflow arthroscope sheath is being used, then the inflow may be via the arthroscope, but otherwise it should be through a separate portal to achieve high flows and high pressure.

The surgeon starts at the anterior border of the acromion and shaves off the insertion of the coraco-acromial ligament from its footprint so that the inferior surface of the acromion is denuded of soft tissue. The bone is then burred down, starting at the front of the acromion and carefully working from the lateral border of acromion to acromioclavicular joint. The process is repeated until a wedge of bone is removed from the anteroinferior acromion, as in the open procedure.

The surgeon takes great care to avoid the acromial artery which runs along the anterior border of the acromion between the coraco-acromial ligament and deltoid. Finally the coraco-acromial ligament is removed, either with the full radius resector or with a duckbill punch.

The acromioclavicular joint may also be excised arthroscopically. This requires great skill and repeated and regular practice. Postoperative rehabilitation is as for the open procedure.

Open subacromial decompression

The Neer anterior acromioplasty is still the 'gold standard' operation for impingement. It is simple, safe, requires a short learning curve, is cosmetically highly acceptable, is extensile should a cuff tear be found, allows easy access to the acromioclavicular joint (should this need to be resected or stabilised) and, in the correctly chosen patient, has a standard 85% success rate with a low incidence of complications.

The shoulder is approached through the Matsen deltoid-on route. The acromial artery is diathermied and divided. The anterior acromion and coraco-acromial ligament are defined. The coraco-acromial ligament is dissected free from its insertion to the undersurface of the acromion but left attached to the coracoid and retracted out of the way. The acromion is resected in two stages. The first is a coronal sawcut to remove any anterior acromion which protrudes forwards in front of the acromioclavicular joint. The second is an axial oblique cut, which removes a wedge of antero-inferior acromion, the full width of the acromion, the full depth of the acromion at the front, and measuring 2 cm in anteroposterior extent. This decompresses the rotator cuff.

There is a disagreement as to whether the acromioclavicular joint should be resected. Some authors state that this is only necessary in 6% of cases and some in 100%, but all agree that any inferior osteophytes should be removed. The joint should be examined and, if the surfaces are very arthritic, then the joint should be excised. The older the patient, the more commonly degenerative change is seen. An excision arthroplasty of the acromioclavicular joint should resect 1.5–2 cm, one-quarter of this resection coming from the acromial side and three-quarters from the clavicular side. Beware that resection of the acromioclavicular joint may expose an occult instability of this joint and for this reason you should perform a Weaver–Dunn reconstruction of the acromioclavicular joint whenever it is excised, using the previously stored coraco-acromial ligament. If the joint is pristine, then the coraco-acromial ligament is excised at this point. The dissection is closed in layers, being very careful to reattach deltoid to the anterior acromion. The skin is closed with a subcuticular suture.

Surgery for rotator cuff tears

Arthroscopic repair

This is an experimental procedure currently under trial by experts. It should not be performed unless as part of a prospective controlled study with the full consent of the patient.

Small cuff tears (less than 1 cm)

These are approached through the Matsen 'deltoid-on' exposure and can usually be trimmed and repaired side to side.

Moderate cuff tears (1–3 cm)

Again the approach is via the Matsen 'deltoid-on' technique. The acromioclavicular joint may be excised for exposure. The rotator cuff is now released. This involves release of the bursa which tethers the cuff to deltoid, the coracohumeral ligament which contracts and tethers the cuff to the base of the coracoid, and an internal release of the cuff from the edge of the glenoid. A very superficial bone trough is now prepared where the cuff has avulsed. This trough should be shallow, just allowing exposure of bleeding cancellous bone. Using stay-sutures, the cuff is advanced and is reattached in the bone trough with interosseous sutures, or suture anchors, or both.

Large cuff tears (3–5 cm)

The approach is as above plus an extension into trapezius. The whole key to such repairs is exposure and release. The repair is as for the moderate tear.

Massive tears (over 5 cm)

Such large tears should only be repaired by a surgeon who is repairing rotator cuff tears every week. Careful consideration should be given before undertaking such an operation because the patient can be made worse by inappropriate surgery which leads to re-rupture or stiffness. The shoulder surgeon may have to use tricks such as scapular osteotomy, local flaps or latissimus dorsi transfer to achieve closure. The coraco-acromial ligament should be Z-lengthened and repaired, for in these patients it is often the only structure preventing antero-superior escape of the humeral head.

Arthroscopic debridement

If a tear is irreparable then debridement of the edges and synovectomy may afford some pain relief. However, repair is better than debridement if the tear is less than massive.

Rehabilitation following acromioplasty and cuff repair

There are three phases to the rehabilitation protocol.

1. Phase one is protective, the goals of which are to protect the cuff repair and the deltoid closure while regaining movement and preventing muscle wasting.
2. Phase two is strengthening, the aims being to regain and improve strength around the shoulder. This phase can only start when there is secure healing of the cuff to the tuberosity and two-thirds of the normal range of movement has been regained in all directions.
3. Phase three is return to work and sport. Entry requirements are full range of movement, no pain or tenderness and the blessing of both physiotherapist and surgeon.

Cuff tear arthropathy

This is the end stage of rotator cuff disease. Fortunately it is rare, occurring in only 4% of people with rotator cuff tears. Clinically the patient is aged 70–80 years and presents with severe pain in the shoulder, weakness and inability to reach. The range of active elevation is only 40–60°. Rotation is markedly limited. On examination there is severe wasting of infraspinatus and supraspinatus. There is usually a large effusion anterior to the shoulder and the head of the humerus is subluxed anterosuperiorly. On attempted movement this subluxation is amplified. The shoulder is extremely weak in all directions. Radiographs show an arthritic humeral head which is subluxed superiorly and is articulating with an eroded and sclerotic acromion. The glenoid is arthritic and shows erosion of the superior rim where it is still articulating with the humeral head. The effusion is either straw-coloured or bloody.

The differential diagnosis is with hydroxyapatite arthritis or 'Milwaukee shoulder', although this may be a variant of cuff tear arthropathy. Syringomyelia or other forms of Charcot shoulder may mimic cuff tear arthropathy.

Treatment is contentious and most difficult. This is a condition without a predictably successful method of treatment. Some surgeons advocate an oversized-head hemiarthroplasty, and some a constrained total shoulder replacement. None of these are spectacularly successful and all have a high incidence of severe complications in such elderly patients.

FROZEN SHOULDER

Frozen shoulder is a comparitively rare condition, accounting for 5% of new referrals to the shoulder clinic. The cause of frozen shoulder is a fibrous contracture of the capsule of the shoulder which literally binds the humeral head to the glenoid, causing stiffness and pain. This contracture is thickest in the rotator interval area of the capsule, tethering the intertubercular groove to the coracoid and acting as a check-rein to external rotation. If this area is examined histologically the contracture is made of thick bands of collagen with fibroblasts and myofibroblasts, an appearance which is identical to that seen in Dupuytren's contracture in the hand.

Definition

Codman coined the term 'frozen shoulder' and his definition is still valid today: 'a slow onset of pain felt near the insertion of deltoid, inability to sleep on the affected side, painful and restricted elevation and external rotation with a normal radiological appearance'. Unfortunately this definition is a bit vague and overlaps with so many disorders of the shoulder that general practitioners would call any stiff shoulder a frozen shoulder. So let us re-define frozen shoulder for the 21st century:

Frozen shoulder is a fibrous contracture of the capsule of the shoulder. Patients present with an insidious onset of true shoulder pain and night pain. The pathognomonic feature is passive limitation of external rotation to less than 30°. There is painful passive limitation of elevation to below 100° and passive limitation of internal rotation to buttock level. Radiographs are normal. Arthrography shows a contracted joint space with obliteration of the subscapular recess and arthroscopy shows a contracted joint with obliteration of the subscapular recess. All other pathology must be excluded.

This last sentence is important, for Wiley was referred 150 patients with a suggested diagnosis of frozen shoulder but at arthroscopy 113 turned out to have another diagnosis.

Natural history

Frozen shoulder runs a course which has three phases: a painful phase, a stiffening phase and a phase of resolution. It is a most protracted disease which lasts at least two years and often five or more years. The textbooks would have you believe that frozen shoulder always gets better and indeed, if you have not been strict in your definition and have erroneously diagnosed many impingement syndromes as frozen shoulder, then you may believe those textbooks yourself. Certainly your examiner will believe those textbooks, so watch out!

It was Codman who stated that 'even the most protracted cases recover … in about two years' and this statement has been copied from textbook to textbook for 65 years. However, if you read his chapter you will see that even he qualifies this recovery for he states that 'it is pretty hard even for the patients to say when they are well'. Against this some of the most powerful voices in orthopaedics have tried in vain to educate the textbook writers but without effect. Simmonds said 'complete recovery … is not my experience'; DePalma said 'It is erroneous to believe that in all instances restoration of function is attained'; Reeves showed that after ten years 25 of 45 patients still had loss of movement, with a functional loss in three; Tibone and Shaffer in the most detailed study of the long-term history of frozen shoulder concluded 'complete resolution is not universal and brings us to question whether this is a self-limiting condition.'

The true natural history of frozen shoulder is that the pain disappears and movement does return as the unaffected shoulder capsule is stretched out, but that some measurable restriction may remain, particularly in external rotation. Most patients compensate well for restriction of external rotation and the deficit, although measurable, is mild and does not affect their function.

Clinical presentation

A 50 to 60-year-old patient presents with an insidious onset of true shoulder pain and severe night pain. The right and left shoulders are equally often affected, as are men and women. The shoulder stiffens rapidly and severely. On examination there is no wasting. Elevation is passively restricted to less than 100°. The pathognomonic sign is the marked restriction of passive external rotation to less than 30°. There are only three conditions which present with such a passive restriction of external rotation: frozen shoulder, arthritis and locked posterior dislocation. The latter two have an abnormal radiograph, whereas the radiograph in frozen shoulder is normal by definition. Internal rotation is passively restricted so that the hand cannot reach above buttock level. There is no crepitus on movement and the power is normal.

Investigation

Haematological and biochemical investigations are normal. Radiographs are normal. This is the one condition in which arthrography is still superior to MRI. Arthrograms show a diagnostic appearance of a contracted joint space with loss of the infraglenoid recess and of the subscapularis recess. MRI shows no significant changes. Arthroscopy shows a consistent abnormality arising out of the subscapularis recess at the base of the long head of biceps: there is a highly vascular villous fronding of the synovium overlying a matted area of granulation tissue which fills the subscapularis recess (*Figure 1.9*). (What is termed the subscapular recess by the arthroscopist looking from the inside is termed the rotator interval by the shoulder surgeon looking from the outside.) The joint capacity is reduced and there are no intra-articular adhesions.

Pathology

Findings at surgery are that the capsule is thickened and contracted. This contraction is maximal at the rotator

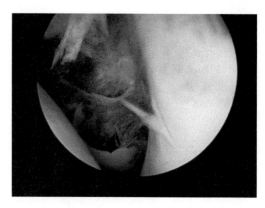

Figure 1.9 Arthroscopic view of the contracted subscapularis recess in frozen shoulder.

interval. The coracohumaral ligament is converted into a tough inelastic band of fibrous tissue spanning the interval between the coracoid process and the tuberosities of the humerus. This acts as a check-rein to external rotation. Division of this contracted tissue restores external rotation.

In the normal shoulder the rotator interval is easily defined. It is the sulcus above the top edge of the subscapularis tendon. It is a triangular sulcus whose margins are the subscapularis tendon at the front, the supraspinatus tendon posteriorly and the base of the coracoid medially. The rotator interval is strengthened by the coracohumeral ligament and the superior glenohumeral ligament which intermingle as they cross from medial to lateral. The long head of biceps lies underneath this sulcus. In a patient with frozen shoulder the rotator interval is no longer a sulcus but is filled with thickened capsule which is highly vascular. No longer can the edges be felt, for the whole area is scarred and indistinct. Thus the usual surgical landmarks (such as the palpable top margin of subscapularis) are lost, which can make surgery difficult in this area. On external rotation of the arm, the thickened coracohumeral ligament sticks out like a cord and can be seen to act as the check-rein to passive external rotation.

We excised the abnormal interval area in 20 consecutive patients with frozen shoulder who failed to benefit from manipulation. Histologically this tissue consists of bundles of collagen fibres. The tissue is highly cellular and highly vascular. Immuno-cytochemistry shows that these cells are mainly fibroblasts and myofibroblasts. The myofibroblast is the contractile fibroblast which is found in Dupuytren's disease and the fibromatoses. Histologically and with immunocytochemistry, this tissue from the shoulder is indistinguishable from Dupuytren's disease of the palmar fascia.

Associated conditions

Diabetes. The relationship between frozen shoulder and diabetes is well established. Diabetic patients have a 10–20% incidence of frozen shoulder, rising to 36% in insulin-dependent diabetics. Diabetics often have a particularly aggressive form of frozen shoulder which may be resistant to manipulation. Diabetes is also common in patients with Dupuytren's disease whose contracture may be particularly severe.

Dupuytren's disease. Patients with frozen shoulder have been found to have evidence of Dupuytren's disease in 18–25%.

Cardiac disease. This is classically associated with frozen shoulder, although this association is not as common as it used to be. Many patients with coronary disease have elevated serum cholesterol and triglycerides. Cholesterol and triglycerides are also raised in frozen shoulder and in Dupuytren's disease.

Minor trauma. Frozen shoulder may be initiated by minor trauma, classically a Colles' fracture. Dupuytren's disease may also be initiated by minor trauma, classically a Colles' fracture.

Treatment

Our generation has a great advantage when it comes to the treatment of frozen shoulder. We know what we are treating, whereas our forbears did not! Treatment must be aimed at stretching, tearing or dividing the fibrous contracture.

Physiotherapy

Mild cases will respond to physiotherapy in the form of gentle passive stretching and mobilisation of the capsule. If the condition is moderate, then it is unlikely that the physiotherapist will be able to stretch the pathological fibrous cord stretching from the coracoid to the humerus, but she may well be able to mobilise and stretch the least affected capsule in the infraglenoid

recess. This will regain elevation, although external rotation will remain restricted. However, most patients can adapt to a loss of external rotation as long as they have regained a functional level of elevation. Most activities can be performed with only 150° of elevation.

Manipulation under anaesthetic

This is the most effective method of treatment. Elevation is restored by tearing the capsule of the infraglenoid recess away from the neck of the humerus. This is felt by the surgeon as a tearing release during forced elevation. Some surgeons prefer to create this tear in the infraglenoid recess by forced passive abduction. If the contracture is mild then the manipulation can break the fibrous cord binding the coracoid to the humerus, and this can be felt by the surgeon as a tearing feeling during forced external rotation.

Some surgeons feel passionately that the manipulation should be performed in a particular sequence. If you come across an examiner with that attitude, just agree with him. However, in reality it is not the sequence that matters; it is knowing what you are doing. The two structures which you set out to tear are the infraglenoid recess (easy), and the fibrous contracture from the coracoid to the humerus (difficult). Arthroscopy following manipulation invariably shows that the capsule of the infraglenoid recess tears away from its insertion into the neck of the humerus. Remember that this is a very vascular area, with the metaphyseal feeders from the posterior circumflex humeral artery entering the humerus at this point: arthroscopically one can not see the tear in the coracohumeral ligament as this is extra-articular, but one may well see haemorrhage in the subscapular recess.

After manipulation, a long-acting local anaesthetic solution should be injected intra-articularly and the patient nursed overnight in a Bradford sling. Urgent physiotherapy starts the following day to prevent the tear which you have created from scarring back up. It takes an average of eight weeks for the pain to settle following manipulation. The patient must be warned of this before the procedure.

Manipulation gained a reputation for causing dislocation and even fracture of the humerus but this was following aggressive manipulation by untrained, mighty men who took the failure of the shoulder to externally rotate as an affront to their manhood. However, we must never overlook an opportunity to learn from history. What this shows us is that the contracted fibrous cord may be stronger than the bone. The bone must never be put in jeopardy and if the contracted cord will not release, then the surgeon should stop and consider open surgical release.

Open surgical release

The patient is placed in the lateral decubitus position and prepared for surgery. A Matsen 'deltoid-on' approach is made to the shoulder. The coraco-acromial ligament is exposed and then excised. The acromial artery is diathermied and divided. The arm is now held in external rotation by the assistant and the fibrous cord is divided using electrocautery. This releases the tether to external rotation and the cord is excised until the shoulder joint is opened. Great care is taken not to damage the tendon of long head of biceps, which lies just below this area and can be tightly applied to the undersurface of the contracture. Once the joint has been entered, the landmarks of the top edge of subscapularis and the forward edge of supraspinatus can be seen, whereas they can not be distinguished from the outside. The whole of the scarred and thickened rotator interval is then excised, taking great care to dissect right down to the base of the coracoid using an arthroscopic duckbill rongeur to clear this area of tethered scar tissue. Finally a manipulation in elevation is performed to release the infraglenoid recess. The joint is filled with 20 ml of 0.5% bupivacaine. No attempt is made to close the defect. The deltoid split is closed and then the skin. The patient is nursed as for a manipulation. This procedure is highly effective, except in insulin-dependent diabetics.

Arthroscopic release

There has been a recent explosion of interest in arthrocopic release of frozen shoulders. Essentially the rotator interval can be excised arthroscopically from within the joint using a combination of electrosurgery and power shaver. The landmarks of the edge of the interval are actually better distinguished arthroscopically than from the outside of the joint and there is less likelihood of damage to long head of biceps. Following the arthroscopic release of the rotator interval, a manipulation is performed to release the infraglenoid recess. This

should not be released arthroscopically (although this has been reported) for the axillary nerve runs just below the capsule and would be endangered by such a manoeuvre.

Over the course of the last decade the enigma which was the frozen shoulder has been unravelled and this has given us a range of effective treatments for this painful and otherwise protracted disease.

SHOULDER REPLACEMENT

Shoulder replacement is now an established and successful method of treatment for the arthritic shoulder. The first recorded shoulder replacement was performed over 100 years ago by Dr Emile Pean of Paris. This shoulder was made of a platinum tube, linked to a vulcanised rubber universal joint, which in turn was attached to the scapula with wire. This device was inserted as a two-stage operation for a tuberculous joint. Surprisingly, it functioned reasonably for two years before it had to be removed. There was a gap of 50 years before further attempts were made at shoulder replacement.

In the USA Dr Charles Neer was the trail-blazer of shoulder replacement. He had to care for patients with severe fracture–dislocations of the shoulder, and found that the results of excision arthroplasty were desperately poor. The modern era of successful shoulder replacement was introduced by Neer with his article on five successful shoulder hemiarthroplasties for fractures in 1955. Neer designed his prosthesis as an unconstrained surface replacement, which was as anatomical as could be engineered at the time. A single diameter of head (50 mm) was chosen. It is a great credit to him that the design of his shoulder has changed little over the course of 40 years, and still remains the basis for our present third-generation modular unconstrained prostheses.

At the same time in Europe, surgeons were working on replacements for tumours around the shoulder. Because the rotator cuff muscles had to be resected in tumour work, constrained devices were designed, but these placed such high loads on the prosthesis-bone interface of the glenoid that they inevitably loosened at this junction. Because of this, constrained shoulder replacements have few indications around the shoulder.

The development of total shoulder prostheses

In 1971 Dr Neer reported upon mating his metal hemiarthroplasty to a polyethylene glenoid. He actually designed the glenoid for difficult shoulders which had erosion or instability, for he felt that the glenoid was not a major pain source. The diameter of the glenoid had to match the head and was also 50 mm. Two glenoids were made, standard and extra small. Two neck lengths of humeral head (15 mm and 22 mm) were manufactured, in order to be able to implant the shoulder replacement in the face of either capsular contracture or glenoid erosion.

The second-generation prostheses were modular, rather than monobloc, and allowed changes in head size. The diameter of the humeral head is highly variable ranging from 36 mm to 56 mm. However, the second-generation prostheses failed to regain a perfectly anatomical result, as they didn't address all the geometrical variables, in particular changes in medial-offset and posterior-offset.

The third-generation shoulder has become far more sophisticated (*Figure 1.10*), in order to be able to vary head diameter, head thickness, facing-angle, medial-offset and posterior-offset. One prosthesis has seven different heads, which can be set at any of eight different positions for posterior-offset; upon one of four different necks, which sit upon one of three different stems. This gives the surgeon 672 combinations to allow for the greatest anatomical match, so he should be able to get it right!

Such sophistication comes at a price. First is the engineering price of three interfaces, two locked with a grub screw, but all of which are vulnerable to loosening, fretting, wear and dissociation. The second price is economic: such a prosthesis is expensive.

Neer introduced his glenoid component in 1971. The first-generation glenoid was a thin polyethylene component with a truncated triangular stem which was cemented into the glenoid.

The first contentious issue on the glenoid side is surface shape. Neer designed his prosthesis with a completely conforming head and socket. However, if radiographs of a shoulder are studied then it can be seen that the glenoid is flatter than the humeral head. Rockwood and Matsen have designed their prosthesis with a glenoid which has a flatter surface shape than the humerus; they have also done cadaver studies which show that there is obligatory antero-posterior motion with elevation of the shoulder, which can only occur with a flatter glenoid than head. Contrary to this, Bigliani has looked not at the bony surface of the glenoid but at the shape of the surface of the cartilage, and has shown this to be thicker at the periphery of the glenoid than in the centre; these studies have shown perfect congruence just as Neer originally stated.

First-generation glenoids were made with a curved back, to match the approximate shape of the glenoid. Inevitably there is a mismatch at the bone–prosthesis interface despite the grouting effect of bone cement. This leads to the 'rocking-horse' effect, warp and deformation. Deformation and warp can be reduced by half through having a second-generation flat back to the glenoid prosthesis, and sawing or routing a flat surface on the glenoid to match the plastic.

Glenoid fixation with cement is particularly difficult. A metanalysis by Brems of 1400 patients showed a 38% incidence of lucent lines at the cement–bone interface. Good cement technique (lavage, drying, pressurisation) is extremely difficult within the tight confines of the glenoid and may be why lucent lines are common. However, cementless designs are also not immune from this problem.

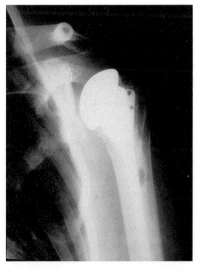

Figure 1.10 Radiograph of a third-generation shoulder replacement.

Indications for shoulder replacement

There are five general indications for shoulder replacement.

Osteoarthritis

Osteoarthritis is the primary indication for shoulder replacement. Compared to the hip and the knee, it is rare. However, as the population ages, and becomes more sophisticated in its medical requirements, the number of people asking for shoulder replacement is growing. Patients are usually in their seventh or eighth decade, and present with increasing pain, stiffness, decreasing independence and radiographs which show a loss of joint space, sclerosis and the tell-tale inferior osteophyte.

One of the interesting features of shoulder surgery is the number of patients who present with secondary osteoarthritis. The proportion of patients with secondary osteoarthritis is far higher in the shoulder than in the hip or knee. Avascular necrosis, acromegalic arthropathy, ankylosing spondylitis, psoriatic arthropathy, haemophiliac arthropathy, pigmented villonodular synovitis, synovial chondromatosis, septic arthritis, arthritis of dislocation and neuropathic arthropathy will all present with secondary osteoarthritis of the shoulder.

Rheumatoid arthritis

The patient with rheumatoid arthritis will often require surgery to the shoulder. Beware; just because a patient has rheumatoid disease, and has shoulder pain, does not mean that he/she needs a shoulder replacement. Patients with rheumatoid arthritis may have referred pain, acromioclavicular pain and rotator cuff disease just like everybody else. There are two different presentations of rheumatoid arthritis in the shoulder. Neer has termed these the 'wet' type and the 'dry' type. The wet type is a very aggressive and erosive arthritis, which progresses very rapidly. The dry type is burnt-out rheumatoid which is less erosive and acts more like a secondary osteoarthritis.

Fracture–dislocations

There is a vogue for attempting biological internal fixation for three and four-part fracture dislocations rather than immediate hemiarthroplasty. The reason for this is the disappointing results seen after hemiarthroplasty in these fracture patients. All too often such a patient will end up with an imperfect or poor result, owing to pain on use and stiffness. Such surgery is difficult, for the soft tissue reconstruction of the shattered tuberosities and mangled rotator cuff requires a degree of obsession rarely found in the trauma surgeon. Whether to opt for internal fixation depends on the blood supply to the humeral head. In this situation the main blood supply to the head, the ascending branch of the anterior circumflex humeral artery, is often ruptured and the viability of the head depends on the small metaphyseal feeders from the posterior circumflex artery. Thus if the calcar is displaced these vessels will be severed and the head is dead. In this situation, internal fixation will turn to avascular necrosis after two years so, it is best to perform a good hemiarthroplasty at the first operation.

Rotator cuff arthropathy

The results of shoulder replacement in this disease are poor. The shoulder usually remains moderately painful and function is not improved over the preoperative state. Even a small reprieve may sway the reluctant surgeon to operate, for the pain can be so severe in this condition. There may be a place for bipolar hemiarthroplasty, giant head hemiarthroplasty or constrained total shoulder arthroplasty in this condition.

Tumour surgery

The results of shoulder replacement are good in tumour resection. However, that is beyond the remit of this chapter.

Contraindications to shoulder replacement

Active sepsis is a contraindication to shoulder replacement. Neuropathic joints such as those affected by syringomyelia are relative contraindications. Shoulder replacement should not be performed in patients with gross instability. The patient must have the will and ability to undertake an active rehabilitation protocol.

Surgery for arthritis

The shoulder is approached using the extended deltopectoral approach with a complete pectoralis major tenotomy. The capsule is opened and the arm is extended and externally rotated to dislocate the head. The osteophyte rim is removed from the circumference of the head. The shaft of the humerus is progressively reamed up and the cutting jig applied. The desired retroversion angle is dialled into the jig and the head sectioned, so that the saw cut exits at the 'key-point': that is the sulcus between the articular surface and the greater tuberosity. The humeral cement plug is inserted into the medullary canal, followed by a temporary tampon and a head protector. The sectioned head is then retracted posteriorly to gain access to the glenoid. The rotator interval and the anterior capsule are released from the glenoid, the inferior capsule from the humerus, and the posterior capsule from the glenoid, in order to rebalance the shoulder and gain good access to the glenoid. The keel-slot is now burred in the glenoid and the bone surface prepared for the glenoid. After trial reduction the glenoid is power-lavaged, dried and cement is pressurised into the keel-slot prior to insertion of the glenoid. After the glenoid cement has cured, a further trial reduction is performed, fine tuning for neck length and head size. The humeral canal is then lavaged, dried and cement is pressurised into the canal using a retrograde-gun technique. The stem is then inserted in the correct amount of retroversion. Finally, the head is applied to the stem, after the humeral cement has cured, and the joint is reduced. Subscapularis is closed, pectoralis major is closed and the wound is sutured.

Rehabilitation following shoulder replacement

The patient is nursed in a sling for the first three days, and then wears the sling at night for a further three weeks. He or she follows a protective-phase physio-therapy regime for the first four weeks, with pendulum, hand and elbow exercises, then starts an active-assisted programme with pulleys to regain the range of motion, and finally undergoes a strengthening programme to regain muscle bulk and control.

Results of surgery

These depend on the age of the patient, their pathology and the amount of preoperative stiffness. There is no benefit in comparing a small study of shoulder replace-ments for osteoarthritis, at an average age of 60 years,

with a small study of 80-year-old end-stage rheumatoid patients. Results must be judged against the disease process and movement expressed as gain in elevation. Apart from Neer's studies there are very few series of shoulder replacement with over 100 cases.

In an analysis of this author's first 140 shoulder replacements, pain was graded on a 30-point score, 0 being severe pain and 30 no pain at all. The results showed that shoulders with osteoarthritis improved from 1.2 to 26, rheumatoid shoulders from 0.3 to 25, those with fractures from 1.2 to 23, and shoulders with cuff-arthropathy from 0 to 15. From this it can be seen that shoulder replacement is an effective operation for pain relief. Gain in elevation was 47° for osteoarthritis, 33° for rheumatoid arthritis, 70° for fractures and just 15° for cuff-arthropathy.

Complications

1. Loosening of components: this is the major long-term complication of shoulder replacement. Loosening usually affects the glenoid component. Cofield reported a 12-year follow-up study, which showed radiolucent lines in 84% of cases and definite loosening in 44%.
2. Instability is the second commonest cause of problems following shoulder replacement.
3. Periprosthetic fracture may occur during the operation or afterwards. Intraoperative fracture is caused by poor surgical technique. Postoperative fracture usually occurs at the tip of the prosthesis, where there is a stress-riser effect.
4. Infection is rare. It may occur primarily or secondarily.
5. Nerve injury may occur to the axillary nerve or the musculocutaneous nerve.
6. Dissociation of modular components may occur, and may be associated with dislocation.
7. Ectopic bone formation has been reported in some series, but is usually a radiological rather than a functional problem.

INSTABILITY OF THE ACROMIOCLAVICULARJOINT

Injury to the acromioclavicular joint in contact sports-people is so common as to be almost normal. Minor injuries occur every weekend, and most sportsmen shrug them off, and forget about them entirely. It can be no surprise that such a small oblique joint, measuring just 9 mm by 19 mm, should be so commonly injured, for it is the weak link when the patient falls on the point of the shoulder. The primary ligamentous restraints against dislocation are the conoid and trapezoid ligaments, which run from the coracoid to the undersurface of the clavicle. These are powerful ligaments, but when they fail they shred and never regain their function, as in anterior-cruciate failure in the knee. Like the cruciate ligaments, there is little point in attempting to suture them back together; reconstruction must depend on bringing in a biological augment. A suitable biological augment is the coraco-acromial ligament.

Classification of instability

Type I

This is the commonest injury. The joint capsule (superior and inferior acromioclavicular ligaments) are sprained. There is no damage to the coracoclavicular ligaments, or to the trapezius or deltoid. This is a minor injury which is treated in a sling for comfort, and the prognosis is for a return to completely normal function.

Type II

Complete disruption of the joint capsule with sprain of the coracoclavicular ligaments. Trapezius and deltoid are uninjured. There is a mild anteroposterior instability, but minimal upward subluxation of the clavicle. (The convention has always been to describe the clavicle as subluxing upward as this is the radiographic appearance, but in reality the clavicle remains in place, and it is the acromion and the whole arm which subluxes downward.) Again this is a relatively mild injury which is treated in a sling for comfort; the prognosis is for a return to completely normal function, although a minor swelling over the joint may remain.

Type III

This is a major disuption. The joint capsule has torn and now the conoid and trapezoid ligaments have totally disrupted, allowing upward subluxation of the

clavicle. The deltoid and trapezius are detached from the distal 2 cm of the clavicle. This joint will never return to normal. However, many powerful sportsmen will accept the deformity (the overlapping of the clavicle over the top surface of the acromion) and the crepitus on movement. The injury is treated with a sling for comfort and 80% regain a normal range of shoulder movement, normal power and accept the mild discomfort as one of the hazards of being weekend warriors.

Conversely 20% will not accept such a result. If, three months after injury, the patient complains of pain, deformity, crepitus, limited function or the arm 'feeling apart', then consideration should be given to reconstruction.

Dozens of operations have been designed for reconstruction of the acromioclavicular joint. These operations fall into four classes: primary acromioclavicular joint fixation (with pins, screws, wires, plates or ligaments), primary coracoclavicular ligament fixation (with screws, wire, fascia, ligament or synthetic material), excision of the distal clavicle, with or without ligament augment, and finally dynamic muscle transfers. The first two methods apply to Type IV dislocations and over, and are discussed below. The last two methods apply to the secondary reconstruction of the chronically symptomatic acromioclavicular disruption. Modern policy is to use the Weaver–Dunn reconstruction as the primary method of repair and to leave the dynamic transfer as a revision procedure.

The Weaver–Dunn operation is a highly successful method of reconstruction for the acromioclavicular joint; so successful that it has superseded all other methods of repair. It is simple, safe and tolerant. The acromioclavicular joint is exposed using the standard Matsen deltoid-on technique. The deltotrapezius fascia is divided over the dislocation, and reveals a pseudo-articulation which is full of synovial fluid. The coracoacromial ligament is fully exposed and released from its insertion into the undersurface of the anterior acromion, but is left attached to the coracoid. The overlapped distal clavicle is exposed subperiosteally, and 2 cm is excised. The joint can now be reduced. Two 2 mm drill holes are made in the distal clavicle, and a number 2 suture is taken through the forward drill hole and weaved down the lateral edge of the coraco-acromial ligament to the coracoid process, and then weaved up its medial border, and taken through the posterior drill hole in the clavicle. A second suture is now similarly placed. The clavicle is reduced both downward and forward and held in position with tension on one of the sutures while the second is tied. The second suture is then tied. The deltotrapezius fascia is repaired. The arm is protected in a sling for four weeks postoperatively.

Some patients undergoing a Weaver–Dunn procedure will not comply with their postoperative regime, and the repair will fail. The author has had patients who have fallen downstairs, gone fishing and fallen in the river or been involved in bar-fighting within two weeks of their repair. Such patients must be carefully counselled before considering further surgery. Dynamic muscle transfers are not as easy in reality as the line drawings in textbooks would have you believe. To get the tip of the coracoid to reach up as far as the clavicle requires extreme elbow flexion and a fair degree of tension. However, as a salvage procedure dynamic transfers do work.

Type IV

The joint capsule is disrupted. The conoid and trapezoid ligaments are torn. The deltoid and trapezius are torn from the distal clavicle and the clavicle is displaced not only upwards but also posteriorly. There is damage to the joint surfaces. The clavicle sits under trapezius, or even button-holed through it. In such a situation, consideration should be given to immediate reconstruction.

There is no point in reducing the joint and fixing it in place with primary acromio-clavicular or coracoclavicular fixation, for as soon as this fixation is removed the joint will once again dislocate. Remember that the conoid and trapezoid ligaments have ruptured. The joint surfaces have also been damaged. The only way to get a good result is by reducing the joint and augmenting the coracoclavicular ligaments, and the best way to do this is the Weaver–Dunn technique.

Because the instability is so great in this situation, some surgeons recommend backing up the Weaver–Dunn with a coracoclavicular screw, of the Bosworth or Rockwood type. As those who have tried this technique know, getting such a screw to hold in the coracoid is difficult. If there is any concern as to whether the repair will hold, a hole can be drilled in the coracoid and a number 2 vicryl taken bone-to-bone, from the clavicle to the coracoid, to back up the ligament whilst it heals and thickens. The repair should be protected in a sling for four weeks.

Type V

The joint capsule is torn, the coracoclavicular ligaments ruptured; the deltoid and trapezius are torn from the clavicle, the clavicle dislocated upwards and backwards. The clavicle is buttonholed through trapezius and is lying subcutaneously. The patient needs an acute Weaver–Dunn procedure.

Type VI

This is academic. You will never see one. However, it is in the books. The distal clavicle is displaced downwards and button-holed through the conjoined tendon or locked under the coracoid. This requires open reduction, excision arthroplasty and Weaver–Dunn reconstruction.

WEIGHT-LIFTER'S OSTEOLYSIS OF THE CLAVICLE

This unusual condition presents in weight-lifters complaining of pain from the acromioclavicular joint. The radiographic findings show a flame-shaped osteolytic area within the distal clavicle, abutting onto the acromioclavicular joint. The acromial side of the joint is normal. There may be bone resorption or tapering of the distal clavicle. The patient may have been on long-term anabolic steroids. Abolition of their pain following a local anaesthetic injection into the joint confirms the diagnosis. Paradoxically, a corticosteroid injection into the joint may be highly beneficial. If surgery is indicated, a simple excision arthroplasty may be all that is required.

DEGENERATIVE ARTHRITIS OF THE ACROMIOCLAVICULAR JOINT

Few designs are perfect. When *Homo sapiens* was designed, a flaw occurred in the blueprint, and this defect is the articular surface of the acromioclavicular joint! The surfaces of the acromioclavicular joint are fibrocartilage and not hyaline cartilage. Early degenerative change of the joint surfaces, and deterioration of the fibrocartilagenous disc within the joint, are normal aspects of ageing. Accelerated wear is found in racquet-sports players. In these patients treatment starts with an intra-articular injection of lignocaine and corticosteroid Should this fail to resolve the patient's symptoms, then a simple excision arthroplasty of 1.5–2 cm of distal clavicle can be undertaken. This procedure can either be performed open, when the superior ligament must be divided but can be repaired, or arthroscopically when the inferior ligament must be opened and cannot be repaired. However, if there is any hint of occult instability (uncovered when the joint capsule is opened), the surgeon must be prepared to stabilise the joint with a Weaver–Dunn procedure.

THE STERNOCLAVICULAR JOINT

Although sternoclavicular disorders are rare, this is a fascinating joint which can not only develop acute or recurrent instability but arthropathies, infections, condensing osteitis and sternocostoclavicular hyperostosis. The ligaments around the sternoclavicular joint are extremely strong. The intra-articular disc ligament and the interclavicular ligaments are very powerful. Grant states that the interclavicular ligament is the analogue of the wishbone of birds. The anterior and posterior sternoclavicular ligaments are weaker.

Acute anterior sternoclavicular dislocation

The patient presents following trauma, complaining of pain and swelling over the sternoclavicular joint. The best radiographic view of the sternoclavicular joint is the 'serendipity view': a 40° cephalad anteroposterior radiograph. Reduction should be attempted, but both surgeon and patient must realise that this is a highly unstable injury and often reduction cannot be maintained; or if it is, it may recur. The surgeon must resist the temptation to attempt open reduction and stabilisation. Pins in this situation are not only dangerous but can be lethal. In Germany two surgeons were charged with manslaughter by negligence following fatal migration of pins. Moreover, scars in this area can be very unsightly, leading to keloid formation over the manubrium. The only tissue available for repair is the tendon of subclavius, which is a pretty poor structure. Remember that in children and adolescents the injury may not be a dislocation but a growth plate fracture which will heal, albeit with a callus bump.

Acute posterior sternoclavicular dislocation

The posterior anatomical relations of the sternoclavicular joint are vital structures. The displaced clavicle may compress the innominate vein, the common carotid and subclavian arteries or the trachea. Reduction should be a matter of urgency. It is polite to inform the on-call vascular team that you have a posterior sternoclavicular dislocation which you are taking to theatre to reduce. The patient should be given a general anaesthetic. A large sandbag is placed centrally on the operating table, between the patient's shoulder blades. The arm is then abducted and put under traction and extension. Usually the joint will then relocate with a satisfactory clunk. Fortunately the reduction is stable. If reduction cannot be achieved, pressure is applied to the anterior aspect of the humeral head forcing the arm into extension. Should this fail, then a towel clip is placed percutaneously around the medial clavicle (but lateral to the vein!) and direct reduction is carried out. Should even that fail, open reduction should be performed. The reduction is stable and no form of internal fixation should be applied. A figure-of-eight dressing is applied.

Sternoclavicular oddities

The middle-aged woman presenting with a painful swelling over the sternoclavicular joint and medial clavicle presents a real diagnostic dilemma. If a serendipity view is inconclusive, then CT scan or MRI of the joint may be valuable.

Arthritis. The swelling and pain may be a primary or secondary arthritis. One particular form is postmenopausal arthritis. Treatment is symptomatic.

Infection. The most bizarre infections seem to have a predilection for the sternoclavicular joint. Although staphylococcal infections are the most common, *Streptococcus, E. coli, Pseudomonas, Pasteurella, Neiserria, Cholera,* spirochaete and tuberculous infections have been reported. Intravenous drug abuse may be a portal of entry.

Condensing osteitis of the clavicle. This unusual condition presents with swelling of the proximal clavicle. The radiograph shows expansion of the medial clavicle with increased sclerosis. Biopsy may be needed for culture and to exclude malignancy. Treatment is symptomatic.

Sternocostoclavicular hyperostosis. This rare condition was first reported in Japan in 1974. Three phases of this disease have been described by Sonozaki. Stage I is mild ossification of the costoclavicular ligaments; stage II shows bony fusion of the clavicle to the first rib; and in stage III the bone mass extends between the clavicle first rib and sternum. It may be associated with pustular skin eruptions on the palm of the hand and the plantar surface of the foot.

CLAVICULAR ODDITIES

Congenital pseudarthrosis of the clavicle

This unusual condition presents in the child with a prominent bony lump in the mid-point of the right clavicle, sometimes associated with pain. The differential diagnosis is between birth fracture of the clavicle, cleidocranial dysostosis and congenital pseudarthrosis. Congenital pseudarthrosis becomes more prominent as the child grows. It always occurs in the right clavicle. Lloyd Roberts suggested that it was caused by pulsation of the subclavian artery, which is always higher on the right, and prevents the ossification centres coalescing. The only case in the world literature of this condition occurring in the left clavicle had dextrocardia! It is usually asymptomatic. When symptomatic the treatment of choice is the use of a small reconstruction plate to hold an intercalary autograft, taken from the pelvic brim, between the freshened ends of the pseudarthrosis. This condition is not associated with neurofibromatosis and heals rapidly after operation.

Birth fractures of the clavicle

This is the most common birth fracture, occurring in 5 per 1000 vertex deliveries and 160 per 1000 breech deliveries. The fracture may present as pseudoparalysis of the arm, with swelling and crepitus at the fracture site. It may present at seven to ten days when the callus lump appears. The fracture is confirmed on radiographs. Birth fractures always heal rapidly and leave no disability. However, they may be associated with obstetric brachial plexus palsy.

Cleidocranial dysostosis

This is an hereditary abnormality of membranous bone formation, in which there is a wide gap in the clavicle and tapered bone ends. The condition is often bilateral. There may be abnormalities of the other membranous bones such as the skull and pelvis. Often there is a family history.

NEUROLOGICAL DISORDERS OF THE SHOULDER

The diagnosis of neurological disorders about the shoulder depends on a comprehensive knowledge of the anatomy of the brachial plexus and its terminal branches, combined with a meticulous neurological examination. Occasionally the help of a neurophysiologist may be required in borderline cases. Although thoracic outlet syndrome and brachial plexus palsy may present to the shoulder surgeon, these are covered in Chapter 7 (pages 219–223).

Winging of the scapula

After referred pain from the cervical spine, winging of the scapula is the commonest neurological presentation to the shoulder clinic.

Pseudo-winging

True winging must be differentiated from pseudo-winging. Pseudo-winging may be due to an abnormal motion of the scapula to protect a damaged area of the rotator cuff, or may be secondary to a space-occupying lesion such as an osteochondroma on the deep surface of the scapula, which pushes the scapula backwards and may cause clicking.

Serratus anterior weakness

This is usually caused by a paralysis of the long thoracic nerve of Bell. This nerve may be injured by pressure (Saturday night palsy) or by surgery such as radical mastectomy or a transaxillary approach for excision of the first rib. The patient presents with weakness of the scapula, and therefore a reduced range of shoulder movement. The deformity is exaggerated by asking the patient to place his hands on the wall in front of him and to lean heavily against the wall. The palsy usually recovers within 18 months; if it persists, a transfer of the sternal head of pectoralis major (lengthened by a fascia lata strip) to the inferior angle of the scapula, may stabilise the scapula.

Neuralgic amyotrophy

Presents with pain, a fever and then weakness of one or more muscles around the shoulder. The long thoracic nerve is often affected by neuralgic amyotrophy. This condition was first described by Spillane in British troops fighting in the Tobruk campaign during World War II, and shares some features with the Gulf War syndrome. It may be associated with inoculation and has also been associated with infection with human parvovirus 19.

Trapezius weakness

Paralysis of trapezius leads to a drooping shoulder and difficulty in shoulder movement. The usual cause is division of the spinal accessory nerve, either by laceration during a fight or inadvertently during surgery. The spinal accessory nerve is a small nerve, just 2 mm in diameter, which crosses the posterior triangle of the neck. It is close to the lymph nodes in this region and is usually injured by inexperienced surgeons biopsying nodes. If the nerve has been divided, the patient usually has severe pain in the shoulder girdle. Repair of the nerve improves movement in most cases.

Fascioscapulohumeral dystrophy

This is an autosomal dominant disease with wide expression. Patients present with symmetrical weakness and winging of the scapulae. They also have weakness of the facial muscles and are thus unable to whistle. They have wasting of the shoulder girdle, but usually have a well-preserved deltoid giving a 'superman' appearance. They are interesting patients to bring up to an examination! The condition can be improved by scapulo-thoracic fusion (Copeland–Howard procedure).

Suprascapular nerve entrapment syndrome

This rare condition presents with pain and marked wasting of infraspinatus in a middle-aged or young patient. The differential diagnosis is a rotator cuff tear. However, patients with suprascapular nerve entrapment syndrome have no tenderness over the greater tuberosity, no sulcus or eminence, no wince on elevation or crepitus and no history of injury. The condition is usually caused by entrapment of the nerve in the suprascapular notch, but it can also be trapped by a ganglion at the spinoglenoid notch. A ganglion will show on MRI scanning. Nerve conduction studies may be needed and show a delayed latency in the suprascapular nerve to infraspinatus. Surgical decompression should be undertaken as soon as the diagnosis is confirmed.

Axillary nerve palsy

The axillary nerve is one of two terminal divisions of the posterior cord of the brachial plexus. The other division is the radial nerve. The axillary nerve is oddly named, for the first thing it does is to enter the quadrilateral space and disappear from the axilla. The nerve supplies the teres minor and deltoid, and its superficial branch innervates the skin over deltoid insertion, the chevron area.

The nerve is most commonly injured by dislocation or fracture-dislocation of the humeral head. Usually this is a contusion of the nerve (a neurapraxia), but the nerve may be ruptured or sustain a neuroma in continuity. The injury to this nerve is not as benign as was previously accepted. If recovery has not occurred in three months, the patient should be referred to a peripheral nerve injury centre for consideration of exploration and grafting.

FURTHER READING

Brems J. The glenoid component in total shoulder arthroplasty. *J Shoulder Elbow Surg* 1993; **2:** 47–54.

Bunker TD, Anthony PP. The pathology of frozen shoulder; a Dupuytren's like disease. *J Bone Joint Surg* 1995; **77B:** 677–683.

Gartsman GM. Arthroscopic acromioplasty for lesions of the rotator cuff. *J Bone Joint Surg* 1990; **72A:** 169–180.

Hovelius L. Anterior dislocation of the shoulder in teenagers and young adults; five year prognosis. *J Bone Joint Surg* 1987; **69A:** 393–399.

Jerosch J, Clahsen H, Grosse-Hackmann A et al. Effects of proprioceptive fibers in the capsule tissue in stabilizing the glenohumeral joint. *Orthop Trans* 1992; **16:** 773.

Neer CS. Anterior acromioplasty for the chronic impingement syndrome of the shoulder. *J Bone Joint Surg* 1972; **54A:** 41–50.

Neer CS, Forster CR. Inferior capsular shift for involuntary inferior and multidirectional instability of the shoulder. *J Bone Joint Surg* 1980; **62A:** 897–908.

Neer CS, Watson KC, Stanton FJ. Recent experience in total shoulder replacement. *J Bone Joint Surg* 1982; **64A:** 319–337.

Ozaki J, Fujimoto S, Nakagawa Y, Masuhara K, Tamai S. Tears of the rotator cuff associated with pathological changes in the acromion. *J Bone Joint Surg* 1988; **70A:** 1224–1230.

Ozaki J, Nakagawa Y, Sakurai G, Tamai S. Recalcitrant chronic adhesive capsulitis of the shoulder. *J Bone Joint Surg* 1989; **71A:** 1511–1515.

Recht MP, Resnick D. Instructional course lectures. Magnetic resonance imaging studies of the shoulder. *J Bone Joint Surg* 1993; **76A:** 1244–1253.

Richards RR, An K-N, Bigliani LU et al. A standardised method for the assessment of shoulder function. *J Shoulder Elbow Surg* 1994; **3:** 347–352.

Turkel SJ, Panio MW, Marshall JL et al. Stabilizing mechanisms preventing anterior dislocation of the glenohumeral joint. *J Bone Joint Surg* 1981; **63A:** 1208–1217.

2

The Elbow

Peter G Lunn

The elbow is not just a simple 'hinge' mechanism; it is a complex joint which is involved in positioning the hand in space either close to, or at a distance from the body, and allows the transfer of a large amount of force. The terms in common parlance in English give an indication of the fact that the elbow is a joint associated with strength; 'elbow grease' and 'power to the elbow', are old sayings which have been passed down through the years and indicate that our forebears certainly appreciated the fact that the elbow is a 'power' joint. In biblical writings over two thousand years ago there are phrases such as, 'Surely the arm of the Lord is not too short to save …?'; the effectiveness of the arm was recognised as being related to its ability to reach out to function over a wide area, so a stiff elbow which limited the span of the arm was equated with weakness and loss of function. In our present-day society terms such as 'elbowed out' indicate the use of the elbow as an instrument of aggression; indeed, the use of the elbow in football is regarded as an aggressive action which is illegal and frequently is the cause of disciplinary action.

The development of elbow arthroplasties has shown that the main problem encountered in their design has been that of loosening, because, although technically a 'non-weight-bearing' joint, the elbow does, in fact, transmit very large forces: up to two or three times body weight under some circumstances, even during normal activities of daily living.

The elbow joint not only transmits a large amount of force but it has to be able to do so throughout its large range of movement; in other words, it has to possess the qualities of flexibility to allow a large range of movement, and stability so that it is functional at any part of the arc of movement. Movement is a vital function of the elbow; if it does not move, the function of the whole of the upper limb is seriously impaired. A stiff elbow is a major handicap whereas other joints such as the wrist or even the shoulder will still allow useful function if stiff but painfree.

It is important, therefore, to always bear in mind that the main function of the elbow is to position the hand and stabilise it so that it can carry out its normal functions. An awareness of hand function is therefore an integral part of assessment of the elbow.

EXAMINATION

This involves the standard approach to examination of any joint, namely; history, inspection, palpation and motion.

History

An accurate history will give much of the information required to make a diagnosis and the clinical examination can then be carried out intelligently in order to see whether or not the relevant physical signs are present to confirm the diagnosis.

Elbow pain may come from the joint itself such as in arthritic conditions, it may come from the adjacent soft tissues as in epicondylitis or ulnar neuritis, or it may be referred from elsewhere, most commonly the neck or shoulder. Elbow pain may also develop secondary to wrist problems particularly if there is pathological shortening of the ulna which can lead to excessive pressure being generated in the radiohumeral joint at the elbow.

Inspection

Look for swelling, deformity or malalignment. The best place to look for joint swelling is on the lateral side of the elbow just distal to the lateral condyle of the humerus. When the elbow is extended there is normally a concavity at this site but if there is swelling of the joint due to effusion or synovitis this will become a prominent convexity which can often be seen clearly or at least palpated. For instance, after a radial head fracture there will be a very tender swelling at this site due to the haemarthrosis.

On the posterior aspect of the elbow, there may be swelling over the tip of the olecranon due to olecranon bursitis, or rheumatoid nodules may be seen on the ulnar border of the forearm. Congenital posterior dislocation of the radial head is often not symptomatic and may be diagnosed by detection of a bony swelling on the posterolateral aspect of the elbow posterior to the normal radiohumeral joint.

The elbow in the extended position normally has a slight valgus alignment (the 'carrying angle') which measures about 10° in males and 14° in females; as the elbow flexes the valgus reduces to approximately a neutral position with the elbow at 90° and slight varus when the elbow is fully flexed (*Figure 2.1*). An assessment of cubitus valgus or varus can therefore only be made reliably when the elbow extends fully. Probably the most common deformity which is seen in general clinical practice is the 'gunstock' deformity (cubitus varus) which occurs as a result of malunion of a supracondylar fracture in a child.

Palpation

The bony landmarks are the medial epicondyle, lateral epicondyle, tip of olecranon and radial head. When the elbow is flexed, the points formed by the medial and lateral epicondyles and tip of the olecranon form an equilateral triangle. When the elbow is extended these points form a straight line.

The medial epicondyle is prominent and readily palpable. On its anterior aspect is the tendon of the flexor muscle origin; on its posterior aspect is the cubital tunnel containing the ulnar nerve. Sensitivity of the ulnar nerve at this site is an important feature of an ulnar compression neuropathy.

The lateral epicondyle is less prominent but can be palpated just proximal to the radiohumeral joint line.

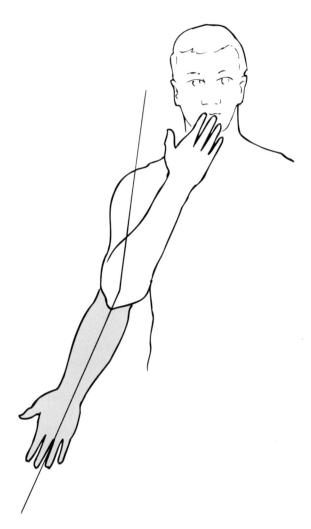

Figure 2.1 'Carrying angle'. Valgus angulation with elbow extended. Varus angulation with elbow flexed.

The radial head can usually be felt, particularly if the forearm is rotated into pronation and supination to confirm its position; it is less easily palpated if there is a joint effusion or haemarthrosis present. An effusion is most readily detected either at the radiohumeral joint line or else in the posterior recess behind the lateral epicondyle, between the radial head and the lateral border of the olecranon.

Motion

Flexion and extension of the normal elbow is from approximately 0–150°; this should allow the patient to reach to the ipsilateral shoulder with his/her fingertips. Some patients will have a few degrees of hyper-extension and in patients with generalised ligamentous laxity this can be as much as 15–20°.

Forearm rotation should be examined with the elbow flexed to 90° and the arm adducted; this ensures that the humerus does not rotate and means that the rotation is only occurring in the forearm. The normal range of rotation is 80° pronation and 80° supination.

The stability of the elbow can be tested by applying varus and valgus stresses with the elbow in extension and also semi-flexed. There are also more complicated posterolateral instability problems which can be tested by the 'pivot shift test'.

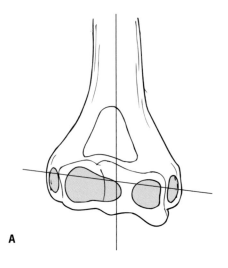

A

OSSIFICATION

Knowledge of the normal ossification centres in the distal humerus is important in allowing interpretation of radiographs in children and even so it is often wise to obtain comparative views of the uninjured elbow as additional assistance.

There are four main ossification centres (*Figure 2.2a,b*):

1. capitellum and lateral part of trochlea
   (appears at 1 year);
2. medial part of trochlea (appears at 10 years);
3. medial epicondyle (appears at 6 years);
4. lateral epicondyle (appears at 12 years).

The epiphysis of the medial epicondyle is the last to fuse and usually does so by 19 years, whereas the other epiphyses are usually fused by 17 years.

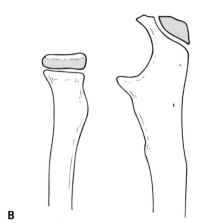

B

Figure 2.2 Ossification centres. (a) Proximal radius and ulna; (b) distal humerus.

ANATOMY

The elbow has two articulations which carry out two separate actions. The ulnohumeral joint has a hinge-like action (known in Greek as a ginglymus) which allows flexion and extension, and the radiohumeral and proximal radio-ulnar joint allow rotational movements (trochoid in Greek) which, in association with the distal radio-ulnar joint result in pronation and supination of the forearm. The elbow is thus classified as a 'trochoginglymoid' joint.

Bony structure

Humerus

The articular condyles are rotated anteriorly at 30° to the longitudinal axis of the humerus (*Figure 2.3*). The trochlea is asymmetrical, with a larger diameter medial flange and a slightly offset transverse axis with a 6–8° valgus tilt (*Figure 2.4*). This, in association with the 4–6° valgus angle of the olecranon accounts for the 10–14° valgus angulation of the elbow in extension, but because of the asymmetry, this becomes a varus angulation of the elbow in full flexion (so that the hand reaches up towards the mouth when the elbow is flexed).

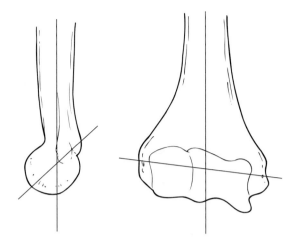

Figure 2.3 Angulation of the humeral articular surfaces.

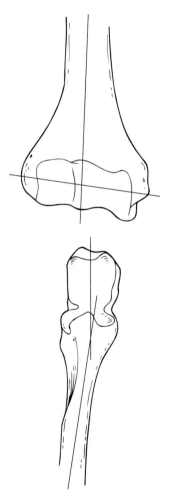

Figure 2.4 Bony alignment of the distal humerus (6–8° valgus) and proximal ulna (4–6° valgus).

Proximal radius

The proximal radius has a shallow concave depression for articulation with the capitellum of the humerus. The major part (240°) of the outer cicumference of the radial head forms an articular surface with the lesser sigmoid fossa of the ulna. The radial neck forms an angle of 15° with the long axis of the radius.

Proximal ulna

The olecranon contains the articular surface for articulation with the humerus (the greater sigmoid notch) and the articulation with the radial head (the lesser sigmoid notch). The greater sigmoid notch forms about a 4° angle with the longitudinal axis of the ulna which contributes to the normal valgus carrying angle of the elbow.

The articular cartilage rarely completely covers the surface of the greater sigmoid notch; there is usually a fissure or 'bare area' (normally covered by fatty tissue) which separates the articular surface of the olecranon from that of the coronoid. This is of practical significance because the olecranon can be divided to allow surgical access to the elbow joint for fixation of complex intra-articular fractures; a chevron-shaped osteotomy can often be fashioned in such a way as to ensure that the osteotomy passes through the 'bare area' so that there is minimal damage to the articular cartilage of the olecranon.

Ligaments

Medial collateral ligament

This has three constituent parts: anterior, posterior and transverse (*Figure 2.5*). The anterior band is the most important for medial elbow stability because it is taut throughout the range of flexion and extension.

Lateral collateral ligament

This shows a significant amount of variation. There are two main parts: the radial collateral ligament and the annular ligament. Some workers have also shown that there is a thickening of the capsule which extends from the lateral epicondyle directly to the ulna and they have termed this part of the lateral ligament complex (correctly, but rather confusingly in my view) the lateral ulnar collateral ligament.

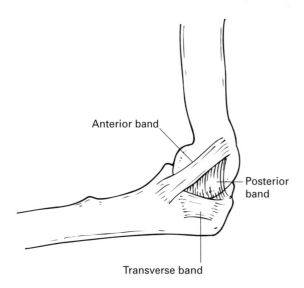

Figure 2.5 The three constituent parts of the medial collateral ligament.

Anconeus muscle

In view of the nature of its attachments, the anconeus is thought to be a dynamic stabiliser of the lateral aspect of the elbow rather than a prime mover; it is functionally more a ligament than a muscle.

Anterior capsule

There is condensation and thickening of the anterior capsule which normally provides a strong restraint to hyperextension of the elbow. Avulsion of the anterior capsule may occur with posterior dislocation and if it is not allowed to heal back strongly it may be associated with recurrent instability, although in practice this is quite uncommon. It is more common for the anterior capsule to heal with considerable scarring and fibrosis which effectively causes some shortening and restriction of full extension.

BASIC BIOMECHANICS

Stability

There is marked bony congruity and stability due to the bony structure. This means that any artificial joint also has to provide a similar level of stability but is

therefore at risk of loosening because the forces taken through the arthroplasty are proportionately greater than the knee, for instance, where the joint surfaces are not particularily congruent and a larger proportion of the forces are taken through the ligaments and other soft tissues.

Medial ligament

This has an important contribution to elbow stability particularly in flexion; the anterior portion of the medial ligament is functionally the most important part of the ligament. When the medial ligament is intact the radial head does not have a significant role in resisting a valgus stress, but when the medial ligament is compromised in some way (as in some forms of fracture-dislocation of the elbow), the radial head does become an important stabilising force to prevent valgus instability.

Lateral ligament

This has three parts: radial collateral ligament, annular ligament, and lateral ulnar collateral ligament. The lateral ligament stabilises the ulna against varus stress and the lateral ulnar collateral component resists rotatory forces.

Anterior capsule

This provides the main soft-tissue stabilisation in full extension.

Forces across the elbow

This is a very complex subject but a simplified analysis shows two things. First, large forces are transmitted across the elbow even in simple day-to-day activities of daily living where up to three times body weight has been measured. Second, the line of action of forces across the elbow is at an angle of 30–40° to the long axis of the arm in an anteroposterior direction. The relevance of this to orthopaedic surgery is that this is the direction in which the humeral component of an elbow arthroplasty will tend to be displaced and it, therefore, requires secure fixation to counteract these forces. A stemmed humeral component will be forced backwards at the joint level and if it loosens, the tip of the stem will be pushed forward and will eventually erode through the anterior cortex of the humerus; this may, in turn, so weaken the bone that a fracture can develop. A humeral component with a stem, therefore, may well erode the distal humerus so much that revision is impossible.

Muscle action at the elbow

The main muscles acting across the elbow as prime movers are the biceps, triceps, brachialis and brachioradialis. Studies of the electromyographic activity of the individual muscles during elbow motion have revealed much information. The anconeus is active in virtually all motion and therefore is regarded as a dynamic stabiliser of the lateral side of the elbow. The action of biceps is of particular interest in that, although it is well recognised as a strong flexor of the elbow and supinator of the forearm, it is also very active during extension of the elbow and functions very much as an 'extension brake'. The biceps has very little flexion activity when the forearm is pronated, however, and the brachialis is regarded as being the 'workhorse' of flexion. In conjunction with brachioradialis these two muscles provide a greater contribution to flexor action than does the biceps alone. The clinical significance of this is that rupture of the biceps tendon will result in more weakness of supination than flexion.

RADIOGRAPHIC EVALUATION

Standard radiographic views give useful information about some aspects of the elbow joint but because of the multiplanar configuration, simple anteroposterior and lateral projections will still leave much of the joint very poorly visualised. For this reason, it can be difficult to detect loose bodies within the elbow joint and assessment of degenerative changes can also be difficult, particularily in the early stages. Some intra-articular fractures of the radial head may not be seen on standard views but can sometimes be shown up with oblique views. Other imaging techniques are also useful to give further information; tomography has always been helpful in the past for the detection of loose bodies, but now computed tomograph scanning gives even more information. Magnetic resonance imaging scanning is indicated more for bony and soft-tissue tumours.

NERVES
Ulnar nerve

This lies in close proximity to the elbow joint in the cubital tunnel and is, therefore, at risk both from elbow trauma and also during surgical exploration. Assessment of ulnar nerve function is an essential part of examination of the elbow. (Ulnar nerve compression neuropathy is dealt with in Chapter 7: pages 231–2.)

Median nerve

The median nerve lies anterior to the joint on the brachialis muscle and is not normally at risk except when an anterior approach to the elbow is being used.

Radial nerve

The radial nerve passes close to the elbow joint, lying on the anterior capsule over the front of the capitellum and radial head, and then it gives off its posterior interosseous branch which passes round the neck of the radius between the two heads of the supinator muscle. It is of significance, therefore, in any surgical approach to the proximal radius and is at particular risk in arthroscopy if the anterolateral portal is not sited correctly.

DISLOCATIONS
Posterior dislocation

This is the most common direction of dislocation of the elbow, usually caused by a fall on the outstretched hand with a semi-flexed elbow. Bony configuration confers much of the stability of the joint, so once the dislocation is reduced it is quite stable unless there is a fracture. The main problem is stiffness so early mobilisation is advisable at about 2–3 weeks, depending on the associated soft-tissue injury. If there is a comminuted fracture of the radial head which requires excision of the bony fragments, a replacement radial head should be inserted in order to maintain the stability of the joint until the soft tissues have healed. If a silastic replacement is used this will fragment with the passage of time and the patient should be warned that it may need to be removed at a later date. A titanium or other type of metallic radial head may have some advantages but, in the long-term, a metal-on-cartilage articulation tends to cause some 'wear' problems in the joint which can cause the patient pain and stiffness. Replacement of the radial head should, therefore, only be undertaken if the joint is unstable and there is no alternative.

Other dislocations

Anterior dislocation is very rare and divergent dislocation is also an uncommon, high-velocity injury in which the radius and ulna are separated. This involves major disruption of the soft tissues including the annular ligament, the interosseous membrane and the distal radio-ulnar joint.

Dislocation of the radial head

Congenital dislocation of the radial head may occur anteriorly, but it is more common posteriorly. Patients with congenital dislocation of the radial head may notice very little functional deficit in the first two decades of life but they can develop osteoarthritic changes in the ulnohumeral articulation in later life. Treatment of congenital dislocation of the radial head is seldom rewarding because the capitellum does not develop normally and is small and dysplastic so that there is very little potential for reconstructing the radio-humeral joint. Treatment is often left until the possible development of degenerative changes in later life.

Reduction of a post-traumatic dislocation of the radial head is worthwhile, however, and may be stable if reduced early but can be associated with some degree of long-term instability which requires reconstruction of the annular ligament.

ELBOW CONTRACTURE
Causes

The common causes encountered in clinical practice are:

1. Trauma.
2. Arthritis: osteoarthris or rheumatoid arthritis.
3. Miscellaneous: infection, haemophilia, burns.

There are also less common causes such as arthrogryposis.

It is helpful also to categorise the contracture as either intra- or extra-articular as this has implications for treatment.

The elbow is one of the commonest joints to develop contractures and loss of full extension is very common after almost any elbow injury. Loss of full flexion is less common but is more serious functionally and is more frequently a cause of a referral for treatment. One of the worst situations to develop is where a patient develops bilateral extension contractures; this can occur in intensive care units with unconscious head injury patients unless particular care is taken to carry out range-of-movement exercises regularly.

Treatment

Conservative

Physiotherapy. This comprises of mobilisation with active movements and gentle passive stretching but avoiding forceful manipulation.

Splinting. Static splinting is best for night-time use. Dynamic splints are helpful but can be bulky and awkward for the patient. An ingenious form of dynamic splintage is the reversed dynamic sling system which has been described for use in haemophilic contractures of the elbow and knee. The main disadvantage is that it needs to be carried out as an in-patient procedure and it is likely to take a week or so to achieve a significant correction.

Surgery

Anterior capsular release is carried out for flexion contracture. There are reports of this being successfully carried out through an anterior approach but this is not an easy exposure of the elbow, and a lateral approach can be used with less risk of complications. If there is also an extension contracture, a modified Kocher incision will allow anterior and posterior releases to be performed through the one incision.

SOFT-TISSUE CONDITIONS OF THE ELBOW
Epicondylitis

This is a common cause of elbow pain, probably the most common, and lateral epicondylitis ('tennis elbow') is the commonest form of the condition and so will be described in greatest detail although many of the features are also characteristic of medial epicondylitis except that this involves the forearm flexor muscles rather than the extensors.

Lateral epicondylitis

Definition

It is a syndrome/symptom-complex characterised by the following clinical features.

1. Pain over the lateral epicondyle and proximal forearm exacerbated by movements involving a combination of gripping of the hand with forearm rotation or elbow movements.
2. Tenderness on palpation over the extensor muscle origin at the lateral epicondyle.
3. Reproduction of pain when the forearm and wrist extensor muscles are stressed actively or passively.

Aetiology

There has been much debate and study of the causes of lateral epicondylitis and although it was originally thought to be an 'overuse' condition it is now clear that there are two main factors involved in the causation of the condition.

Trauma. The condition was originally described in tennis players and it is still common in those who undertake frequent vigorous sporting activities particularily in racquet and throwing sports at a high level (professional or semi-professional). There is also a small number of cases in which the condition appears to develop after a direct blow to the lateral epicondyle although it is not clear whether this is the prime cause of the condition or whether this is a 'trigger' mechanism in a vulnerable patient.

Constitutional factors. A proportion of patients, and probably the majority seen in standard clinical practice, have a constitutional tendency to develop this condition and they may also develop other similar conditions such as rotator cuff tendonitis, medial epicondylitis ('golfer's elbow'), carpal tunnel syndrome, de Quervain's tenovaginitis and trigger finger. The rheumatological screening tests are normal and there is no specific test which will identify susceptible patients. This has been described as the 'mesenchymal syndrome' because of the observation that some patients are prone to several or all of these conditions which all have a similar pathology.

It appears, therefore, that many of these conditions are brought to light by physical activity but not actually caused by it. This is supported by epidemiological studies which have shown that the incidence of lateral epicondylitis is similar in those undertaking heavy manual labour and those in sedentary occupations.

Pathology

There have been a large number of opinions given on the pathology of epicondylitis; it has been described as a bursitis, tendonitis or synovitis, depending on which author you read. However, papers published more recently show that the changes seen in tennis elbow are not primarily those of an inflammatory process, but more those of degeneration. Characteristically, there are macroscopic changes in the central portion of the tendon where there is a shiny, 'ground-glass' appearance with oedema and gelatinous material. Microscopically, there are changes of hyaline degeneration with an absence of inflammatory cells, but large numbers of fibroblasts and vascular granulation tissue which Nirschl describes as 'angiofibroblastic tendonosis'.

The relevance of this information is that it suggests that the process is not so much a traumatic one which causes the typical signs of injury followed by inflammation and repair, but more an avascular degenerative process which is very similar to the changes seen in other situations such as rotator cuff tendonitis, Achilles tendonitis and plantar fasciitis. Strictly speaking, therefore, these conditions would be more correctly described as being cases of 'tendonosis' rather than 'tendonitis'.

Clinical features

History. There is usually a gradual onset of pain over the lateral epicondyle with radiation down the proximal forearm in the line of the extensor muscles. The pain is provoked or worsened by movements of the forearm or elbow associated with gripping of the hand. For instance, lifting a shopping-bag by the handle may well cause discomfort, whereas lifting a similar weight such as a tray with the hand supinated and the fingers stretched out in full extension may not cause any discomfort.

Physical signs. There is localised tenderness over the lateral epicondyle and pain in the same area when the extensor muscles are tensioned actively by resisted wrist or finger extension, or by making a fist and gripping strongly. Passive tensioning of the extensor muscles by extending the elbow, pronating the forearm and flexing the wrist will also provoke discomfort at the tendonous origin of the extensors at the lateral epicondyle.

Treatment

The majority of cases resolve with conservative treatment which includes rest, modification of activities, anti-inflammatories, physiotherapy, use of an epicondylitis clasp and cortisone injection. Surgery is reserved for the small proportion of cases which fail to respond to conservative treatment and surgery. The clasp or brace is thought to act by providing a counterforce so that when the extensor muscles contract the non-elastic brace dissipates the energy which is generated to help protect the osseotendinous junction at the muscle origin. There is evidence to suggest that there is some objective benefit from the use of this type of epicondylitis clasp in some situations.

Surgery. Release of the extensor muscle origin at the lateral epicondyle is the standard surgical procedure. It is recognised that the main site of the pathology is in the tendon of origin of extensor carpi radialis brevis (ECRB) and in order to release this much of the remainder of the extensor muscle which overlies it must also be released. Other techniques which have been described include release of a portion of the annular ligament, lengthening of the ECRB in the distal forearm, anterior capsular release, localised denervation of the lateral epicondyle and decompression of the posterior interosseous nerve.

Results. A study of 185 articles on lateral epicondylitis indicates that the understanding of this condition and its treatment does not readily stand up to conventional statistical analysis. It seems that most treatment measures have a reasonable success rate but no one form of treatment is significantly better than the others and so one has to keep an open mind about the best treatment for an individual patient. On balance, therefore, it is customary to use conservative measures initially and only resort to surgery when other (conservative) measures fail. The surgical treatment is also dependent on individual preference to a certain extent, but it seems that most authorities accept that release of the ECRB tendon at the lateral epicondyle is an essential part of the procedure and the results show that the majority of patients do benefit from this. On average, the published results suggest that approximately 85% of patients will get complete relief of symptoms after surgery, about 5% will have no benefit and the remaining 10% will still have some discomfort with certain vigorous activities. It is likely that at least a proportion of the failures can be attributed to the fact that the wrong diagnosis has been made and in this respect a bone scan can be helpful in confirming the diagnosis.

Medial epicondylitis

This is seven to ten times less common than lateral epicondylitis. The features are similar to those of lateral epicondylitis except that the flexor group of muscles is involved. The main difference, however, is that it is quite often also associated with ulnar nerve symptoms due to compression of the nerve in the cubital tunnel.

ARTHRITIC CONDITIONS OF THE ELBOW

There are a number of inflammatory arthropathies which may afflict the elbow such as psoriatic arthropathy, systemic lupus erythematosus and gout but rheumatoid arthritis is the most common and can affect almost any age group.

Rheumatoid arthritis

Juvenile rheumatoid arthritis

The main difference between the effects of rheumatoid arthritis in the juvenile and the adult is that in the juvenile it tends to cause marked joint stiffness and may even progress to complete bony ankylosis. The joint pain and swelling can be helped by a combination of anti-inflammatory medication, physical therapy and splintage. Surgery is rarely indicated but in some cases synovectomy can be of benefit, although the outcome is rather unpredictable. It is likely that synovectomy is most effective if carried out at an early stage of the disease before there has been irreversible damage to the joint surfaces, but there are not many surgeons who feel that they have sufficient experience of this procedure to know which cases are likely to benefit and therefore it is not frequently performed. The greatest experience and the best results seem to be from Scandinavian countries where the procedure is carried out more frequently.

In some children with Still's disease, the disease destroys the joint and it becomes completely ankylosed. These are the patients who may require elbow arthroplasty because bilateral stiff elbows constitute a severe functional problem and it is preferable to try and retain motion in at least one elbow if at all possible. This is obviously somewhat controversial as elbow replacement arthroplasty is not yet established as a standard orthopaedic procedure; however, it is now being done in a number of specialist centres on a regular basis and it is therefore worthy of consideration in such a centre on the rare occasions when this situation does occur.

The results of the different forms of arthroplasty show that total elbow replacement is more successful and predictable in terms of pain relief and range of movement than the other recognised arthroplastic techniques such as excision or interposition arthroplasty. There are significant risks of long-term problems which may require revision of the arthroplasty in the future and these are discussed more fully below under 'elbow arthroplasty'.

Adult rheumatoid arthritis

It is relatively uncommon for a patient with rheumatoid arthritis to present with elbow involvement as the first joint affected by the rheumatoid arthritis. More commonly a patient first requires treatment to the lower limbs (hips and knees) before developing disabling problems with their elbows.

The main symptom is pain in the elbow, which is a constant ache made worse by lifting objects. Often the pain is worst when the elbow is stressed in extension, such as when pushing open a spring-loaded door or pushing up from an armchair. The main problem is that the elbow becomes unpredictable and it can 'give way' when the patient is lifting a hot drink to her mouth or carrying out other similar activities.

Treatment. As with any rheumatic condition the primary treatment is medical and surgery is only indicated

if medical treatment is failing. The options for surgical treatment are either synovectomy or some form of arthroplasty: excision arthroplasty, interposition arthroplasty or total elbow replacement. Arthrodesis is not a reasonable option because the function of the arm is so poor with an arthrodesed elbow that, in my view, it should virtually never be performed. An arthrodesis may well relieve the pain from an arthritic elbow joint but patients are unlikely to thank you for fusing their elbow any more than they would if you fused their temporomandibular joint to try and help relieve jaw pain. The elbow must move.

Synovectomy. This is indicated for florid recurrent synovitis which is not responding to medical treatment but which has not yet caused any serious damage to the articular cartilage. Ideally, the radiographs should be essentially normal, without any joint space narrowing and in theory, the joint should then regain good function once the inflamed synovium has been removed. In practice, there are not many British surgeons who either see patients at this stage or are prepared to carry out a synovectomy at an early stage, although this is certainly the logical thing to do. Part of the reason for this is that the results of synovectomy are rather variable and unpredictable. It is a painful operation with a difficult postoperative course of rehabilitation and it often results in some loss of motion; it may therefore compromise the result of any further surgery, particularly a total elbow replacement. As yet, there is no reliable marker to indicate which patients are likely to benefit from synovectomy and this is certainly an area for research. If there were a blood test such as the ESR or rheumatoid factor which could be used quantitatively to identify patients who are likely to have a good result from synovectomy, the procedure might well make a come-back into the surgical armamentarium, whereas at present it is kept very much in reserve and used for only a very limited number of patients.

Excision arthroplasty. Various techniques have been devised but the main principle is that the articular surfaces are excised in such a way that the olecranon can fit into a 'trough' in the lower end of the humerus and form a fibrous pseudarthrosis which allows a functional range of movement with some degree of stability (*Figures 2.6 and 2.7*). Unfortunately, the stability that can be achieved with these techniques is rather variable

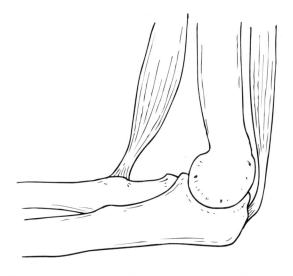

Figure 2.6 Lateral view of excision arthroplasty of the elbow.

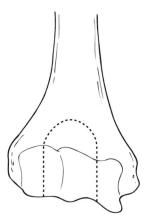

Figure 2.7 Line of excision of the distal humerus for excision arthroplasty. Anteroposterior view.

and this is what determines their effectiveness. The triceps must be functioning to achieve satisfactory stability, so some cases with extensive scarring or soft-tissue loss on the extensor aspect of the elbow may well be unsuitable for excision arthroplasty.

Interposition arthroplasty. Many different materials have been used as interposition membranes in the elbow. The advantages of this procedure are that the joint stability may not be compromised in the same way as with an excision arthroplasty. The joint is still suitable for salvage by other techniques (excision arthroplasty or

total elbow replacement) and it should allow some joint motion with some degree of pain relief. The main problems are that the range of movement which is achieved may be limited and the pain relief may be incomplete or temporary; the interposition material usually fragments with the passage of time because of the forces which pass through the elbow and the symptoms may well then recur. Synthetic materials such as silastic sheeting are particularily vulnerable in this respect and are no longer used, but biological materials are more reliable. Various autologous tissues have been used as interposition membranes, including skin, fat, fascia lata and muscle; animal tissues have also been used including pig's bladder. However, probably the best available technique is that in which a portion of the triceps tendon is interposed between the joint surfaces while still left attached proximally so that it retains its blood supply.

Total elbow arthroplasty. Upper limb arthroplasty techniques have been developed but they are not yet at the stage to produce the same level of results as are achieved with lower limb arthroplasties except in a few specialised centres. One of the main landmarks in the development of elbow arthroplasties was by Souter (1973). He studied the results of hinged elbow arthroplasties in a group of rheumatoid patients and noted that the initial results were excellent both in terms of pain relief and also in terms of range of movement. This was therefore a great advance in the treatment of these patients for whom there had previously been very little to offer surgically once the joint had degenerated beyond the stage at which soft-tissue procedures such as synovectomy were indicated. However, the important points which this study showed were that, although the early results were good there was then a significant failure rate from about two years onwards, and what was worse was that following failure by loosening or infection, the elbow became virtually unsalvageable because the stems of the prostheses eroded through the bone causing considerable weakening of the bone, fragmentation and occasionally, fractures.

Subsequently, elbow arthroplasties were designed in order to try and minimise the complications of the stems and, as in knee arthroplasties, stemless components were developed. One of the earliest of these designs was the Liverpool elbow, which was a small surface replacement requiring minimal bone excision. If these components did loosen, it was readily salvageable and therefore constituted an important advance on previous designs but it was only suitable for a limited number of patients with rheumatoid arthritis and could not be used in cases with more extensive bony erosion (Larsen V).

Souter, therefore, in conjunction with the bio-engineering department in Strathclyde University, studied the anatomy and biomechanics of the elbow with particular reference to the erosive changes that occur in rheumatoid arthritis, and devised a total elbow arthroplasty with minimal stems. The humeral component has a 'stirrup' configuration which allows fixation with rotational stability in the only residual area of reliable cortical bone, which is in the epicondylar ridges. Because of the long lever-arm effect of the humerus and forearm, and the ability of the arm to function in abduction, there is considerable rotational stress on the fixation of elbow arthroplasty components and this can be a significant factor in the initiation of loosening of the humeral component in particular. The Souter–Strathclyde system addresses this problem and also has other components which can be utilised in more complex situations where the bone at the joint level is not adequate for stemless fixation and a stem has to be used.

The Coonrad–Morrey arthroplasty deals with the problem of fixation at the joint level in a different manner by utilising an anterior flange to try and prevent posterior migration of the humeral component and give some degree of rotational control. It also has an intramedullary stem and although the published results on the whole have been good there is concern over how salvageable it would be if the prosthesis should loosen or fail for any other reason.

The main options for elbow replacement at present are between linked and unlinked, constrained or semi-constrained, and stemmed or stemless arthroplasties. Most of the arthroplasties developed after the failure of the original fixed hinges were unlinked and semi-constrained, but because of instability problems the designs became more constrained and some linked prostheses were also developed with 'sloppy' hinge mechanisms which allowed flexibility at the linkage and so reduced the risk of loosening, as some of the angulatory and rotational stresses are taken by the ligaments and other soft tissues.

In Britain, the commonest arthroplasties of the semi-constrained unlinked type are the Souter which is stemless and the Kudo which is stemmed. The Coonrad–Morrey is a linked prosthesis which is useful for cases where there may be some deficiency of the epicondylar ridges; the anterior flange gives some rotational control as well as providing additional resistance to posterior displacement. It is my view that, as far as possible, an unstemmed prosthesis should be used for a primary arthroplasty and stemmed arthroplasties reserved for salvage or revision procedures.

Osteoarthritis

Osteoarthritis may develop as a primary arthritic condition with the typical gradual progressive onset, usually in men in about the fifth or sixth decades of life with complaints of aching discomfort, stiffness, restriction of movement and, sometimes, intermittent locking and effusions. Alternatively, it may develop as a secondary condition due to damage to the articular surfaces of the joint, usually as a result of fractures or dislocation. There are also less common causes of secondary osteoarthritis such as septic arthritis and even in a small number of cases, osteochondritis dissecans.

Clinical features

The patients usually complain of discomfort and stiffness in the elbow; the pain is often most painful with forced extension such as when carrying a weight in the out-stretched hand or when trying to throw a ball. The pain is usually at the back of the elbow, in the region of the olecranon fossa, and patients may lose some flexion movement which can affect their ability to reach to the mouth with the hand or to reach to the collar to knot their tie. They also commonly lose some extension although they rarely regard this as being much of a functional problem and, in fact, on some occasions the extension deficit has to be drawn to the patient's attention as they have not been aware of it. Many patients also experience intermittent locking of the elbow due to loose bodies and this can be associated with swelling and joint effusion.

Treatment

In the early stages of osteoarthritis, symptomatic measures such as physiotherapy and cortisone injections can be helpful. With further progression, more radical measures will be required such as arthrotomy and removal of loose bodies. Joint debridement is also beneficial in moderately severe cases provided there is still some articular cartilage present; the procedure described by Outerbridge and Kashiwagi (the 'OK' procedure) is an ingenious and effective means of debriding the osteophytes and removing loose bodies from all compartments of the joint through a single posterior triceps-splitting incision. This can give modest improvements in the range of movement and quite good benefit in terms of pain relief. It seems that the fenestration of the olecranon has an 'osteotomy' effect which gives more pain relief than would otherwise have been anticipated.

BURSITIS AND MYOSITIS

Bursitis

The commonest bursa at the elbow is the olecranon bursa which overlies the subcutaneous border and tip of the olecranon. There are also less common deep bursae associated with the biceps tendon, close to its insertion on the radius, and the triceps tendon on its deep aspect close to the tip of the olecranon. These bursae may become inflamed and painful and sometimes become infected; with the bursa associated with the biceps tendon at its insertion it is important to differentiate between a simple cubital bursitis (which is the term for inflammation of this bursa) and a partial tear of the biceps tendon, which can also present with similar symptoms although there is usually a history of a strain or some other form of trauma in the case of a partial rupture. However, it is also the case that a cubital bursitis can develop as a result of degeneration of the biceps tendon insertion which may be a preliminary to rupture.

Myositis ossificans

The elbow has long been recognised as a joint which is at risk of developing ectopic bone formation. However, it is important to differentiate between calcification and ossification. Calcification occurs frequently after injury, such as a dislocation of the elbow, where there is calcific deposition (calcium pyrophosphate) in the collateral ligament(s). Ossification is where ectopic bone

forms and this is often seen most dramatically after head injury. Myositis ossificans is where ectopic bone forms within muscle tissue. This is sometimes seen in the elbow in the brachialis muscle which lies directly over the anterior capsule of the elbow and has a large surface area as well as a very large origin from most of the anterior surface of the distal end of the humerus. The incidence of myositis ossificans at the elbow is very low, however, and does not justify the traditional teaching that patients should not undergo passive exercises after elbow surgery or injury for fear that this might provoke the development of myositis.

RADIO-ULNAR SYNOSTOSIS

This condition may be either congenital or acquired; in the latter case it develops as a result of bony or soft-tissue injury.

Congenital

Congenital cases are frequently bilateral and there is very little functional deficit because the child grows up without any forearm rotation, it is usually not detected until they are a few years old and sometimes not even until teenage or adult life. The position of the forearm is variable. Some patients have a fixed pronation deformity and in others the forearm is in almost neutral rotation; only in a minority is there fixed supination. Treatment is only required if there is sufficient functional deficit and more commonly for a severe pronation deformity.

Treatment

Rotational osteotomy is the most common treatment, either by a proximal osteotomy through the synostosis in younger children (with K wire fixation) or by more distal osteotomies of both the radius and ulna with compression plating in adults.

Attempts to regain active and passive forearm rotation are less predictable. It is necessary to excise the synostotic bony bridge and then to insert some form of interposition membrane (such as fascia lata) between the radius and ulna, but in order to achieve a reasonable range of rotation it is usually also necessary to excise the radial head and incise the full length of the interosseous membrane. Not surprisingly, it is very difficult to maintain the range of movement post-operatively because of the extent of the scar tissue, so the end result can be unrewarding except in a child who is able to co-operate with an exercise programme. Older patients (teenagers and older) are better served by a rotational osteotomy.

Acquired

Post-traumatic synostosis can occur after either bony injury or soft-tissue injury in the forearm. A congenital synostosis invariably affects the proximal radio-ulnar joint but a post-traumatic synostosis may occur anywhere along the length of the forearm. The disability is much more marked in post-traumatic cases and there is, therefore, a greater indication for reconstitution of the forearm rotational mechanism rather than a fusion in a functional position. The results are better than in the congenital cases, probably at least in part due to the fact that the proximal and distal radio-ulnar joints have been functioning prior to the accident and therefore at least have the potential for recovery. In addition, the interosseous membrane will allow rotation of the radius unless it has become scarred and contracted as a result of the trauma.

A bony bridge can join the radius and ulna either following a closed fracture treated conservatively or after open reduction and internal fixation. The principles of treatment are the same, namely to try and prevent bony bridging if possible and secondly to remove the bony bridge if it has already developed.

Prevention

The two measures which are likely to help prevent ectopic bone forming between the radius and ulna are the same as those for the prevention of ectopic bone elsewhere.

1. *Drug treatment:* non-steroidal anti-inflammatory drugs, particularily indomethacin, have been shown to be of benefit in reducing the rate of formation of heterotopic bone after hip replacement. Diphosphonates also have a beneficial effect in slowing down the formation of heterotopic bone, although it may be that this effect is only temporary and further heterotopic bone may form once the drug is stopped.

2. *Physical therapy:* it has long been taught that passive stretching exercises, particularly of the elbow, may increase the risk of ectopic bone formation and stiffness but active movements do not have this detrimental effect. This has not been explained scientifically and it will be interesting to see if this is still held to be the case in the future with the increasing use of mechanical methods of constant passive motion which are used in some units for patients after injuries and surgery to the elbow.

It may well be that there are some situations such as burns which do carry a particularly high risk of elbow stiffness due to ectopic bone formation. The extensive soft-tissue component of the injury could render these patients more susceptible to these problems than patients with other forms of elbow trauma.

Radiotherapy has also been advocated for the prevention or reduction of heterotopic bone but this has the theoretical risk of formation of post radiation sarcoma and therefore is not widely used.

UNCOMMON CAUSES OF ELBOW PAIN

Ostechondrosis and osteochondritis dissecans

These conditions affect children, mainly boys, during their growing years. They are both causes of pain in the elbow.

Osteochondrosis usually occurs after the age of 5 and before the teenage years. It is a form of avascular necrosis of the capitellum and has some features similar to Perthes' disease of the hip. It goes through a degenerate, necrotic phase followed by regeneration, but it is rarely associated with deformity and collapse and the prognosis is generally good.

Osteochondritis dissecans also commonly affects boys but in the early teens (13–16 years). They usually experience aching discomfort and develop a slight flexion contracture which causes pain if they try and force the elbow into full extension such as when throwing during sporting activities. A proportion of patients also develop signs and symptoms of a loose body. The prognosis is variable and whereas most suffer only temporary discomfort, a proportion experience continuing problems and may go on to develop degenerative change in later years.

Olecranon 'impingement'

Some sportsmen develop pain on the region of the olecranon fossa when the elbow is forcibly extended. This particularly affects throwers and bowlers in cricket. The condition may be eased by a posterior injection of steroid but if it recurs, surgical exploration through a small posterior triceps-splitting approach reveals an inflamed synovium in the region of the olecranon fossa and sometimes with loose bodies. There is often an impingement osteophyte at the tip of the olecranon where a bony spur develops in response to the repeated impingement of the tip of the olecranon against the fossa. The normally thin sheet of bone across the fossa also thickens up considerably, to more than 1 cm thick, and may need to be trimmed.

Dislocating ulnar nerve

The ulnar nerve normally passes through the cubital tunnel at the elbow and is held in position by the overlying fascia formed between the two heads of the flexor carpi ulnaris muscle. In a significant proportion of the general population, however, the ulnar nerve does not stay in the cubital tunnel during flexion and extension movements of the elbow; one study has shown that 16.2% of the population demonstrate subluxation or dislocation of the nerve.

When the nerve subluxes during elbow flexion it is more vulnerable to trauma and those that dislocate completely can develop a friction neuritis due to the repeated trauma and resulting fibrosis in the nerve. This is a condition which causes pain, whereas a simple compression neuropathy of the ulnar nerve is associated with sensory and sometimes motor changes but is not usually painful.

'Snapping' triceps

Painful clicking or 'snapping' over the medial epicondyle can occur due to hypertrophy of the medial head of triceps seen in some sportsmen, particularily weight-lifters, and this may or may not be associated with ulnar nerve symptoms due to irritation or compression of the ulnar nerve. Similar symptoms can occur due to an abnormal insertion of the triceps or an anomalous tendon of the medial head. These patients also develop painful 'snapping' of the medial triceps

tendon which can only be relieved surgically by transferring the medial portion of the tendon insertion laterally at the olecranon.

FURTHER READING

An KN, Morrey BF. Biomechanics of the elbow. In: Morrey BF (ed.) *The Elbow and Its Disorders*, Philadelphia: WB Saunders, 1993.

Brattstrom H, Khudairy HA. Synovectomy of the elbow in rheumatoid arthritis. *Acta Orthop Scand* 1975; **46:** 744.

Buxton JD. Ossification in the ligaments of the elbow joint. *J Bone Joint Surg* 1938; **20:** 709.

Childress HM. Recurrent ulnar nerve dislocations at the elbow. *Clin Orthop* 1975; **108:** 168.

Coonrad RW, Hooper WR. Tennis elbow: its course, natural history, conservative and surgical management. *J Bone Joint Surg* 1973; **55A:** 1177–1182.

Dickson RA. Reversed dynamic slings: a new concept in the treatment of post-traumatic flexion contractures. *Injury* 1976; **8:** 35.

Dimberg L. The prevalence and causation of tennis elbow (lateral humeral epicondylitis) in a population of workers in an engineering industry. *Ergonomics* 1987; **30:** 573.

Funk DA, An KN, Morrey BF, Daube JR. Electromyographic analysis of muscles across the elbow joint. *J Orthop Res* 1987; **5:** 529.

Hamilton PG. The prevalence of humeral epicondylitis: a survey in general practice. *JR Coll Gen Pract* 1986; **36:** 464.

Karanjia ND, Stiles PJ. Cubital bursitis. *J Bone Joint Surg* 1988; **70B:** 832.

Kashiwagi D. Intra-articular changes of the osteoarthritic elbow, especially about the fossa olecrani. *Jpn Orthop Assoc* 1978; **52:** 1367.

Labelle et al. (Montreal) *J Bone Joint Surg* 1992; **74B:** 5.

Laine V, Vainio K. Synovectomy of the elbow. In: Hijmans W, Paul WD, Herschel H (eds) *Early Synovectomy in Rheumatoid Arthritis*. Amsterdam: Excerpta Medica Foundation, 1969; 117.

Major HP. Lawn-tennis elbow. *Br Med J* 1883; **2:** 557.

O'Driscoll SW, Bell DF, Morrey BF. Posterolateral rotatory instability of the elbow. *J Bone Joint Surg* 1991; **73A:** 440.

Ritter MA, Sieber JM. Prophylactic indomethacin for the prevention of heterotopic bone formation following total hip arthroplasty. *Clin Orthop* 1985; **196:** 217.

Souter WA. Arthroplasty of the elbow with particular reference to metallic hinge arthroplasty in rheumatoid patients. *Orthop Clin North Am* 1973; **4:** 395.

Spinner RJ, Davids JR, Goldner RD. Dislocating medial triceps and ulnar neuropathy in three generations of one family. *J Bone Joint Surg* 1997; **22A:** 132–137.

Stover SL, Niemann KM, Miller JM. Disodium etidronate in the prevention of postoperative recurrence of heterotopic ossification in spinal cord injury patients. *J Bone Joint Surg* 1976; **58A:** 683.

Urbaniak JR, Hansen PE, Beissinger SF, Aitken MS. Correction of post-traumatic flexion contracture of the elbow by anterior capsulotomy. *J Bone Joint Surg* 1985; **67A:** 1160.

Wadsworth CT, Nielsen DH, Burns LT, Krull JD, Thompson CG. The effect of the counterforce armband on wrist extension and grip strength and pain in subjects with tennis elbow. *J Orthop Sports Phys Ther* 1989; **11:** 192.

Wilson FD, Andrews JR, Blackburn TA, McClusky G. Valgus extension overload in the pitching elbow. *Am J Sports Med* 1983; **2:** 83.

3

The Wrist

Nicholas Barton and Tim Davis

ANATOMY

Readers of this book will be familiar with the bony anatomy of the carpus so it will not be described here, except to emphasise that a large proportion of the surface of each carpal bone is articular. None (except the pisiform) has a tendon inserted onto it, so the position of the bones is controlled by their shape and by ligaments. Damage to these ligaments allows abnormal movements between the carpal bones (carpal instability).

You should therefore have some knowledge of the ligaments, which are fully described and illustrated in Taleisnik's book on the wrist.

The *intrinsic ligaments* connect adjoining carpal bones: they are very short and not amenable to direct surgical repair. The scapholunate ligament, which lies between the scaphoid and lunate bones is the most commonly injured. It does not fill the space between these two bones but forms a horseshoe around their anterior, proximal and posterior aspects. Thus, contrast medium injected into a normal mid-carpal joint will track proximally between the scaphoid and lunate but will not pass into the radiocarpal joint; the same applies to the lunotriquetral ligament. Both these ligaments allow some movement between the proximal carpal bones, in contrast to those between the bones of the distal carpal row which are held together so firmly that they move as one.

The *extrinsic ligaments* are longer and connect carpal bones to the radius or metacarpals. They are intra-capsular and are not easily visible from the outside of the joint: they are best seen from inside, through an arthroscope, though they are not always as clear-cut as drawings suggest. Those on the dorsum, which converge towards the triquetrum, are less substantial than those on the front of the carpus, of which the most important are three radiating from the radial styloid process (Figure 3.1).

1. The misleadingly-named 'radial collateral' ligament runs distally from the front of the radial styloid to the tuberosity of the scaphoid.
2. The radio-scaphocapite ligament runs obliquely to the long axis of the arm across the waist of the scaphoid, to which it has some attachment. This strong ligament is seen in anterior approaches to the scaphoid and when excising volar wrist ganglia.
3. The radiolunate ligament runs almost transversely across the wrist.

In addition there is, more centrally and deeper, the radio-scapholunate ligament of Testut, reinforces anteriorly the intrinsic scapholunate ligament.

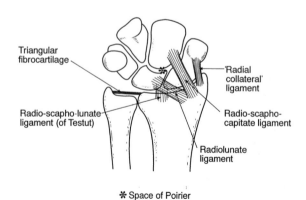

Figure 3.1 The most important of the anterior ligaments of the wrist.

There is no ligament running from the centre of the distal end of the radius to the capitate and this leaves an area of weakness, the space of Poirier, over the front of the lunocapitate joint.

The triangular fibrocartilage lies between the flat distal end of the ulna and the triquetrum and is the most important part of a more complicated structure known as the triangular fibrocartilage complex (TFCC). It joins the medial (or ulnar) border of the radius (sigmoid notch) to the base of the ulnar styloid and allows the radius to swing around the fixed ulna in pronation and supination. In addition there is an ulno-carpal meniscus homologue attached to the radius and ulna, though this may merge with the triangular fibrocartilage. These two structures, together with the dorsal and anterior radio-ulnar ligaments, the rather indefinite ulnar collateral ligament and the sheath of the tendon of extensor carpi ulnaris, comprise the TFCC.

There is no real collateral ligament on either side of the wrist.

The flexor retinaculum is familiar as the roof of the carpal tunnel. Its function is to prevent bow-stringing of the tendons and it is incorrect (though common, especially in the USA) to call it the transverse carpal ligament. After surgical release of the carpal tunnel, the cut edges heal together so that the retinaculum is restored though slightly wider (from radial to ulnar) than before; indeed, if you operate again it may be hard to believe that anything was done the first time.

MECHANICS

Barnes Wallis, designer of the Wellington bomber and inventor of the dambuster bomb, conceived in 1946 the idea of an aircraft in which the relationship between the wings and fuselage could be changed, as in birds, according to the needs of different situations. The carpus is also a structure of variable geometry.

Before considering this, we had better mention the terminology. It is perfectly acceptable to speak of flexion, extension, abduction and adduction of the wrist; indeed it is preferable as it is simpler and follows the usage for other joints. However, the terms palmar-flexion, dorsiflexion, radial deviation and ulnar deviation have become so embedded in the literature that it seems best to use them here. Radial and ulnar do have the advantage that they apply whichever way the wrist is viewed, whether in pronation or supination. Similarly, anterior and posterior are correct terms, but palmar and dorsal are more usual. Volar (from the Latin *vola*, the hollow of a hand or foot) is also widely used, but palmar is considered preferable.

In palmar- and dorsiflexion, about half the movement takes place at the radiocarpal joint and half at the mid-carpal joint. This means that arthrodesis of one of those joints, but not the other, should leave about half the normal wrist movements; in practice, it is usually rather less.

In radial deviation, the trapezium must approach the radial styloid and, to accommodate this, the scaphoid effectively shortens by flexing. With the wrist in a neutral position, the scaphoid is normally flexed at an angle of 40–60° to the long axis of the arm. In radial deviation it flexes more and in ulnar deviation it partially extends. (That is why radiographs for fractures of the scaphoid are taken in ulnar deviation, when the scaphoid is more extended and more perpendicular to the X-ray beam.) This flexion in radial deviation involves all three bones of the proximal row of the carpus, partly driven by the slightly helical shape of the joint between the triquetrum and hamate. If the scapholunate ligament or, less commonly, the luno-triquetral ligament is torn, then the bones ulnar to the tear do not flex in radial deviation but remain in a fairly neutral position.

We have spoken of the proximal and distal rows of the carpus but Taleisnik (who was brought up in Argentina and therefore speaks Spanish) has revived the columnar concept of Navarro, according to which the wrist consists of three longitudinal columns: a lateral or mobile column (which is the scaphoid), a central column (comprising the lunate and the distal row) and a medial column (the triquetrum). Lichtman proposed a sort of compromise in which the carpus is considered as a ring. Much argument has taken place between supporters of these theoretical concepts, but it may be that some wrists function more like rows and others more like columns; in the latter, there will be more flexion of the proximal row during sideways movements.

HISTORY

Pain is the most common complaint and one must ascertain its severity, quality and location and whether it is aggravated by particular activities or movements. If the patient can point with one finger to the painful spot, then there there is a good chance of finding an organic cause which can be cured.

The nature of any *swelling* will emerge on examination. As in other parts of the body, a complaint of 'swelling' where none can be found on examination may indicate a psychological problem. However, a feeling of swelling of the hand, as though it would burst, is a common complaint in carpal tunnel syndrome.

Stiffness is common in arthritis or after injury but is seldom a complaint except in sportsmen. In ordinary life one only uses about half the full range of movement of the wrist: indeed patients whose wrists have been arthrodesed are usually happy with the outcome.

Clicking may be of little significance or great importance (see below).

'*Weakness*' must be defined. It usually means that pain on trying to lift something prevents the patient from doing so. This may also be described as 'giving way'.

EXAMINATION
Look

One should look at the wrist from all four sides. If you simply turn the hand over from palm-down to palm-up, you must realise that you have altered not only the aspect which you are inspecting but the anatomical relationships, because you have changed the position of the forearm from pronation to supination and the radius has rotated around the ulna. The lower end of the ulna may sublux dorsally in pronation (as in rheumatoid disease) but not in supination; less commonly it displaces anteriorly in supination but not in pronation.

The most common localised swellings are ganglia, but a lump on the back of the second or third carpometacarpal joint may be a carpometacarpal boss; to make life more complicated there may be a ganglion overlying a boss. Small dorsal ganglia are only visible when the wrist is flexed. De Quervain's stenosing tenovaginitis also produces a localised swelling which is often visible if compared with the other wrist.

A more diffuse swelling is likely to be tenosynovitis. If this term is used, as it should be, in its true pathological sense, it is virtually confined to rheumatoid disease and infections such as tuberculosis; the appearance at operation of these two conditions is identical and,

although in Britain it is usually rheumatoid, you should not take this for granted. Tenosynovitis of the flexor tendons may cause a 'compound palmar ganglion' bulging out proximal and distal to the inextensible flexor retinaculum (beneath which it may compress the median nerve). The same thing may happen to a lesser extent with the extensor retinaculum, but on the back of the wrist one usually just sees a diffuse swelling over the carpus and carpometacarpal joints. Synovitis of the wrist joint itself is very difficult to detect clinically as the joint is surrounded by other structures.

Remember to look for scars, which may be important clues to old injuries or operations.

Feel

The single most important part of the examination is precise localisation of tenderness. Every carpal bone except the trapezoid is palpable and you should practice on your own wrist until you can feel them (see *Table 3.1*).

Similarly, many of the joints are palpable and, if you know where the bones are, then you should be able to identify the joint between them to detect tenderness arising from that joint. The scapholunate joint is in the *centre* of the back of the wrist. The pisotriquetral joint, sometimes the seat of osteoarthritis, can easily be balotted from the ulnar side. The trapeziometacarpal joint is often osteoarthritic and tenderness over it may be the only clinical sign. (This must be distinguished from the other common causes of tenderness on the radial side of the wrist: a fractured scaphoid and de Quervain's disease.) You also need to identify the trapeziometacarpal joint to inject it though this is not easy; distraction helps, but a bit of poking around may be needed.

When palpating, start where you don't expect it to be tender and work towards where you think it will be. Use one fingertip and be systematic, working right round the wrist at four levels: the distal end of the radius and ulna, the proximal row of the carpus, the distal row of the carpus and the carpometacarpal joints.

Move

It is wise to start with the *distal radio-ulnar joint* so that you don't forget it. Do this by asking the patient to pronate and supinate actively. If your assistance is

Table 3.1 The palpable bones of the wrist

Scaphoid	*Tuberosity*: anteriorly (e.g. in Kirk Watson's test). *Waist*: in the snuffbox, but always compare with other wrist as pressing firmly in the snuffbox normally causes pain due to pressure on the terminal branches of the radial nerve. *Proximal pole*: dorsally and more central than you might think, distal to Lister's tubercle on the radius where the EPL tendon changes direction
Lunate	Dorsally and centrally, especially when the wrist is flexed. There is a tendency to feel too far distally, so identify the dorsal lip of the radius
Capitate	Dorsally, distal to the lunate, especially in full flexion when the head of the capitate becomes prominent
Triquetrum	Dorsally and on the ulnar side, especially in radial deviation
Pisiform	Anterior and ulnar, just proximal to the hypothenar eminence. You can trace the flexor carpi ulnaris tendon distally to it
Hamate	*Body*: dorsally and on the ulnar side, especially in radial deviation. *Hook*: anteriorly and deeply. Press firmly about 1.5 cm distal and radial to the pisiform
Trapezium	Just proximal to the base of the first metacarpal, which can be identified by moving that bone. Easiest to feel on the radial side

required, grasp the mid-forearm as holding the patient's hand to rotate the forearm involves the wrist joint and may confuse the issue.

Movement of the *wrist joints* is also best done actively, comparing both wrists. Measure dorsiflexion by placing a small goniometer (which will fit in your pocket) on the front of the wrist; for palmar flexion, put it on the back.

Abnormal movements are of two types. The first is one in which the patient complains, when the bones suddenly move from one position to another, of with a click or clunk which may be painful (see below). Ask the patient to demonstrate it to you; pay attention the first time as it may be too painful to repeat. The other type requires passive movements to detect ligamentous laxity. One of the examiner's hands holds the bone or bones on one side of the joint to be tested, while his

other hand holds the bone or bones on the other side of the joint. Stress is then applied in each direction. The most important are:

1. anterior–posterior (AP) drawer
2. scapholunate ballotment
3. triquetrolunate ballotment
4. pisotriquetral ballotment
5. Kirk Watson's test (see below)

Listen

Four different sounds have been described as emanating from the wrist. If a sound is painless, it is unlikely to be significant.

1. A vacuum click. This low-pitched sound is of no importance and cannot be repeated for 20 minutes.
2. A 'catch-up clunk'. When ligamentous damage or laxity allows one carpal bone to linger behind its moving neighbours, that bone suddenly has to move fast to catch up, causing a clunk which may be painful. The most common example of this important physical sign is Kirk Watson's test, with which you must be familiar. Watson himself calls it the scaphoid shift test: 'The patient is approached by the examiner as if to engage in arm wrestling, face to face across a table with diagonally opposed hands raised (right to right or left to left) and elbows resting on the surface in between. With the patient's forearm slightly pronated, the examiner grasps the wrist from the radial side,' "placing his thumb on the scaphoid tuberosity (as though pushing a button to open a car door)" and "wrapping his fingers around the distal radius. The examiner's other hand grasps at metacarpal level, controlling wrist position. Starting in ulnar deviation and slight extension, the wrist is moved radially and slightly flexed with constant thumb pressure on the scaphoid.' As described earlier, this radial deviation causes the scaphoid to flex. 'The examiner's thumb pressure opposes this normal rotation, causing the scaphoid to shift in relation to the other bones of the carpus. This scaphoid shift may be subtle or dramatic.' A truly positive test requires both pain on the back of the wrist (not just where you are pressing on the scaphoid tuberosity) and a click, and comparison with the opposite wrist is essential.

3. A repeatable snap may be caused by a loose flap of cartilage.
4. Tendons slipping over a bony prominence may produce a high-pitched click.

Light

Large ganglia are transilluminant. Have a throat torch in your pocket.

Function

If the patient has complained of pain or difficulty in performing particular tasks such as lifting a teapot or using a screwdriver, get him to do it while you are watching. This often enables you to define what the problem is. In the Hand Clinic one should have a variety of objects available for such tests, but this may not be possible when you are doing the clinical part of the FRCS Orth. examination.

INVESTIGATIONS

It is unintelligent to go through the same list of investigations in every patient. The nature of the symptoms and signs suggests possible diagnoses and indicates the direction in which the investigation should go. Nevertheless, most patients should have the wrist radiographed. This is wise even with a simple ganglion, if there is any doubt as to whether the ganglion is causing the pain. However, the radiographic views which you order should depend on the clinical findings; if you just ask for radiographs of the wrist, that is what you will get and serve you right. For example, special views are required to show a fracture of the scaphoid, osteoarthritis of the pisitriquetral joint, a fracture of the hook of the hamate or a carpometacarpal boss.

The routine views of the wrist are posterior-anterior (not AP) and lateral. It is assumed that you can unhesitatingly identify each bone on the PA view but on the lateral you should also be able to trace the outline of the scaphoid, lunate, capitate and trapezium (*Figure 3.2*). On both views you should look for the two concentric Cs formed by the radiocarpal and mid-carpal joints (*Figures 3.2 and 3.3*). If the C is not a smooth curve or the two sides are not concentric, something is wrong. On the lateral view (*Figure 3.2*) you should also check that the distal row of the carpus is in line with the base of the metacarpals; carpometacarpal dislocation is still frequently missed, as are dislocation of the lunate and perilunar dislocation.

The lateral view should be taken with the wrist in a neutral position, neither flexed nor extended. Unfortunately many radiographers are still taught to have the wrist extended, which makes it impossible to assess whether it is significant if the lunate is tilted into extension (or dorsiflexion); if the wrist is straight,

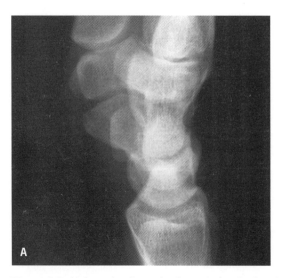
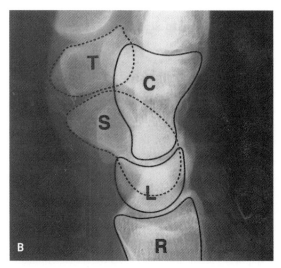

Figure 3.2 (a) Lateral radiograph of a normal wrist showing the radiocarpal and mid-carpal joints as concentric Cs. (b) the outlines of the scaphoid, lunate, capitate and trapezium.

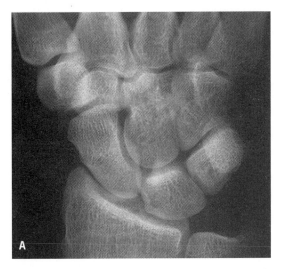 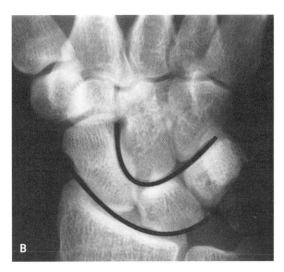

Figure 3.3 PA radiograph of a normal wrist showing the radiocarpal and mid-carpal joints as concentric Cs.

such extension of the lunate indicates dorsal inter-calated segment instability (DISI), which is considered below.

The PA view is normally taken with the wrist straight unless a fracture of the scaphoid is suspected, in which case the wrist is ulnar-deviated to extend the scaphoid. On a PA radiograph of the wrist, the ulnar styloid is out to the ulnar side as you normally see it in the radiograph for a Colles' fracture. The wrist is radio-graphed PA because it is easier to put the wrist on the plate with the palm down (forearm pronated). In contrast, radiographs of the whole forearm are taken AP, with the forearm supinated, so that the radius and ulnar are parallel instead of crossed: on this view the ulnar styloid projects beyond the *centre* of the head of the ulna.

A few years ago, there was a vogue for 'carpal insta-bility views' taken at the extremes of movement in all directions, plus an AP view with the patient gripping tightly to try and elicit any scapholunate separation. We have found that these seldom yield useful informa-tion, as the abnormal relationship between the carpal bones may only appear in an intermediate position (e.g. partial radial deviation), not at the extreme. Nevertheless it is sometimes useful to obtain PA views in radial and ulnar deviation. As described above, the position of the proximal row changes from one to the other and you should be familiar with these appear-ances. In radial deviation the scaphoid looks shorter and the cortex around its tuberosity may present a

signet-ring appearance; the lunate, in addition to moving more ulnarwards in relation to the radius, looks triangular compared to its four-sided shape in ulnar deviation; the triquetrum has a tubercle at the corner which is closest to the capitate★. A full, helpful and illustrated account of these changes and those on stress views was given by Schernberg.

Where abnormal movements are suspected, *screening* is the best way to demonstrate them. The surgeon and radiologist should both be present and the examination should be recorded on video tape so that it can be studied repeatedly at leisure. First move the wrist slowly to each of the four extremes in turn. Then invite the patient to make the movement required to produce any click or pain. Finally apply AP and lateral stresses. Examine the other wrist too for comparison.

Arthroscopy is also useful for suspected mechanical abnormalities and can demonstrate changes in cartilage which can be detected in no other way. However, it is more difficult than arthroscopy of the knee as there is less room and it takes considerable experience to become familiar with the appearances. It is often difficult, especially in older patients, to decide whether the changes seen are normal degeneration, 'chance' findings or the cause of the patient's symptoms. One

---

★A mnemonic for these is STT (shorter, triangular, tubercle): those are the appearances in *radial* deviation and the STT joint (scaphoid-trapezium-trapezoid) is on the *radial* side of the wrist.

should never consider the arthroscopic findings in isolation. They should always be considered with the clinical findings.

If the history, examination and radiographs do not suggest a mechanical problem, a *bone scan* is wise. In a normal person very little of the isotope is taken up by the soft tissues, but if they are damaged or diseased they can take up appreciable quantities so that an abnormal area is identified: thus the term 'bone scan' is slightly misleading and it can be used as a general screening test to exclude anything nasty. If one specifically suspects infection, one can ask for a gallium scan which detects pooling of white blood cells; nowadays the radiologist would probably employ a scan using the patient's own blood which has been withdrawn, labelled with indium (which attaches itself to the white blood cells) and is then injected back into the patient. In Keinböck's disease, where one might expect to see reduced uptake, there may in fact be increased uptake due to revascular-isation and deposition of new bone. A 'bone scan' is also useful in those patients, usually young women, with rather ill-defined symptoms around the wrist; rarely is an abnormality detected but, if not, the normal scan can be used as reassurance.

Arthrography has largely been superseded by arthroscopy and magnetic resonance imaging (MRI). If employed, the contrast medium should be injected in three phases★. The first injection is into the mid-carpal joint: the contrast medium may track proximally between the scaphoid and lunate and between the lunate and triquetrum but should not enter the radio-carpal joint. Second the radiocarpal joint is injected and third the inferior radio-ulnar joint. Having demon-strated a communication, it may be hard to decide whether it is degenerative or traumatic and sympto-matic or asymptomatic.

It is neither good medicine nor efficient use of resources to employ computed tomography (CT) and MRI in all patients with painful wrists but in selected cases they can yield priceless information. With further refinement and experience, MRI may provide the answer to many questions. Both investigations are

difficult to interpret and you will need a report by a radiologist with a special interest in this area. One thing MRI can certainly do is to show the avascularity of the lunate in Keinböck's disease before changes become apparent on ordinary radiographs.

INJURIES OF THE DISTAL RADIO-ULNAR JOINT

Dislocation of the distal radio-ulnar joint

Distal radio-ulnar joint dislocations only rarely occur in isolation: they are more often seen in association with fractures of the distal radius or the shaft of the radius (Galeazzi fracture). Isolated dislocations may be either palmar or dorsal and are frequently missed on standard radiographs. The diagnosis is suspected when, after a wrist injury, the forearm is locked in supination or pronation and cannot be passively rotated; attempting to do so is most painful. On palpation, the ulnar head may be tender and prominent palmarly or dorsally. Careful examination of the PA wrist radiographs should show incongruity of the distal radio-ulnar joint, often with overlap of the two articular surfaces (*Figure 3.4*). Acute dislocations should be reduced closed and immobilised in an above-elbow plaster with the forearm in mid-rotation for six weeks.

Instability

This follows injuries to the ligaments of the joint and allows the ulna to slip forwards and backwards during pronation and supination: another cause of painful clicking of the wrist. Various ligament reconstructions have been recommended but, in our opinion, none is wholly satisfactory; if they are tight enough to prevent instability, they may also limit rotation of the forearm. We believe the best solution for *disabling* instability is a Kapandji operation (see below); less troublesome insta-bility is probably best left untreated.

CARPOMETACARPAL JOINT DISLOCATIONS

These injuries usually affect the fifth, or fourth and fifth, carpometacarpal joints but may involve all the finger rays. Furthermore, dislocation of the thumb

---

★Although three-phase arthrography is the gold standard, our radiologist now only injects contrast medium into the radiocarpal joint. This shows most triangular fibrocartilage complex and intercarpal ligament tears and is much quicker and cheaper than 'three-phase' arthrography.

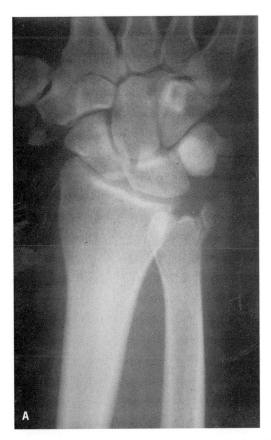 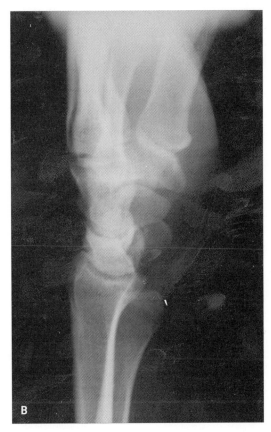

Figure 3.4 Palmar dislocation of the distal radio-ulnar joint. (a) The articular surfaces of this joint are overlapped on the PA view (not a true PA, as the forearm was locked in supination). (b) The lateral view is a good one as the metacarpal shafts are all in the same plane; thus the palmar displacement of the distal ulna is significant and indicates a palmar dislocation.

carpometacarpal joint may occur in isolation, though the 'Bennett's' fracture–dislocation is more common. The dislocations are dorsal and are characterised by tenderness over the affected joints and prominence of the involved metacarpal bases on the back of the hand. However, the prominence of the metacarpal bases may be obscured by soft-tissue swelling. The PA radiograph shows the involved metacarpal bases overlapping the hamate and/or capitate and does not show the carpo-metacarpal joint spaces. The lateral view shows dorsal displacement of the metacarpal bases and palmar angulation of the involved metacarpals; furthermore on this view the metacarpal shafts no longer lie in the same line as the radius and capitate (*Figure 3.5*). Unfortunately these injuries are often missed, even by orthopaedic surgeons; this is either because a lateral radiograph is not taken or because it is taken but not studied carefully enough.

These dislocations, in contrast to fracture–dislocations, are usually stable once reduced and can be managed satisfactorily by closed reduction and immobilisation of the wrist in 30° extension in a below-elbow plaster for three weeks★. If one is concerned that the reduction is unstable, then percutaneous Kirschner wires may be passed across the involved joints under fluoroscopic control.

★After you have reduced a dislocation of any joint, you should always stress the joint in order to assess the stability of your reduction and record your findings clearly in the notes. You should then always obtain check radiographs to confirm that the joint is reduced, however confident you feel; these may show persistent dislocation/subluxation or an associated fracture which makes the injury unstable. If you do not do these checks, the doctors in the Fracture Clinic will not know (a) whether they need to obtain serial check radiographs and (b) when they can safely mobilise the joint.

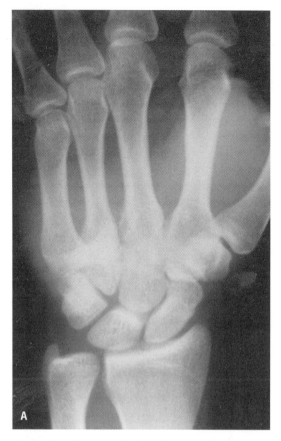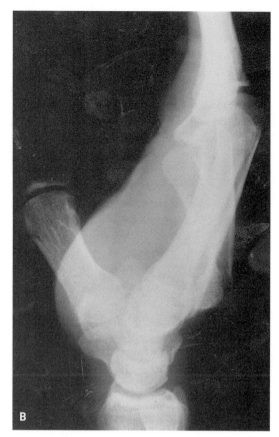

Figure 3.5 (a) PA and (b) lateral radiographs showing dislocations of the fourth and fifth carpometacarpal joints.

INJURIES TO THE CARPAL JOINTS

Dislocations

Fractures of the carpal bones are covered in another volume of this series but we will briefly deal with dislocations and ligamentous injuries. In fact, most dislocations are accompanied by fractures of small fragments of bone, especially from the radial styloid, though these may not be apparent until the dislocation has been reduced. Sometimes the bony fragment is larger and important.

Any pattern of dislocation is possible and all require a violent force to produce them. They have been classified into those where the dislocation occurs along a 'lesser arc' around the lunate and those involving a 'greater arc' which includes the lunate and part or all of one or more other carpal bones. In practice these injuries are uncommon and you will seldom encounter any but the following four (*Figure 3.6*):

1. perilunar dislocation ⎫
2. dislocation of the lunate ⎬ lesser arc
3. trans-scaphoid perilunar dislocation (known in some countries as de Quervain's injury) ⎫ greater arc
4. transcapitate perilunar dislocation ⎭

Changes are clearly visible on both PA and lateral radiographs although they are often overlooked by junior doctors. Radiographs of these injuries are often shown in the clinical and oral parts of the FRCS Orth examination, leading to discussion about complications and management.

Management of lesser arc injuries

It is thought that these two injuries represent two stages of the same process. First there is perilunar dislocation, but in some cases the rest of the carpus

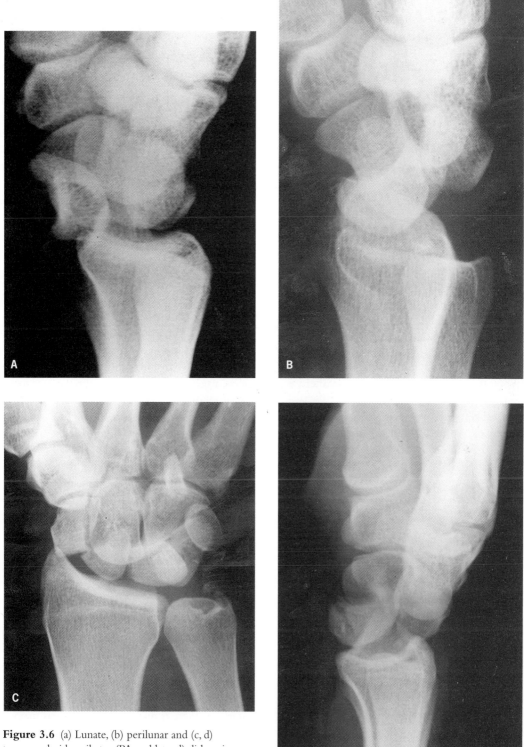

Figure 3.6 (a) Lunate, (b) perilunar and (c, d) trans-scaphoid perilunar (PA and lateral) dislocations of the wrist.

then moves forward (in a palmar direction) again and pushes the lunate out into the carpal tunnel. Surprisingly this does not always cause compression of the median nerve, nor does it often cause avascular necrosis of the lunate because a flap of capsular attachment remains intact and presumably carries a blood supply.

Various manoeuvres are described to achieve reduction and these should be undertaken by an experienced orthopaedic surgeon in theatre under general anaesthetic in case open reduction is required. The traditional approach was to get the bones roughly back to their positions and then keep the wrist in plaster for two or three months.

It is now considered that more attention should be paid to exact reduction. For example, a persisting gap between the scaphoid and lunate is not accepted. Open reduction is carried out and Kirschner wires stuck into the carpal bones are used as joysticks to get them into perfect alignment; other Kirschner wires are then driven across the injured joints to maintain reduction and the joysticks are removed. The ligaments are repaired as best one can; often the carpus needs to be exposed both from the back and the front for this purpose. A prolonged period in plaster afterwards is required.

The aim of this modern approach is to avoid later carpal instability (see below) but in practice follow-up of patients treated in the old-fashioned way has found that the wrists are not unstable but stiff. It remains to be shown that they will be better following operative treatment.

Management of greater arc injuries

If there is no major fracture they can be treated like lesser arc injuries. A fracture across the waist of the scaphoid with a dislocation is, however, a definite indication for open reduction and internal fixation. This is because there may be torn ligament or capsule lying within the fracture, which is unstable because of the ligamentous damage. If treated conservatively the fracture has a 50% chance of non-union, which can probably be reduced by accurate open reduction and fixation, preferably with a Herbert screw.

Alternatively, or in addition, a perilunar dislocation may be accompanied by a fracture of the neck of the capitate, whose head may then rotate through 180°

so that its convexity faces distally rather than proximally; unfortunately this element of the injury may be overlooked. This rare event requires open reduction and internal fixation.

Torn ligaments

Individual ligaments in the wrist can be torn in an injury which falls short of dislocation. These are usually missed because the radiograph is normal, but can sometimes be detected by a careful examination.

As an example, a general practitioner was lifting an arthritic patient onto the examination couch when he felt a sudden pain in his own wrist. A radiograph in the local A & E Department was normal and he was reassured, but his wrist remained painful and he telephoned one of us for advice. He said that the pain had felt just like a previous occasion when he had dislocated his shoulder. Examination revealed tenderness precisely over the scapholunate ligament and Kirk Watson's test was strongly positive. Radiographs showed *dorsal intercalated segment instability* (DISI); the lunate was extended and the scaphoid flexed, thus increasing the scapholunate angle (see below pages 71–2). There was also a slight increase in the scapholunate gap. At exploration next day, the scapholunate ligament was found to have torn in a step-shape. Using Kirschner wires as joysticks, the scaphoid was extended and the lunate flexed back to their normal positions; other Kirschner wires were then driven across to maintain this reduction. Because of the shape of the tear in this case, it was possible to suture it. The wires were removed after six weeks and the plaster cast after eight weeks. He made an excellent recovery and resumed playing tennis.

This story has been told because if the patient had not been a doctor himself and had not telephoned a consultant whom he knew, the diagnosis would not have been made until much later, when repair is impossible and one has to choose between ligamentous reconstruction or limited carpal fusion, neither of which is entirely satisfactory. This, unfortunately, is what usually happens in Great Britain where it often takes a long time to see an experienced orthopaedic surgeon if there is no fracture or obvious major injury. If you are lucky enough to see such patients early, be sure you remove any plaster cast so that you can make a very careful clinical examination.

Sprains

Think of all those patients with painful wrists after an injury in whom repeated radiographs are normal. What is the cause of the pain? It may be an occult fracture, visible only on CT, but whose presence can be detected by a bone scan. It may be a torn ligament, as in the GP described above. In most cases, however, it is surely a sprain, that is to say a tearing of a few fibres in a ligament but not enough to tear it right across and disrupt it. Such injuries settle with a few weeks of immobilisation.

However, sprained wrist is a diagnosis which can only be made in retrospect, after two sets of radiographs a fortnight apart and a bone scan. In the early stages, it is wise to follow the old adage 'sprained wrist does not exist'.

CARPAL INSTABILITY

This is a difficult subject, but not as difficult as it is made to seem by unnecessarily complicated terminology. Unfortunately these terms are now established and you will be expected to know them and, worse still, their abbreviations. However, we shall start by discussing the matter in plain English.

The concepts are straightforward. The bones of the carpus may assume abnormal positions or alignments, either between the two rows (if the extrinsic ligaments are abnormal) or between the bones of one row (if the intrinsic ligaments alone, or in conjunction with the extrinsic ligaments, have been torn). This may come on immediately after an injury or later, or may be due to inherent ligamentous laxity. The abnormal position may be present all the time, or intermittently when it is induced by a particular position or activity. The latter is, like an intermittent fault in any machine, difficult to detect and thus to correct; in practice this is one of the main problems in diagnosing carpal instability. Intermittent instability may also be a party trick, like voluntary dislocation of the shoulder, where surgery is best avoided.

The carpometacarpal joints of the fingers allow little movement (30° at the fifth, 15° at the fourth and virtually none at the third and second) so the main part of the distal row of the carpus is held fairly firmly to those metacarpals. In contrast, the proximal

row to some extent floats free between the radio-carpal and mid-carpal joints; it is an *intercalated segment* (intercalated = inserted between different items or layers). The position of the proximal row, lacking any muscular control, is determined partly by the concave shape of the radiocarpal and mid-carpal joints but mainly by ligaments, especially the strong anterior ligaments.

In normal flexion and extension of the wrist, the movement takes place simultaneously and about equally at the radiocarpal and mid-carpal joints. However, if the proper constraints are lacking it is possible for the radiocarpal joint to extend while the mid-carpal joint flexes, or vice versa. This is called *intercalated segment instability*, which usually affects the whole of the proximal row (scaphoid, lunate, triquetrum) but is most easily assessed by the position of the lunate on a lateral radiograph taken with the wrist in a neutral position. If the proximal row (judged by the lunate) is extended, or inclined dorsally, in relation to the long axis of the radius and capitate, the situation is called dorsal intercalated segment instability (DISI for short). Flexion of the proximal row, with the lunate inclined towards the volar aspect, is called volar intercalated segment instability (VISI) and is much less common.

Other elements of the official terminology are shown in *Table 3.2*.

Kirk Watson (quoted by Taleisnik) has compared the carpal joints to a Jack-in-the-box, spring-loaded but kept under restraint. 'A ligament tear is akin to releasing the Jack-in-the-box, allowing it to assume a different, paradoxically more stable, but abnormally aligned position.' The key bone, centrally situated in the carpus and representing the Jack-in-the-box, is the lunate, whose natural inclination due to its shape is to lie in

Table 3.2 Elements of the official terminology

Plain English	Official
Constant	Static
Intermittent	Dynamic
Between bones of the same carpal row (in practice, the proximal row)	Dissociative
Between the proximal and distal rows, or between the proximal row and distal radius	Non-dissociative

dorsiflexion. It is normally held in a state of potentially unstable equilibrium by:

1. its own shape and position as an intercalated segment between the forearm and hand;
2. the shape of the surrounding articular surfaces (particularly that of the distal radius);
3. pressures exerted by neighbouring carpal bones;
4. the guiding and restraining support of carpal ligaments.

Changes in any of these characteristics can potentially lead to unstable alignments:

1. when the lunate collapses, as in Kienboch's disease (pages 87–9);
2. when the radiolunate relationship is reversed after mal-union of fractures of the distal radius;
3. when scaphoid action on the lunate becomes abnormal after unstable scaphoid fracture;
4. after various types of ligamentous tears.

This introduces another type of carpal instability called adaptive, which is the consequence of deformity in the distal radius. This deformity is usually angulation into dorsiflexion following an old Colles' fracture which carries the lunate into dorsiflexion and obliges the patient, if he wishes to have his wrist straight, to keep his mid-carpal joint fully flexed, which sometimes causes aching and a feeling of weakness relieved by extending the wrist.

Finally, there are forms of carpal instability due to combinations of the above or defying other classification, which are called complex.

Thus we are left with an array of indigestible labels with rather similar abbreviations (two of them being those of law enforcement agencies), any of which may be either static or dynamic:

1. carpal instability, dissociative   (CID)
2. carpal instability, non-dissociative   (CIND)
3. carpal instability, complex   (CIC)
4. carpal instability, adaptive   (CIA)

Green, who himself wrote the chapter on this difficult subject in the third edition of his book on *Operative Hand Surgery*, added a fifth type:

5. carpal instability longitudinal (or axial). This is the consequence of rare injuries, often associated with fractures, in which carpal bones are separated from their neighbours by longitudinal tearing of the ligaments which normally hold them together from side to side, e.g. the hamate and the capitate. The best treatment is to detect the injury early, approach it from the front and back, stabilise the carpus with Kirschner wires and repair the ligaments as best one can.

Now let us look at some specific examples of carpal instability. The most important is scapholunate dissociation.

Scapholunate dissociation

The acute injury has already been mentioned and may represent the first stage of a lesser arc injury. The chronic form may follow this (especially in a patient with a tendency to lax ligaments) or a dislocation of the wrist with tearing of the scapholunate ligament. It also occurs in rheumatoid disease and idiopathically. It may be 'static', in which case a PA radiograph will reveal the Terry-Thomas★ gap of more than 2 mm between the two bones, or 'dynamic' in which case the gap only exists in certain positions of the wrist. The scaphoid, its proximal pole no longer restrained by attachment to the lunate, moves into more flexion by rotating around an axis across its waist from side-to-side (marked by a large spot on *Figure 3.7a*) and the line on *Figure 3.7b*. This is a form of DISI due to CID. To understand what is really happening, you must realise that the axis around which the scaphoid flexes is transverse to the long axis of the scaphoid but oblique to that of the arm and hand. Seen from the back, the more flexed scaphoid looks shorter and there appears to be a gap between it and the lunate (*Figure 3.7* and *3.8*). However, this is not because the scaphoid and lunate have moved apart from side-to-side, but because the scaphoid has flexed (*Figure 3.7c*). If, at operation on a fresh case, you push the proximal pole of the scaphoid anteriorly, it rotates back into its normal relationship with the lunate and the gap disappears. This is sometimes called 'rotary subluxation of the scaphoid', a radiological term which may cause confusion because it seems to suggest rotation of the scaphoid about its long axis (like rotation of the forearm) which is not

---

★Terry-Thomas was not a surgeon but an actor with a gap between his two front teeth.

Normal position **Scapholunate dissociation**

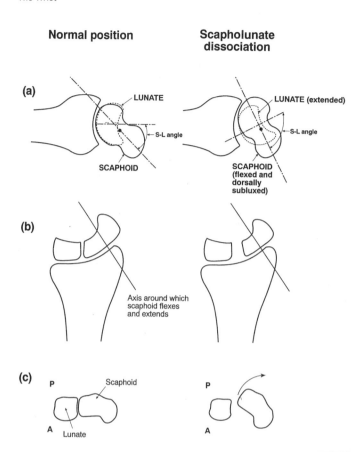

(a)

(b)

Axis around which
scaphoid flexes
and extends

(c)

Figure 3.7 Diagrams showing the positions of the scaphoid and lunate in normal circumstances (left) and in scapholunate dissociation causing DISI (right). (a) Lateral view: the normal scapholunate angle is 45–60°; in scapholunate dissociation the scapholunate angle is increased because the lunate has extended and the scaphoid has flexed further. The large dot indicates the axis around which the scaphoid flexes and extends. (b) PA view: in scapholunate dissociation there appears to be a gap between the lunate and scaphoid. This is caused by flexion of the scaphoid around the axis marked on the diagram. The removal distance between the adjacent articular surfaces of the lunate and scaphoid should be less than 2 mm. (c) Oblique lateral view, in the line of the axis around which the scaphoid flexes and extends, as marked on (a) and (b). In scapholunate dissociation, the scaphoid flexes so that its proximal pole rotates dorsally and away from the lunate. Restoration of the normal alignment is achieved by pressing the proximal pole of the scaphoid in a palmar direction, not by pushing the scaphoid and lunate together.

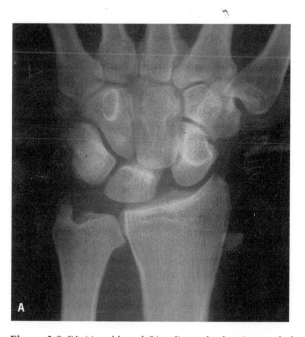

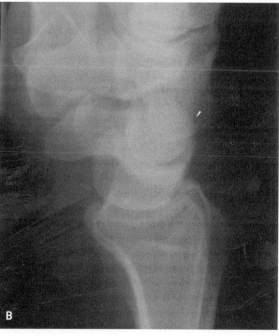

Figure 3.8 PA (a) and lateral (b) radiographs showing scapholunate dissociation; the lateral view shows that the scapholunate angle is increased, due to extension of the lunate and flexion of the scaphoid.

what is meant. Occasionally the scaphoid may actually snap from one position to another: from normal flexion to excessive flexion. Usually the flexed position is constant or the change more gradual, but Kirk Watson's test encourages the scaphoid to move with a sudden, clinically detectable and painful snap.

The obvious treatment is reconstruction of the scapholunate ligament but in late cases this does not work well. Fusion of the scaphoid to the lunate would hold it, but it is difficult to achieve because the area of bony contact is small. It is easier to fix the other end of the scaphoid by fusing it to the trapezium and trapezoid (STT fusion: the foolish term 'triscaphe fusion' should not be used) or to fuse the scaphoid to the capitate. We have found that neither ligamentous reconstructions nor limited carpal fusions, even if technically successful, can be relied on to give good results; furthermore, limited carpal fusions have a significant non-union rate. Another way to prevent excessive flexion of the scaphoid is to hold its distal pole dorsally by Blatt's capsulodesis, in which the bones are restored to correct alignment using Kirschner wires as joysticks and then a dorsal flap of wrist capsule, based proximally, is advanced into a groove on the back of the distal pole of the scaphoid to keep it pulled dorsally. (Recently Herbert has modified this by basing the flap distally and attaching it to the distal radius, which is easier.) Afterwards, as in any form of soft tissue reconstruction of carpal ligaments, the bones must be held in their correct alignment by Kirschner wires for two or even three months until the soft tissues have healed strongly enough to take the load.

Triquetrolunate dissociation

This is rare but similar in principle. The difference is that the scaphoid and lunate are both flexed, leaving the triquetrum extended; an example of VISI due to CID. It can occur in rheumatoid disease.

Mid-carpal subluxation

The frequency and types of carpal instability seen in the UK seem to differ from the USA whence most of the literature emanates. In our experience one of the more common varieties is laxity of the mid-carpal joint, allowing the head of the capitate to slip out of the socket formed by the distal end of the lunate. This

can be seen on screening, especially with AP stress, and it produces a painful click. The other wrist often has similar laxity though this is not painful. (Here one should issue a word of warning, as many wrists can be made to show mid-carpal instability if the wrist is subjected to axial compression and AP stress. Thus the mid-carpal instability may not be the cause of a patient's wrist pain, especially if there is no history of painful clicking.) The trouble seems to be caused by some quite minor injury in a person with lax ligaments. It can be alleviated by mid-carpal fusion, at the expense of wrist motion. This is an example of dynamic non-dissociative instability.

According to Taliesnik a similar phenomenon may occur in patients with mal-union of the distal radius so that the mid-carpal joint is flexed and the head of the capitate is almost subluxed dorsally and poised to pop out.

Triquetrohamate instability

Mulligan has described another form of mid-carpal instability, occurring particularly in young women, where there is abnormal and painful movement between the triquetrum and hamate, again sometimes following a minor injury. He elicits this by ulnar-deviating the wrist, pronating the hand and pushing the ulnar side of the dorsum of the carpus anteriorly. The symptoms may be cured by fusing those two bones together; a trial can be made by holding them together with staples introduced by a stapiliser.

Ulnar translocation of the carpus

In rheumatoid disease, and sometimes after injury, the whole carpus may translocate ulnarwards on the radius, leaving a gap between the scaphoid and radial styloid. It used to be said that this was promoted by excision of the distal end of the ulna, but in most cases that is excised when it has already displaced dorsally and ceased to support the carpus. This sideways displacement of the carpus can be controlled by radiolunate fusion (the Chamay procedure) or, of course, radiocarpal fusion.

Summary of carpal instability

In practice, carpal instability concerns the proximal row, i.e. its relationship to the distal radius and the distal row of the carpus, or the relationship between the bones which compose the proximal row.

Whatever words are used, the questions to be answered are:

1. What bone or bones are abnormally placed or aligned?
2. What direction or angle do they adopt?
3. Are they like that all the time or only intermittently?
4. What is the cause of the instability?
5. Is this the cause of the pain? (Not every alteration in carpal alignment is pathological and some pathological malalignments may be assymptomatic. For example congenitally lax wrists may be mal-aligned but work well and without symptoms.)
6. How can it be prevented?

GANGLIA

Ganglia are by far the most common soft tissue tumours of the wrist and hand and are usually found in specific locations around the wrist and in the hand. They are three times as common in females as males and are most often found in the 10–40 age group, but can occur at any age. Approximately 10% of ganglia are first noticed after a specific definite injury but there is no proven association with any particular occupation, work practice or 'repetitive activity'.

Pathology

Ganglia are either single or multiloculated translucent cysts which arise from either the capsule of a joint (most commonly the wrist and distal IP joints) or a tendon sheath. Those arising from a joint remain attached to this structure by a thin pedicle. Their thin walls consist of compressed collagen fibres and sparse flattened cells and they have no synovial or epithelial lining. About 70% arise from the scapholunate ligament on the dorsum of the wrist joint and 20% arise from the flexor surface of the wrist joint, either from the radiocarpal or scaphotrapezial joint capsules. The pathogenesis of ganglia is uncertain but theories of joint capsule synovial herniation and mucoid degeneration have been proposed. A minority develop as a secondary feature of a metacarpal boss, joint osteoarthritis or de Quervain's tenovaginitis.

Presentation

Most ganglia present as swellings which appear suddenly or gradually develop over a period of months. They may be painful in the early stages, presumably due to stretching of soft tissues, but large ones are often painless. Thus, if a patient presents with wrist pain and a ganglion, do not assume that the pain is due to the ganglion; there may be a different cause. Typically, they become firmer, larger and more painful with activity. Deep ganglia may compress surrounding structures and cause secondary symptoms. For example a ganglion lying next to the superficial branch of the radial nerve may cause paraesthesiae and pain on the extensor surface of the first web space. Very rarely palmar wrist ganglia may compress the median nerve in the carpal tunnel or the ulnar nerve in Guyon's canal.

The diagnosis is usually immediately apparent but in cases of uncertainty, ganglia can be distinguished from solid soft-tissue tumours by transillumination and aspiration. The 'occult' dorsal wrist ganglion which arises from the scapholunate ligament and only attains a diameter of 2 or 3 mm, requires specific mention as it does not become sufficiently large to cause an obvious swelling but may cause most troublesome dorsal wrist pain. These ganglia are usually detected by palpating the dorsal surface of the fully flexed wrist joint and comparing its contours with those of the contralateral wrist. A prominent proximal pole of the scaphoid or capitate head is sometimes mistaken for a dorsal wrist ganglion but in cases of uncertainty the presence of a ganglion can usually be confirmed by ultrasonography (MRI).

The commonest finger ganglion arises from the A1 pulley of the flexor tendon sheath. The patient describes it as like a small pebble or pea which causes discomfort when gripping objects.

Conservative treatment

Sensible conservative treatment options include reassurance, aspiration alone, aspiration with multiple puncture of the ganglion wall or aspiration with injection of steroid. The natural history of ganglia is that the majority resolve spontaneously within a period of one or two years, so simple reassurance is all that is required if a ganglion is causing few symptoms; this is particularly the case in children, who do not like needles! Simple aspiration using a wide-bored hyperdermic needle cures 30% of ganglia and in a further 40% either settles the symptoms or reassures the patient sufficiently so that no further treatment is required. One should not forget that the immediate concern of many patients who develop a ganglion is that they have a cancer and nothing is so reassuring as an aspiration which removes the swelling and allows the patient to see the harmless jelly within the syringe. Some doctors recommend multiple puncture of the ganglion wall or inject steroid into the ganglion following aspiration, but neither measure improves the results of simple aspiration.

Surgical treatment

Surgery should be reserved for ganglia which persist for many months and cause troublesome symptoms. Properly performed surgery has high success and low recurrence rates but inadequate surgery, which fails to trace the pedicle down to the joint capsule, has a high recurrence rate. A tourniquet must be used and general or regional anaesthesia is recommended for all ganglia arising from the wrist joint. Wrist ganglia are best exposed through transverse incisions. First the cyst is exposed and then its pedicle, which may be long and tortuous, is identified and traced down to the joint capsule which is incised around the base of the pedicle and excised with the ganglion. Great care must be taken not to damage surrounding tissues. Volar wrist ganglia frequently lie between the terminal branches of the radial artery; the terminal branches of the radial nerve and the palmar cutaneous branch of the median nerve are also in close proximity and are thus 'at risk'*. If it is adherent to the artery, leave that part of the ganglion wall attached to the artery; if you remove the rest, and especially the pedicle, it should not recur. In the case of dorsal wrist ganglia, which arise from the scapholunate ligament, excision of the capsule around the pedicle often leaves a 1 cm diameter defect in the dorsal wrist capsule. Indeed if you do not see the

---

*Most surgeons take great pride in excising ganglia without bursting them. However the dissection and surgery are much easier and safer if large ganglia are purposefully burst. The authors, who are both highly skilled and technically brilliant surgeons, far prefer to announce loudly at the beginning of the operation that they are about to burst the ganglion on purpose, rather than hear the theatre staff snigger when they accidentally burst it during a difficult and tedious excision – of course we could have removed it intact if we wanted to!

proximal pole of the scaphoid, you have not done an adequate excision. However, it is not necessary to close or repair this capsular defect and to do so may cause joint stiffness. The skin wound should be closed with particular care as these patients are often sensitive to cosmetic defects. Postoperatively it is not necessary to immobilise the wrist in plaster and we advise a bulky dressing which restricts wrist movements but is only worn for five days.

Ganglia sometimes disappear for periods of time, only to reappear at a later date. If a patient presents for surgery at a time when his ganglion cannot be palpated, the surgeon should not be tempted to proceed with surgery. Although the patient may reassure him that this has happened in the past, only for the ganglion to recur, it may never recur. Furthermore, although no trace of the ganglion may be found at surgery, it may recur a few weeks later.

OSTEOARTHRITIS

The wrist joint (the radiocarpal and mid-carpal joints) and the distal radio-ulnar joint can both become osteoarthritic, either in isolation or combination. The osteoarthritis may be primary or secondary to trauma or an inflammatory arthropathy such as gout. Long-standing mal-union of intra-articular fractures of the distal radius, non-union of scaphoid fractures and wrist ligament injuries may all cause painful wrist osteo-arthritis, but this is by no means an inevitable consequence of these injuries.

Wrist joint (as opposed to distal radio-ulnar joint) osteoarthritis

Pathology

Osteoarthritis may be *generalised* and involve many of the radiocarpal and mid-carpal articulations or *localised* and involve only selected articulations, usually those around the scaphoid which is the most mobile carpal bone. Watson assessed 210 osteoarthritic wrists and found the *scapholunate advanced collapse* (SLAC) pattern in 57% and localised osteoarthritis of the articulation between the scaphoid and the trapezoid and trapezium (STT osteoarthritis) in 10% (*Figure 3.9*). This analysis excludes the trapeziometacarpal joint which we will not consider here as it is described in Chapter 4 (pages 161–6).

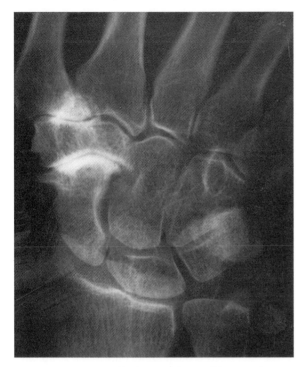

Figure 3.9 Radiograph of osteoarthritis of the articulation between the scaphoid and the trapezoid and trapezium. This lady also has trapeziometacarpal joint osteoarthritis.

The SLAC wrist describes a relatively common pattern of osteoarthritis (*Figure 3.10*) which used to be considered the inevitable end-stage of scapholunate dissociation. In this condition the structures which maintain the normal scapholunate alignment (the wrist capsule and the scapholunate ligament) fail, either due to trauma or spontaneous osteoarthritic degeneration. This allows the lunate to extend and the scaphoid to flex, thus reducing the *carpal height* (*Figure 3.11*). Either as a result of this 'carpal collapse' or as an accompanying degenerative change, the articulation between the distal scaphoid and the radial styloid process becomes osteoarthritic. Later on, the articulation between the proximal part of the scaphoid and the distal radius also becomes osteoarthritic and the lunocapitate and lunohamate joints may eventually become osteoarthritic. However, the radiolunate joint is usually, though not inevitably, well-preserved (*Figure 3.10*).

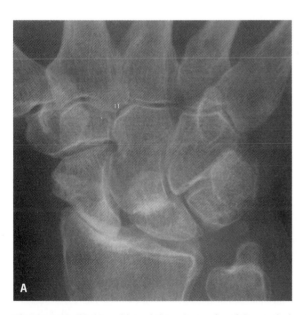

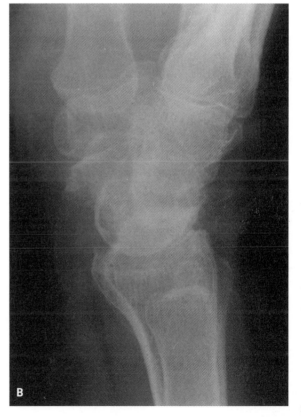

Figure 3.10 PA (a) and lateral (b) radiographs of the scapholunate advanced collapse (SLAC) pattern of wrist osteoarthritis showing advanced radioscaphoid and lunocapitate joint involvement and scapholunate separation. The radiolunate joint is well preserved.

(a)   *(b)*

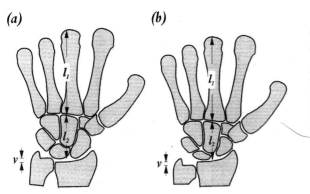

Figure 3.11 The **carpal height ratio** is used to assess **carpal collapse**. This is determined on a PA radiograph by dividing the height of the carpus (l_2) by the length of the third metacarpal (l_1): l_2/l_1. In scapholunate dissociation (b), the capitate migrates proximally between the lunate and the scaphoid, thus reducing the height of the carpus and the carpal height ratio. The normal limits for the carpal height ratio are 0.46–0.61. [I (TRCD) do not think that you need to know this for the FRCS (Orth) exam but then I am not an examiner! My co-author is an examiner but I have never seen him calculate the carpal height ratio and doubt whether he knows the normal range! However, he says that other examiners do ask about carpal height.]

Ulnar variance is the difference (v) between the height of the articular surface of the distal ulna and that of the adjacent ulnar border of the distal radius, measured in millimetres on special standardised radiographs. In (a) the ulna extends beyond the radius and thus there is ulna-positive variance. In (b) the ulna is shorter than the radius and thus there is ulna-negative variance.

With a long-standing non-union of the scaphoid, its proximal pole behaves like a little lunate and osteo-arthritis develops between the radial styloid process and the distal fragment of the scaphoid, but not between the radius and the proximal fragment. This is sometimes called *scaphoid non-union advanced collapse* (SNAC).

Presentation

Wrist osteoarthritis usually presents with pain on use, which is often remarkably well localised to the affected joints in localised wrist osteoarthritis. The patient may also complain of restricted wrist movements which are painful at their extremes and the wrist may be diffusely swollen or exhibit localised swelling over osteoarthritic articulations. The hand is usually weak and the patient may feel crepitus on wrist movements.

The wrist may be diffusely swollen and tender osteophytes may be palpable, particularly on the dorsum of the radiocarpal joint and over the radial styloid process. Wrist movements are usually restricted and painful at their extremes. In STT osteoarthritis, the patient frequently has localised swelling and tenderness over the scaphotrapezial joint but wrist flexion may be the only movement which is restricted and painful at its extreme.

Investigations

Plain PA and lateral wrist radiographs usually identify wrist joint osteoarthritis and allow the surgeon to assess whether this is generalised or localised to specific joints. CT scans and arthroscopy are sometimes used to assess the extent of the osteoarthritis if limited wrist fusions are being contemplated.

Treatment

Wrist osteoarthritis often causes only minor symptoms, in which case all that is required is advice and analgesia. Strong leather wrist supports may allow patients with troublesome osteoarthritis to return to, and stay in, manual labour for many years.

Surgery for generalised osteoarthritis.

Total wrist fusion. The standard surgical treatment for generalised wrist osteoarthritis is a total wrist fusion in which the radiocarpal, mid-carpal and third carpometacarpal joints are fused. Unless it is also osteoarthritic, the distal radio-ulnar joint is retained and thus forearm rotation is preserved. Osteoarthritis, as opposed to rheumatoid arthritis, is usually unilateral, so movement of the other wrist will be retained. Before deciding to operate, it is wise to immobilise the wrist in a below-elbow plaster for one or two weeks so that the patient can assess the likely functional outcome of his surgery.

Wrist fusion is normally performed through a dorsal approach: the dorsal 50% of the articular surfaces of the radiocarpal, mid-carpal and third carpometacarpal joints are resected down to cancellous bone and cancellous bone graft (usually harvested from the iliac crest) is then packed into these joints. The wrist joint is then stabilised with a strong plate (usually a small dynamic compression plate, though a special titanium plate has been designed for this purpose) which extends from the distal radius to the third metacarpal shaft. Care should be taken not to fuse the wrist with the lunate and scaphoid compressed down onto the distal radius as the distal ulna may then impact on the triquetrum, causing pain during forearm rotation; instead, the normal height of the radiocarpal articulation should be maintained with bone graft. The ideal position of fusion is debated but most surgeons either fuse the wrist in neutral alignment or in slight extension (20°) which may improve grip strength. It is important to fuse the third carpometacarpal joint as the dorsal plate sometimes irritates the finger extensor tendons, causing pain and is therefore subsequently removed. If this joint has not been fused, it is then subjected to high forces when the hand is used and may become very painful*.

Postoperatively the wrist is initially immobilised in a plaster backslab and finger movements are encouraged. The great advantage of stabilising the fusion with a strong plate is that after one or two weeks the wrist need only be supported with a wrist splint until the fusion is solid (usually within ten weeks). This surgery requires an extensive dorsal approach and many patients experience considerable pain and difficulty in regaining finger flexion; a vigorous programme of physiotherapy is necessary. Although hand strength may take many

*When I (TRCD) arrived as a new consultant in Nottingham, the other author (NJB) 'kindly' offered to let me take over some of the patients on his waiting list. One of these patients was a young man (I hope I will eventually forget his name) who NJB had already operated on three times, all unsuccessfully, trying to get his scaphoid fracture to unite! I fused this man's wrist using a small dynamic compression plate but did not bother to fuse the middle finger carpometacarpal joint as, in 'my experience' (in retrospect, what experience?) the plate never needed to be removed, so long as it was put on properly. The wrist fused without problem but the patient complained of persistent hand pain which I was forced to attribute to the plate, even though I had put it on correctly! I thus removed the plate, whereupon the patient started to complain of even worse pain, directly over the middle finger carpometacarpal joint. I tried to fuse this joint without applying a plate but this did not work, so I then fused it using bone graft and a dynamic compression plate. This carpometacarpal joint fusion was successful, but the patient then complained of dorsal hand pain which I was again forced to attribute to the plate, even though I had again applied it correctly. I therefore removed the plate: Barton 3 – Davis 5!

months to recover, the long-term results of total wrist fusion are good and this operation is usually recommended for young manual workers who require a stable, rather than a mobile, wrist joint. It is often stated that a total wrist fusion causes little disability to manual and sedentary workers but it undoubtedly creates some disability. For example, a car mechanic will have difficulty using his hand in narrow spaces in and around engines and a butcher will have trouble cutting meat (try cutting meat on a benchtop without ulnar deviating your wrist).

Total wrist arthroplasty. Total wrist joint replacement has a high complication rate in osteoarthritis and the five-year failure rate, in particular the loosening rate, remains unacceptably high.

Wrist denervation. This procedure is indicated for patients with generalised osteoarthritis who wish to retain wrist movements. The aim is to create a painless wrist joint by dividing all its sensory nerves: the posterior and anterior interosseous nerves and the fine (often invisible) articular branches of the superficial radial and other small nerves which cross the wrist joint. Several incisions around the wrist are needed and useful (though not complete) pain relief is probably achieved in 40% of cases. If a wrist denervation does not relieve the pain, then nothing is lost and a wrist fusion may be offered.

Surgery for localised osteoarthritis.
Symptomatic STT osteoarthritis. This can be treated by either an STT joint fusion or excision arthroplasty.

STT joint fusion requires resection of the articular surfaces through a dorsoradial incision, cancellous bone grafting and stabilisation of the STT joint with two Kirschner wires. A below-elbow cast is worn until union, which usually takes eight weeks. This procedure prevents most mid-carpal joint movement but does not impede radiocarpal joint movement. Postoperatively, most patients retain 50% of normal wrist movements, though they often experience some residual wrist pain.

In excision arthroplasty of the STT joint, the osteoarthritic articulations of this joint are excised, though the important intercarpal ligaments are preserved so that the scaphoid retains its normal alignment. The pseudarthrosis thus created may be left empty or filled with a rolled-up length of palmaris longus tendon.

Excision arthroplasty preserves wrist movements though, as with STT fusion, the patient often complains of some residual discomfort.

Isolated radio-scaphoid osteoarthritis. This may be treated by radial styloidectomy, though the results of this procedure are unpredictable. Care should be taken not to excise too much of the radial styloid process as the important radial collateral, radioscaphocapitate and radiolunate ligaments are attached to its base, and excessive resection can result in wrist instability and ulnar translocation.

The SLAC wrist. This can be treated by a 'four corner fusion' of the mid-carpal (lunocapitate and triquetro-hamate) joint and excision of the scaphoid. This is usually performed through a transverse dorsal incision and the mid-carpal fusion is bone-grafted and stabilised with K wires until union. In the SLAC wrist the luno-capitate joint subluxes dorsally as the lunate extends, so it is important to restore the normal alignment of this joint at surgery or wrist extension may be limited postoperatively. This procedure preserves some wrist movement, though in our experience the pain relief and wrist stability produced is not as satisfactory as a total wrist fusion. In the past the scaphoid was replaced with a silastic prosthesis, but this is unnecessary and the implants are no longer available.

Distal radio-ulnar joint osteoarthritis

Primary osteoarthritis of the distal radio-ulnar joint is unusual, though this joint frequently becomes deranged and osteoarthritic following fractures of the distal radius. Whereas one can perform most activities satisfactorily with a stiff wrist, restricted forearm rotation is much more disabling*.

Presentation

Patients with distal radio-ulnar osteoarthritis present with restricted and/or painful forearm rotation. They often have difficulty carrying trays and receiving change in shops and complain of pain on the ulnar border of the wrist on use. On examination, the distal radio-ulnar joint is usually tender and the patient's pain is reproduced by

---

*An eminent colleague who fractured his wrist tells us that flexion and extension of the wrist are luxuries: he says that life is really about pronation and supination!

forearm rotation, especially if the radius and ulna are compressed together. Distal radio-ulnar joint pain may also be provoked by ballotting the joint and crepitus can sometimes be detected. The diagnosis is usually confirmed on standard plain wrist radiographs.

Treatment

Mild cases of distal radio-ulnar osteoarthritis are managed conservatively with advice and analgesia. However, painful forearm rotation and restricted fore-arm rotation can cause considerable disability and surgical treatment is often required (*Figure 3.12*).

Excision of the distal ulna. Excision of the distal ulna (Darrach's procedure: *Figure 3.12a*), though excellent in rheumatoid arthritis, is no longer widely used for post-traumatic and primary osteoarthritis. This is because of concern that excision of the distal ulna may allow the radiocarpal joint to sublux gradually to the ulnar side. However, the reader should recall that the strong extrinsic wrist ligaments, which are found in the palmar capsule of the radiocarpal joint, run in an ulnar direction from the distal radius to the carpal bones and thus resist ulnar translocation. We have never seen significant ulnar translocation or subluxation following a Darrach's procedure for osteoarthritis but this operation does not always produce a good result, especially in younger active non-rheumatoid patients. This is because instability of the stump of the ulna produces discomfort on rotation of the forearm and a feeling of weakness in the wrist.

One of Dr Darrach's former residents told us that Darrach himself did not excise the whole of the ulnar head but preserved a strip of bone on the ulnar side, including the styloid, and the ligaments joining this

(a)   *(b)*   *(c)*

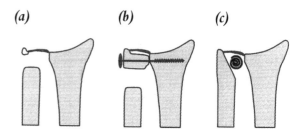

Figure 3.12 Surgical options for osteoarthritis and post-traumatic disruption of the distal radio-ulnar joint. (a) Darrach's resection of the distal ulna, (b) the Kapandji procedure, (c) Bower's hemi-resection interposition arthroplasty.

to the ulnar side of the carpus. This modification is essentially the fore-runner of Bower's 'hemi-resection arthroplasty' and Kirk Watson's 'matched distal ulnar resection'. These procedures seem to us similar in principle, as both excise the articular portion of the distal ulnar but not its medial side. Bowers combines this with soft-tissue interposition of a ball of rolled-up tendon or muscle (*Figure 3.12c*), a type of procedure popular in the USA. Neither of these procedures is common in Europe, where the Kapandji procedure is favoured.

Kapandji procedure. This operation (*Figure 3.12b*), which has superseded Darrach's procedure in post-traumatic and osteoarthritic cases, preserves the distal ulna and thus 'prevents' ulnar translocation of the radiocarpal joint. The distal radio-ulnar joint is fused by resecting its articular surfaces and compressing the distal ulna and radius together with a lag screw. A 1 cm segment of the distal ulna, just proximal to the distal radio-ulnar joint, is then resected in order to restore forearm rotation. Postoperatively, the wrist is mobilised in a below-elbow plaster for three weeks and the patient is then encouraged to rotate the forearm and mobilise the wrist. Satisfactory forearm function is regained in 80% of patients following the Kapandji procedure, but 20% complain of painful and troublesome clicking, giving way and instability during forearm rotation; this also occurs following Darrach's procedure. After both procedures most patients experience relatively painless clicking during forearm rotation which is due to the extensor carpi ulnaris tendon slipping over the proximal ulnar stump. However, painful clicking and giving way, which occurs in 20% of cases, is due to abutment of the proximal ulnar stump on the distal radial metaphysis. This *ulnar abutment* pain is most difficult to treat; various tendon slings have been suggested though none is regularly successful. Furthermore, although fusion of the ulnar stump to the radial metaphysis (an operation requiring a large bone graft and having a significant failure rate) cures abutment pain, it prevents forearm rotation, so may be more disabling than the abutment pain.

WRIST PAIN FOLLOWING COLLES' FRACTURE

Colles' fractures are through cancellous bone and often heal with some collapse, so that the distal radius is shortened and tilted dorsally. The inferior radio-ulnar joint, which is hemicylindrical in shape, is thus distorted so that its convex and concave sides are no longer in the same axis; furthermore, the distal ulna now protrudes into the wrist joint and may cause ulnar impaction (see below). Inferior radio-ulnar joint incongruency may cause pain on the ulnar side of the wrist, especially on pronation and supination. Such pain is fairly common shortly after the fracture but frequently settles down after a few months, so we advise no surgical treatment for six months. However, the pain persists in 30% of cases and, if severe, can usually be successfully treated in the elderly (aged 60 +) by excising the distal end of the ulna. In young patients, it is not so easy because Darrach's procedure in these circumstances does not always produce a good result (see above). A 'hemi-resection arthroplasty' or 'matched distal ulnar resection' may produce better results. It is also possible to realign the articular surfaces of the inferior radio-ulnar joint by a corrective 'open-wedge' osteotomy of the distal radius, but it is difficult to get it exactly right as to length and tilt. In these younger post-traumatic patients, we have found that the Kapandji procedure produces good results in 70% of cases.

If the fracture of the distal radius extends into the radiocarpal joint and unites with a significant articular step (> 2 mm), a second possible cause of continuing symptoms is introduced. These intra-articular mal-unions are difficult to correct, so every effort should be made to obtain an accurate reduction at the outset (reduce articular steps of more than 2 mm; smaller steps are well tolerated in the radiocarpal joint), if necessary using external or internal fixation in younger patients. If there is a single step in the distal articular surface of the radius it is possible, though not easy, to take it apart and restore correct alignment. If painful post-traumatic osteoarthritis develops, the best solution is radiocarpal fusion with or without a Kapandji operation, depending on the state of the inferior radio-ulnar joint.

RHEUMATOID ARTHRITIS AT THE WRIST

Rheumatoid arthritis presents with wrist pain in only 20% of patients, but sooner or later the wrist and/or the distal radio-ulnar joints are involved in 90%. The inflammatory synovitis causes ligamentous laxity, destroys articular cartilage and invades bone, causing cyst formation and bone destruction. The end-stage of this disease is either spontaneous fusion of the wrist joint or palmar dislocation and ulnar translocation of the radiocarpal articulation. The radiocarpal joint eventually dislocates so that the distal radius lies palmar to the distal ulna.

Presentation

These patients are usually referred to an orthopaedic surgeon with pain rather than deformity, stiffness or persistent swelling. Though many wrists with advanced joint destruction causes surprisingly little pain and don't need surgery. It is important to assess the whole patient and assess accurately his or her functional disabilities and expectations of treatment. The surgeon must ascertain that the wrist problem is of major concern to the patient, who may be much more disabled by restricted walking or rheumatoid disease of the hand, elbow or shoulder, which therefore have more pressing needs. Ill-advised surgery to the wrist may make matters worse, particularly if the patient has to use sticks or crutches to walk. The wrist joints (radio-carpal and mid-carpal) and the distal radio-ulnar joints must be examined and assessed separately and the surgeon must decide whether any pain and disability is arising from the wrist joint, the distal radio-ulnar joint or both. This is done by assessing each joint for tenderness, swelling, subluxation or dislocation, restricted movements and pain during and at the extremes of joint movement.

Radiography

PA and lateral wrist radiographs are required and it is also advisable to obtain a PA view of the whole of the hand so as to assess the severity of the arthritis throughout the hand. Larsen has devised a method which we find useful for staging the radiological appearances of the rheumatoid joints which has been modified for the wrist by considering dislocation and ankylosis (*Table 3.3*). It is not necessary to know or use the numbers of the stages but you should be aware that these stages exist, as treatment depends on the stage of the disease.

Alternatively rheumatoid wrist disease can be graded according to the Wrightington classification (*Table 3.4*), which is used by many British surgeons, including some examiners in the FRCS Orth.★

Table 3.3 Modified Larsen classification of rheumatoid wrist radiographs

Stage 0	Normal radiographs
Stage 1	One or more of: periarticular soft tissue swelling, bone demineralisation and slight joint space narrowing
Stage 2	One or more of: marginal erosions, joint space narrowing and subluxation or dislocation of the distal radio-ulnar joint
Stage 3	Articular erosions and/or joint space narrowing, dislocation of the distal radio-ulnar joint, ulnar translocation of the carpus
Stage 4A	Mid-carpal ankylosis and radiocarpal subluxation
Stage 4B	Radiocarpal ankylosis
Stage 5A	Destruction of the carpus and radiocarpal joint dislocation
Stage 5B	Destruction of the carpus with radiocarpal and mid-carpal ankylosis

Table 3.4 Wrightington rheumatoid wrist radiographic classification

Grade 1	Architecture of wrist preserved apart from: Peri-articular osteoporosis and erosions Early cyst formation Slight flexion of the scaphoid (DISI)
Grade 2	The radioscaphoid and mid-carpal joints are well preserved but one or more of the following are present: Ulnar translocation of proximal carpal row Marked palmar flexion of the lunate Gross flexion of the scaphoid Radiolunate joint degeneration
Grade 3	The bony architecture of the distal radius is well-preserved apart from pseudocyst formation on its palmar and distal surface. One or more of the following are present: Mid-carpal joint degeneration Radioscaphoid joint erosion Palmar subluxation of the radiocarpal joint
Grade 4	Significant loss of bone stock from the distal radial articular surface. Gross erosion of the medial side of the radius at the level of the distal radio-ulnar joint

★You need not know both classifications.

Treatment

Early disease

Larsen Stage 1–3 wrist rheumatoid arthritis is usually managed conservatively with analgesics, non-steroidal anti-inflammatory drugs, intra-articular steroid injections and wrist splints. Some doctors recommend wrist joint synovectomy at these stages in the belief that this arrests the progression of the rheumatoid disease process. However, most surgeons only do this in rare instances, when a patient has persistent painful synovitis which has not responded to conservative measures.

Wrist joint synovectomy. This is performed through a dorsal approach and both the wrist and distal radio-ulnar joints are cleared of inflammatory synovium. A complete wrist joint synovectomy cannot be performed through this approach as the palmar surface of the wrist and distal radio-ulnar joints cannot be reached. An *extensor tendon synovectomy* is often performed at the same time and, if the extensor carpi ulnaris tendon has subluxed palmarly, this should be replaced in its normal position and held there with a sling created from a strip of the extensor retinaculum, because palmar subluxation of this tendon encourages palmar subluxation of the ulnar border of the carpus and dorsal subluxation of the distal ulna.

Synovectomy with radio-lunate fusion (Chamay procedure). Some surgeons recommend that the lunate is fused to the radius at the same time as synovectomy to prevent subsequent palmar dislocation and ulnar subluxation of the radiocarpal joint and radial deviation deformity of the metacarpals (and thus also prevent finger MP joint ulnar deviation deformities). Provided the mid-carpal joint is still functioning, this procedure preserves some wrist extension and flexion.

Radiocarpal fusion. This goes one step further than the Chamay procedure but allows preservation of the mid-carpal joint and its movement, if the disease has not already diminished this. It seems particularly appropriate if the other wrist needs a complete fusion.

Advanced disease (Larsen Stages 4–5)

Distal radio-ulnar joint. The distal radio-ulnar joint is commonly involved in rheumatoid arthritis and frequently subluxes or dislocates. Painful distal radio-ulnar joint destruction is usually treated by excision of the distal end of the ulna (Darrach's procedure). This osteoporotic bone should be divided with a power saw because bone-cutters cause splits and splinters: any sharp edges or spikes should be smoothed off with a bone nibbler to protect the tendons. Some surgeons prefer the Kapandji procedure or recommend a synchronous radiolunate fusion to prevent the theoretical risk of ulnar translocation, but we do not think that either has any advantages over the Darrach's procedure. In rheumatoid arthritis, excision of the distal ulna usually restores a virtually full range of painless forearm pronation and supination, though patients are sometimes troubled by painful clicking during forearm rotation (see above).

The wrist joint. When the articular surfaces are severely damaged and considerable joint destruction has occurred, the choice of operations lies between arthrodesis and arthroplasty.

Arthrodesis. Arthrodesis of the wrist is a popular procedure for advanced rheumatoid arthritis. It provides lasting pain relief though, of course, abolishes all wrist (though not radio-ulnar) movements. In rheumatoid arthritis, as opposed to post-traumatic and primary osteoarthritis, there is a natural tendency to bony ankylosis of the wrist and all the surgeon has to do is encourage this. It is not unknown for the wrist joint to fuse spontaneously and become painless while on the waiting list for surgical fusion, so make sure to see your patients preoperatively!

Wrist arthrodesis is performed through a straight longitudinal dorsal skin incision and the dorsal halves of the carpal bones and the distal radius are fragmented with bone nibblers. The bone fragments are then packed into the wrist joint which is usually stabilised with a Steinmann pin or Stanley intramedullary nail. This is normally inserted through the third MP joint and passed down the metacarpal shaft and across the wrist joint into the distal radius. Alternatively, damage to the MP joint can be avoided by introducing the intramedullary nail between the bases of the second and third metacarpals, but this gives less good fixation. Other stabilisation techniques, such as staples or plaster immobilisation alone, may be used but the great advantage of intramedullary nail fixation is that it provides immediate solid fixation and supplementary external splintage is only needed for one or two weeks. Thus, it reduces the risk of postoperative hand stiffness which can develop if the wrist is immobilised in plaster for six or more weeks. The fusion rate is high and few complications occur provided the soft tissues are treated carefully. With the intramedullary nail technique, the wrist is inevitably fused in neutral alignment unless the nail is purposefully bent after insertion. Fusion in extension, though often recommended for osteoarthritis, should be avoided in rheumatoid arthritis as this will prevent the patient from using this hand to wipe her bottom. This is true even when the other wrist and hand function well, as their function may deteriorate later as the disease progresses. Despite the concerns of some surgeons, we feel that bilateral wrist fusions are acceptable in rheumatoid arthritis.

Wrist arthroplasty. Several total wrist replacements have been designed and used in rheumatoid arthritis, but none produces reliable lasting results. The Swanson silastic arthroplasty usually preserves a 40–60° arc of wrist flexion and extension, which many patients find beneficial. This prosthesis is inserted through a dorsal approach after excision of the proximal carpal row. Silastic wrist implants can fracture and the wrist joint may subsequently dislocate. For these reasons and because the results of wrist arthrodesis are satisfactory, silastic implants are not widely used, and are contraindicated if the wrist joint is subluxed or dislocated.

Extensor tenosynovitis

Presentation

Inflammation of the tenosynovium surrounding the extensor tendons of the fingers and wrist as they pass under the extensor retinaculum is common in rheumatoid arthritis. The synovial swelling, which can be very large, has well-demarcated margins and may be nodular and fluctuant. It may have a bilobed appearance, with fusiform swellings proximal and distal to the extensor retinaculum which prevents any swelling directly over the wrist joint. Tenosynovitis around the extensor pollicis longus tendon presents as a fusiform swelling on the radial border of the wrist.

Treatment

Extensor tenosynovitis usually responds to conservative measures such as anti-inflammatory medication and steroid injections. The indications for surgery are:

- persistent tenosynovitis despite adequate medical treatment;
- extensor tendon rupture.

Extensor tenosynovectomy. This is performed through a straight longitudinal incision★. The extensor retinaculum is elevated, either as an ulnar- or radially-based flap and the tenosynovium is carefully dissected off the tendons, including the extensor carpi ulnaris and radialis longus and brevis if necessary. The extensor retinaculum is then placed under the extensor tendons to reduce the risk of subsequent tendon rupture.

Extensor tendon rupture. Long-standing extensor tenosynovitis may rupture the finger extensor tendons, either by synovial invasion into the tendon or increasing the pressure under the extensor retinaculum and thus decreasing tendon blood flow. Extensor tendons may also fray and rupture if they lie against and rub on bony prominences which have become roughened and eroded by the rheumatoid disease process. Thus the little and ring finger extensor tendons may rupture on the distal ulna if this has protruded through the dorsal wrist capsule.

Clinical features. Finger extensor tendon rupture causes an extensor lag at the MP joint which may develop suddenly or gradually over a period of weeks. The interosseous muscles extend the interphalangeal (IP) joints, so these joints do not develop extensor lags and their active and passive ranges of extension are equal. There are three important differential diagnoses for finger extensor tendon rupture. The first is palmar

---

★A note about incisions on the back of the wrist in rheumatoid patients. Some years ago, two of the world's leading rheumatoid surgeons went ski-ing together in the Alps. Norbert Gschwend went down first and was followed by Al Swanson, who came to a stop with a flurry of snow, turned to his companion and said 'Norbert, what incision do you use on the back of the wrist in rheumatoid arthritis?'

We tell this story not only to remind you that ski-ing is inherently boring and should not distract you from your revision for the FRCS Orth; but also to show that there is a real problem which preys upon the minds of even the most distinguished surgeons. The skin here is thin, especially in rheumatoid patients on steroids, and healing may be delayed; we have known it to take months. S-shaped incisions give good access but produce more problems in healing. The older we get, the more we favour straight longitudinal incisions on the back of the wrist when access to tendons is required.

subluxation of the finger MP joints, which causes fixed flexion deformities rather than extension lags of these joints. The second is ulnar subluxation of the finger extensor tendons at the MP joints; this is detected by asking the patient to extend his fingers actively and observing that the finger extensor tendon passes ulnar to, rather than directly over, the MP joint. The third differential diagnosis is posterior interosseous nerve compression secondary to elbow joint synovitis; wrist extension is retained in this condition, as the motor branch to extensor carpi radialis longus arises from the radial nerve above the elbow. Posterior interosseous nerve compression should be suspected when:

- there is active elbow joint disease;
- both the extensor pollicis longus and finger extensors are affected;
- the extensor carpi ulnaris is paralysed (often difficult to detect);
- the loss of finger extension has developed slowly over several weeks.

Rupture of the extensor pollicis longus tendon is usually secondary to tenosynovitis but may occur due to fraying on a roughened Lister's tubercle. It is not always immediately apparent, as the thumb intrinsic muscles can extend the IP joint to neutral, though not into hyperextension. The patient not only complains of loss of IP joint hyperextension, but also of weakness of thumb adduction, extension and supination, so that he cannot place his thumb alongside his index finger. Frequently he is also unable to fully extend the MP joint, as the extensor pollicis brevis tendon is often congenitally inadequate. A simple test for extensor pollicis longus function is to place the patient's hand palm down on a flat surface and ask him to lift his thumb off this surface. If he is unable to do this then the extensor pollicis longus may be ruptured, but the surgeon should confirm that the thumb can be passively lifted off the flat surface and that its IP joint can be passively hyperextended; if not, these clinical findings are probably attributable to joint contracture.

Rupture of both extensor tendons to the little finger is the most common finding, though the little and ring finger extensor tendons frequently rupture simultaneously or sequentially. Less often patients present with loss of little, ring and middle finger extension but rupture of the extensor tendons of all four fingers is most uncommon. If the extensor digitorum communis tendon ruptures in isolation, the patient presents with middle and ring finger extensor lags, as the extensor indicis proprius and extensor digiti minimi tendons are still able to extend the index and little fingers.

Treatment. The aims of treatment are to restore finger extension and prevent rupture of further extensor tendons.

Further tendon ruptures are prevented by addressing the cause of the initial tendon damage. Thus if the rupture is secondary to tenosynovitis, a tenosynovectomy is performed and the extensor retinaculum is released and placed under the remaining intact tendons. With the ulnar finger extensors, we believe that the tendon damage is usually due to fraying on a sharp prominence between erosions on the the ulnar head, so the distal ulna must be excised (Darrach's procedure).

The extensor tendons cannot be repaired as they are frayed and their proximal ends retract into the forearm. The results of tendon grafting are unpredictable. Rupture of the little finger extensor tendons is therefore usually treated by suturing the distal tendon ends to the intact ring finger extensor tendon or by transferring the extensor indicis proprius tendon. If both the ring and little finger extensor tendons are ruptured, the distal end of the ring finger extensor tendon is buddied to the middle finger extensor tendon and extensor indicis proprius tendon is transferred to the little finger extensor tendons (this may already have been transferred to the thumb, but that is surprisingly uncommon; most patients either rupture the extensor pollicis longus or the finger extensors). The situation is more difficult if the middle, ring and little finger extensor tendons are all ruptured. In this situation, the extensor indicis proprius tendon may be transferred to the little finger (assuming that the index finger extensor digitorum communis is intact) and the ring finger flexor digitorum superficialis tendon is transferred (through the interosseous membrane or around the radial border of the wrist) to the distal ends of the middle and ring finger extensor tendons. Setting the correct tension in all these tendon transfers is critical; it is imperative that they are not too tight as this will restrict finger flexion which is much more disabling than restricted finger extension. Usually the tension is set so that the transfer is tight when the wrist is fully extended and the fingers are fully flexed. If the tension is not enough, the operation fails; if it is too much, flexion of the fingers is restricted, which is worse still. Postoperatively the tendon repairs or transfers are protected by immobilising the wrist and hand on a volar slab with the wrist in neutral and the finger MP joints extended for three weeks. The results of these tendon transfers are variable; they are much better when the wrist has a full range of movement and can amplify the transfer's action. Wrist flexion, through its tenodesis effect, tightens the transfer and aids extension of the MP joints whereas wrist extension relaxes the transfer and allows full finger flexion.

Extensor pollicis longus tendon rupture is usually treated by an extensor indicis proprius transfer, whose tension is set so that the thumb can be fully flexed with the wrist extended and is fully extended with the wrist flexed. One of the several abductor pollicis longus tendons or the palmaris longus tendon may be used as an alternative if extensor indicis proprius is unavailable. The results of surgery for extensor pollicis longus tendon rupture are also dependent on the range of wrist movement but are usually good.

Flexor tenosynovitis at the wrist

Rheumatoid tenosynovitis may also develop around the wrist and finger flexor tendons as they pass through the carpal tunnel. This may cause swelling, carpal tunnel syndrome, weakness, or loss of flexion of the IP joints of the digits (remember that the interosseous muscles flex the MP joints). This loss of IP joint flexion may be due either to the actual mass of the synovitis restricting tendon excursion (causing a *reduced* range of active flexion) or flexor tendon rupture (causing *complete* loss of active flexion).

Flexor tendon rupture may be secondary to synovial invasion of the tendon(s), but is usually due to mechanical attrition on a bony spur on the flexor surface of the wrist joint. Typically the flexor pollicis longus and the index profundus tendons fray on the rough surfaces of the distal pole of the scaphoid and the scaphotrapezial joint which protrude into the carpal tunnel. The differential diagnosis for combined flexor pollicis longus and index finger profundus tendon ruptures is an anterior interosseous nerve palsy in the proximal forearm. In this nerve palsy there may be localised tenderness over the median nerve in the proximal forearm and the thumb IP joint usually passively extends and flexes during wrist flexion and extension as a result of the tenodesis effect of the intact flexor pollicis longus tendon. Furthermore, if the flexor pollicis longus tendon is intact, the IP joint of the thumb can be passively flexed by using your thumb to apply firm localised pressure over the tendon in the distal forearm. If only a single digit's flexor tendon(s) has ruptured, this may have occurred within the fibrous digital flexor sheaths, rather than at the wrist. In this instance the finger flexor sheath may be swollen and tender due to tenosynovitis and both the profundus and superficialis tendons may be inactive.

Treatment

Flexor tenosynovitis at the wrist is usually treated conservatively but surgery is indicated if there is:

- persistent painful tenosynovitis despite appropriate conservative measures;
- persistent carpal tunnel syndrome;
- flexor tendon rupture.

The management of ruptured flexor tendons at the wrist is similar to that of extensor tendon ruptures. Further tendon damage is prevented by exploring and decompressing the carpal tunnel, performing a cautious flexor tenosynovectomy and trimming any bony prominences. The tenosynovectomy should be undertaken with care, as scarred tenosynovium may be holding together the ruptured ends of the tendons and removing it produces a lot of unattached ends and a problem in restoring continuity. Superficialis tendon ruptures (rare at this level) cause little if any functional disability and do not require treatment. Loss of active flexion of the thumb IP joint is disabling because the joint hyperextends during pinch, but loss of active flexion of the distal interphalangeal joint of the fingers does not always cause disability if the superficialis tendon is intact. Flexor pollicis longus and profundus tendon ruptures are not amenable to direct repair and single profundus ruptures (usually index) are best treated by attaching the distal end to the adjacent (usually middle) profundus tendon. Flexor pollicis longus ruptures may be reconstituted with a tendon graft or treated with a ring finger superficialis transfer. Alternatively the thumb IP or finger distal IP joint may be fused, in which case the surgeon has to decide whether or not to explore the carpal tunnel to find and address the cause of the injury and prevent further tendon ruptures.

As with the extensor tendons, the results of tendon transfers and grafts are influenced by the mobility of the wrist.

KIENBÖCK'S DISEASE

Kienböck's disease of the lunate bone (lunatomalacia) was first described by Kienböck, a radiologist in Vienna, in 1910 when radiographs were just coming into use. (All the osteochondritides were described around the same time and for the same reason.) Most surgeons have a radiograph showing Kienböck's disease and they often show it if they are examining in the FRCS Orth. This leads on to questions about classification and treatment.

Pathology

The whole of the lunate bone shows the characteristic changes of avascular necrosis and the progression and staging of this disease are similar to those of avascular necrosis at other sites. Kienböck's disease was staged by Lichtman (*Table 3.5*) according to the radiological appearance of the lunate bone (*Figure 3.13*).

Table 3.5 Radiographic staging of Kienböck's disease

Stage 1	Normal lunate architecture and bone density except that there **may** be either a linear or compression fracture. In the absence of a fracture the condition is diagnosed by bone scan or MRI. The articular cartilage, which receives nutrients from the synovial fluid, is normal. There may be an associated wrist joint synovitis.
Stage 2	The lunate shows increased radiodensity but retains its normal outline. Cysts may be present within the lunate but its articular cartilage is normal. The increased radiodensity is due to revascularisation and new bone deposition on dead trabeculae.
Stage 3	The lunate has collapsed and fragmented. Although the articular surfaces are no longer smooth, the articular cartilage is still alive. Stage 3 Kienböck's disease is often subdivided into **Stage 3A** (no carpal collapse) and **Stage 3B** (carpal collapse) according to whether there is associated *carpal* collapse, with proximal migration of the capitate, scapholunate dissociation and scaphoid rotation.
Stage 4	As a result of lunate and carpal collapse, the wrist has become osteoarthritic.

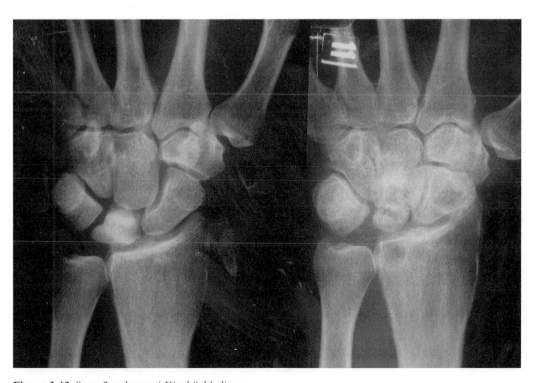

Figure 3.13 Stage 2 and stage 4 Kienböck's disease.

Kienböck's disease does not necessarily progress from stage 1 to stage 4. If the lunate retains its normal architecture during revascularisation (stage 2), a complete recovery can occur and some sufferers probably never complain of any symptoms. However, the usual natural history is for the lunate bone to fragment and collapse over a period of time, possibly as long as several years. Lunate collapse is probably due to normal forces causing microfractures within trabeculae weakened by bone resorption during revascularisation.

Aetiology

The cause of Kienböck's disease is uncertain. Although it has been proposed that it may occur as a result of a definite single, though forgotten, wrist injury or repeated minor injuries, there is no strong evidence to support either hypothesis.

It has been reported that some of the lunate bone overlies the ulna in patients with Kienbock's disease, whereas in normal wrists the whole of this bone overlies the radius. Furthermore, Kienböck's disease is more common in wrists with _ulna-negative variance_, in which the ulna is shorter than normal so that the articular surface of the distal ulna lies proximal to that of the distal radius (_Figure 3.11_). This may cause abnormal shear forces within the lunate bone, with force transmitted only in the portion articulating with the distal radius. This could cause microfractures in the lunate, but it fails to explain why in Kienböck's disease the whole lunate bone becomes avascular before collapsing. Ulna-negative wrist variance may be a consequence rather than a cause of Kienböck's disease and cases undoubtedly occur in ulna-positive wrists.

Presentation

Kienböck's disease usually occurs in young adults, though it can present in later life. The patient may complain of only mild wrist pain and slightly restricted wrist movements; sometimes the symptoms are so mild that the patient does not seek medical advice and the condition is only picked up as a chance finding. There may be few clinical signs but there is usually tenderness over the dorsal pole of the lunate. Wrist movements, in particular dorsiflexion, are reduced and painful at their extremes. If osteoarthritis has developed then the clinical findings are more generalised.

Radiography

Kienböck's disease is usually diagnosed and staged on plain radiographs though these are normal in the very earliest stages of the disease. Ulnar variance (_Figure 3.11_ on page 78) is measured on special PA views of both wrists, each of which is taken with the forearm in neutral rotation, the elbow flexed to 90° and the shoulder abducted 90°. This is important because the apparent length of the ulna in the same patient varies according to the angle of the film and the position of the forearm (the ulna is relatively longer in supination and relatively shorter in pronation); one cannot make a firm statement about ulnar variance from a single standard radiograph.

No further investigations are usually required, though a bone scan will show increased radioactive uptake (due to revascularisation and new bone deposition) within the lunate bone in the earliest stages of Kienbock's disease, when the plain radiographs are normal (stage 1). Ordinary and computed tomography accurately detect lunate collapse which may not be discernible on plain radiographs and MRI scans clearly show the avascular changes within the lunate.

Treatment

The reader should remember that Kienböck's disease often causes little disability and that the severity of symptoms and the radiological appearances do not correlate well. Furthermore, it does not always progress from stage 1 to stage 4 and carpal collapse (_Figure 3.11_) and osteoarthritis may take many years to develop or never occur. As no surgical procedure has been conclusively shown to prevent the progression of Kienböck's disease, it is both authors' opinion that surgery should only be performed when a patient's pain and disability cannot be managed conservatively by reassurance, analgesia and splintage. The authors advise caution when considering surgery, as this may actually reduce the patient's likelihood of returning to his previous occupation and the long-term results of operative and non-operative treatment may be identical.

Numerous operations have been suggested for Kienböck's disease. These can broadly be divided into procedures for stage 1 and 2 disease which aim to prevent lunate collapse and fragmentation, procedures for stage 3 disease which attempt to restore or retain normal carpal height and alignment following lunate collapse, and salvage procedures for stage 4 disease when the wrist is osteoarthritic.

Kienböck's disease without lunate collapse (stages 1 and 2)

The intention of surgery at these stages is to prevent lunate collapse, either by correcting ulnar negative variance and thus reducing the biomechanical shear stresses within the lunate or by encouraging rapid revascularisation.

Ulna-minus variance, if this is present, is corrected either by shortening the radius or lengthening the ulna. The intention is to produce 'ulna-neutral' variance with the surfaces of the distal radius and ulna at the same level so that the ulnar portion of the lunate is supported by the distal ulna. Thus the radius is shortened or the ulnar is lengthened by an amount equivalent to the preoperative ulna-minus variance. Ulnar lengthening osteotomies, which are bone grafted and stabilised in distraction with a plate, have a significant non-union rate. Radial shortening osteotomies, which are performed through the distal radial metaphysis and are usually stabilised with a buttress plate, have a lower non-union rate and for this reason are usually preferred.

The second surgical option is to encourage revascularisation of the lunate, usually by a pedicled vascularised bone graft which may be harvested with part of the origin of the pronator quadratus muscle from the flexor surface of the distal radius. The portion of the pronator quadratus muscle which is attached to the graft is mobilised, carefully preserving its insertion (and thus the bone graft's blood supply) onto the ulna. The graft is then placed within the lunate, which has previously been 'hollowed-out' with a curette. An alternative technique of revascularisation is to mobilise a dorsal digital artery which is then divided distally and placed within a drill hole on the dorsum of the lunate. The value of these revascularisation procedures (especially the dorsal digital artery technique) is uncertain and one should remember that avascular bone usually collapses during revascularisation when it is weakened by the resorption of dead trabeculae. Furthermore surgical trauma may itself weaken the lunate.

Pain is decreased in about 70% of cases by radial shortening, ulnar lengthening or vascularised bone graft procedures and it is attractive to attribute this to the theoretical premise for the surgery (correction of lunate bone shear stresses or revascularisation of the lunate). However, the pain relief may have occurred for other reasons; osteotomies modify bone blood flow and partial denervation is an inevitable consequence of all wrist joint surgery. Moreover, some surgeons claim improvement from shortening the radius even when there is neutral ulnar variance to start with.

Kienböck's disease with lunate collapse (stage 3)

At this stage, correction of ulna-minus variance and lunate revascularisation are unlikely to be beneficial. Excision and replacement of the lunate with a silastic prosthesis was once popular and appeared to produce satisfactory results. However, silastic lunate prostheses are no longer marketed as silicone wear particles can cause 'silicone synovitis'. Titanium lunate implants can be purchased and sometimes produce reasonable short-term results; they have to be sutured in place. If carpal collapse has occurred, and the scaphoid lies in excessive flexion, some surgeons recommend that carpal height is restored by performing a limited wrist fusion (scapho-capitate or scaphotrapezial-trapezoid) at the same time as inserting a lunate prosthesis. Other operations include:

- limited wrist fusion without excision of the lunate;
- limited wrist fusion with excision of the lunate;
- wrist denervation;
- proximal row carpectomy;
- total wrist fusion.

If limited carpal fusions are performed, then the range of wrist movements will inevitably be reduced to at most 50% of normal. This in itself may be as disabling to the patient as his preoperative pain, especially as pain relief is often incomplete.

Stage 4 Kienböck's disease

At this stage the wrist is osteoarthritic but pain may be relieved by a strong leather wrist splint, wrist denervation or total arthrodesis.

TRIANGULAR FIBROCARTILAGE COMPLEX TEARS

Triangular fibrocartilage complex (TFCC) tears are a relatively rare cause of wrist pain and are classified according to their location. Peripheral tears are usually post-traumatic and can occur:

- at the insertion of the TFCC into the sigmoid notch of the radius;
- at the TFCC insertion into the base of the ulnar styloid process;
- in the dorsal and palmar radio-ulnar ligaments which constitute the palmar and dorsal edges of the TFCC.

Central tears are usually degenerate and are often found in association with ulna-positive variance (the opposite of what is often present in Kienböck's disease). In this condition the triangular fibrocartilage is squashed between the prominent distal ulna proximally and the triquetrum and lunate distally during ulnar deviation, thus causing a central defect. In addition, the prominent distal ulna may damage the adjacent articular surface of the lunate, on which it abuts during ulnar deviation. When this is painful, the condition is called *ulnar impaction.*

Presentation

Triangular fibrocartilage tears are frequently asymptomatic but can cause ulnar wrist pain and restrict forearm rotation. On examination there is often tenderness over the triangular fibrocartilage and forearm rotation may be reduced and painful at its extremes. The patient's pain may be reproduced by ballottment of the distal radio-ulnar joint and resisted forearm rotation.

In ulnar impaction, forearm rotation is painless when the wrist is held in radial deviation but is painful when it is held in full ulnar deviation. Forced ulnar deviation also usually exacerbates the patient's pain.

Investigations

Plain wrist radiographs do not show the TFCC but in ulnar impaction they may show ulna-positive variance and a localised subchondral defect in the part of the lunate which impacts on the distal ulna during ulnar deviation (*Figure 3.14*).

Triangular fibrocartilage tears are usually diagnosed arthrographically or at arthroscopy. However, it must be stressed that triangular fibrocartilage tears are often asymptomatic and may be coincidental 'chance' arthrographic or arthroscopic findings. Thus the presence of a

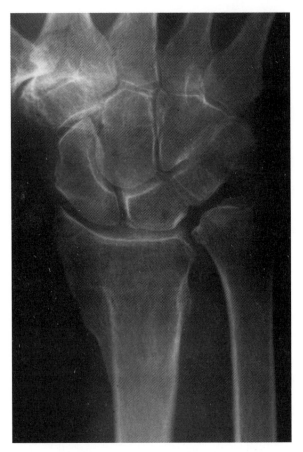

Figure 3.14 This man sustained a fracture of the distal radius which united with shortening, producing ulna-positive variance. The distal ulna is now impacting on the lunate, causing a sclerotic rim at the site of abutment.

triangular fibrocartilage tear is only of significance when the clinical picture is consistent with this diagnosis. Arthrography demonstrates leakage of dye between the radiocarpal and distal radio-ulnar joint but does not accurately locate or assess the size of the tear. In contrast, arthroscopy allows direct visualisation and accurate assessment of the tear's size and location.

Treatment

Many triangular fibrocartilage tears respond to conservative treatments such as restriction of activities, splintage and steroid injections. They can be trimmed arthroscopically which sometimes produces symptomatic relief.

Peripheral tears causing persistent pain may be repaired arthroscopically or at open operation, though this is not easy as the triangular fibrocartilage is small and the exposure is restricted. As with knee menisci, the healing potential of peripheral triangular fibrocartilage tears is uncertain.

Large central flap tears will certainly not heal; they may be trimmed arthroscopically but this is ineffective if there is associated ulnar impaction as the ulna still abuts on the lunate. Ulnar impaction is treated with good results by shortening the ulna, either through a shaft osteotomy or by trimming the distal end of the ulna beneath the TFC (the wafer procedure of Feldon). The ulna only needs to be shortened 1–2 mm and it is not necessary to repair or resect the TFC tear.

PISOTRIQUETRAL JOINT DISEASE

The pisotriquetral joint may become painful as a result of localised pisotriquetral osteoarthritis, chondromalacia, pisiform fracture or a pisotriquetral joint sprain; we have once seen avascular necrosis of the pisiform in a surgical registrar.

Presentation

Patients with pisotriquetral joint pain present with pain on use felt directly over the pisiform bone. The pain is reproduced by:

- pressing the pisiform bone firmly against the triquetrum during active wrist flexion and extension;
- moving the pisiform from side to side while compressing the pisotriquetral joint.

Investigations

The pisotriquetral joint is not visible on standard wrist radiographs, but is clearly seen on special views, including the carpal tunnel and 30° supinated 'lateral' views. The features of pisotriquetral joint osteoarthritis are similar to those of other joints. A bone scan may show a localised hot spot over the pisotriquetral joint but this investigation is not indicated if the clinical findings are strongly suggestive of pisotriquetral joint pathology. The clinical diagnosis can be confirmed by injecting a small volume of local anaesthetic into the pisotriquetral joint (not always an easy procedure) and observing the result.

Treatment

Pisotriquetral joint pathology often responds to conservative measures including a period of restricted activities and intra-articular steroid injections. If these measures are unsuccessful, the condition is readily treated by excision of the pisiform bone. This causes virtually no disability, provided that the pisiform bone is carefully 'shelled out' of the flexor carpi ulnaris tendon, maintaining its continuity. The bone is bigger than you expect, especially if it is enlarged by osteophytes.

UN-UNITED SCAPHOID FRACTURE

Scaphoid non-union may start to cause wrist pain many years after the fracture and sometimes there is no recollection of a previous fracture. The treatment of the scaphoid non-union depends on numerous factors, including the presence of secondary wrist osteoarthritis. This subject will be covered in the future WB Saunders volume on trauma.

INTRA-OSSEOUS GANGLIA

A ganglion which develops within the scapholunate ligament may erode and expand into the adjacent surfaces of the lunate and scaphoid, rather than passing dorsally and presenting as a dorsal wrist ganglion. These intra-osseous ganglia are most commonly found within the lunate bone but sometimes in the scaphoid and can destroy significant portions of this bone. However, they do not cause collapse of the bone or damage its articular surfaces.

Presentation

Intra-osseous ganglia are often detected as chance findings on radiographs but can cause persistent dull central wrist pain which is aggravated by use. Wrist movements are usually full and painless. The diagnosis is usually made after radiographs have been taken and should be regarded as a *diagnosis by exclusion*. In other words one should exclude all other possible causes before attributing the pain to the ganglion, which may be asymptomatic. One differential diagnosis of intra-osseous lunate ganglia is Kienböck's disease but the

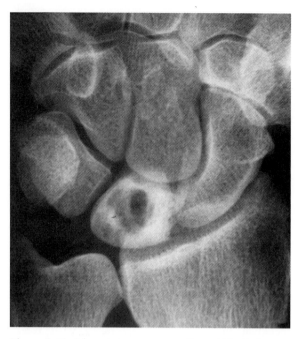

Figure 3.15 A large intra-osseous ganglion within the lunate.

radiological appearances of these two conditions are quite different (*Figures 3.13 and 3.15*). Tiny round translucencies in carpal bones are common but they are only significant and a potential cause of pain when they have a sclerotic margin and communicate with the articular surface.

Treatment

Intra-osseous ganglia are treated with reassurance if they are asymptomatic or only causing minor symptoms. If they cause persistent and troublesome pain they may be treated surgically, with curettage and bone grafting through a dorsal wrist exposure. This surgery does not reliably relieve the pain (which may be due to another undiagnosed pathology) and collapse of the lunate can occur following curettage of a large ganglion.

The commoner causes of wrist pain are summarised in *Table 3.6*.

MANAGEMENT OF CHRONIC WRIST PAIN

As your career progresses, it will become increasingly apparent that one is often unable to diagnose the cause of a patient's wrist pain. This fact is driven home when

Table 3.6 Summary of the commoner causes of wrist pain (not including recent injuries or rheumatoid arthritis which may affect any or all parts of the wrist)

Location	Cause of pain
Radial	De Quervain's stenosing tenovaginitis Osteoarthritis of the trapeziometacarpal joint Osteoarthritis of the scaphotrapezial joint Un-united scaphoid fracture Ganglion
Dorsal and/or central	Ganglion (may be occult) Kienböck's disease Scapholunate dissociation Intra-osseous ganglion Scapholunate advanced collapse
Ulnar	Distorted inferior radio-ulnar joint after fracture of the distal radius Arthritis of the inferior radio-ulnar joint Torn TFCC with or without ulnar impaction Unstable inferior radio-ulnar joint Piso-triquetral osteoarthritis Un-united fracture of hook of hamate

one is asked to see increasing numbers of secondary and tertiary referrals. The management of chronic wrist pain depends on two important decisions. First the surgeon must decide whether a patient's pain exhibits the typical characteristics of physical pain. Physical pain is consistently localised and described by the patient and is usually aggravated by use and eased by rest. Furthermore, the clinical findings (tenderness and painful movements) are consistent between appointments. If the location and quality of the pain and the clinical findings vary from time to time, then the pain is probably not due to physical disease and is unlikely to respond to any orthopaedic treatment.

Second, it is important to recognise when the time has come to stop carrying out further and increasingly invasive investigations in the hope of finding a treatable cause for a patient's pain. This is in part determined by the severity of the pain and the extent of the disability, which must always be carefully assessed. It is probably wise to perform a bone scan, but wrist arthrograms and nerve conduction studies are uncomfortable, wrist arthroscopy is undoubtedly painful and MRI and CT scans are expensive. None of these investigations should be performed on the 'off-chance' that they will produce an unsuspected diagnosis. They should only be used to confirm or refute a suspected clinical diagnosis, and only then if the surgeon considers that the patient will benefit from appropriate treatment. For example, is the pain sufficiently troublesome to warrant a limited wrist fusion which restricts wrist mobility and requires a period of sick leave? However, when all is said and done, many patients find one or two 'normal' simple investigations (plain wrist radiographs and simple blood tests) much more reassuring than a doctor's opinion, based solely on an unremarkable medical examination, that there is 'nothing seriously wrong'. A bone scan, which is quite an impressive 'high-tech' procedure in the eyes of the patient, is also valuable for this purpose though the result is almost always predictably normal; alternatively you may find a 'red-herring'.

The more one investigates a patient, the more one reinforces his belief that something serious may be wrong. Furthermore, the surgeon becomes increasingly at risk of performing inappropriate surgery. For example, if a patient with radial border wrist pain who 'will try anything' has an arthrogram or an arthroscopy which shows a triangular fibrocartilage tear, even the most hardened surgeon will sometimes reassess the situation and convince himself that treating the tear will cure the pain, even though it is immediately obvious to others that this is not the case. It is also easy to over-diagnose and over-treat new diagnoses such as odd carpal instabilities; if one is uncertain as to the cause of a pain, it is usually best to avoid surgery. The patient can always return later if he or she develops new symptoms and signs which allow the doctor to make a confident diagnosis, but a limited wrist fusion, once performed, can never be undone. This and other wrist procedures have a significant morbidity (restricted movements) which may compound the pain, which inevitably persists if the operation did not address the true cause of the wrist pain.

Chronic pain is hard to tolerate and when one tells a patient that one cannot diagnose the cause of his/her pain, it is important to stress that this does not mean that you necessarily think he or she is malingering or exaggerating, or that their pain is of a psychological nature. This will only make the patient resentful and make the pain more difficult to bear. We think that patients with well-localised wrist pain and no inappropriate findings almost certainly have physical pain, but due to a condition not yet commonly recognised by the medical profession. Furthermore, just because patients are seeking compensation does not mean that they are necessarily overstating their disability or malingering.

Fortunately, most undiagnosed *physical* wrist pains are transient, but some persist and cause permanent disability. In these patients the key is to encourage the patient to accept that the wrist pain is undiagnosable, treat the pain rather than its cause, offer referral to a pain clinic when appropriate, and encourage the patient to alter his or her lifestyle so as to cope with the pain.

CLINICAL QUESTION

A 62-year-old obese lady with rheumatoid arthritis presents with a three-month history of inability to extend the ring and little fingers of her dominant hand. Six months previously she suffered a myocardial infarct and ever since she has complained of shortness of breath on walking. On examination the IP joints of all the fingers extend fully but the MP joints of her ring and little fingers have 60° extension lags.

Question 1. What is your differential diagnosis?

On further examination, a soft tissue swelling is detected over the extensor tendons at the wrist and the distal ulna is prominent dorsally. Furthermore, painful crepitus is elicited from the distal radio-ulnar joint during forearm rotation. The extensor tendons of all the fingers lie in the correct position, dorsally over the MP joints and there is no swelling around the elbow which has a full range of movement.

Question 2. How would you treat this lady's hand?

Three months later this lady attends for her preoperative assessment and reports that she is now unable to extend any of the fingers of her right hand. Examination confirms 60° extension lags of the MP joints of all the fingers. Crepitus is elicited from the distal radio-ulnar joint but this is no longer particularly painful. Wrist movements are reduced to only 20° flexion and 30° extension.

Question 3. How would you now treat this lady's hand?

Answers

Question 1

Closed rupture of the ring and little finger extensor tendons, subluxation of the ring and little finger extensor hoods at the MP joints and partial interosseous nerve palsy. Rheumatoid arthritis affecting the MP joints cannot account for these extension lags; this would cause fixed flexion deformities.

Question 2

The most likely cause of tendon ruptures is erosion on the dorsally subluxed distal end of the ulna. Thus the surgical treatment should include:

- excision of the distal ulna and extensor tenosynovectomy with release of the extensor retinaculum, which is then placed deep to the extensor tendons (to prevent further tendon ruptures); and
- extensor indicis proprius transfer to the little finger extensor tendons and buddying of the middle and ring finger extensor tendons (to restore active extension of those fingers).

The lady's general health is poor but these operations are warranted as the results are usually good and they should prevent further tendon ruptures. Furthermore, they can be performed under a Bier's or an axillary block.

Question 3

The further (middle and index finger) extensor tendon ruptures must have occurred as a result of the persistent tenosynovitis as these tendons do not lie directly over the distal ulna, even when it is subluxed. As direct tendon repair is impossible and tendon grafts do badly in this instance, tendon transfers are the only method of restoring MP joint extension; transfer of the middle finger superficialis tendon (FDS) to the index and middle finger and the ring finger FDS to the ring and little finger extensor tendons is the usual transfer but the results are not particularly good, especially when the wrist joint has a reduced range of movement and cannot amplify the excursion of the transfer. Furthermore, this would take too long to perform under a Bier's block and would probably require a general anaesthetic.

The lady was questioned about her disabilities and reported that she could perform most of her daily activities, though she had trouble putting her hand round large objects such as jam jars. In view of the anaesthetic risk, the unrelible nature of the proposed surgery and the fact that reasonable hand function was retained, the hand was left untreated. One should remember that, as there are no remaining intact extensor tendons to any of the fingers, excision of the distal ulna or an extensor tenosynovectomy are unnecessary (indeed the tenosynovitis had settled when all the extensor tendons had ruptured).

The key lessons are: (1) extensor tendon ruptures should be treated promptly because the remaining intact extensor tendons may be at risk; (2) extension of the IP joints (by intrinsic muscle action) is retained after rupture of the long extensor tendons and in many instances this allows reasonable hand function.

FURTHER READING

Angelides AC, Wallace PF. The dorsal ganglion of the wrist: its pathogenesis, gross and microscopic anatomy, and surgical treatment. *J Hand Surg* 1976; **1:** 228–235.

Green DP. Carpal dislocations and instabilities. In: Green D (ed.) *Operative Hand Surgery*, 3rd edn, vol. 1. New York: Churchill Livingstone, 1993: 861–928.

Hodgson SP, Stanley JK, Muirhead A. The Wrightington classification of rheumatoid wrist X-rays: a guide to surgical management. *J Hand Surg* 1989; **14B:** 451–455.

Larsen C, Amadio P, Gilula L, Hodge J. Analysis of carpal instability: 1. Description of the scheme. *J Hand Surg* 1995; **20A:** 757–764.

Lichtman DM, Mack GR, MacDonald RI, Gunther SF, Wilson JN. Kienböck's disease: the role of silicone replacement arthroplasty. *J Bone Joint Surg* 1977; **59A:** 899–908.

Palmer AK. Kienböck's disease – the influence of arthrosis on ulnar variance determination. *J Hand Surg* 1987; **12B:** 291–293.

Palmer AK, Werner FW. The triangular fibrocartilage complex of the wrist – anatomy and function. *J Hand Surg* 1981; **6:** 153–162.

Schernberg F. Roentgenographic examination of the wrist: a systematic study of the normal, lax and injured wrist. *J Hand Surg* 1990; **15B:** 210–228.

Taleisnik J. *The Wrist.* New York: Churchill Livingstone, 1985.

Watson HK, Ashmead D, Makhlouf MV. Examination of the scaphoid. *J Hand Surg* 1988; **13A:** 657–660.

Watson HK, Ballet FL. The SLAC wrist: scapholunate advanced collapse pattern of degenerative arthrosis. *J Hand Surg* 1984; **9A:** 358–365.

4

The Hand

4A

Examination of the Hand

Nicholas Barton and Patrick Mulligan

The hand is not a joint and not just an assemblage of joints, but a complicated motor and sensory organ. To examine it so that you don't miss anything, you need a *scheme*.

It is possible to adapt the late Alan Apley's admirable 'Look, feel, move', making sure that you test active as well as passive movements and that 'feel' includes not only what you can feel (palpation) but what the patient can feel (sensation).

However, it is better to use a rather different scheme for the hand. No patient ever has a full physical examination, including all that would be done by a neurologist, a proctologist, an ENT surgeon and every other kind of specialist. Patients are examined in a selective way, based on what has been revealed by the history and by the early part of the examination (indeed, the examination may discover something which causes you to go back to the history and start asking more questions). What is needed is to be comprehensive in the *relevant* examination.

This applies particularly to the hand. A full examination would take about half-an-hour, but this is seldom necessary: patients with rheumatoid arthritis are those who come closest to needing such a complete examination. However, if you have a scheme, you can make the appropriate parts of the examination in full consciousness that you are leaving out the others. A trigger

finger is a trigger finger and it is not necessary to spin it out, though it is wise to make sure there are no signs of rheumatoid arthritis.

This selective examination also applies to the clinical parts of the FRCS Orth exam, where you will encounter hands either as part of a complicated long case (e.g. rheumatoid arthritis) or as short cases (Dupuytren's contracture and nerve palsies being especially favoured) and in this limited time you have to concentrate on the relevant features. Patients with recent injuries are unlikely to appear in this context, but are such an important part of hand surgery that they must be considered in this section.

The fingers should always be identified by name, not number. 'The third finger' is ambiguous because some people count the thumb and some don't. This leads to mistakes. Every year the Medical Defence Union reiterates the importance of *naming* the fingers.

LOOK

As in Apley's system, start by taking a general look or you may miss something important. In particular, look at the *posture* of the hand: for example, a hyperextended metacarpo-phalangeal (MP) joint of the thumb is often secondary to an adduction contracture at the carpometacarpal joint which is the real seat of the pathology. Similarly, a clawed hand indicates interosseous paralysis. Muscle wasting and scars may also be obvious at a glance, though you will soon study them more closely. One finger may be more or less flexed than its neighbours and this can be an important sign ('straight finger points to a cut flexor tendon'). Rheumatoid arthritis can cause a variety of Z-deformities in the hand. Remember the medical conditions which may be revealed by examination of the hand, such as liver palms and abnormalities of the nails (see below).

INDIVIDUAL TISSUES

We have found it best to examine each layer of tissue in the order in which one encounters them surgically in, for example, an operation for Dupuytren's contracture which also requires release of a contracted joint.

Skin

Look especially for scars, which can be very difficult to see on the palmar surface of the hand. A scar overlying a lump suggests that it is an inclusion dermoid cyst. The position of the scar suggests the underlying anatomical structures which might have been damaged: there may be a scar from a wound in which a nerve or tendon has been divided and which, remarkably enough, the patient has forgotten (or avoids mentioning because it was incurred in a discreditable way).

Excessive sweating is usually due to nervousness, but may be caused by thyrotoxicosis or alcoholism; lack of sweating follows division of a sensory nerve, because the sympathetic fibres travel with the sensory ones.

In ordinary practice, and especially in medicolegal practice, the soft clean skin of one finger, in contrast to the others which are thick-skinned and grimy, shows that this finger is not used much: this is usually because of sensory impairment. At the other extreme, callosities indicate that the hand is used, even if the patient denies this.

Knowledge of palmistry is not required in the orthopaedic fellowship but it is worth noticing abnormal skin creases. The creases develop in the embryo at the same time as the joints: if a joint does not develop, nor does the crease. If a joint is not used, the crease may become less prominent but does not disappear completely. It is important to realise that the flexion crease for the MP joints of the fingers is that formed by the proximal and distal transverse palmar crease, *not* the crease at the base of the fingers which overlies no joint. (Patients with Down's syndrome have a single transverse palmar crease, but you will already have recognised the facies.) The flexion creases within the fingers do mark the position of the interphalangeal joints.

Tumours of the skin are usually referred to plastic rather than orthopaedic surgeons.

Psoriasis and the café-au-lait patches of neurofibromatosis are relevant but seldom seen on the hand itself. Haemorrhages in the nail-folds may be due to rheumatoid disease, scleroderma or dermatomyositis.

Nails

These are a specialised type of skin but should be examined. There are two main causes of abnormality.

1. Medical conditions: clubbing, koilonychia, splinter haemorrhages, the pitting of psoriasis.
2. The consequences of an old injury: transverse grooves* (which grow out), longitudinal splits (which don't), detachment of the leading edge of the nail from the underlying tissues (onycholysis), excessive thickness of the nail, or the parrot-beak deformity which occurs after loss of the soft tissues on the tip of the finger.

Onycholysis also occurs in psoriasis and fungal infections: the latter may cause white streaks on the nail.

Subcutaneous tissues

What is the next thing you see when you cut through the skin? Blood! That is why surgery of the hand must always be done under tourniquet (unless there is an ischaemic condition, sickle-cell anaemia, or an arteriovenous shunt for renal dialysis) so that you get a clear view of the structures you are about to divide. Under these conditions, the next thing you see beneath the skin is fat. Examination of the skin was done by

---

*These also develop in periods of illness or malnutrition. They may be accompanied by transverse white lines known by physicians as Beau's lines.

inspection, but for abnormalities in the subcutaneous tissues you need to palpate.

Probably the most common is Dupuytren's disease, which arises in the longitudinal fibres of the palmar fascia but spreads superficially into the fat and is often adherent to the skin, which may be drawn down into pits. This must be distinguished from callosities which are thickening of the skin itself from repeated pressure on the same spot, usually by a tool used at work.

Apart from Dupuytren's disease, lumps in the subcutaneous tissues are most often ganglia; they arise deeply but bulge out, especially around the wrist, on the front of the fingers, and near the base of the fingernail where they may actually rupture through the skin. (Ganglia at this site are called mucoid cysts and, unlike ganglia elsewhere, are associated with osteoarthritis in the underlying joint.) Ganglia in the hand (as opposed to the wrist) are usually too small to transilluminate, but the faintly blue colour may be detectable. The second commonest lump in the hand is pigmented villonodular synovitis (also known by a host of other names, mostly misleading and therefore best avoided). This condition arises in synovium, either of a joint or of the flexor tendon sheath. The lump is multilocular and has an orange or brown colour which is sometimes visible through the skin. The third most common lump in the hand is an inclusion dermoid cyst, following an old penetrating injury, so look for an overlying scar which may be tiny. (Pathologists prefer to reserve the term 'inclusion dermoid' for a congenital condition in the face and call these pilar cysts.) Presumably one could get a sebaceous cyst in the hair-bearing area on the back of the hand, but we have never seen one. Lipomata are very rare below the elbow, though occasionally seen in the thenar or hypothenar regions where there is a lot of fat.

Blood vessels

This part of the examination is only required in trauma and in patients complaining of circulatory problems. Look at the colour of the skin. In patients with dark or black skin, this is easiest to assess under the nail or on the front of the digits. Capillary return is not necessarily a good sign; it can be seen in venous occlusion, such as that due to thrombosis after a replantation. What you want to see is normal colour and temperature,

compared to the patient's other digits or other hand which you believe to be normal. Both hands are affected in Raynaud's disease and the colour change can be provoked by immersion in cold water.

The hand actually receives most of its blood through the ulnar artery, which you can feel pulsating at the wrist if you obliterate the radial pulse by pressing on it.

Allen's test examines both arteries as follows.

1. The patient makes a tight fist to exsanguinate the hand.
2. You press with one of your thumbs on the ulnar artery and your other thumb on the radial artery to occlude them both.
3. The patient straightens his fingers, which now look rather white.
4. You release *one* artery and watch whether the colour returns immediately.
5. Repeat, releasing the other artery.

This is not wholly reliable and a serious investigation of vascularity requires arteriography, but you will be expected to know how to perform Allen's test.

A similar test can be used to assess the patency of the digital arteries on each side of the finger.

Nerves

A hand without feeling is as though it were blind. There are two levels of examination of sensation.

It is wise in all patients to do a quick screening test by lightly stroking with your finger some area of the patient's skin which you are entitled to consider normal and then similarly stroking the front of the index finger (median nerve), front of the little finger (ulnar nerve) and the back of the hand (radial nerve). The question which you ask must be 'Does that feel the same?' (as the normal area). It is no use saying 'Can you feel that?', as a patient who has cut his median nerve may reply 'Yes', presumably because the examination produces some movement or slight pressure on the back of the hand. Ideally you should use a wisp of cotton-wool, but for simple screening most surgeons just use their own fingers.

Patients with nocturnal symptoms of carpal tunnel syndrome usually have normal sensation at the time of examination and there is no need to indulge in more complicated methods of clinical sensory examination, except for provocative tests such as Phalen's test, which consists of flexing the wrist for 60 seconds to see if that reproduces the symptoms.

A serious sensory examination is required in neurological conditions and, in orthopaedic practice, after nerve injuries. Even if exploration is obviously necessary, you should try to define the site and extent of the injuries first to decide how experienced a surgeon should do the operation and how long it is likely to take. It is very unsatisfactory to start operating under local anaesthetic in the Accident and Emergency Department and then find that the injury is too complicated to deal with there.

A proper sensory examination takes some time. Sticking needles in the hand causes pain and bleeding. It is better to cover the patient's eyes and ask him to distinguish between the sharp and blunt ends of a safety-pin (the sharp end is not as sharp as a needle). Two-point discrimination (2 PD) is fairly quick, requires no special tools (you can open out a paper-clip, but make sure it has not got a little hook on the end from faulty manufacture) and is quantitative; the drawback is that this seductively appealing measurement may bear little relation to whether the digit is actually used or not. The paper-clip can be applied to one spot (static 2 PD) or drawn across the finger-tip (moving 2 PD); the former tests slowly adapting nerve fibres and the latter rapidly adapting fibres, which recover more quickly after injury and are of more practical use in feeling things. The fact is that we have no reliable way of measuring sensation. After a nerve injury, adult patients do not recover 40% or 70% of normal sensation; they develop a different kind of sensation, which we cannot quantify and which is often unpleasant. Functional tests are the most helpful; if there is reasonable motor function, then the patient's ability to pick up a normal paper-clip from a flat surface depends on sensation in the digits involved. Picking up a pin provides a more difficult test.

The best tests have the patient blindfolded and any normal digits covered by a rubber glove from which the parts over the abnormal digits have been cut off. The patient is then asked to identify by touch various textures and shapes. This takes too long to do in the clinic (let alone in the FRCS Orth exam) and is best delegated to an occupational therapist who is experienced in this type of assessment.

When examining any patient with sensory symptoms, remember two things.

1. The symptoms may be referred from the neck. If you do not examine the neck, you will fail the clinical and, if you fail the clinical, you will (under the present rules) fail the whole examination. An orthopaedic surgeon making a neurological examination should THINK ROOT (*Table 4A.1*). You also need to know the dermatomes (*Figure 4A.1*) but realise that they do vary from person to person.
2. Although you must have clear and certain knowledge of the distribution of the nerves in the hand, few patients have read *Gray's Anatomy* and are aware that the ulnar nerve should supply $1^1/_2$ digits and the median nerve $3^1/_2$. One patient in five has a sensory distribution which does *not* conform to this textbook normality (the same applies to the motor distribution of these two nerves).

The most important indication for sensory examination in orthopaedic practice is after a cut which has damaged a nerve, and this means any cut on the hand or arm, as the cutting agent may go in obliquely and deep. The commonest reasons for missing a nerve injury are:

1. failure to examine sensation in each of the ten digital nerves;
2. failure to examine it properly (e.g. 'Can you feel this?');
3. the casualty officer putting in local anaesthetic;
4. abnormal nerve distributions;
5. a nerve which has been cut cleanly and has its ends still in contact may continue to conduct electrical impulses for a few hours before it starts to degenerate.

The last must not be used as a convenient excuse: most failures are due to the first two causes.

At a later stage, lack of sweating is a valuable sign and can be elicited by the 'pen test'. The side of an ordinary plastic ball-point pen, held very lightly by you between your thumb and one finger, is drawn across the patient's finger. Normally there is some resistance due to moisture on the surface of the skin; the lack of resistance on dry denervated skin is easy to feel.

In small children who cannot co-operate in an intelligent way, the wrinkling test is useful, though not applicable during the FRCS Orth examination. The patient's hands are placed in a bowl of water as hot as can comfortably be tolerated and kept there for

Table 4A.1 Main nerve root supply of key muscles in the upper limb. This is a simplification of the true situation, intended to help you assess each nerve root. In the muscles which move the hand, variations are frequent and the roots, shown in brackets, supply that muscle in about 30% of cases. We gratefully acknowledge the help of Mr Rolfe Birch, whose huge experience in treating brachial plexus lesions gives him unique knowledge of distributions from each root.

	Muscle	Main root supply	Peripheral nerve
Shoulder	Deltoid	C5	Axillary (circumflex nerve)
	Infraspinatus	C5	Suprascapular nerve
	Latissimus dorsi	C7★	Posterior cord of brachial plexus
Elbow	Biceps	C6	Musculocutaneous nerve
	Brachioradialis ('supinator jerk')	C6	Radial nerve
	Triceps	C7	Radial nerve
Wrist	Extensor carpi radialis longus	C6	Radial nerve
	Extensor and Flexor carpi ulnaris	C7	Radial and ulnar nerves
Fingers	Extensor digitorum	C7 (or C8 or T1)	Radial nerve
	Flexor digitorum profundus and Superficialis	C8 (or T1)	Median nerve (except ulnar half of profundus)
Thumb	Abductor pollicis brevis and usually Opponens pollicis	T1 (or C8)	Median nerve
	Interossei, Adductor pollicis, Hypothenar muscles	T1 (or C8)	Ulnar nerve

★In contrast, pectoralis major may take contributions from all five roots C5 to T1.

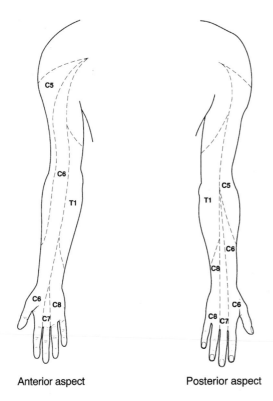

Figure 4A.1 Sensory nerve root distributions in the upper limb. Again we thank Mr Rolfe Birch for his advice.

15 minutes; they are then examined *immediately* after coming out of the water. Normally innervated skin wrinkles up, as it does if you stay too long in a hot bath. Denervated skin does not do this: the reason is not known, but may involve the sympathetic nervous system.

In nerve injuries, the level of the lesion is usually obvious (unless there are injuries at two levels). In nerve compression syndromes, the level can usually be determined clinically if you know the branching pattern of the nerves, with which you must therefore be familiar. To take the ulnar nerve as an example, its dorsal cutaneous branch leaves the main nerve a few centimetres above the wrist and supplies the ulnar part of the back of the hand and the back of the little and ring fingers. An ulnar neuropathy at the elbow (which is the most common level) will affect that area, whereas compression at the wrist, which may be due to a ganglion so deep-seated that it cannot be felt from outside, will not. Such a ganglion compressing only the deep branch of the ulnar nerve will not affect the sensory branches and, if it is distally placed, will be beyond the branch to abductor digiti minimi which is therefore spared.

Tinel's sign assesses the progress of a recovering nerve. It is essential to start *distally* to avoid flooding the hand with paraesthesiae. Then work proximally until paraesthesiae are elicited: this indicates the part which the regenerating nerve fibres have reached.

Temperature and vibration sense are important to neurologists but seldom to us.

The motor function of nerves is tested by examining the muscles which they supply.

Muscles

Nerves also supply muscles though, as has been said, not always strictly according to the anatomical text-book. Don't be misled by an adduction contracture of the carpometacarpal joint of thumb causing an abnormal position of the first metacarpal into thinking that there is thenar wasting, though there may be both. Wasting is detected by inspection, and power by contraction against resistance. You must, of course, know the MRC scale of muscle power from 0 to 5.

The lumbricals cannot be tested in normal circumstances and there are no muscles in the digits (so it is a mystery why digits occasionally become thinner after a nerve injury), but there are three groups of muscles in the hand, each containing one muscle which is easiest to examine.

1. *Thenar muscles.* Flexor pollicis brevis is usually supplied jointly by the median and ulnar nerves, so testing it is of no value for diagnostic purposes. Opponens pollicis is important functionally but ulnar-innervated in 20% of people: it may, therefore, continue to work after the median nerve has been cut. Abductor pollicis brevis is almost always pure median and is therefore the one to test when assessing that nerve. The patient's hand rests palm-up on a table and he is asked to lift his thumb up towards the ceiling against the gentle resistance of your finger. (This movement is usually called palmar abduction of the thumb to distinguish it from radial abduction, though that might equally well be called extension.)
2. *Hypothenar muscles.* Abductor digiti minimi is easy to test. If unilateral, this can be done by the patient pressing both his little fingers side-to-side against each other and seeing which gives way.
3. *Interossei.* The first dorsal interosseous is visible and palpable. It abducts the index finger away from the middle finger. A crude but simple check on the interossei, which you can use in children, is to ask the patient to cross his fingers for luck.

Adductor pollicis is examined by Froment's test: take a large piece of paper or folder of notes and hold one side between both your thumbs (keeping them straight) and the sides of your index fingers. Ask the patient to hold the other side in the same way and pull it away from you. If his adductor pollicis is paralysed, he will try to hold the paper by flexing the interphalangeal (IP) joint of his thumb, using flexor pollicis longus. You can test adductor pollicis and the first dorsal interosseous simultaneously by asking the patient to keep his thumb and index finger straight but bring them together: if the ulnar nerve is working normally, the first dorsal interosseous can be seen to bulge out as it contracts (Semple's test).

Grip strength is quite a good measure of intrinsic function, as the interossei flex the MP joints of the fingers.

Another important indication to examine muscles is paralysis. Here you must establish not only what muscles are paralysed or weak, but which muscles are acting normally and can be considered as donors for tendon transfer. This includes all the muscles in the forearm and, since you cannot distinguish between their muscle bellies by palpation, you must use one of your hands to provide the resistance and the other to palpate the *tendon* of the muscle being examined and feel whether it stands out. (It is impossible to distinguish in this way between extensors carpi radialis and brevis, but you can pick out the other wrist tendons individually.)

In paralysis of the anterior interosseous branch of the median nerve (which supplies FPL and the radial half of FDP), the patient cannot make an 'O' between his thumb and index finger: the IP joint of the thumb and the distal interphalangeal (DIP) joint of the index finger hyperextend instead. (If this test is attempted in ulnar paralysis, the opposite happens: the MP joints hyperextend and the IP joints flex more than usual.)

Figure 4A.1 shows the nerve roots supplying the key muscles in the upper limb. It is simplified to give one main root for each muscle, though actually most of the more proximal muscles are supplied from several root levels. (This is of practical importance in polio: muscles supplied from several levels may continue to function but those with a limited source are paralysed.) This is for reference and to remind you to think about it, but you are not expected to keep all this in your mind. Again, there are individual variations, revealed by detailed examination of patients with brachial plexus injuries.

Tendon sheaths

The next structures you encounter as you explore the hand more deeply are the tendons in their sheaths: paratenon for the extensors and synovial and fibrous sheaths for the flexors and the tendons around the wrist.

Be accurate in your terminology for conditions affecting the tendon sheaths. Tenosynovitis means inflammation of the synovial sheath; in practice we only see this in rheumatoid disease or acute and chronic infections. Thickening of the fibrous sheath (e.g. trigger digits and de Quervain's disease) should be called stenosing tenovaginitis because the synovium is normal. If you tell a patient that he or she has tenosynovitis, then he or she will go straight to a solicitor because most people have been led to believe – quite wrongly – that tenosynovitis is caused by their work.

A third condition, seldom seen by orthopaedic surgeons, is peritendonitis crepitans or intersection syndrome, which affects the radial wrist extensors about 5 cm above the wrist where they are crossed by APL and EPB, at this point there is palpable and sometimes audible crepitus when the wrist is flexed. There is no tenosynovium at that level, so this is not tenosynovitis either.

DeQuervain's thickening is palpable and sometimes visible, but there is seldom clicking. In contrast, trigger fingers and thumb have palpable and sometimes visible clicking, but one can seldom distinguish the thickening from the normal anterior prominence of the metacarpal head.

Rheumatoid tenosynovitis may cause typical triggering or may herniate through the fibrous sheath within the finger and obstruct movement of the flexor tendon at that level. In severe cases, the fingers are thick like sausages and for that reason difficult to flex. Less obvious cases can be detected by pinching up the skin on the front of the proximal phalanx, when you feel more than the usual two thicknesses of skin.

Tendons

Start by asking the patient to make a full fist and then to straighten the hand out completely. Similarly, check active flexion and extension of the thumb. If you have any doubt as to whether any joint is moving fully, you need to make a more detailed examination and this certainly applies if there is a recent cut on the hand, wrist or forearm, when there is no excuse for failure to examine every tendon which might be damaged. On the palmar surface, there are two wrist flexors, one thumb flexor and two flexors in each finger. On the extensor side there are nine muscles: three wrist extensors, three thumb extensors (including abductor pollicis longus, which is really the extensor of the carpometacarpal joint) and three finger extensors (extensor indicis proprius, extensor digitorum with four tendons[*] and extensor digiti minimi which usually has two tendons).

Do not forget that tendons may be partly cut so that some movement is possible but painful; this is an indication for surgery, as you cannot tell clinically whether it is 10% cut (which can be left) or 90% cut (which needs repair). Partial division is particularly common in flexor pollicis longus, which may rupture completely a few days or weeks later when the patient starts using it normally again.

It is easy to eliminate the action of flexor digitorum superficialis (in this case the modern name is better than the old 'sublimis', which should be discarded) by holding the proximal interphalangeal (PIP) joint straight with your own finger on the patient's middle phalanx so that you can test whether profundus is flexing the DIP joint, though it cannot do so fully in that position.

It is not so obvious how to eliminate the action of profundus to examine superficialis but, as you probably know, it can be done. The key is that profundus can be regarded as one muscle with four tendons so that, if any finger is prevented from flexing, the muscle belly cannot contract fully.[†] Superficialis, in contrast, can be regarded as four muscles, each with its own tendon. To test superficialis, you therefore eliminate profundus contraction by holding three fingers straight: one finger

---

[*]The old name extensor digitorum communis was much better. There is normally no extensor digitorum brevis in the human hand (there is in the foot) but it occasionally occurs as an anomaly and may be diagnosed as a ganglion or extensor tenosynovitis.

[†]Another and important consequence of this anatomical arrangement of profundus is that, after a finger is amputated, the cut end of its profundus tendon may become adherent so that grip with the intact fingers is also weakened.

is left free and the patient asked to bend it, which he can only do at the PIP joint, using superficialis. If you are not familiar with this, practise it on yourself. Many people do not have an effective superficialis to the little finger; in contrast, some do have an independent profundus to the index finger.

Rheumatoid disease causes rupture of tendons, so here too each must be examined. Although it is not possible to stretch a tendon, in rheumatoid disease a tendon may rupture within its synovial sheath which remains in continuity and, as it scars up, provides partial function of that tendon. Tendons may become adherent to other structures following injury, so that their excursion is limited. On the back of the hand this limits overall flexion rather than extension, though individually each joint can be flexed fully if the others are extended.

The success of flexor tendon surgery is measured by the total active movement (TAM), which is the sum of the active range of movement at each of the three joints (i.e. total active flexion minus lack of active extension). This should be at least 160°. A rough measure, the flexion deficit, is the distance by which the tip of the flexed finger falls short of the proximal or distal palmar creases; this does not take into account lack of extension, which may be a greater problem.

Joints

Start by looking and feeling for swelling of the joints, which can be detected on their dorsal and lateral aspects, and feeling for tenderness, especially at the carpometacarpal joint of the thumb where tenderness may be the only clinical sign of osteoarthritis, which is common in that joint. While examining the tendons, you asked the patient to flex and extend his or her digits fully. (People of Oriental origin can often hyperextend the joints of the fingers.) If this was possible, then you already know that all the MP and IP joints have full ranges of movements.

If not, you need to find out whether this is a musculotendinous problem or a joint problem or, to put it another way, if active movements are limited you must find out whether passive movements are limited too.

Each of the relevant joints should be examined and its range of movement measured with a small goniometer (which will fit in your pocket). This does not apply to the carpometacarpal joints, because the

second and third have no movement and the fourth and fifth very little; that only leaves the first (the carpometacarpal joint of the thumb) whose movements are very important but hard to measure. Opposition is strictly speaking, as its name suggests, a position rather than a movement; a combination of movements is required to produce it. Normally the thumb lies at right-angles to the fingers: in opposition it rotates almost another 90° to bring the pulp of the thumb to the pulp of the fingers. Ask the patient to bring the tip of his thumb to the base of the little finger: it should rotate so that the thumb nail faces away from the finger. Try it on yourself. Lack of movement at the base of the thumb may be concealed by increased movement at the MP joint: ask the patient to move his thumb in a circle and watch the movement of the first metacarpal. If that appears normal but you suspect the first carpometacarpal joint, try passive movements with compression (the grinding test) which may elicit pain.

The IP joints are pure hinges and the MP joints mainly hinges so, if appropriate (which it is after injuries and in rheumatoid disease), these must be tested for abnormal sideways movements. The classic cause of this is a torn ulnar collateral ligament of the MP joint of the thumb.

Bones

Fractures, bony prominences and congenital abnormalities can often be detected clinically but the way to find out about the bones is by looking at radiographs. Whenever possible, these should be centred on the area concerned, so that it is shown as well as possible. Radiographs of the whole hand are only centred on the MP joints of the fingers. Insist on both postero-anterior (PA) and lateral views.

Malrotation in a finger, usually due to a recent or mal-united fracture, is not obvious on radiographs (unless it is very severe) and must be looked for clinically, especially if there is a spiral fracture. If you flex any one finger it will come down towards the scaphoid tuberosity, but if you flex them all together, they should come down parallel to each other. Get the patient to do this and notice whether one finger tends to cross over or under the others. Also look at the finger-nails end-on and compare them to those in the other hand.

The carpometacarpal joint of the thumb is set obliquely to the others, so PA and lateral views of the hand provide two oblique views of this joint. If you want to see it properly you must order special views: those described by Gedda were devised for just this purpose but PA and lateral views centred on the *metacarpophalangeal* joint of thumb will, if large enough, include the carpometacarpal joint and show it at more or less the correct angle.

Other investigations are seldom needed, as examination of the hand is essentially clinical: even radiographs are unnecessary in many cases (e.g. trigger fingers, carpal tunnel syndrome, Dupuytren's contracture) though, of course, you do need them for injuries and arthritis.

FUNCTION

Just as a proper examination of the foot includes standing and walking, so a proper examination of the hand includes function.

In most orthopaedic conditions the complaint is pain: in the hand, this is less often the case and the complaint is often loss of function. However 'loss of function' by itself is so broad a term as to be meaningless and what you have to do is to find out what function is lost and why.

There are three main types of grip:

1. Pinch grip: tip of thumb to tip of finger.
2. Key grip: tip of thumb to side of index finger.
   This is stronger than pinch grip.
3. Grasp with whole hand.

If the patient complains of difficulty in performing a particular task, the best way to define the problem is to get the patient to perform that task in front of you. To that end we have in our hand clinic a variety of objects to be manipulated, including a cup, coffee jar, a brick, a teapot, some knitting and a steering wheel. These are not likely to be available in the somewhat artificial circumstances of the FRCS Orth examination, though you will probably have coins, keys and a pen in your pocket. However, even if it is not very applicable to the examination hall, it should be firmly established in your routine as one of the most important parts of the examination in your clinic. It comes at the end but must not be forgotten.

Measurement of grip and pinch strength, though again not appropriate in the FRCS Orth exam, are valuable in assessing disability and observing progress. The best instrument is a Jamar dynamometer on which the patient cannot feel how hard he is squeezing, so genuine maximal grip will be consistent on several squeezes, whereas patients who are not really trying will produce variable results.

Having thus reviewed the examination of the hand and suggested a scheme or, in computer jargon, a menu from which you can pick the appropriate parts, you can move on to the sections which follow and describe different disorders within the hand. They may repeat some of what has been said here, but that is no bad thing as a way of hammering home certain key points.

FURTHER READING

Gedda KO. Studies of Bennett's fracture: anatomy, roentgenology and therapy. *Acta Chir Scand Suppl* 1954; **193**: 37–49.
(This supplement has 114 pages. You are not expected to read them, but this reference is given so that your radiographers can consult the relevant section if they wish.)
McGrouther DA. Examination of the hand and management of hand injuries. In: Hobsley M, Johnson AG, Treasure T (eds) *Current Surgical Practice*, Vol. 6. London: Edward Arnold, 1993: 160–178.

4B

Deformities

Patrick Mulligan and Michael Waldram

CONGENITAL ANOMALIES

In the Intercollegiate Examination, you may meet these uncommon conditions as short cases and as a topic in the hand surgery viva. There is opportunity to discuss the development and the function of the hand, as well as indications for surgery. Musculoskeletal and general embryology may be a part of this.

The conditions are listed in the agreed International Classification. This is not entirely satisfactory but is the best we have.

1. Failure of formation of parts:
   (a) transverse arrest;
   (b) longitudinal arrest.
2. Failure of differention of parts:
   (a) soft tissue involvement;
   (b) skeletal involvement;
   (c) congenital tumorous conditions.
3. Duplication (polydactyly).
4. Overgrowth.
5. Undergrowth.
6. Congenital constriction band syndrome.
7. Generalised skeletal anomalies.

In each of these anomalies it is likely that the questions will be directed to certain aspects of the condition. These are:

- incidence
- associated visceral anomalies
- heredity
- functional disability
- surgical intervention (timing, indication and outcome).

There are numerous and bizarre congenital anomalies. Not all will be discussed here, only some of the more common ones of which you should have a working knowledge. It is not expected that every candidate will have in-depth experience of managing such conditions, or have even seen them.

The congenital hand clinic requires the input of surgeons with technical skills in plastic and orthopaedic aspects of hand surgery. Experience only comes over many years of seeing sufficient numbers of these children. The anxious parents also need help from paediatricians, geneticists, therapists and self-help groups. At first the child is often too ill to be submitted for surgery. This is frequently because of visceral involvement which can delay matters for months or years. Full paediatric assessment of the cardiovascular, renal and haematological systems must be undertaken before surgery. Even where the anomaly is apparently minor in the hand, the related associated anomalies can be severe and dangerous. However, in most cases presenting later in childhood, the abnormality is confined to the hand.

The timing of surgery is frequently within the first year of life. Most surgical procedures should be undertaken before the age of four, if possible. After this time, when going to school, it is difficult for the child to re-learn manual skills as central cortical representation of the deformity has already become well established. In some cases, however, the anomalies are best left until the child has gone through all the growth periods. In such cases supervision is required during childhood to prevent any untoward development.

Incidence

It is impossible to know the exact incidence of hand anomalies in the population. There is no study which has been able to show this accurately. It has been said to be between 1 and 2% of live births. Birch-Jensen (1949) suggested 1 in 1000 live births; Conway and Bowe (1956) estimated 1 of every 626 live births.

In 1982, Lamb found 18 deformities per 10,000 of the population, with 10.9 per 10,000 having more than one deformity and an incidence of 11.4 if stillborns were included. These figures are quoted from David Green's book '*Operative Hand Surgery*'; it is concluded there, and from others, that polydactyly is probably the most common deformity. In others, syndactyly seems to head the list.

Embryology

Limb buds are thought to form between the 25th and 55th days of gestation. In the hand the critical area is the apical ectodermal ridge (AER), where, in the mesenchyme, blood vessels appear as well as the primordium to the skeleton. Physiological cell death in the tissues between the digits brings about their separation. Failure of this can stop separation and cause syndactyly. Complete failure means absence, over-activity can mean duplication. Haemorrhage can lead to a more confused pattern where there is failure of development and separation as seen in acrosyndactyly. More recently, fibroblastic growth factors (FGFs) have been isolated and are shown to play a vital part in the localisation and development of the limb bud. There are a number of different growth factors involved.

The three main areas of development have traditionally been referred to as central, pre-axial and post-axial in the forearm and hand. Disturbance of any one of these gives well-recognised deformity.

FAILURE OF FORMATION OF PARTS

Transverse arrest

This can take place at any level from the shoulder to the distal phalanx. Within the hand these can be abnormalities of the length of digits, a metacarpal hand or a carpal hand (*Figure 4B.1*). In shortened digits, the presence or absence of components of the joints or the

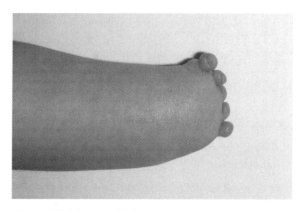

Figure 4B.1 Longitudinal transverse arrest.

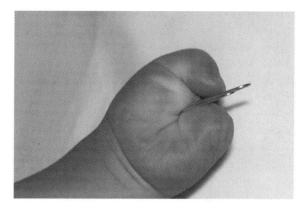

Figure 4B.2 Longitudinal transverse arrest – thenar/hypothenar grip.

capacity to grow are vital in decision-making for reconstruction. In the first twelve months of life, phalangeal transfer from the toes can allow growth in the remnants of absent digits. These are free unvascularised transfers of the proximal phalanges of the affected toes. Where there is one mobile digit present, perhaps the thumb, then composite toe transfer into the hand can be considered using microvascular techniques. This will give a pillar providing grip strength, sensation and growth. Where there is an adequate metacarpal base on which to position this, there has been considerable benefit (*Figure 4B.2*).

Where there is absence of all digits and metacarpals, then the help of prosthetic planning is required. The balance must be achieved for the child to allow adequate cortical development. The prosthesis should not inhibit this but be applied carefully with clear functional benefit. Children frequently achieve remarkable function in even the most bizarre handicap and unless the prosthesis is of clear advantage then it will be discarded. The drawback of a prosthesis is that it has no sensation. The shorter the limb, the more likely it is to help. Bilateral defects can benefit most.

Longitudinal arrest

Failure of formation of radius (pre-axial): radial hemimelia

This is no longer called radial club hand. The pre-axial failure of development frequently involves not just the radius but also the radial carpus, with a hypoplastic or absent thumb. In the fully developed classic deformity there are degrees of radial deficiency from minimal shortening to complete absence (four grades). In the carpus, scaphoid, trapezium and trapezoid may be absent or small and there will be carpal tilt to the radial side. The thumb is floppy (pouce flottante) or absent. The fingers are poorly developed with little or no active flexion in the interphalangeal joints (*Figure 4B.3*).

The incidence varies from 1 in 50,000 to 1 in 100,000 live births. About 50% of these are bilateral. There are no clear hereditary factors implicated, so it was previously considered to be autosomal dominant deformity. This is now disputed and environmental factors are thought to be more responsible. The incidence, therefore, is sporadic. Toxic insults to the embryo, such as thalidomide, commonly cause this deformity.

There are many associated anomalies, some of which are very serious. These can prevent the child from having treatment or, more frequently, delay intervention in the

hand deformity. Many other systems are implicated and some of the common syndromes are as follows:

- Fanconi anaemia – haemopoietic system
- thrombocytopaenia absent radius syndrome (TAR) – haemopoietic system
- Holt–Oram syndrome – congenital heart lesions
- Vater syndrome – alimentary and skeletal mal-development.

In mild cases, manipulation and control with strapping, plaster or brace is generally sufficient. The most severe anomalies can be considered for correction of wrist deformity and provision of a thumb. This is prevented where the child is too ill. There should always be normal elbow flexion. Surgery gives poor results when undertaken in adults. In some children the deformity is so severe that correction cannot be achieved for fear of vascular disturbance. It is best done early in life, even in the first year.

It must be impressed on the parents that complete normality can never be achieved in these cases and the child will still have significant deformity, although with some improvement of function and appearance of the hand. There is very disturbed anatomical distribution of nerves and arteries in these deformities. This should be fully appreciated and assessed before surgery. The main arterial supply and innervation from nerve trunks should be identified. Treatment entirely by passive stretching is difficult.

Correction of wrist/forearm deformity: (Figure 4B.4) The term for this has become centralisation. In many cases it is, in fact, fusion where the ulna is put into a slot in the carpus. This was favoured by Lamb and has given very good results after follow up of over 20 years. Radialisation was introduced by Buck-Gramko (1985); in this, the hand is put further over the ulna so that most of the radial metacarpal is in line with the ulna, though this may not be possible where there is severe deformity. Considerable muscle re-balancing is required. Osteotomy of the ulna is also necessary. In each of these, the position is held by a wire or a pin (*Figure 4B.5*).

More recent developments have introduced external fixation or circular frame techniques. These have allowed correction of the deformity after stretching. The deformity needs to be held throughout the rest of childhood

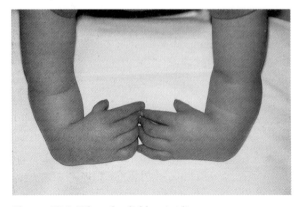

Figure 4B.3 Bilateral radial hemimelia.

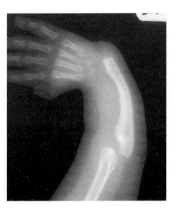

Figure 4B.4 Radial hemimelia – before wrist correction.

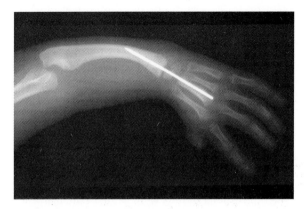

Figure 4B.5 Radial hemimelia – traditional correction.

by adequate bracing techniques. It is now considered that the lengthening of such forearms might be undertaken later in childhood. At the present time the results using external fixators have resulted in some complications and are still less predictable than the traditional methods.

Thumb reconstruction (pollicisation) Children who are left with the wrist uncorrected will develop grip in the ring and little fingers (postaxial grip); that is why the centralisation should be done first. It is then necessary to provide pre-axial grip and this means a thumb. There are many techniques but that introduced by Buck-Gramcko is the most frequently used. Essentially, this is transfer, shortening and rotation of the index finger. The digital artery to the middle finger on the radial side is ligated, allowing the transposed index finger to take the supply from that side, having made sure the middle finger has an ulnar digital artery. Enough venous drainage is important. The common digital nerve to the adjacent sides of the index and middle fingers 5 split back to the palm. The proximal four-fifths of the metacarpal is resected through the epiphyseal plate and the metacarpal head, which is retained, becomes equivalent to the trapezoid. It is rotated, hyperextended at the metacarpo-phalangeal joint and placed in the soft tissues at the carpal level on the radial side. The intrinsics are released and re-attached to the level of the neck of the proximal phalanx. This is done by using small wings from the dorsal hood. The position requires *more* than 90° rotation for opposition. The new thumb is sutured in position using the flaps which have been designed at the beginning of the procedure.

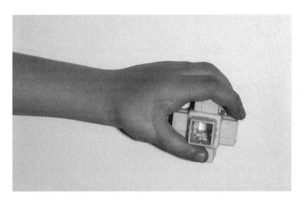

Figure 4B.6 Pollicisation from index.

The tension and position of these flaps is the most critical point in the eventual function and position of the thumb. The flexor tendon is left intact but the extensor tendons are shortened. Cosmetically, the thumbs can be very acceptable and most children find excellent function (*Figure 4B.6*). There should be 40° of palmar abduction and 150° of rotation in order to achieve a final functional position of 120°. When this procedure is undertaken in the presence of radial hemimelia, it must be realised that the fingers have poor function in the proximal interphalangeal joints, so the transposed digit in this case should be longer than it would be when transposed for other reasons.

Failure of formation of ulna (postaxial): ulnar hemimelia

This is a very rare deformity, involving the failure of formation of parts on the ulnar side of the forearm. It is combined with a more serious hand anomaly and results in a short forearm with progressive bowing of the radius in many cases. Very few people have the opportunity of seeing such a case and it behaves completely differently from the radial hemimelia described above (p. 106). You should not be expected to develop the management of such a condition but it may be useful to recognise it if shown a radiograph (*Figure 4B.7*).

Central deficiency: cleft hand

The nomenclature is difficult. True cleft hand is a deep split in the tissues, through the middle of the hand down to the level of the carpus, with a central absence of at least one digit (*Figure 4B.8*). This should be distinguished from symbrachydactyly, where digits are present but fused and very short. This is more complex and variable. There may also be absence of the second and fourth rays and even the first, so that the hand is not actually cleft. Varying degrees of severity occur in the same family and even the same patient so they are clearly manifestations of the same condition. Transverse bands may be present. Other terms for this are ectrodactyly and lobster-claw hand. This is regarded as 'atypical cleft hand'.

Cleft hand is frequently seen bilaterally, it is more common in boys and can involve the feet. The typical deformity has dominant inheritance; some skip a generation. The atypical deformity is thought to be sporadic and has many associated anomalies which can be cardiac and alimentary.

Treatment: typical cleft hand. In some, the fingers are completely mobile and when grip is attempted they fall together with an excellent position. No surgery is required. Flatt described this as a functional triumph from a social disaster. In others, the two sides of the cleft are held widely apart and, with resection at the base and approximation of the two sides, the deformity can be lessened and function improved. At metacarpal level, interweaving of tendons provides a transmetacarpal ligament. When the cleft is eccentric, transfer of one metacarpal across the hand gives better balance. Deepening of the thumb web space is frequently required, or even creation of a thumb.

Treatment: atypical cleft hand. In this condition, any synostosis is separated and metacarpal resection may be required. In hypoplasia, metacarpal or phalangeal lengthening can be considered. Toe to hand transfer is also available.

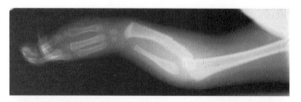

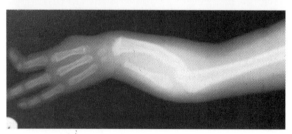

Figure 4B.7 Ulnar hemimelia – forearm and hand deformity.

Intersegmental deficiency (intercalary deficiency): phocomelia

In this failure of formation of parts, there is a hand but a variable length of arm has not developed so the hand is too proximal; there can be extreme shortening with development of hand components at the level of the shoulder. Three types are described:

1. hand attached to shoulder;
2. forearm present;
3. arm present.

This deficiency forms 8% of all congenital upper limb anomalies. About 60% of these were the result of thalidomide use. It can be associated with other skeletal anomalies in the forearm on the other side and many

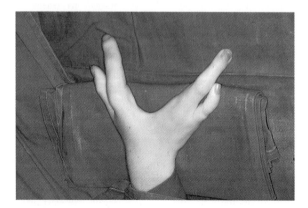

Figure 4B.8 'Typical' cleft hand.

other visceral anomalies may be involved. There is no indication for surgery and most often a prosthesis is required. These patients develop very considerable facility for function in the hands. In the past, most surgery has been unsuccessful and it is frequently better to leave patients to their own devices.

FAILURE OF DIFFERENTIATION OF PARTS

Syndactyly (webbed finger)

There are two main groups in this condition. In the first group, 'simple' syndactyly, there is soft tissue fusion between two digits or more which can be complete or incomplete. In the second, 'complex' syndactyly may just represent distal bony fusion or a fibrous synostosis at the distal phalanx (Figure 4B.9). In the more complicated complex syndactyly the bony architecture is severely disturbed and can include hypoplasia and duplications within the composite.

Syndactyly is said to occur in 1 in 2000 births and is more common in males and is as frequently bilateral as unilateral. It is probably the commonest congenital abnormality of the hand, although not in orthopaedic practice as most cases are referred to plastic surgeons. A clear family history is found in 10%. Flatt reported that, when it occurs alone, it is always a part of an inherited autosomal disorder. It can, however, be sporadic and part of a syndrome. It is a common presentation in associated anomalies such as Apert or acrocephalosyndactyly (Apert's syndrome). There are many conditions in which syndactyly may or may not be present and where there are other congenital anomalies. Partial syndactyly of the toes is very common and needs no treatment.

Treatment. The presence of webbing alone is not an indication for surgery, particularly when it is incomplete. However, separation allows the digits to function separately (e.g. on keyboards) and normal gloves can be worn. When there are discrepancies in length between the two digits or there is presence of a bony fusion, then the indications are clear. The shorter digit will deform the longer one and cause progressive deformity. Release at an early stage is essential to correct this, even if only the distal ends are separated.

In simple syndactyly, and in distal complex syndactyly, separation is undertaken using multiple zig-zag

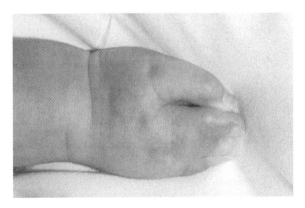

Figure 4B.9 Complex syndactyly – Apert's syndrome.

incisions across the cleft from finger to finger and immediately identifying the level and distribution of the neurovascular bundle to each digit. The position and level of the web space is critical and a basal rectangular flap should be adequate to take through the web. It is essential that this is wide enough and secure in order to achieve a good result and prevent web creep. Gaps are presented which are completed using skin grafts, preferably of full thickness. In the more complex syndactyly, excision of bone and a more extensive flap creation is required. Normally one would not separate both sides of one digit for fear of jeopardising the blood-supply. Immobilisation to prevent contracture is important. The skin graft should be taken as full thickness from a glabrous area.

Arthrogryposis

This is a very severe and generalised type of soft tissue anomaly. Arthrogryposis multiplex congenita comes into this classification of failure of differentiation of parts. The exact nature of this condition is not well understood. It appears to involve connective tissue and also has a neurogenic component. It may have an environmental cause, perhaps from toxic drugs or chemicals causing mutation, and neurovascular blocking agents have also been blamed. There is abnormality in endplate transport and changes within muscles. The contracture of muscle and joint brings about the deformity.

In the upper limbs, a severe deformity shows flexion at the wrist and fingers (*Figure 4B.10*). There is frequently an extension deformity of the elbow and internal rotation of the shoulder, again supporting a possible neurogenic distribution. When all of the upper

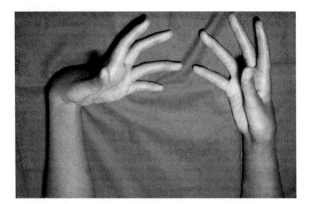

Figure 4B.10 Arthrogryposis – one wrist corrected.

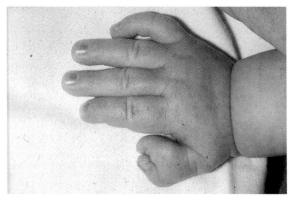

Figure 4B.11 Pre-axial polydactyly.

limb is involved there is very severe loss of function. In such cases, no abduction of the shoulder, flexion of the elbow or extension of the wrist is possible. It can also affect the lower limb and sometimes all four limbs are affected. There is no development of the muscles involved. Sharrard believed this to be consistent with localised lesions in the anterior horn cell columns. He considered orthopaedic treatment should take account of the paralytic nature of the deformities.

In some milder forms, release of the thumb and palmar deformity can be achieved with skin release and tendon transfers. If this is not possible then, at a later age, metacarpophalangeal fusion of the thumb may be employed. The flexion deformity of the wrist can be extremely severe and, at the end of growth, arthrodesis may help function but will also certainly improve the cosmetic aspect of the condition (Figure 4B.10). Proximal row carpectomy is an alternative. Release of flexion of the fingers in the clutched hand deformity is very difficult and unlikely to improve function. Flexion deformity of fingers can be helped by interphalangeal joint arthrodesis, when bone deformity with ulnar drift of the digit can be considered for soft tissue release of the intrinsic in connection with metacarpal oseotomy. In many cases, however, the deformity of the fingers is best left alone and the patient should be helped to develop finger function as best they can.

DUPLICATION (POLYDACTYLY)

Duplication can be anything from the whole limb, which is exceedingly rare, to a digit which is quite common. It is very uncommon proximal to the hand.

In the digits, polydactyly is regarded as being:

1. radial (pre-axial)
2. central
3. ulnar (postaxial).

Pre-axial polydactyly (i.e. duplication of the thumb)

A classification of this duplicated thumb was provided by Wassel. There may be duplication of the distal phalanx or at any level, proximally occurring either within the length of the bone, partial or complete, or at the joint level (*Figure 4B.11*).

In the Wassel classification there are seven different levels with subgroups in levels four and seven where the triphalangeal element is found. It is not essential for you to know these: you can simply describe the level at which the bifurcation occurs. It is thought to occur in 0.8 per 1000 live births, is said to be higher in American Indians and Orientals and is more than twice as common in males than females. Type four is the most common.

Associated anomalies are more serious when there is triphalangism but one should look carefully for cardiac anomalies such as Holt–Oram syndrome, Fanconi pancytopenia, Blackfan–Diamond anaemia and hypoplastic anaemia. It can also be associated with other severe anomalies.

Treatment

The operation is not just removal of the extra thumb, but making one thumb out of two. The relative size of one element to the other, the level at which duplication takes place or the angulation of the various components makes the planning for correction of duplication important and difficult. The child must be studied carefully, first to decide which thumb is used most and, therefore, to be retained. The aim should be to reconstitute at the joint level and undertake tendon transfer to provide re-balancing of the digit and the capsule. If necessary, osteotomy can be undertaken to realign the abnormal joint.

The more common symmetrical deformity allows excision of the lesser digit and transfer of skin flap and spare tendons to provide ligaments and digital balance.

Lastly, transferring one digit to another can also be considered, the aim being to correct the deformity and stabilise the joint.

Postaxial polydactyly

Frequently this is a small nubbin of skin on the ulnar side of the hand which is taken care of in the obstetric nursery by tying a ligature around it.

Type II postaxial polydactyly, which is rare, shows a portion of digit with normal components with an enlarged or bifid metacarpal. Type III consists of a complete digit with its own metacarpal and soft tissues and is very rare (*Figure 4B.12*).

Postaxial polydactyly is ten times more common in blacks than whites; 1 in 3000 live births in whites. The true incidence in whites is not known because frequently the little skin tags are removed. It is probably the most common congenital anomaly. There is a strong genetic inheritance pattern. It has many associated anomalies which can affect any system, including alimentary, skeletal, neurological, cardiac, renal, eyes or ears. There are also many chromosomal abnormalities associated with this condition.

Duplication of the ulna is associated with mirror hand deformity. It is thought to be a spontaneous genetic mutation passed on as an autosomal dominant trait. Because of its rarity it is really a curiosity.

OVERGROWTH

Overgrowth can take place in any part of the limb and frequently extends from the hand proximally into the wrist. This is called macrodactyly. It is frequently present at birth and certainly develops in early

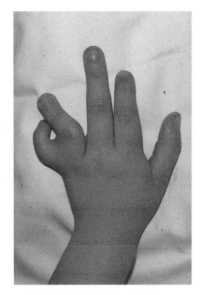

Figure 4B.12 Postaxial polydactyly.

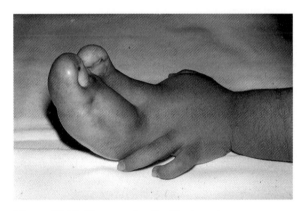

Figure 4B.13 Overgrowth – lipofibromatosis.

childhood. If present at birth it can keep the same growth.

In the second type, where it appears after birth, it accelerates in growth compared to the other digits (*Figure 4B.13*). It is very uncommon and is mostly unilateral. It is most frequently seen in the index finger but when two fingers are involved there is associated deviation. It is said to have an incidence of 0.9%, the most common type being lipofibromatous, i.e. there is excessive fat and connective tissue. However, the phalanges may be too long. It is associated with neurofibromatosis, hyperostosis and hemihypertrophy.

It does not seem to be inherited and the cause is not known. Ingalls suggested abnormal nerve supply, abnormal blood supply and abnormal humoral mechanisms. There is evidence that nerves have effect by their growth factors and impaired nerve function seems to stimulate the growth of other tissues. It may be associated with Von Recklinghausen's disease. A very rare association is Proteus syndrome. In this, the tissue is completely different and rather primitive cartilage-type tissue and there are a number of other associated anomalies. It is easily distinguished from neurofibromatosis.

Treatment

In lipofibromatosis, the distribution may be on one or both sides of the digits. Frequently it comes proximally through the palm and magnetic resonance imaging (MRI) has been very useful in identifying the extent and size of the lesion and it is particularly helpful when the lesion penetrates through the palmar spaces into the dorsum of the hand or comes proximally through the carpal tunnel.

Treatment, by de-bulking the digit, is done in stages. Sometimes the deformity is so gross that the digit is amputated; if so, transfer of one digit across the palm gives a better balance. In due course a second digit can be de-bulked or reduced by bony excision at a later date. Fusion of epiphyseal plates can also be considered. This is difficult to be certain of as growth rate within these phalanges can not be clearly assessed. Occasionally there is a vascular pattern in this condition. This is much more difficult to deal with and frequently only requires to be treated in the presence of pain. Despite attempts to reduce the length and width of the finger, it may remain so unsightly, and also stiff, that it has to be amputated.

UNDERGROWTH (BRACHYSYNDACTYLY)

This is often difficult to classify as it seems to come into many of the other groups (*Figure 4B.14*). Because of this, it has many associated anomalies. Treatments include correction of synostosis, lengthening, toe phalangeal transfer, metacarpal or carpal lengthening by distraction of graft.

CONGENITAL CONSTRICTION BAND SYNDROME

These can be simple constriction rings, associated with deformity of the distal part, which is bulbous (*Figure 4B.15*). When there is failure of separation of fingers as well, this is acrosyndactyly. Patterson reported constriction band syndrome to be present in 1 in 15,000 live births. Most are sporadic and the aetiology is controversial. The most extreme example of this is interuterine amputation of a formed limb. It is thought, therefore, to happen later in pregnancy than the normal timing of other congenital anomalies.

It is said to occur more frequently in young mothers in their first pregnancy or in problem pregnancies with premature birth that is not related to drugs. It can be

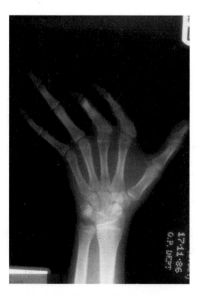

Figure 4B.14 Undergrowth – brachysyndactyly.

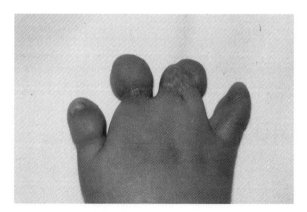

Figure 4B.15 Constriction band syndrome.

associated with neural tube defects, craniofacial anomalies, abdominal and thoracic wall defects. Many other hand deformities may be involved. Club foot, cleft palate and scoliosis can also be associated with this condition. Neurological or vascular impairment is common.

Treatment

Treatment of this syndrome is according to the defect present. Constrictional rings are lengthened by Z-plasty of the bands. This may have to be repeated and good knowledge of skin flaps is essential for this type of surgery.

GENERALISED SKELETAL ANOMALIES

Madelung's deformity

It most commonly presents in adolescence; I have seen it more in females. The presentation is frequently because of the protrusion of the distal ulna. The distal radius articular surface is grossly angled and there is limitation of movement. There are often cystic changes around the distal radial epiphysis which appears to have closed at one side (*Figure 4B.16*). It is said to be associated with median nerve irritation and there can be pain in the wrist. It can be genetic with autosomal dominant trait. Other associated anomalies include Langer syndrome, dwarfism and Turner syndrome. It is associated with skeletal dysplasia. Because it gets worse with growth, the deformity is progressive, but not after skeletal maturity. It seldom causes pain.

The principle of correction of the deformity is to increase the length of the ulna and change the angulation of the distal radial epiphysis. Sometimes the ulna is resected and in others arthrodesis is the option chosen. In severe cases, a normal wrist cannot be provided. Vickers, in his series, found that none got worse and most had improved symptomatically and, as shown by radiography, some even had an increase in movement. It is likely that external fixators using distraction-correction techniques will change the approach to this condition.

Clinodactyly

This is a description of a deformity where the finger is bent from side to side; there is no rotational element.

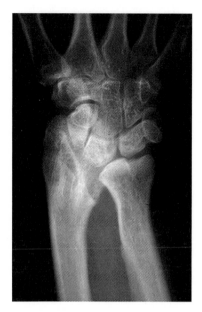

Figure 4B.16 Madelung's deformity – sloping radius, subluxed ulna.

Most common in the little finger, it can appear in early childhood but most frequently presents in adolescence with a lesser growth spurt. In most cases, there is thought to be an abnormality in the direction of the epiphyseal growth of one of the phalanges. This can be mild, producing a trapezoidal bone but in the more severe cases there is a triangular or delta bone. Light and Blevins give a classification of the delta bone, describing three groups.

In some patients there is a strong family history and it can, therefore, be regarded as an autosomal dominant trait. There are many associated anomalies including syndactyly, polydactyly and symphalangism. In the little finger, Down syndrome is a common accompaniment. It can be associated with many other severe visceral anomalies (*Figure 4B.17*).

Treatment

Delta bone. Ppening wedge osteotomy reverse wedge graft can be used. Another technique is to divide the abnormal growth plate at an earlier stage and pack it with fat, this is the Langenskiold operation. The epiphyseal bracket must be interrupted, then growth can take place longitudinally. This procedure is technically more difficult. I have undertaken it using a very fine

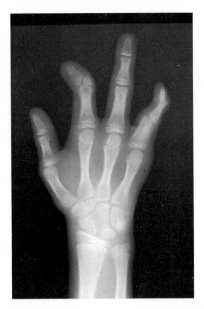

Figure 4B.17 Clinodactyly of index finger with delta bone.

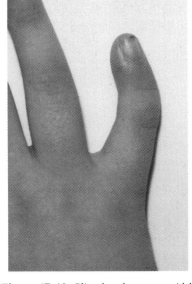

Figure 4B.18 Clinodactyly – trapezoidal.

pair of bone cutters of a fashionable manicure set, which are really excellent. Re-alignment of capsule in tendons is frequently required.

Trapezoidal bone. (*Figure 4B.18*) This only needs treatment if there is overlapping of the fingers or there is progressive deformity. A closing wedge osteotomy through the neck of the middle phalanx is held with a Kirschner wire.

Triangular bone, not extending right across finger. If this is incorporated, then an osteotomy is required. If it is free, it can be excised and the capsule of the joint resected. In the thumb, this is known as hitch-hiker's thumb; it can be corrected by a closing osteotomy.

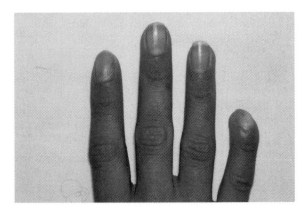

Figure 4B.19 Kirner's syndrome.

Kirner's deformity

This is a flexion deformity of the distal phalanx which presents towards the end of childhood. It can be bilateral but is seldom progressive (*Figure 4B.19*). The incidence is said to be sporadic but can be inherited. There is an association with Cornelia-de-Lange syndrome and Turner syndrome.

The curved sclerotic distal phalanx is underdeveloped. Treatment is normally avoided. If it is very severe, osteotomy can be considered but the results are variable.

Camptodactyly

This is a deformity seen in the little finger with flexion at the proximal interphalangeal joint. It varies from a very mild deformity to one that can go beyond a right angle. Children present at an earlier stage and it is progressive. It is frequently bilateral but not symmetrical. In the younger age group it is equal in boys and girls but in adolescence it is mostly girls. It appears in 1% of the population. There is no clear inheritance but it can be autosomal dominant and involve more than one finger. Other cases are sporadic. It is associated with

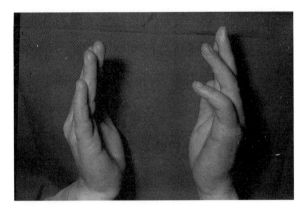

Figure 4B.20 Camptodactyly.

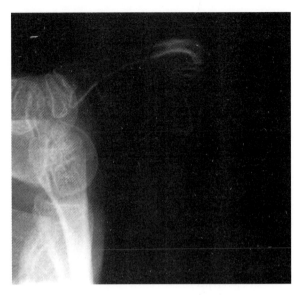

Figure 4B.21 Camptodactyly – deformity at PIP joint.

other connective tissue contractures such as Dupuytren's disease, Marfan's syndrome, arthrogryposis or absence of extensor tendons. It can also be associated with many other genetic syndromes (*Figure 4B.20*).

The mechanism of deformity is not clear. There seems to be a generalised absence of all tissue development in the little finger, from the skin to the capsule and tendons. There is an abnormality in the direction of the flexor creases and a very short gap between the metacarpo-phalangeal and proximal interphalangeal flexor creases.

Even at an early age, the severe cases are not correctable and lateral radiographs show early changes in the neck of the proximal phalanx and the flexor aspect of the base of the middle phalanx which is enlarged (*Figure 4B.21*). Only if there is passive correction should any surgery be considered. Surgery is best in young patients who have full correction when the metacarpophalangeal joint is flexed. In these cases there is often an abnormal insertion of the lumbrical muscle, so that it fails to extend the proximal interphalangeal joint; it may have a fibrous band in the superficialis which may itself be short. Any of these could be released and, in some cases, very good results are achieved. The superficialis can be transferred to improve extension, or extensor indicis proprius used for the same purpose. In general, most children, until the end of childhood, are treated with corrective splintage to hold the position so that it does not become severe. It may get worse in the adolescent growth spurt (and sometimes first presents at that stage, mostly in girls) but not afterwards. Flexion is full and function, therefore, normal.

In general terms surgery is best avoided. Splintage, when applied, should be done carefully so that the three-point fixation encourages correction of the flexion deformity without putting an extension stress across the distal interphalangeal joint.

Surgery in adolescence and beyond is normally contraindicated unless there is a clear identifiable causative structure. In such cases, the statement of Smith and Kaplan should be remembered: 'Every structure about the base of the finger has been implicated as a determining factor.'

DUPUYTREN'S CONTRACTURE

DEFINITION

Proliferative fibroplasia of the palmar fascia forming nodules and cords with secondary flexion contracture of the finger.

HISTORY

Felix Plater of Basel in 1614 described in the third volume of his 'observations' a stonemason with a condition drawing in the little and ring fingers with ridging of the palmar skin. Plater believed the tendons had pulled out of the fibrous sheath and were bow-stringing across the palm, an interpretation error that persists some 300 years later especially among medical students!

In the Western Isles of Scotland "The Curse of the MacCrimmons" made playing of the bagpipes impossible.

The hand of Papal benediction deriving from the position of Dupuytren's contracture has not been substantiated. Early ecclesiastical traditions holding the fingers flexed may predate any classical hand posture of the ring and little fingers from Dupuytren's contracture.

Henry Cline was lecturer of anatomy at St Thomas' Hospital in 1777. He was one of John Hunter's pupils and is credited with first dissecting a cadaver with this condition. Sir Astley Cooper learnt from Cline and lectured in London to many trainee surgeons. He described the condition clearly, well before Dupuytren who visited him in London in 1826.

Guillaume Dupuytren performed his first palmar fasciotomy on a coachman at the Hotel Dieu in Paris in 1831. He was a true general surgeon of astounding clinical practice. His name became attached to the condition which he published and demonstrated widely. He was in death, as in life, a colourful character who insisted that his post-mortem be performed in front of his own medical staff and published in the local weekly journal.

KEY FACTS

Dupuytren's contracture is seen in 4–5% of the population and is ten times commoner in men. It is common in those of Scandanavian and Celtic origin. It is seldom seen before the fifth to seventh decade of life, but affects 17% of men over 65 and 30% of those over 85 years. It is rarely reported in black or oriental races and there is a strong hereditary link. There is a prevalence of 68% in first degree relatives. The inheritance pattern suggests an autosomal dominant mechanism. Dupuytren's occurs in 42% of epileptics and has a lower than average incidence in patients with rheumatoid arthritis. It is commoner in diabetic patients and those suffering from alcohol excess.

About 5% of patients have a lesion in the medial plantar fascia of the foot (**Ledderhose's** disease) and 3% of patients have induration of the penis making it crooked when erect (**Peyronie's** disease). Thickened

knuckle pads occur on the dorsum of the proximal interphalangeal joints. Any of the above associated factors comprise a strong **diathesis** and such patients are more prone to recurrence and progressive disease.

AETIOLOGY

The cause of Dupuytren's contracture remains unknown. The possibility that trauma and manual labour are causative has been extensively investigated, but the disease is no more common in manual than office workers. The presence of haemosiderin in the Dupuytren's lesion suggests haemorrhage from tears, but in whites the lesion occurs as often in the non-dominant hand.

In 1972 Gabianni and Majno implicated the *myofibroblast* as the dominant cell type. The myofibroblast is a contractile cell possibly originating from a transformed perivascular smooth muscle cell. The fibroblast is not in itself abnormal but produces increased type III collagen when there are a lot of fibroblasts together (high cell density). One mechanism for fibroblast stimulation may be *oxygen free radicals*, although it is still not known whether the presence of these is cause or effect.

Dupuytren's tissue is formed by fibroplasia and hypertrophy of the palmar fascia. Two theories exist on the mechanism of pathological change. In the *intrinsic theory* the concept is metaplasia of the existing fascia and not the formation of new tissue. Subcutaneous nodules develop first and later mature to become cords. In the *extrinsic theory* diseased tissue arises in the fibro-fatty subdermal plane and attaches itself to and grows on the underlying fascial bands. Contracture of the proximal interphalangeal joints and displacement of a neurovascular bundle in a digit results from one pattern of contracture of the fascial bands. The disease follows existing anatomical pathways. It is the widely accepted norm that normal anatomical fascial condensations are known as *bands* and pathological tissue of Dupuytren as *cords*.

SYMPTOMS

The ulnar fingers get in the way when

- washing the face
- combing the hair

- putting on make–up
- putting the hand in a pocket
- putting hands in gloves
- may affect racquet sports and golf.

Pain or parasthesiae are rarely seen. Nodules may be painful in the early stages when surgically they are best left alone, although injection of steroid has been claimed to help.

PROGNOSIS

Recurrence rate after operation varies between 5 and 50%. Such a wide variation is partly due to the difficulty of making the clinical distinction between recurrence and extension of the disease. Recurrence is more likely when the following factors are present:

1. Hereditary: if there is a history in the family or first degree relatives the chance of recurrence is higher.
2. Female: in women the disease usually begins later in life and progresses more slowly but the results of surgery are worse and the chance of a postoperative flare reaction is twice as common as in men. Do not operate on women unless it is really necessary.
3. Alcoholism or epilepsy.
4. Knuckle pads.
5. Bilateral: symmetrical disease is less common than unilateral disease. It usually progresses more on the ulnar side of the hand than on the radial side.
6. Previous surgery with early recurrence.

Exam tips

History: check	*Examination:* check
a) dominance	a) sex
b) family history	b) nodules and cords site
c) rate of progression	c) MCP angle (measure)
d) diabetes?	d) PIP angle (measure)
e) epilepsy?	e) knuckle pad (Garrod)
f) alcohol?	f) secondary boutonnière?
g) foot involvement?	g) previous surgical scars and sensation
h) smoking?	h) increased sweating, high sympathetic tone, risk of reflex sympathetic dystrophy.
i) trauma?	

SIGNS

The table top test of Hueston (1992) involves placing the fingers and hand prone on a table top. The test is positive when the hand will not go flat. If it is negative, surgery is probably not indicated. Metacarpophalangeal (MCP) joint contracture usually is correctable with surgery but proximal interphalangeal (PIP) contracture is often not correctable. The optimum time to operate is when MCP contracture is established and before PIP joint contracture is greater than 45°. In a number of cases PIP joint contracture can be compensated by MCP hyperextension.

STAGING

There is nothing worse than a well-intentioned specialist registrar picking a case from the waiting list in the consultant's absence, only to find an elderly man with advanced recurrent contracture and fingers in the palm.

Luck described three stages of Dupuytren's contracture in 1959: *proliferative, involutional* and *residual*, but this does not really help sort out which cases are difficult and need a more experienced surgeon. A suggested staging for practical purposes is included below, but would need explaining for exam purposes (Woodruff, 1998).

Stage I	Early palmar disease with no finger contracture: leave alone.
Stage II	One finger involvement with only MCP contracture: ideal for surgery.
Stage III	One finger involvement at both MCP and PIP joint level: surgery not easy.
Stage IV	Features of stage III but with more than one finger involvement: surgery prolonged and only partly successful.
Stage V	Finger in palm deformity: consider amputation.

CONSENT

It is suggested that preoperatively you should mention the following to the patient:

1. Surgery is not curative: there may be recurrence.
2. The small possibility of digital nerve damage, and the importance of surgical repair if recognised at the time of surgery. Transient numbness as a result of neurapraxia of the digital nerves should also be discussed.

3. The possibility of a stiff hand (recurrence, flare reaction, reflex sympathetic dystrophy). Patients like to know details of the anaesthetic, time of operation and how long before they can drive. It is important to emphasise the time taken for healing (e.g. skin at least two weeks, loss of grip six weeks).
4. If a postoperative splinting regime is employed, then it should be emphasised before surgery.

TREATMENT

Non-operative treatment

X-ray therapy is no longer employed and extension splinting is rarely successful. Spontaneous resolution has been described, but the natural history in most cases is for the contracture to progress. Gradual soft tissue distraction for advanced cases has been reported, but is not commonly employed, and is usually followed by surgery at the end of distraction.

Surgery

Anaesthesia. Axillary or supraclavicular regional block is very suitable. Bier's block anaesthesia will not usually give enough operating time.★

Tourniquet. 100 mm above systolic pressure, recording tourniquet time in the operating theatre. Use the Esmarch bandage rather than a Rhys Davis exsanguinator to give good exsanguination in the palm.

Diathermy. Use bipolar cautery (extremity surgery near end arteries).

Magnification. Two to three times loupe magnification is recommended. An operating microscope is not required, but would be recommended in the unlikely event of digital nerve damage.

Procedure. There are six surgical options:

1. subcutaneous fasciotomy (after Luck)
2. partial selective fasciectomy (after Skoog)
3. complete fasciectomy

★August Karl Gustav Bier (1861–1949) was assistant to Van Esmarch (of the exsanguinating bandage) and later Professor of Surgery in Berlin. He gave the first spinal anaesthetic and introduced the time hat to the German Army in World War I.

4. fasciectomy with skin grafting (Dermofasciectomy) (after Hueston)
5. external fixator
6. amputation at the PIP joint or metacarpal neck.

Incisions

There are two types of incision that are generally used. A linear with Z plasty, this is the commonest and has the advantage of interruption of the longitudinal cord. The Z plasties are made at an angle of 60° and sited at the level of the transverse creases of the finger. The ends of the oblique cuts should be opposite each other. The Z plasties should not be cut until after the removal of the Dupuytren's tissue as finger position can affect skin tension. Draw them out on the skin first (*Figure 4B.22*). The disadvantage of this incision is the difficulty of matching up the skin incisions in two-finger disease (*Figure 4B.23*) Bruner's zig-zag incisions give good exposure but it can be difficult to raise the flaps if the skin is thin and the zig-zags large, as suggested by Bruner, can lead to troublesome scarring at the sides and base of the finger. McCash (1984) described an open palm technique whereby the fairly large defect made by using a transverse incision and correcting the contracture is left open to heal by secondary intention. The results are good, but it is important to explain the process to the patient who may get alarmed at seeing an open wound in the dressing.

Subcutaneous fasciotomy (after Luck). This is useful in the very elderly or frail patient. It consists of division of palmar cords only and can normally be adequately performed under local anaesthetic. Put the tenotome between skin and cord and press down do not saw to and fro. This procedure cannot be performed for finger disease because of the risk of digital nerve damage. Extension splinting is useful to reduce the risk of recurrence.

Partial selective fasciectomy (after Skoog). Here the aim is removal of the longitudinal contractile cords and nodules. This is the commonest surgical procedure for Dupuytren's disease.

Start at the distal end of the carpal tunnel. Define the palmar fascia and create a dissection to either side of the longitudinal cord between the cord, which lies superficial, and the neurovascular plane which lies deep. Dissect out the cord, turning it distally like the tongue of a shoe. Various 'foot processes' will pass

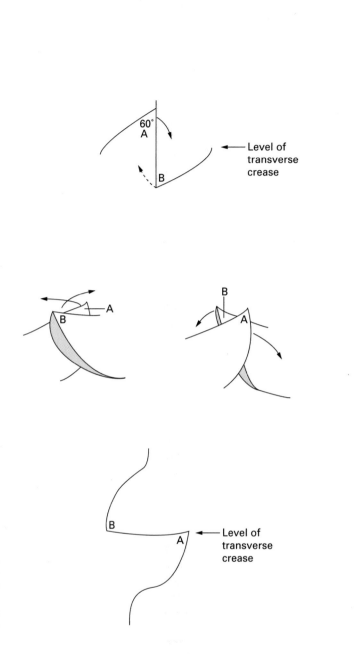

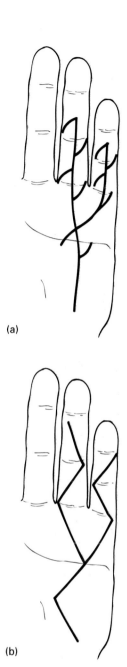

(a)

(b)

Figure 4B.22 A 'Z' plasty is fashioned by cutting two triangular skin flaps of equal base length. The angle at the apex should be no less than 60° and the sides slightly curved. Some subcutaneous fat should be preserved to prevent ischaemia. Cut one side and pull it over to the other before that is cut. The end result should interrupt the longitudinal scar line like a step.

Figure 4B.23 The two common incisions used for Dupuytren's. (a) Linear with 'Z' plasty. The Z plasty is made at the level of the transverse creases, and is less necessary in the proximal palm. The Z plasties should not be cut until the end of the procedure as finger position can influence skin tension. Care should be taken in the finger to avoid cutting the digital nerves. (b) Bruner's zig-zag incision. This gives good exposure, but raising the skin flaps can be difficult if the palmar skin is thin. The angle should not be less than 90°.

down either side of the flexor tendon and these may be cut transversely at their root by sharp dissection. At the level of the transverse crease, the transverse fibres of the palmar aponeurosis (sometimes called the superficial transverse ligament) will appear and these can normally be preserved as they are not involved in the contracture, and play an important role in preserving palmar grip and preventing palmar flexor tendon bowstringing. At the level of the metacarpal head, the digital neurovascular bundles must be carefully displayed by blunt transverse scissors dissection. This is the danger area for digital nerve damage (*Figure 4B.24*). A spiral band may pull the neurovascular bundle away from its normal anatomical position in the gutter beside the flexor sheath.

The distal dissection is often difficult, with Dupuytren's tissue ending directly under the skin or in a large subcutaneous nodule. There is no natural plane between the skin and the Dupuytren's tissue and this has to be created by sharp dissection. It is useful to develop a constant awareness of the position of both the radial and ulnar digital nerves, but they may be displaced by disease from their normal position, even to the other side of the finger (*Figure 4B.25*). Dissection beyond the middle of the middle phalanx is difficult and may prove unprofitable in correcting extension: moreover, it increases the risk of nerve damage with additional risks of difficulties with skin closure. If, after removal of contractile tissue, the finger still remains flexed at the PIP joint then cautious release of the PIP joint capsule and check-rein ligaments, that pass down either side of the volar plate may be performed. Volar plate or full collateral release is not recommended, especially in the elderly when postoperative stiffness is more likely. Kirshner wires across the PIP joint may have the same result.

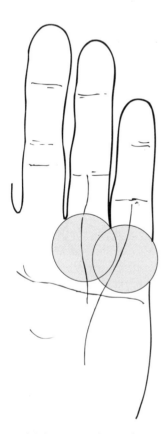

Figure 4B.24 The danger area during dissection is at the level of the metacarpal head where abnormal cords can displace the neurovascular bundle from its normal position in the gutter adjacent to the flexor tendon. Scissor dissection is recommended here.

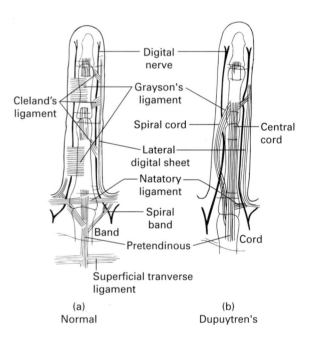

Figure 4B.25 (a) Parts of the normal digital fascia that become diseased. The superficial transverse ligament lies at the level of the transverse palmar crease and is not involved in the Dupuytren contractile cord. The natatory ligament lies at the base of the finger. Grayson's and Cleland's ligament are shown in the finger; they hold the skin during flexion and extension of the finger. (b) The spiral cord of Dupuytren's tissue develops in the pretendinous band, the spiral band, the lateral digital sheet and Grayson's ligament. With contraction it straightens out and displaces the neurovascular bundle.

At the end of the procedure both digital nerves should be clearly seen from proximal to distal, although excessive dissection around the nerve causes devascularisation. Tourniquet release, either temporary or full is preferred by many surgeons to ensure capillary return to the finger-tip. After skin closure, a bulky hand dressing is applied and the forearm and hand elevated.

Complete fasciectomy (removal of the whole of the palmar aponeurosis). This is rarely, if ever, indicated since it is associated with complications of both nerve damage and haematoma formation. The healing time is longer and such radical surgery does not prevent recurrence.

Dermofasciectomy (after Hueston). This was described for patients with a strong diathesis and poor prognosis. Some of the skin overlying and attached to the disease is excised and replaced by a skin graft which acts like a 'fire-break' in the contracting process. This technique is useful for recurrent contracture when the skin is densely involved, or when the skin is badly devitalised during surgery. Hueston recommended grafting of full thickness skin which can be taken from the upper arm. Tonkin found that skin replacement does not jeopardise hand function. The kind of patient warranting primary dermofasciectomy would be a young epileptic alcoholic with bilateral severe disease and Ledderhose's disease of the foot! In recurrent disease it is more often indicated.

External fixator (after Messina). This new technique involves attaching an external fixator to the fifth metacarpal shaft with a cumbersome outrigger system applying longitudinal traction by a transverse Kirshner wire through the middle phalanx. It is suitable for grade V disease. After two weeks of distraction surgical release is performed. This is a promising new technique which could have profound implications for understanding Dupuytren's disease at a cellular level, as under distraction it appears the phenomenon of regression occurs.

Amputation. This is suitable for grade V disease, especially if the palmar skin is macerated. Removal at the PIP joint level or fifth metacarpal neck should be considered. Preservation of the whole of the metacarpal head leads to a cosmetic deformity and awkward handshake with no obvious advantage. PIP joint fusion could be considered but would require shortening of the phalanges with loss of bone stock, and the stiff finger may still get in the way. If an amputation through the metacarpal neck is considered then this is best performed with an oblique cut using a fine oscillating saw. Amputation neuromata can be reduced by sharp nerve division under tension so that the proximal nerve ends retract away from the stump. A filleted finger skin flap can be used to cover palmar defects as a turnover flap if palmar skin needs to be removed. It should not be made too long, preserving good blood supply to the tip.

COMPLICATIONS

Early complications include:

- digital nerve damage
- haematoma
- wound breakdown or infection
- vasospasm and digital ischaemia.

Late complications include:

- flare reaction (tenderness, red wound, swelling probably a mild form of reflex sympathetic dystrophy, commoner in women)
- reflex sympathetic dystrophy, commoner after nerve injury
- recurrence
- breakdown of palmar skin in the form of fibrotic clefts.

TUMOURS

OSSEOUS TUMOURS IN THE HAND

Benign tumours

Enchondroma

Enchondroma is the most common tumour within the bones of the hand. The hand is also the most common place to find this tumour of cartilage. Most patients are young people who present with a fracture. In others this is an incidental finding. Patients occasionally complain of pain or swelling (*Figure 4B.26*). The ulnar side of the hand in the phalanges is the most common site. When seen as multiple lesions, they can be part of Ollier's disease involving one limb. This has a poorer

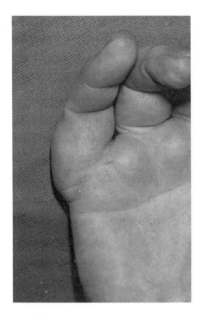

Figure 4B.26 Enchondroma.

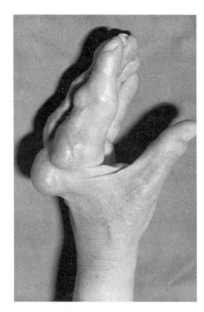

Figure 4B.27 Multiple enchondromata – Ollier's disease.

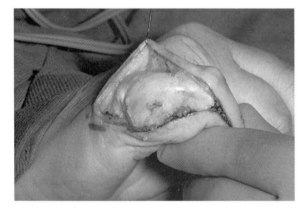

Figure 4B.28 Enchondroma. Biopsy – diagnosis in doubt.

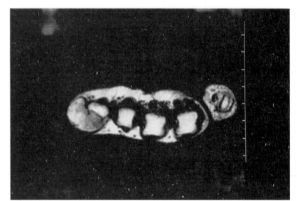

Figure 4B.29 MRI of enchondroma breaching cortex of little finger.

prognosis in terms of malignant change, which is worse in multiple enchondromatosis which is polyostotic. The single enchondroma is so unlikely to undergo malignant change that this can be disregarded in treating the chondroma (*Figure 4B.27*).

The lesion is in the metaphysis adjacent to the epiphyseal plate. It is normally said that lesions which enlarge or become painful should be submitted to biopsy because of the rare chance of malignancy. Biopsy is only undertaken to avoid a misdiagnosis (*Figure 4B.28*). If there is a clear decision by the surgeon and radiologist that this is a benign enchondroma,

then there is no need for surgery. MRI is likely to be helpful in confirming the diagnosis (*Figure 4B.29*). If there is a fracture, it should be rapid to heal. The normal treatment is excision and curettage. Bone graft is necessary when structural support is required. Many cases are well looked after by simple observation. After removal there is a recurrence of 2%.

Osteochondroma

Osteochondroma is a very uncommon tumour in the hand and more commonly seen proximal to the wrist.

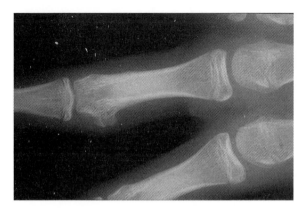

Figure 4B.30 Osteochondroma of phalanx.

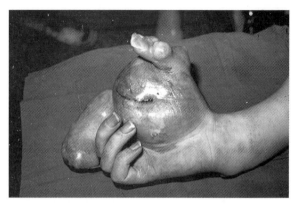

Figure 4B.31 Chondrosarcoma.

It can sometimes be part of diaphyseal aclasis. Pain, increase in size or interference of local structures is the main reason for excision. Change in size after closure of epiphyses is a warning sign (*Figure 4B.30*).

Other benign bone tumours

These are only seen very occasionally in the hand. They include unicameral bone cyst, aneurysmal bone cyst, chondromyxoid fibroma and osteoid osteoma. Each behaves as elsewhere in the skeleton and is treated along the same lines. Giant cell tumour in the phalanges is extremely uncommon but has a high local recurrence rate and should always be excised.

Malignant bone tumours

Primary malignant bone tumours, such as osteosarcoma or Ewing's tumour, are again very rare in the hand. Histology is difficult. Block excision is undertaken and adjuvant therapy, such as chemotherapy or radiotherapy, should be undertaken in conjunction with oncological support.

Chondrosarcoma

Malignant cartilage tumour can be a primary lesion and was first reported in 1943 by Liechtenstein and Jaffe. There are only 85 cases in the literature. It is more likely to happen in older people. Some (27%) chondrosarcomas are secondary to a benign cartilage lesion. It is very rare, and may never be seen in a single finger enchondroma (0–2%). The malignancy rate in multiple hereditary exostoses, is not agreed

and is variable in the literature (1–25%). Again, the histological grading can be difficult and some just require watching. Local excision by curettage has a high recurrence rate, so block excision is preferable. Overall, there are thought to be 5% metastases from this lesion (*Figure 4B.31*).

Bone metastases

Less than 1% of skeletal metastases occur in the hand; the most common sources are the lung, kidney and breast. They are more commonly seen in the later stages of malignancy. The distal phalanges are the most common site. Bone metastasis can be confused with a benign tumour with infection, but there is usually no periosteal reaction. Treatment is in conjunction with the management of the primary tumour.

Other malignant tumours

Soft tissue tumours of the hand are extremely rare. Rhabdomyosarcoma is a very malignant tumour, but it can respond to block excision and multiple lesion chemotherapy. It has only been recognised in the last 30 years.

Malignant change in benign bony tumours in the hand

Enchondroma

- Solitary: less than 1%
- Multiple: Ollier's; Maffucci; Skeletal
          Varies from 15% (Lewis and Ketcham)

20% (Schajowic)
22% (Mayo Clinic)
32% (Dahlin)
50% (Jaffe)

Osteochondroma

- Solitary: >1% Mayo;   >1% Shajowic
- Multiple: 11% Jaffe;   20% Mayo;   15% Shajowic

HAND GANGLIA

Definition

A ganglion is a mucin-filled cyst usually attached to an underlying synovial cavity of joint or tendon. Histology shows that it can be simple or complex (multiloculated).

The wall consists of compressed collagen and flattened cells with no epithelial or synovial lining. The root consists of interconnecting clefts with a tortuous duct connecting the main cyst to the underlying synovial cavity.

Ganglia contain mucin which is a mixture of glucosamine, albumin, globulin and a high concentration of hyaluronic acid. Sometimes the mucin is blood-stained.

Flexor sheath ganglion

Key facts

The flexor sheath ganglion is the third most common ganglion in the hand after the dorsal wrist and volar radial ganglion. It occurs at the base of the finger and is invariably small (3–8 mm) and tender on compression. Because of its size it is sometimes known as a 'pearl' ganglion.

Clinical features

Examination reveals a tender pea-sized lump at the base of the finger. It is attached to the tendon sheath (*Figure 4B.32*) but does not move with finger flexion, unlike the flexor tendon nodule seen with trigger finger.

Surgery

Consent should include mention of possibility of recurrence (10–20%). Regional or general anaesthetic may be employed. Bier's block anaesthesia is quite

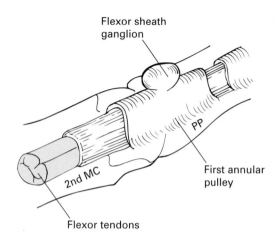

Figure 4B.32 A flexor sheath ganglion arising from the dorsal surface of the first annular pulley. It will not move with digital flexion. MC, metacarpal; PP, proximal phalanx.

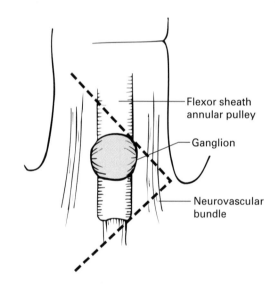

Figure 4B.33 Skin incision used for a flexor sheath ganglion crossing the basal finger crease. The ganglion is removed with an ellipse of annular pulley.

satisfactory. A tourniquet with Esmarch bandage and preferably loupe magnification two to three times should be used. The incision is 'V'-shaped across the basal finger crease (*Figure 4B.33*). Excision, as with any ganglion, should include the root down to the origin, in this case the flexor sheath. Do not suture the hole as this increases the recurrence rate by encouraging more connecting ducts to form from daughter cysts which may be present. This technique of ganglion excision was first described by Angelides and Wallace and is not widely known, even by examiners! A soft dressing may be applied postoperatively.

Mucous cyst

The mucous cyst is a ganglion as an expression of osteoarthritis at the distal interphalangeal (DIP) joint (see page 167).

Key facts

The cyst tends to lie to one side of the extensor tendon or the other. The earliest expression may be ridging of the nail-plate. Heberden's nodes are often present. Radiographs show degenerative change, especially on the lateral view. Symptoms may include recurrent discharge, possibly with infection (*Figure 4B.34*).

Surgery

Consent should include the mention of the possibility of recurrence. This can only be prevented for certain by joint fusion, but most patients do not want to consider this initially, so excision is the normal first line of treatment. Regional anaesthesia (Bier's block) or finger anaesthesia (metacarpal block) with a finger tourniquet may be used. The glove technique can be used for both finger exsanguination and tourniquet; the finger of a sterile surgical glove is placed over the affected finger. The tip of the rubber finger is cut off and rolled down like a condom. This has the purpose of both exsanguination and tourniquet, but avoids the excessively high pressures created by tight red rubber tubing. Remember to place an artery clip on the rubber as the colour is very similar to exsanguinated skin. The tourniquet time should be recorded as in any other surgical procedure.

The incision is difficult, as care must be taken of the germinal matrix of the nail bed that lies beneath the eponychial skin-fold. For this reason it is best to use an 'H' - or 'L' - shaped incision. Involved skin may require elliptical excision. The ganglion cyst is mobilised and traced back to the joint. A bilobed or horseshoe ganglion may grow out around both sides of the extensor tendon. All tissue between the extensor tendon and the

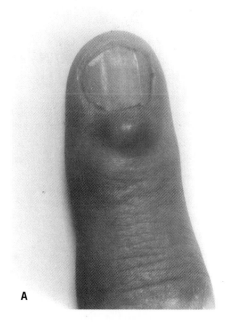

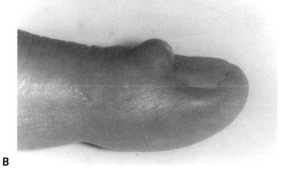

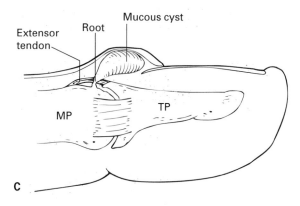

Figure 4B.34 Photographs (a,b) and drawing (c) of a mucous cyst at the distal interphalangeal joint, an expression of osteoarthritis at the distal interphalangeal joint. MP, middle phalanx; TP, terminal phalanx.

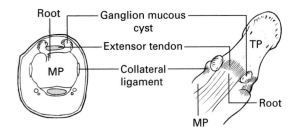

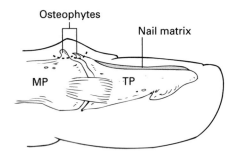

Lateral View (at DIPJ)

Figure 4B.35 Mucous cyst at the distal interphalangeal joint (DIPJ). The cyst may present on both sides of the extensor tendon in a horseshoe manner. Surgery consists of trimming the dorsal osteophytes, and tracing the ganglion root back to the joint. MP, middle phalanx; TP, terminal phalanx.

collateral ligament is removed and osteophytes are trimmed (*Figure 4B.35*). Sometimes a small loose osteophyte can be found close to the joint.

Other hand ganglia

PIP joint ganglia occur between the central slip and the lateral band. Their treatment consists of surgically tracing the root back to the joint according to the Angelides principle.

Extensor tendon ganglia occur on or within the tendons and always move with tendon excursion. They usually occur at the metacarpal level and are well defined, unlike a rheumatoid swelling. The patient may complain of aching or snapping.

Carpometacarpal boss occurs at the base of the second metacarpal. This may be an expression of osteoarthritis at the second carpometacarpal joint, and frequently has

an associated ganglion, which may cause the underlying boss to be overlooked. It is twice as common in women and usually occurs in the third to fourth decade. It is often confused with dorsal wrist ganglion. Surgery is not very successful but consists of excision of the bony spurs with the associated ganglion. Beware of the branches of the superficial radial nerve.

Ganglia can occur at the carpometacarpal joint of the thumb in association with osteoarthritis, over the first dorsal extensor compartment in association with de Quervain's tenosynvaginitis, in the carpal tunnel producing median nerve symptoms, and in Guyon's canal producing ulnar nerve symptoms. Intra-osseous ganglia rarely produce symptoms unless the surrounding sclerosis reaches the articular surface.

INCLUSION DERMOID

This the result of implantation of keratinised skin into the subcutaneous tissue by injury. A cyst forms, lined with squamous epithelium and filled with keratin and cholesterol. The palmar aspect of the hand is a common site and there may be a small scar over the lump. Surgery consists of elliptical excision.

GIANT-CELL TUMOUR OF TENDON SHEATH (PIGMENTED VILLONODULAR SYNOVITIS)

After ganglion this is the second most common tumour found in the hand and a classic favourite with examiners.

This condition is known under a variety of names, none of which is entirely satisfactory. You may find examiners with a strong preference for one of the following:

- giant cell tumour of tendon sheath
- pigmented villonodular synovitis
- benign synovioma
- xanthoma of tendon sheath.

Key facts

Giant-cell tumour of tendon sheath is a benign lesion that possesses the capacity for local recurrence (10–20%). A very rare malignant variant of this tumour has been described. It can occur in adults of any age but is commoner between the ages of 30 and 50 years, and is more frequently seen in women. The tumour develops slowly over a long period of time, and may remain the same size for many years. It must not be confused with its namesake giant-cell tumour of bone, which is different in both behaviour and histology.

Clinical features

There is a well-circumscribed lobulated firm mass, normally situated over the flexor aspect of the finger near a joint but not growing from the joint (*Figure 4B.36*). It is attached to deep structures and does not transilluminate. The skin is normally mobile over the mass, although it may be stretched tight over the dorsal extensor surface at the end of the digit. There may be a brown or orange tinge visible through the skin. Remember to check sensation if the swelling is near a

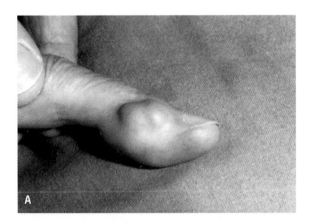

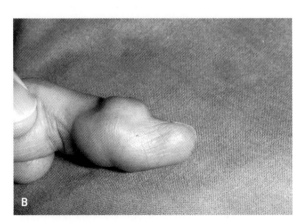

Figure 4B.36 a,b Appearance of giant-cell tumour of tendon sheath. A firm mass fixed to deep tissues.

digital nerve. Radiographs are usually normal; cortical erosion is seen in only a small number.

Types

The commonest type seen in the hand is *localised* and arises from a tendon sheath or adjacent joint. Microscopically there are proliferative spindle fibroblastic cells which are 'bland' (lacking malignant features of nuclear atypia). There are a few multinucleate giant cells, inflammatory cells and xanthoma cells. There is a dense collagenous capsule, but nests of tumour cells can be found outside this. Some examiners may call giant-cell tumour of tendon sheath a 'benign synovioma', as distinct from a synovial sarcoma. This is an unfortunate term as there are few similarities between giant-cell tumours of tendon sheath and synovial sarcomas.

A *diffuse* form of giant cell tumour not seen in the hand occurs in areas adjacent to large weight-bearing joints such as the knee and ankle, either directly connected to the joint or growing from a bursa. Diffuse giant-cell tumour of tendon sheath is synonymous with the extra-articular form of *pigmented villonodular synovitis* (PVNS), but note this does *not* occur in the hand, where the giant cell tumour of tendon sheath is 'localised' (see paragraph above). PVNS normally grows within a joint and is full of haemosiderin and villous synovial hyperplasia.

For a more full explanation see Further Reading and remember tact when attempting to educate a worn out examiner!

Differential diagnosis

- foreign body granuloma
- fibroma of tendon sheath
- fnclusion dermoid
- xanthoma tuberosum (diffuse tendinous deposits seen in patients with familial hyperlipidaemia)
- digital lipoma (rare).

Surgery

Consent should always include mention of recurrence (10–20%). Careful planning of skin incisions is important, particularly if the tumour is large. The tumour is nodular and has deep clefts across its surface. Protection of the digital neurovascular bundle is important, as it

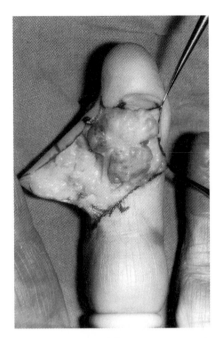

Figure 4B.37 Appearance of the same tumour as in *Figure 4B.36* at operation. Macroscopically there was a golden-brown appearance. Note that the digital nerve in close proximity to the tumour.

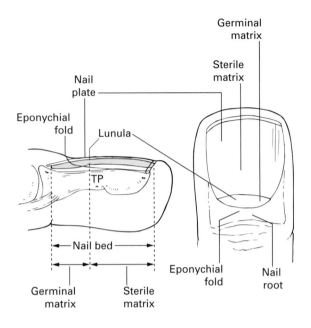

Figure 4B.38 An appreciation of the anatomy of the nail-bed and surrounding structures is vital to understanding the acute and reconstructive treatment options after fingernail injury. TP, terminal phalanx.

frequently lies across the tumour like a rope across a balloon. Macroscopically the mass has a golden-brown appearance (*Figure 4B.37*). Dissection is not difficult as there is normally a well-circumscribed capsule, although sometimes the mass needs to be taken out piecemeal. Tumour tissue may be found extending around the digit, or on the back of the skin. A pressure dressing is usually required to prevent haematoma.

In summary, localised giant cell tumour of tendon sheath occurs in the hand. It is benign and nodular with a surrounding capsule. It shells out easily and is distinct from extra-articular PVNS or diffuse giant-cell tumour of tendon sheath which occurs near a large weight-bearing joint. It is not malignant but hard to excise completely so may recur locally.

FINGERNAIL

Post-traumatic deformities of the fingernail are very difficult to reconstruct. The cosmetic deformity is obvious and, for the female patient especially, the ugliness of a deformed nail is socially distressing. The best way to avoid the problem is correct treatment in the first place. This relies on a sound understanding of the anatomy of the fingernail and surrounding structures matched with an aggressive primary surgical treatment of most nail-bed injuries (*Figure 4B.38*). Finger-tip injuries are common and frequently undertreated in casualty departments, but orthopaedic surgeons seldom pay much attention to the nail either.

The commonest missed injuries are *dorsal proximal dislocation of the nail-plate*, when the lateral skin is torn and the proximal nail-plate avulsed so that it lies on top of the eponychial skin fold. A new nail tries to grow up, but meets resistance resulting in an ugly lumpy deformity. Initially the torn nail-bed should be repaired and replaced under the eponychial fold together with the nail plate.

Untreated *nail-bed injuries involving the germinal matrix* result in scarring of the germinal portion of the nail-bed. Subsequent growth results in a ridged nail or, if the skin of the eponychial fold adheres to the underlying nail-bed at the time of injury, then a skin bridge (*pterygium*) can result in a split nail. Initial treatment consists of suture of the torn nail-bed with some fine dissolvable suture (e.g. 6 Ocatgut) and replacement of the nail-plate back under the eponychial fold. Anchoring sutures are not necessary as sterile Histoacryl glue (sterile 'superglue') is less traumatic and carries no additional risk of tissue damage if used sparingly. If the nail-plate has been lost at the time of the injury then some aluminum foil from the end of a suture packet is quite satisfactory as a temporary stent to prevent a pterygium.

Non-adherence of the new nail occurs when the germinal matrix produces a new nail without difficulty, but the sterile matrix is either deficient or scarred, and has become epithelialised. The nail-plate lifts off and is frequently caught on clothing. This is a difficult problem. In the foot you would recommend obliteration of the germinal matrix with phenol, but in the hand this is not cosmetically acceptable. The only other treatment is a nail-bed graft from the great toe, but these are not always successful and can get infected.

Nail remnants occur after amputation, when there are nests of germinal matrix still producing spicules of nail normally from the corners of the eponychial fold. They are best treated by re-exploration and surgical ablation, or phenol ablation of the germinal nail-bed remnants.

A *hook-nail deformity* occurs when the germinal matrix produces the new nail, which has nothing to grow out onto, as a result of fingertip loss. The fingernail grows right over the fingertip in an unsightly deformity like an animal's claw. Early treatment consists of soft tissue advancement from the volar side in the form of a V-Y Atasoy advancement flap or a reconstruction of the lateral pulp using a Kutler flap. Late reconstruction consists of the *antenna procedure* when most of the curved nail is removed and the pulp and sterile matrix is then split open like a fish's mouth (*Figure 4B.39*). Three small Kirshner wires 'kebab' the pulp in the elevated position and a cross-finger flap is then used to fill in the defect.

Non-traumatic nail deformities are less common than traumatic ones, but infection of the subungual area is the most common of hand infections and frequently fungal in origin.

A *paronychial infection* requires removal of the nail plate for adequate drainage of pus. Removal of only the lateral margin of the nailplate is acceptable if the infection is well localised. Fungal infections require removal of the whole nail plate and topical application of antifungal agents to the nail-bed.

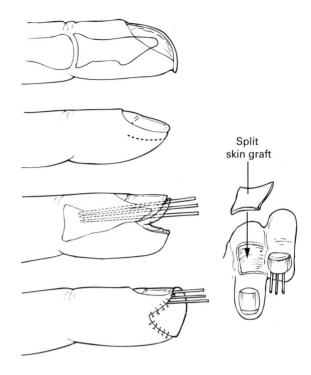

Figure 4B.39 The antenna procedure for hook-nail deformity after Atasoy. The nail-plate is partly removed and the pulp opened like a fish's mouth. Stabilisation with K wires is followed by soft tissue reconstruction with a cross-finger flap.

Pyogenic granuloma is a red elevated collection of granulation tissue. It can arise from the nail when there has been a perforation of the nail plate, usually iatrogenic, and is best treated with topical silver nitrate.

Subungual glomus tumours (Masson's tumours) are unusual. They present as discoloured areas under the sterile matrix, with exquisite tenderness, and have a vascular-neural origin. Excision consists of removal of the nail plate and shelling out the tumour from the surrounding nail-bed.

A *subungual exostosis* is a 'bony diverticulum' from the terminal phalanx and has the typical cartilaginous cap seen with exostoses elsewhere in the body. This elevates the nail plate, with subsequent ridging if the germinal matrix is involved. Excision may be accompanied by nail-bed reconstruction if there is a large defect. *Subungual melanoma* carries an even worse prognosis than melanoma elsewhere in the body. The diagnosis may be delayed as the picture may mimic infection. It is commoner in the thumb or big toe, and in those of fair complexion. Nodal involvement is present in 40% of patients at first presentation. After a biopsy is taken, including sampling of the lymph nodes, then the tumour can be staged before definitive treatment which usually consists of ray amputation.

Most nail deformities can be avoided by correct initial management. A new nail grows in approximately four months in the adult. After a major nerve injury, e.g. median, a transverse ridge can be seen on the growing nail in the territory of that nerve. This is known as Beau's line, and is rather like the rings seen on a cut tree representing its history. In reflex sympathetic dystrophy, nail hypertrophy can occur but the exact neural mechanism by which this happens is poorly understood.

CLINICAL PROBLEM

EXAM SHORT CASE

An 88-year-old right-handed woman presents in outpatients with a seven-year history of an atraumatic painless swelling of the left middle finger (*Figure 4B.40*). There is no history of numbness or past history of gout. She had a previous bilateral mastectomy for carcinoma many years ago. She says that the swelling of the finger has enlarged in the last year.

Question 1. What would you look for in the examination?

Question 2. What investigations would you request?

Question 3. What is your differential diagnosis?

Question 4. What treatment would you recommend?

Answer to question one

1. Local examination, texture (i.e. cystic, firm, etc.), attachment to deep structures, skin adherence, tenderness.
2. Sensation (two-point discrimination) distal to the lesion.
3. Movement, flexor tendon function, grip (whilst doing this it is acceptable to ask the patient how it bothers her).
4. Transillumination: this will tell you whether it is cystic, lipoma or solid.
5. Distant examination: look for lymph nodes in the elbow and axilla. (Ask the patient whether she has any other similar swellings.)

Exam tip

Remember to go at the speed the examiner wants you to; that is, be methodical, explaining why and what you are doing. Move on to the diagnosis if you know it; if not, a safe approach is more important than the right answer. There are always key words that seem to unlock an impasse and bring a smile to the examiner's face. Sometimes finding these is frustrating and difficult for both sides. If you don't understand the question, say so. It is better to say you don't know than to waste point-scoring minutes in silence, but too many 'don't knows' are an admission of defeat! Getting on to the examiner's wavelength is perhaps the most difficult

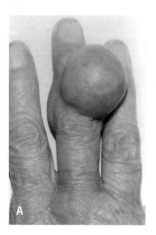
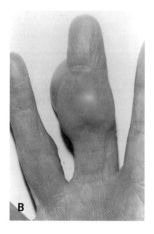
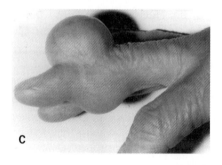

Figure 4B.40 Clinical problem: 88-year-old female with a seven-year history of swelling on the middle finger.

'art' of the viva experience. Some like to go fast, whereas others appear painstakingly slow. Remember the examiner's style is no indication of your performance or score. If the questions are getting difficult he may be impressed and be probing the extent of your knowledge!

Answer to question two

1. Plain radiographs (*Figure 4B.41 a,b*). These are normal and make a secondary deposit unlikely.

2. Bloods: full blood count normal; erythrocyte sedimentation rate 18; alkaline phosphatase 436 (normal); rheumatoid factor <40; serum urate normal. This excludes rheumatoid arthritis, gout, secondary deposit or infection.

3. Magnetic resonance scan (*Figure 4B.41 d,e*). This suggests a fatty lesion, especially seen on the STIR sequence (Short Tan Inversion Recovery sequence).

Answer to question three

The differential diagnosis includes giant cell tumour (although the surface looks too smooth), lipoma, digital fibroma (unlikely on the MRI). There was no tenderness to suggest. Schwannoma, and there are no vascular features. The size suggests a benign process.

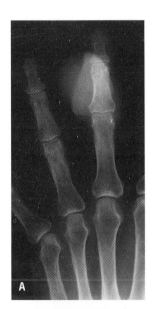
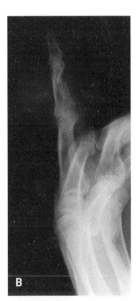
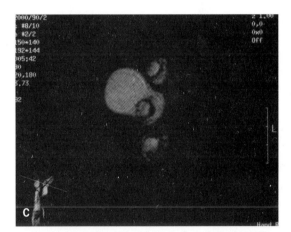
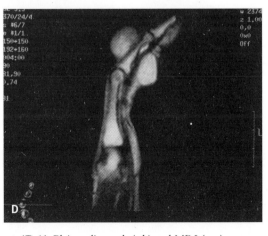
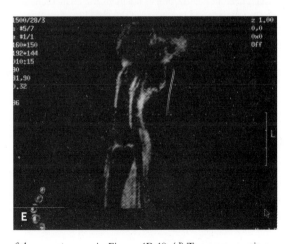

Figure 4B.41 Plain radiograph (a,b) and MRI (c–e) appearance of the same case as in Figure 4B.40. (d) Transverse section showing solid lesion. (e) STIR sequence showing fatty lesion.

Answer to question four

Recommendation; symptoms must be clearly defined, i.e. functional loss, discomfort, cosmesis, fear of cancer. Surgical options include incisional biopsy to establish the diagnosis and excisional biopsy; this would almost certainly carry risk of skin or neurovascular damage and could result in finger amputation which should therefore be mentioned preoperatively. This would probably have to be at a level proximal to the proximal interphalangeal joint and would result in a 'battlement' deformity with adjacent fingers being longer. This makes the holding of small objects difficult, i.e. coins or buttons. Ray amputation is functionally better, but is a bigger operative procedure for an elderly person to withstand. Elective amputation can result in neuroma on the digital nerves and this should be explained in the consent. Primary amputation should not be undertaken without first making a histological diagnosis.

I would recommend incisional biopsy first, and after histological diagnosis, excision via a volar Bruner's incision and dorsal elliptical incision, if the patient was prepared to accept the possibility of amputation through the proximal phalanx if the fingertip was not viable after tourniquet release.

The patient refused surgery!

FURTHER READING

Deformities

Buck-Gramcko D. Pollicization of the index finger: methods and results in aplasia and hypoplasia of thumb. *J Bone Joint Surg* 1971; **53A**: 1605–1617.

Buck-Gramcko D. Radialisation as a new treatment for radial club hand. *J Hand Surg* 1985; **10A**: 964–968.

Dobyns SH, Wood VE, Bayne. Congenital hand deformities. In: Green DP (ed.) *Operative Hand Surgery*, Vol. I. Edinburgh: Churchill Livingstone, 1993; 251–528.

Flatt AE. *The Care of Congenital Hand Anomalies*. St Louis, MO: Quality Medical Publishing, 1994.

Kay SP, Wiberg M, Bellew M, Webb F. Toe to hand transfer in children: functional and psychological aspects. *J Hand Surg* 1996; **21B**(6): 735–745.

Lamb DW, Scott H, Lam WL, Gillespie WJ, Hooper G. Operative correction of radial club hand. *J. Hand Surg* 1997; **22B**(4): 533–536.

Strickland, Kleinman. Thumb reconstruction. In: Green DP (ed.) *Operative Hand Surgery* Vol. II. Edinburgh: Churchill Livingstone 1993: 2043–2156.

Swanson AB, Swanson G de G. A classification for congenital limb malformation. *J Hand Surg* 1983; **8**: 693–702.

Tickle C. Experimental embryology as applied to the upper limb. *J Hand Surg* 1987; **12B**(3): 294–300.

Dupuytren's contracture

Hueston JT. The table top test. *The Hand* 1982; **14**: 100–103.

McCash CR. The open palm technique in Dupuytren's contracture. *Br J Plastic Surg* 1964; **17**: 271–280.

Woodruff MJ, Waldram MA. A clinical grading system for Dupuytren's contracture. *J. Hand Surg.* 1998; **23B**. 303–305.

Tumours

Angelides AC, Wallace PF. The dorsal ganglion of the wrist: its pathogenesis, gross microscopic anatomy and surgical treatment. *J Hand Surg* 1976; **1**: 228–235.

Castelló JR, Garro L, Romero F, Campo M, Nájera A. Metastatic tumours of the hand. *J Hand Surg* 1996; **21B**(4): 547–550.

Enzinger FM, Weiss SW. *Soft Tissue Tumours* St Louis, MO: CV Mosby, 1988: 638–657.

Noble J, Lamb DW. Enchondromata of the bones of the hand. *The Hand* 1974; **6**: 3.

Peimer, Moy, Dick. Tumours of bone and soft tissue. In: Green DP (ed.) *Operative Hand Surgery* Vol II. Edinburgh: Churchill Livingstone, 1993: 2225–2250.

Saunders C, Szabo RM, Mora S. Chondrosarcoma of the hand arising in a young patient with multiple hereditary exostoses. *J Hand Surg* 1997; **22B**(2): 237–242.

Schajowic F (ed.). *Tumours and Tumour-like Lesions of Bone.* Berlin: Springer, 1994.

Tordai P, Hoglund M, Lugnegard H. Is the treatment of enchondroma in the hand by simple curettage a rewarding method? *J Hand Surg* 1990; **15B**(3): 331–334.

Xarchas K, Papavassiliou N, Tsoutseos N, Burke FD. Rhabdomyosarcoma of the hand. *J Hand Surg* 1996; **21B**(3): 325–329.

Fingernail

Atasoy E, Godfrey A, Kalisman M. The "antenna" procedure for the "hook nail" deformity. *J. Hand Surg.* 1983. 8(1): 55–58

Kleinert HE, Putcha SM, Ashbell ST, Kutz JE. The deformed fingernail, a frequent result of failure to repair nail bed injuries. *J Trauma* 1967; **7**: 177–189.

4C

Arthritis in the Hand

Michael Craigen

RHEUMATOID ARTHRITIS

Rheumatoid arthritis is a chronic systemic autoimmune inflammatory disease. The orthopaedic surgeon's involvement in rheumatoid arthritis often represents a minute part of a period of time extending over decades of gradual worsening disability. It is important to remember that patients have often learnt to accommodate their disability long before they seek orthopaedic help, so the surgeon's involvement in their treatment should be specifically aimed at improving disability without believing it is possible to return these patients to a completely normal existence. In fact attempts to do this may only worsen the psychological adjustment to the condition.

Initial involvement with the disease is said to involve the hand in nearly 15% of patients, although it is common for patients to present late to orthopaedic surgeons, as their functional deficit is often less severe than the deformity that is apparent.

PATHOLOGY

Rheumatoid arthritis predominantly affects the synovium. The joint tissue damage is caused by neutrophils that ingest immune complexes and release hydrolytic enzymes, oxygen radicals, thromboxanes, leukotrienes and arachidonic acid metabolites that include prostaglandins. These promote the inflammatory reaction and release of degradative enzymes that damage articular cartilage, ligaments, tendon and bone. The pathological process includes synovial hypertrophy and hyperplasia associated with the proliferation of fibroblasts, small vessels and inflammatory cells which result in pannus

(granulation tissue) formation. This pannus destroys the cartilage by producing collagenase and prostaglandins. The joints are also damaged by increasing joint fluid volume and pressure associated with the mechanical forces applied across the joints. Microscopically this results in swelling around the joints and also of the synovial which surrounds tendons where they pass under retinacula.

CLINICAL COURSE

The disease goes through three stages in its clinical course.

Proliferative phase

This involves the development of acute synovitis that produces warm, swollen, painful joints. There is tendon sheath involvement, often more affecting the extensors than the flexors, and patients in this phase can develop carpal tunnel syndrome and trigger fingers. Treatment in this phase tends to be predominantly medical but sometimes surgical involvement is required if medical treatment fails.

Destructive phase

During this phase, chronic synovitis develops which can often cause irreversible damage to tendons and joints. Joint effusions occur which stretch soft tissues, particularly the ligaments and produce joint instability. There is involvement of the articular surface and the classical deformities start to develop. Tenosynovitis is again a major problem, along with triggering and tendon rupture.

Reparative phase

In this phase there is diminution of the acute synovitis, producing the so-called 'burnt out' type of arthritis. The chronic inflammation is replaced by fibrous tissue and this produces joint ankylosis. There is a decrease in tendon excursion and a tendency for the patient to develop a fixed position, although this is often painless.

The surgeon can be involved at any stage in these three processes but it is common in hand surgery not to see patients until at least the destructive, and often the reparative phase.

PATTERN OF DEFORMITY

In contrast to the weight-bearing joints, the pattern of deformity in the hand and the wrist is very much dependent on the direction of pull of the tendons that cross the joints. There is normally a delicate balance between the flexor and extensor mechanisms. This can be disrupted as a result of damage, particularly to the ligaments supporting the individual joints. Despite the difference from the lower limb, the pattern of deformity occurs in a similar fashion producing the classical zig-zag deformity. This pattern, however, can be either in the coronal or sagittal planes. It is important to remember this zig-zag pattern, as one deformity in a joint is usually mirrored by a deformity in a proximal

or distal joint. For example, deformity in the wrist very much dictates the pattern of deformity in the metacarpophalangeal (MP) joints (*Figure 4C.1*). Failing to deal with the more proximal joint deformity is likely to result in recurrence or persistence of deformity in the joint you are treating.

CLINICAL ASSESSMENT OF THE RHEUMATOID HAND

In the lower limb the major disability associated with arthritis is an inability to bear weight and this is usually directly related to the level of pain in individual joints. However, in the upper limb and particularly in the hand, although pain is an important feature, the maintenance of function of the hand and its associated upper limb is often more important than simple pain relief. Therefore, decisions on treatment must ensure that the function of the hand is at least not compromised by the treatment and preferably it should be improved. In addition, surgeons should not underestimate the cosmetic appearance of the hand; improvement in appearance often influences a patient's decision in favour of surgery and this works in the surgeon's favour when the functional results are not as good as he would like them to be.

Clinical assessment is crucial in deciding what, if any, treatment is appropriate. It is helpful to see the patient

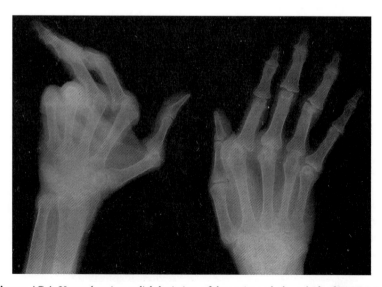

Figure 4C.1 X ray showing radial deviation of the wrist and ulnar drift of MCP joints.

on two occasions before making a definite decision on surgery, though in an exam setting this is obviously not possible. (Rheumatoid patients are commonly shown in examinations as they have multiple joint involvement and stretch the candidates in their clinical and decision-making abilities.)

You should concentrate on assessing how the disease is affecting both the patient and the function of the hand, as well as being certain that the surgery intended should do what both the surgeon and the patient desire. Consideration must be given to the function of other joints in the upper limb that may affect the outcome of the surgery. (For example, surgery to enable a patient to hold a hairbrush may be useless if the patient's shoulder prevents the hand reaching the head).

HISTORY

The three major symptoms complained of by arthritic patients are pain, loss of function and deformity, although patients are often unwilling to admit that the cosmetic appearance of their hand is a significant problem.

Pain

The pain in rheumatoid arthritis of the hand is caused by two main pathological processes.

Synovitis

The synovitis can be either acute or chronic and can often cause severe pain, both in individual joints and in the hand as a whole. This synovitis can also affect the tendons and synovitis at either site can cause loss of motion in the hand. It is important to differentiate which area the pain is coming from, as the presence of synovitis in joints without pain is not unusual. Careful clinical examination can differentiate between synovitis arising from joints and tendon-sheaths and the outward clinical appearances can often differentiate between the acute and chronic forms.

Secondary osteoarthritis

In the reparative or third stage of rheumatoid arthritis joint destruction leads to loss of articular cartilage and causes a condition resembling secondary osteoarthritis. Often these patients have reached the 'burnt out' phase and have little sign of acute synovitis. It is common for patients reaching orthopaedic surgeons to have already developed the secondary osteoarthritic changes, as many rheumatologists persist with medical treatment in the face of continued synovitis. As in idiopathic osteoarthritis, the major clinical feature is pain localised to the joints, which is made worse by activity. The treatment of these joints is rather more predictable as the cause of the related loss of function is reasonably easy to ascertain. The pain in the hand is not quite so characteristically associated with motion as in the lower limb, as the hand particularly can be load-bearing in many relatively minor activities often not associated with motion, such as holding a pen or using a knife and fork.

Loss of function

This is a very personal symptom. Loss of function in the hand can often result from loss of function in a more proximal joint. There is little point in correcting the range of movement and deformity in the MP joint when it is impossible to place the hand in a useful position because of arthritis involving the distal radio-ulnar joint, wrist, elbow and shoulder. Similarly, the loss of function in the hand is not always related to joint involvement; it may be due to tendon synovitis or rupture.

In the exam setting, assessment of loss of function can be quickly performed by a shortened 'activities of daily living' assessment. This involves specific questions about activities such as ability to use a toothbrush, a hairbrush, a knife and fork, problems with dressing (particularly pulling up trousers and underwear and in doing up bra straps and pulling up tights). Questions should also assess the ability to hold small objects such as a cup, and to manipulate fine objects as in writing, operating a remote-control, sewing and knitting. Assessment of function should include asking about activities involving both range of movement, power of movement, precision of movement and sensation. In this way, one can rapidly gain an appreciation of the patient's own assessment of the areas in which they are disabled and therefore the areas to which clinical treatment should be addressed if possible.

Cosmesis

It would be wrong to underestimate the effect of the cosmetic appearance of the hands on the patient's perception of their own disability. The hand is constantly exposed and the deformities associated with rheumatoid arthritis often create significant reactions in 'normal' people. This can cause embarrassment as well as a tendency for the patient to be labelled 'disabled' and treated accordingly. Although patients are unwilling to admit it, often the improved appearance of the hand after surgical treatment is the reason why the patient is satisfied with the result. Although in the clinical assessment the cosmetic appearance must be secondary to the symptoms of pain and loss of function, concurrent surgical treatment of rheumatoid nodules, the correction of swollen joints and removal of extensive synovitis can often have significantly beneficial effects.

EXAMINATION

Examination of the rheumatoid patient can at first seem overwhelming because of the number of joints affected by the disease. Assessing which areas of the hand are causing the most disability often seems quite daunting.

Because of this, there is a temptation to rush ahead and start to examine individual joints because of the lack of time. However, a lot of information can be gained merely by looking at the natural posture of the patient's hand and this can be done while taking the history. This observation must be performed in a systematic fashion. It is also important to reiterate that the examination of the rheumatoid hand should include the examination of the wrist, elbow and shoulder. Particular attention should be paid to the wrist and also to the function of the distal radio-ulnar joint, especially in supination. The examination should, as in all situations, be divided into the 'look, feel, move' method popularised by Apley.

Look

The classical appearance of the rheumatoid hand is of a rather swollen wrist, probably in radial deviation with a prominent distal ulna, the MP joints in ulnar deviation and the thumb in some form of zig-zag deformity, either in the coronal or sagittal planes. The PIP joints may be in either a swan-neck or boutonnière type deformity. It should be possible to see if the long extensor tendons are ruptured by the appearance of drooping fingers at the MP joint, though severe ulnar deviation at the MP joint can give a similar appearance. The history should help in differentiating these two possibilities. Looking at the flexor aspect of the wrist usually provides less information, although the appearance of swelling proximal to the distal wrist crease might suggest the presence of flexor tenosynovitis. Wasting of the thenar eminence should routinely be looked for, as carpal tunnel syndrome is a common abnormality in rheumatoid arthritis. Although flexor tendon rupture is less common, it may often be apparent by the posture of the finger, as with a cut tendon.

Other features include the presence of rheumatoid nodules, and signs of other inflammatory arthritides such as the nails and psoriatic plaques in psoriasis, calcific deposits or gouty tophi and skin changes in scleroderma and systemic lupus erythematosus (SLE).

Feel

Palpation of the rheumatoid hand can often differentiate synovitis from joint effusions, and indicate whether synovitis is acute or chronic. The consistency of rheumatoid nodules, as well as their site, usually differentiates them from other diagnoses.

Sensation should be checked routinely.

It is also important to assess the stability of joints, particularly in psoriatic arthritis and SLE. In rheumatoid arthritis the ulnar collateral ligament of the MP joint of the thumb is often lax. The absence of ligamentous support to joints will usually preclude arthroplasty as a method of treatment.

The passive correctability of deformed joints should also be assessed, as it is often a guide as to whether soft-tissue surgical procedures are likely to be successful. This correctability must be tested with the ligaments in maximum tightness (with the MP joints this is in flexion).

Move

A combination of joint and tendon disease makes assessment of movement in the hand difficult. It is quite common to find individual joints affected by both tendon disease and joint disease, as in a long-term flexor tenosynovitis resulting in secondary proximal interphalangeal joint contractures.

It is usually easier at this stage to get the patient to try to extend all joints fully, to flex all joints fully and to oppose the thumb fully to get a general impression of the range of movement of the individual joints. It is more common for the MP joints to lose extension and the PIP joints to lose flexion.

As the tendons are often forgotten, it is probably helpful to assess their function first. The flexors should be assessed in standard fashion and the extensors carefully assessed to ensure that any extensor lag is caused by extensor tendon damage rather than subluxation of the extensor tendons into the ulnar gutters. Tightness in the intrinsic muscles is common in rheumatoid arthritis and is assessed by maintaining the MP joint in full extension and assessing whether full flexion of the PIP joint is possible: the so-called intrinsic tightness or Bunnell's test (*Figure 6.2* on page 195). If the MP joint is deformed, this test should be performed with the joint in both deformed and corrected positions to assess both the ulnar and radial intrinsics. Loss of flexion may be due to flexor tenosynovitis or possibly a locked trigger finger distal to the A2 pulley. Similarly inability to extend at the PIP joint may be caused by the same pathology. Assessment of joint movement is reasonably straightforward in a passive fashion although inability to extend the PIP joint can be due to tendon pathology.

CLINICAL FEATURES OF OTHER INFLAMMATORY ARTHRITIDES

The most important other arthritides to consider in these patients are gout, SLE, systemic sclerosis (scleroderma) and psoriatic arthritis.

In gout, the distal interphalangeal (DIP) joints are usually affected and the classical tophi are seen. (These should not be confused with mucus cysts associated with osteoarthritis at the DIP joint.) However, gout can also affect other joints, producing a similar acute synovitis to that in rheumatoid arthritis (*Figure 4C.2*).

In SLE, the ligamentous laxity is the major pathology, often with radiological preservation of joint surfaces.

In psoriatic arthritis, considerable destruction of joints can occur, particularly of the DIP and PIP joints, producing gross multi-directional instability but with significant radiological changes.

In scleroderma, the arthritis is often similar to that in rheumatoid arthritis but the deposition of calcium

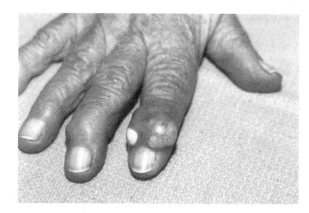

Figure 4C.2 Gouty tophi in DIP joints.

within the skin helps to make the diagnosis. The skin in these patients is often very tight and it is unlikely that the range of movement will be greatly improved by surgery due to soft tissue contractures, rather than due to any failure of the surgical procedure. Specific features in individual joints will be considered under each joint.

GENERAL MEDICAL ASSESSMENT

In the FRCS Orth examination, a patient seen as a long case may be assumed to be under consideration for surgery; thus a general physical examination should at least be contemplated, even if you have not enough time to do it. In rheumatoid arthritis, where multi-system disease is common, specific attention should be paid to the cervical spine and the temporo-mandibular joint (both of which may compromise intubation) and any pulmonary involvement. Restriction in movement of the upper limb should also be recorded to prevent injury while establishing venous access.

If possible, patients with SLE should be identified and this can often be done from the classical ligamentous laxity associated with this condition.

INVESTIGATIONS

Patients with rheumatoid arthritis require a full medical work-up, first to confirm the diagnosis and second to ensure that other systems are not affected either by the disease or the treatment.

Medical assessment of inflammatory arthritis should, from a surgeon's point of view be used predominantly to ensure the correct diagnosis, particularly in differentiating rheumatoid arthritis from SLE, gout and psoriatic arthopathies as the pathology and destructive changes are often very different and the results of surgery also vary.

In principle, all patients should have radiographs taken of the joints affected. Don't be tempted to ask for 'hand' radiographs as these often fail to visualise the PIP and DIP joint spaces; specify which joints you are interested in.

Before surgery, the white cell count (which can be reduced in Felty's syndrome), platelet count (which can be reduced with non-steroidal anti-inflammatory drugs) and liver function tests (which can be affected by methotrexate) should be measured. If appropriate, radiographs should be taken of the cervical spine.

When other joints of the upper limb are involved it is often helpful to have a formal activities-of-daily-living (ADL) assessment by an experienced hand or occupational therapist as a way of assessing which joints are causing the most disability. Other more specific tests for the hand include the Jebson test which uses various different activities to assess hand function. These include seven sub-tests:

1. writing
2. turning over 3 × 5-inch cards
3. picking up common small objects
4. simulated feeding
5. stacking chequers (draughts)
6. picking up large light objects
7. picking up large heavy objects.

Another well-established test for neurological function is Moberg's pick-up test, which measures the speed with which certain small common objects, such as coins and paper-clips, can be picked up. These types of test take a long time and are really only suitable outside the out-patient clinic and examination hall. They are often performed by therapists as part of an ADL assessment.

PLANNING TREATMENT

The planning of treatment in the rheumatoid patient is extremely complex. Decision-making requires consideration of the way the disease is affecting the patient as a whole and also careful assessment of the level of disability that an individual joint or set of joints is causing. There are several different methods of making this decision simpler, but it is finally up to the individual surgeon to develop a degree of experience and a feel for the assessment of these patients. Souter has produced a useful and reliable method of deciding what should be treated and when treatment should be performed. It may be helpful to stage the disease. This has been done in several different ways; one of the more useful is shown in *Table 4C.1*.

There are some specific classifications, such as Nalebuff's classification of the thumb and of swan neck and boutonnière deformity, that are useful in deciding treatment of these individual problems. These are considered below.

The goals of treatment should be:

- pain relief
- improvement in function
- prevention of further damage
- cosmesis.

In general, drug treatment is used in the first instance and especially for patients who are multiple acute inflammatory involvement with severe synovitis, swelling and pain of an acute or chronic nature. Once joint damage starts to occur, the role of drugs is merely in controlling pain and possibly preventing progression of disease.

If surgery is contemplated, the more proximal joints should generally be operated on before more distal joints, and tendons should be dealt with before joints. This enables mobilisation to its fullest extent by daily

Table 4C.1 Staging of rheumatoid arthritis

Stage	Clinical findings	Treatment
I	Early or acute synovitis	Non-operative medical management/splinting
II	Persistent acute or chronic synovitis	Synovectomy
III	Specific deformation	Reconstructive
IV	Severe crippling	Salvage

use and prevents joints becoming stiff because it is impossible to move them.

FLEXOR TENOSYNOVITIS

Before considering the joint deformities and malfunctions that are so common and so problematical, it is important to consider the pathological changes that are often difficult to diagnose but yet vital to the results of treatment of the more obvious deformities. Tenosynovitis is the hallmark of the rheumatoid hand, but the most obvious site on the extensor part of the wrist often distracts the examining surgeon from the flexor side of the wrist and 'more importantly' the flexor side of the hand.

Symptoms

Flexor tenosynovitis, if present in the carpal tunnel, can cause carpal tunnel syndrome and overall loss of finger motion.

In the palm and the fingers it can cause slightly less atypical clinical presentations such as triggering, loss of active finger flexion or passive finger extension. Sometimes loss of passive finger flexion can mislead the surgeon into thinking that the joints are the cause of loss of function rather than the tendons.

Inevitably flexor tenosynovitis can coexist with any related joint problems in the hand. Therefore the clinical presentation can often be obscured and not typical of acute tenosynovitis.

Examination

As the assessment for the presence of flexor tenosynovitis is difficult, it is vital that it is carried out carefully. It is standard practice to look for the presence of carpal tunnel syndrome, although often clinical tests such as Phalen's test are difficult to perform because of the arthritic joints. When in doubt, nerve conduction tests are useful. The presence of carpal tunnel syndrome, or at least its symptoms, must lead the surgeon to consider the presence of flexor tenosynovitis.

Examining the tendon function is more difficult. For example swan-neck deformities can often be due to an isolated rupture of the flexor digitorum superficialis.

Examination should proceed in the normal fashion of look, feel and move.

Look

Observe the overall posture of the hand, looking particularly for evidence that tendon ruptures may have occurred and the presence of isolated swan-neck deformities. The shape of the fingers should also be closely examined, as significant swelling over the volar side is sometimes a little difficult to see. The flexor aspect of the fingers can appear bulky due to chronic synovitis. As in all examinations, the other hand, if relatively unaffected, can be used for comparison.

Feel

Palpation is also equally important in this aspect of rheumatoid disease. A thickened sensation around the distal palmar crease area at the entrance to the A1 pulleys may indicate the presence of synovitis and the rather puffy thick feel to the rheumatoid hand is a strong indicator of the presence of such pathology. Similarly palpation of the fingers may also indicate the presence of nodules or again diffuse synovitis. Normally you can pinch, between your own finger and thumb, two thicknesses of skin in front of the patient's proximal phalanx. Thickened tenosynovium bulges out through defects in the fibrous sheath and creates a wodge of tissue instead. (This is sometimes called the pinch test.) At the wrist, swelling is often found proximal to the carpal tunnel in the distal forearm indicating synovitis: again the other side can be used for comparison for this purpose.

Move

Examination of the tendon function should be performed in the standard fashion for both FDS and FDP. Do not assume that inability to flex the finger at the DIP joint is due to tendon rupture; this can be caused by adherence of FDP to FDS and therefore the natural posture of the hand is often a guide as to whether the tendon is intact or merely adherent.

As the fingers are moved, the area of both the entrance to the A1 pulley and around the A2 pulley area should be palpated for nodules which might be causing triggering. These can lock the finger in flexion or sometimes in extension if it lies distal to the A2 pulley. Finally, on moving the joint you may often feel crepitation over the tendons which may again indicate the presence of tenosynovitis.

The most common flexor tendons to rupture following flexor tenosynovitis are FPL and the index finger FDP. Function of these can be tested for by asking the patient to pinch, which is normally done tip-to-tip, but in the presence of a ruptured FDP to the index, or FPL to the thumb, the pinch becomes pulp to pulp.★ (This, however, can also indicate the presence of an anterior interosseous nerve compression and if there are potential signs of this it may be better to do nerve conduction tests first.)

Treatment

Conservative

Sometimes, in the acute phase splintage and medical treatment (such as non-steroidal anti-inflammatory drugs or steroids) can be used successfully. However, it is unkind to the patient to persist with such treatment if the flexor tenosynovitis is quite obviously affecting the function of the hand. Steroid injections into the carpal tunnel or into the fingers can also be used, but these should be reserved for the acute phase rather than for chronic tenosynovitis.

Stanley has stated that if chronic synovitis has been present for more than four months or if conservative treatment fails to resolve it within such a period, it is probably better to proceed to surgery. In general, when in doubt it is better to perform a tenosynovectomy to prevent flexor tendon rupture rather than to persist with medical treatment.

The presence of tendon rupture is an absolute indication for surgery.

Surgery

Synovectomy. Synovectomy is the most effective form of treatment for acute flexor tenosynovitis. Notwithstanding the beneficial effect of synovectomy on tendon (and thus hand) function, if consideration is being given

to joint surgery then it is crucial to ensure that the flexor tendons are running freely. This is particularly the case at the MP joint but also at the PIP joint. Failure to attend to the flexor tendons is likely to result in poor function following surgery to both MP and PIP joints.

Flexor tenosynovectomies should not just be restricted to the carpal tunnel. The three main sites for surgery are likely to be the carpal tunnel, the palm at the level of the mouth of the A1 pulley, and the fingers at the level of the PIP joint just distal to the A2 pulley. The surgeon should be prepared to open all three sites, although in general I tend to start either in the carpal tunnel or at the distal palm depending on the most likely site of the synovitis. This is decided by the site of the swelling and the presence or absence of carpal tunnel syndrome.

Assuming that surgery is instigated in the palm, a zig-zag incision is made at the distal palmar crease level and the flexor tendons identified at the mouth of the A1 pulley (*Figure 4C.3*). Using a blunt hook, the

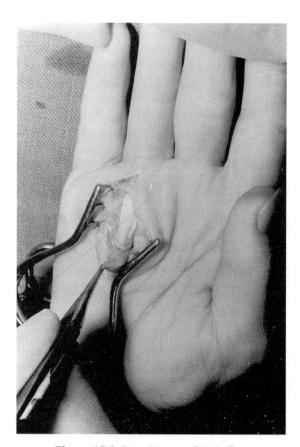

Figure 4C.3 Synovitis around A1 Pulley.

★ Confusingly, this may also be called the pinch test; in this case the pinching is done by the patient rather than the doctor.

tendons should be retracted and full synovectomy performed both proximally and distally. At this level the FDP and FDS tendons should be drawn simultaneously in opposite directions in order to break down any adhesions between the two sets of tendons; sometimes these can be quite dense adhesions and may need to be divided surgically, although some surgeons have recommended excision of the FDS if these adhesions are severe.

If it appears obvious that there is tenosynovitis both proximally and distally, additional incisions may need to be made in the fingers distally and in the carpal tunnel proximally. It is essential that you should be able to demonstrate at the time of surgery full extension and full flexion when pulling on the tendons either in the carpal tunnel or in the palm.

Some surgeons will then continue with other procedures such as MP arthroplasties at the same sitting; most will mobilise the hand first and proceed to other surgery when full movement is achieved. The problem with both courses is that sometimes the mobilisation needs of the flexor tenosynovectomy are different from the needs of the joint surgery and these decisions need to be made in individual cases.

Tendon rupture. Tendon rupture is an absolute indication for surgical intervention in flexor tenosynovitis. It is sometimes difficult to diagnose tendon rupture, particularly if it is an isolated superficialis tendon or if there is extensive joint disease as well as tendon inflammation. The commonest tendons to rupture are the profundus tendons, particularly the ones on the radial side where there is often a bony spur from the scaphoid that can cause an attrition rupture. Surgical treatment of tendon ruptures inevitably requires tenosynovectomy in the first instance but the treatment of the rupture is often difficult. The options include the following.

Primary tendon repair. This is rarely if ever indicated in rheumatoid arthritis, as the tendon ends are usually ragged and inflamed and the tissue inappropriate for primary repair.

Primary tendon graft. The passage of a long flexor tendon graft is fraught with considerable difficulties, as the graft is being expected to pick up its blood-supply from diseased and inflamed synovium and bare bone around it. For this reason tendon grafts in rheumatoid arthritis have poor results, although in a young patient they

should at least be considered. However, bridging small defects in tendons with tendon grafts can be effective, though this is usually only helpful in the carpal tunnel or palm where there is more room for bulky repairs.

Tendon transfer. Unlike the extensor aspect, there is a limited number of tendon transfers available. Brachioradialis and palmaris longus have been used but the results are quite variable. In the thumb it might be possible to use one of the abductors but this is probably not very suitable in elderly patients, as an extensor tendon is used to replace a flexor.

Side-to-side suture. This is particularly good in older patients, in whom side-to-side suture seems to produce excellent function, bearing in mind the severity of the disease. Obviously the more flexors that are involved the less suitable this is, but certainly this should be considered for ruptures at the wrist level.

Arthrodesis. Fusion of the DIP joint is particularly good, especially in elderly patients with a ruptured profundus but an intact superficialis. When both profundus and superficialis tendons are ruptured, it may be appropriate to fuse the DIP joint and reconstitute the superficialis rather than expect the longer excursion of the profundus to work. This is particularly useful in the index finger where stability for pinch grip is more important than full flexion for power grip.

Summary of operative options. In tendon rupture there are many choices available and it is up to the surgeon to apply whichever seems the most appropriate in the individual situation. The operation should be tailored to the patient and the severity of his or her disease, as well as to the extent of the rupture and the quality of the tendons left behind. The severity of the joint disease governs how effective tendon surgery for rupture can be. It must be emphasised that full synovectomy should be performed simultaneously with any tendon repairs as re-ruptures are not uncommon. (Extensor tenosynovitis is covered in Chapter 3 on pages 84–86).

THE METACARPOPHALANGEAL JOINTS

The metacarpophalangeal joints are probably the most common joints in the hand to be affected by rheumatoid arthritis. Initially the synovitis causes stretching of the soft tissues, which can affect the extensor hood, the collateral ligaments and the volar plate, and indirectly can be responsible for the development of the classical ulnar drift noted in this condition (*Figure 4C.4*). Several theories are put forward as to the cause of the ulnar drift and it is likely that all these factors have a role in the production of the deformity.

- The tendency of the wrist to go into radial deviation. As the extensors and the flexors of the fingers cross both joints and approach the MP joints from a slightly ulnar direction, there is an ulnar deviation applied by both the flexor and extensor mechanisms. The combination of this with the weakness of the collateral ligaments results in gradual drifting of the fingers to the ulnar side.
- A similar pathological process causes weakening of the volar plate and the collateral ligament stabilisation of the flexor sheath and A2 pulley, thus allowing ulnar deviation of the flexor tendon pull which exacerbates the drift.
- Stretching of the extensor mechanism by the synovitis can cause the extensor mechanism to sublux to the ulnar side, again making the deforming force increase. The laxity of the collateral ligaments as a result of the synovitis allows this deforming force to have further effect.
- Erosion of the metacarpal heads underneath the insertion of the collateral ligaments on the radial side

removes the tensioning effect of the shape of the metacarpal head on the radial collateral ligament, allowing it to sublux into a synovitic hole which allows increasing deformity with reducing resistance.

Thus over a period of time the ulnar drift can gradually increase and once commenced it is almost impossible to stop without surgical intervention. Over a period of time the extensor mechanism subluxes into the gutter between the MP joints making the problem worse. At the same time the ulnar collateral ligament becomes scarred and tightens, as does the interosseous muscle on the ulnar side of the joint. At this stage passive correction of the joint is almost impossible, thus making splintage ineffective.

Symptoms

Patients with rheumatoid arthritis often have severe deformity in the MP joint, but the function of the hand remains relatively good. The ulnar drift and subluxation of the extensor tendon does result in loss of active extension at the MP joints which can become quite severe, but there is rarely loss of flexion in the joint as the strength of the flexors overcomes the extensors. The loss of mechanical advantage in the extensors due to ulnar subluxation helps the flexion, although often this can result in volar subluxation of the base of the proximal phalanx.

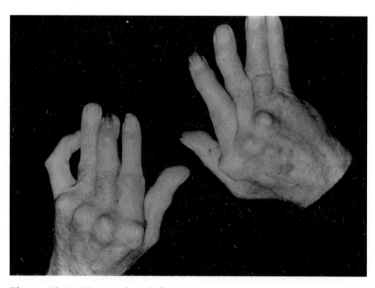

Figure 4C.4 MP joint ulnar drift.

Patients will tend to present with three main problems.

1. The deformity of the hand. There is reasonably strong anecdotal evidence that the patient's satisfaction with surgery to the MP joints may be directly related to the cosmetic improvement following surgery. The patient's concern with the cosmetic appearance of the hands should not be underestimated.
2. Pain. This is usually due either to the chronic synovitis which has been unresponsive to medical treatment or, more commonly, to significant damage to the joints resulting in effectively a secondary osteoarthritic process. Not surprisingly this pain tends to be worse on movement, although if only due to synovitis it can be quite severe at rest as well.
3. Loss of function. The commonest problem here is inability to extend the MP joint sufficiently to open the hand to receive any large articles. The ability to flex the MP joints is rarely lost, although often disease in the PIP and DIP joints can affect finger function.

To decide which (MP, PIP or DIP) joint dysfunction is causing symptoms, it is useful to have a collection of items of everyday nature of varying sizes which patients can be asked to manipulate so that their function can be observed and the particular problems identified more clearly. In the exam setting, a pen and coin can serve a similar purpose without using too much time.

Examination

Having decided that the indications for treatment are fulfilled on the history, there are certain factors within the examination that need to be emphasised as this significantly affects what treatment can be offered. As in the examination of all joints, assessments of other joints in the hand, particularly the PIP and DIP joints, should be made, as well as the function of the wrist joint.

In the MP joints certain features require specific assessment.

1. The passive range of movement at the MP joints and whether lifting these joints into greater dorsiflexion than the patient can actively achieve produces significant pain.
2. The ability to passively correct the ulnar drift. If the ulnar drift is not correctable, then only surgical treatment will correct the deformity.

3. Whether the MP joints can be actively extended if the ulnar drift is corrected passively.
4. The presence of synovial swelling around the MP joints. It is important to differentiate synovial swelling from merely a prominent metacarpal head due to volar subluxation of the volar phalanx.
5. The ability to reduce the volar subluxation if present.
6. The presence of intrinsic tightness, tested by passively extending the MP joint and then assessing whether the PIP joint can fully flex without resistance (*Figure 6.2* on page 195). It is important to ensure that the PIP joint itself has normal range of movement before assuming this test is positive.
7. The integrity of the flexor and extensor tendons, particularly checking the extensor mechanism at the wrist and the flexor tendons in their synovial sheath and in the carpal tunnel. The presence of extensive tenosynovitis requires simultaneous or prior treatment to MP joint surgery or stiffness will recur due to inability to mobilise the joints.
8. All patients should be assessed for the presence of carpal tunnel syndrome.

Investigations

Radiographs of the MP joints are vital in deciding what types of treatment are likely to be useful (*Figure 4C.5*). If this is an early presentation, then assessment of the overall rheumatoid status and referral to a rheumatologist may be indicated. Radiographs will tell you how badly destroyed the MP joints are and can particularly show the degree of volar subluxation, erosion of the base of the proximal phalanx and ulnar drift. All these factors may make surgery technically more difficult.

Treatment

As in all arthritic joints, treatment can be divided into medical treatment, splintage surgery or a combination of all three.

Medical treatment

Medical treatment is certainly appropriate in the acute and to a lesser extent the chronic synovitic stage in rheumatoid disease, particularly when there is multiple joint involvement throughout the body. It is in some

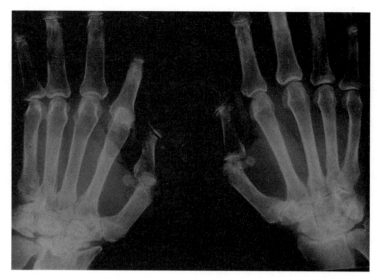

Figure 4C.5 X-ray showing MP joint disease.

ways unfortunate that there is a tendency among rheumatologists to persist with medical treatment when it is obviously failing to prevent progression of the disease. However, this may, to some extent, be realistic in that surgical treatment does have an uncertain outlook.

Splintage

Splintage is useful in the early stages of ulnar drift. It will not correct the deformity, but merely prevent its progression, although it does help to place the fingers in a more functional position for use. However, the splints are often bulky and are commonly unacceptable to the patients. Correcting the ulnar drift by night splintage is tolerated better and may be effective in preventing progression. Splintage can be combined with medical treatment in the acute synovitic phase to protect the soft tissues, particularly the collateral ligaments and volar plate, from further unnecessary stretching.

Therapists can also educate patients to avoid unnecessary stress on the MP joints (so-called joint protection methods). For example when unscrewing a jar by right-handed patients there is a significant ulnar deviating force applied to the MP joints and patients have to be taught to prevent this. Unnecessary power pinching of thumb to index finger may also worsen the problem or possibly precipitate it.

Surgical treatment

Unfortunately, the commencement of ulnar drift is merely the start of a slippery slope. A small amount of deformity causes ulnar displacement of the pull of the flexors and extensors, thus causing extra stress on the joint in an ulnar direction, and making the deformity worse.

The decision on what type of surgery is indicated depends entirely on the presenting complaint of the patient and the state of the MP joints. The presence of deformity without significant pain or loss of function is an area of some contention, although there is some reasonable evidence to suggest that at some stage surgery is likely to be required in patients with even quite early features of ulnar drift.

Flatt maintains that the presence of even a small amount of ulnar deviation radiologically at the MP joint with ulnar subluxation at the base of the proximal phalanx indicates that ulnar drift deformity is an inevitable sequel. However, it is impossible to predict the time-scale in which this will occur. This justifies recommending some sort of stabilisation procedure in patients with ulnar drift, but it is sometimes difficult to persuade both the rheumatologist to refer the patients, and the patients to undergo what is quite major surgery in order to prevent a potential problem in the future. The other conundrum is that patients with severe ulnar drift often have quite satisfactory function and do not feel their symptoms justify surgery. The main operative techniques fall into three main categories:

1. soft tissue balancing
2. synovectomy
3. MP arthroplasty

Soft tissue balancing. It is reasonable in those patients with minimal synovitis, but with ulnar drift, to suggest rebalancing the MP joints as a means of preventing further deformity. Some patients with ulnar drift do have significant symptoms despite little or no destructive changes on radiography. However, there is no guarantee that progression will occur at a particular rate or that symptoms will become serious in the future, which makes it slightly more difficult to sell the suggested procedure to the patient. Prior to deciding whether to proceed with surgery it is vital to ascertain what structures are tight, particularly assessing both the radial and ulnar intrinsic muscles by testing in both ulnar deviation and radial deviation.

Surgery, as in all approaches to the MP joint, can be performed either through longitudinal incisions over each joint or a single transverse incision approximately 1 cm proximal to the metacarpal heads. The extensor hood has been approached in three different ways and candidates should be aware of the different reasons given for the different types of approach.

- Flatt describes a radial incision, with mobilisation of the radial interosseous of the index finger which allows the hood to be reefed on the radial side to prevent recurrence of the drift and then further repair of the extensor mechanism in order to centralise the extensor hood. This is certainly reasonable in the early stages, but in later stages the extensor hood is very thin and there is little to re-attach the extensor tendon to.
- Others describe a central split in the extensor mechanism, providing better tissue to suture and allowing a double-breasting repair to centralise the tendon. This is the technique that I personally use, as the quality of the tissues is pretty good even in the most severe deformities.
- Others divide the ulnar side of the extensor mechanism (*Figure 4C.6*), thus freeing up the extensor mechanism and allowing it to sit more dorsally. This prevents the ulnar tightness of the extensor hood pulling the extensor tendon into

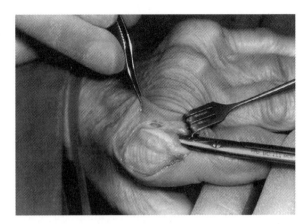

Figure 4C.6 Approach to MP joint.

the gutter between the MP joints. The only problem that I have had with this technique is that, if simple release fails to centralise the tendon, then it becomes very difficult to hold the tendon in the mid-line and prevent further ulnar subluxation.

Having divided the extensor mechanism a plane is developed between that and the capsule and the capsule is then either opened longitudinally, which I favour, or transversely to inspect the joint and perform any synovectomy that may be necessary. At this stage the ulnar intrinsic should be released by dividing it under direct vision, level with the joint on the ulnar side where it is separate from the extensor hood. It is then important to assess whether the joint can be corrected without release of the ulnar collateral ligament. The patients that I see usually have more severe deformity and therefore usually require release of the ulnar collateral ligament.

Having obtained correction of the joint, it is then necessary to maintain this correction. Several different techniques have been described to achieve this:

- reefing of the extensor mechanism;
- use of an ulnar strip of extensor mechanism based proximally, which is passed through the radial capsule and then reefed onto itself or passed through the dorsal cortex at the base of the proximal phalanx;
- reinforcement of the radial collateral ligament, as in MP joint replacement, by detachment of the radial collateral ligament and re-attachment into drill holes on the radial side of the metacarpal;
- crossed intrinsic transfer.

Crossed intrinsic transfer is an attractive solution which utilises the divided ulnar interosseous to reinforce the radial side of the finger next to it. Thus the ulnar interosseous of the index finger is used to reinforce the middle and so on. Inevitably this leaves the index finger without protection, but the first dorsal interosseous can be advanced more dorsally into the extensor mechanism and reefed, to provide a similar effect. There are advantages and disadvantages of inserting the intrinsic transfer either into the radial collateral ligament of the adjacent joint or into the lateral band of the adjacent joint. Although insertion into the lateral band does provide a greater mechanical advantage to the correction, there are concerns that crossed intrinsic transfer can cause later development of swan neck deformity. The results of Straub would confirm this, the swan-neck deformity often occurring several years after the crossed intrinsic transfer. As a result, many others have recommended transferring the intrinsic, not to the lateral band, but into the radial collateral ligament of the adjacent joint.

One report of a long-term review of crossed intrinsic transfer with an average follow-up of 12.7 years, showed reasonably well that the operation does prevent progression of ulnar drift despite progression of the systemic disease. Various examples are quoted of unilateral surgery to support this.

Synovectomy. Synovectomy for rheumatoid arthritis is not a curative procedure. For this reason many surgeons have become disenchanted with it, and although there is some anecdotal evidence that it does arrest local disease or at least slow progression of the disease, there are no controlled trials to support this. These anecdotes may falsely attribute improvement to surgery, in that 30–50% of patients with rheumatoid arthritis will have spontaneous remission.

Some surgeons recommend a period of six to nine months of conservative treatment prior to performing synovectomy. However, others feel that the speed at which the MP joint can deteriorate is such that even time on the waiting-list for operation may lose the opportunity for surgically-useful synovectomy. The presence of pain with intermittent swelling uncontrolled by medical treatment or permanent swelling is likely to be the best indication for synovectomy. It may be that with intermittent symptoms medical treatment in the form of local injections may help the

situation. The author's only experience of this method is in using steroid injections and in these situations multiple steroid injections might suppress the synovitis to some extent. Chemical synovectomy has been performed using various materials such as thiotepa or nitrogen mustard. The author has no personal experience of these materials but they are said to produce some suppression of synovitis, although this may only be temporary.

Assessment of the degree of joint destruction is always difficult and radiographs rarely reflect the degree of joint damage found at surgery. The degree of synovial erosion can often be seen more clearly using the Brewerton radiographic projection, in which the MP joints are flexed 65° and the tube is angled 15° to the ulnar side of the hand. This throws the area of insertion of the collateral ligaments into profile and may show erosions around these insertions characteristic of an aggressive synovial infiltration.

In general the patient's symptoms govern the surgery required. Usually some deformity is present in patients requiring synovectomy, so you should be prepared to perform soft-tissue releases, along with the synovectomy. The incision and approach for this procedure is the same as above (*Figure 4C.7*). A particular area to look for synovial infiltration is just distal to the collateral ligaments in the metacarpal head. There are often little pockets of very aggressive synovitis that can rapidly cause severe soft-tissue damage and thus deformity; these can be curetted out. In addition the area proximally on the volar side of the metacarpal head, beneath the volar plate, may also hide a significant pocket of

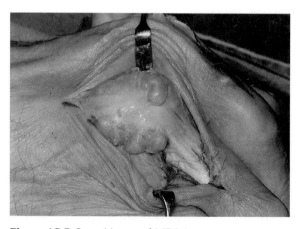

Figure 4C.7 Synovitis around MP joint.

synovial tissue. Flatt claims that at least 80% of the total synovial tissue requires to be excised. He states that if 40% of the synovial lining of the joint remains, this is capable of producing recurrence of the synovitis which is enough to cause persistent joint destruction.

It is unrealistic to expect a 100% synovectomy, which is why recurrence does occur following this operation. Flatt reviewed 67 patients receiving synovectomy for multiple joints over a ten-year period and found that the chances of recurrence directly related to the severity of disease at the time of operation, especially in patients whose systemic disease activity persists postoperatively. However, there is some evidence that a total early synovectomy in patients without severe disease may prevent rheumatoid disease recurring locally in that individual joint.

Metacarpophalangeal arthroplasty. Metacarpophalangeal arthroplasty is one of the commonest operations performed in the fingers of the rheumatoid hand. The types of arthroplasty can be divided into the excisional arthroplasties, using some form of soft-tissue interposition or stabilisation, and joint replacement arthroplasties of which there are many different types.

The clinical indications for arthroplasty are similar to those for synovectomy. If the joint surfaces are denuded of cartilage, the pain is now emanating from the joint surfaces rather than from the inflamed synovium. Often this decision can only really be made at the time of surgery. Patients in whom the appearances on radiography are borderline should be warned that an arthroplasty may be necessary.

Excisional arthroplasty. This is a procedure of which I have had no experience, but basically involves excising either or both the head of the metacarpal and the base of the proximal phalanx. The proximal phalanx is then shaped into some form of point to provide some stability (variations on Fowler's operation) or soft tissue is interposed between the cut bone ends (interposition arthroplasty) using either part of the extensor mechanism or, in the Tupper arthroplasty, the volar plate.

It appears that those excisional arthroplasties without soft tissue interposition allow better movement but unfortunately little stability in radio-ulnar, dorso-volar or rotational planes making the function of the fingers poor. The best results are in those in which soft tissue interposition is performed, which provides greater stability but less movement. Over a period of time

excisional arthroplasty appears to cause gradual absorption and shortening of the metacarpal shaft and, in general, the results are worse than those procedures using some form of replacement arthroplasty.

Prosthetic replacement. Prosthetic replacement is one operation in rheumatoid arthritis that has stood the test of time, particularly with Swanson silicone-rubber flexible implants (*Figure 4C.8*), though many other designs of prosthetic replacement have been used, from unconstrained to fully constrained hinge-type prostheses. Because of the damage caused to the soft tissues by the synovitis, the use of unconstrained prostheses, unlike in most other joints, has not met with great success. The problem with prosthetic replacement in the fingers is that the joints are subject to stresses in all planes: flexion, extension, abduction and adduction. Unlike the knee, the collateral ligaments are usually of such poor quality that stability in the coronal plane is insufficient to allow the fingers to function satisfactorily. In some ways this is the same problem as found with excisional arthroplasty. Although some semi-constrained total joint arthroplasties have been designed, nothing so far has superseded the functional results obtained with Swanson silicone arthroplasty. It is important to realise that this arthroplasty is not truly a joint replacement and functions merely as a spacer with some stabilising features. The fact that the stems are allowed to piston in and out of the bone and that flexion of the prosthesis occurs throughout the length of it rather than at a central hinge, seem to help rather than hinder its function. Also the degree of rotational instability inherent in the construct allows the natural movement of the MP joint

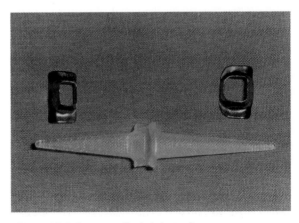

Figure 4C.8 Swanson silastic joint replacement.

to take place. It must also be remembered that by the time most patients with rheumatoid arthritis get to prosthetic arthroplasty of the MP joint, the normal kinetics of the joint have long since been lost. Even re-alignment of the joint often fails to completely return the soft tissues around the joint to their normal position. It is likely that after metacarpophalangeal joint arthro-plasty there will still be a tendency for the joint to sub-lux volarly, so release of all soft tissue contractures that might cause persistence or recurrence of such defor-mity should be performed as part of the procedure.

The approach to the MP joints is the same as that previously described for soft-tissue release. The struc-tures that have to be released to allow the joint to re-align itself are the ulnar collateral ligament, the ulnar intrinsic and the volar plate insertion on the base of the proximal phalanx. The bony resection consists of excision of the head of the metacarpal, leaving some of the flare of the metacarpal intact, preferably with some of the radial collateral ligament insertion. Often the radial collateral ligament has to be elevated in order to imbricate it and to prevent recurrence of the ulnar drift. The metacarpal head excision should be done in a slightly radial direction in relationship to the shaft of the metacarpal. This is often quite difficult to judge as the metacarpals converge towards the carpometacarpal joints. The proximal phalanges are merely reamed, unless there are large osteophytes that might impinge on the prosthesis. It is not unusual to find considerable dorsal erosion of the base of the proximal phalanx, and the temptation to square off the end of the proximal phalanx by resecting the volar aspect of the bone should be resisted. The reaming of the canals is nor-mally performed with the Swanson rectangular ream-ers, but often the base of the proximal phalanx is more easily reamed using a powered burr. Considerable care requires to be taken to avoid breaching the cortex. It is recommended that a rectangular hole should be made, supposedly to provide rotational control. In view of the amount of rotational movement taking place between the stem and the bone, it is likely that this contributes little, but most surgeons (including myself) continue to do this.

In the little finger it is important to differentiate between the abductor digiti minimi, which should always be divided, and the flexor digiti minimi which should be preserved. After preparation of the metacarpals and ensuring that there is full correction of the volar

subluxation of the proximal phalanx, the trial prosthesis is inserted using the biggest possible prosthesis which will fit into the space. At this stage it must be checked that the prosthesis sits comfortably within the joint, that full correction of the ulnar drift has been performed, and that on extension the prosthesis does not buckle and the proximal phalanx try to sublux volarly again.

Having ensured that the soft tissue correction is adequate, the radial collateral ligament for each joint should be re-constructed. This can be done using crossed intrinsic transfer, by reinforcement of the radial collateral ligament (as described under the soft-tissue correction) or by using the radial half of the volar plate. This latter technique requires a longitudinal incision of the volar plate and mobilisation from the proximal end which is then inserted into the head of the metacarpal to replace the radial collateral ligament. All these different techniques have their proponents. I tend to reef the radial collateral ligament of the index finger, using part of the volar plate, and for the other three joints to perform crossed intrinsic transfers to the joint capsule rather than into the neighbouring intrin-sic. Following insertion of the correct prosthesis using the no-touch technique and using blunt instruments, the extensor mechanism is closed in the method previ-ously described.

Postoperative management is as important as the surgery itself. I normally apply a volar plaster slab holding the fingers in their corrected position. The plaster extends beyond the PIP joints and should be well padded to prevent skin problems. On the first or second postoperative day an outrigger splint is con-structed by the occupational therapist. This consists of a dorsal orthoplast base with an outrigger splint and elastic slings under the proximal phalanges of the fingers. The angle of the pull of these elastic bands should apply a radial-deviating force but the tightness of the rubber bands should not prevent full active and passive mobilisation, although they must be strong enough to passively extend the MP joint. This balance is extremely difficult to achieve, particularly in the little finger; Swanson's therapists recommend that the little finger should merely be taped to the ring finger and no rubber band should be applied to the little finger. The dynamic splint should if possible, be kept in place for 12 weeks following surgery. The patient wears a static splint at night that extends to the end of the fingers, maintaining the MP joints in extension.

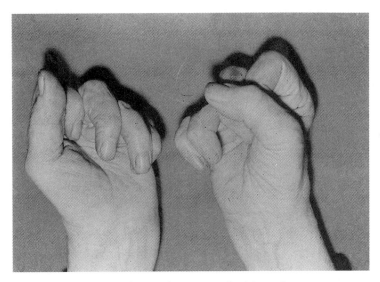

Figure 4C.9 Range of Flexian of MP joints after joint replacement.

Results. The results of MP arthroplasty are reasonably consistent whatever prosthesis is used. In general, the active range of movement achieved is approximately 50°, patients not usually achieving full extension but having approximately 70° of flexion (*Figure 4C.9*). Compared to before the operation, there is more extension and less flexion. In all papers published of long-term follow-up, there is gradual decrease in the range of movement, mirroring the progressive nature of the disease. Despite the rather poor range of movement, the patients are almost universally delighted with the results and this may be due to the improvement in appearance, as often the joints had ceased to be painful before the operation.

Complications. With all silicone arthroplasties, there appears to be a significant but maybe unimportant fracture-rate. This is increased in those in which the soft tissue release is inadequate, but often the fracture of the prosthesis does not produce any significant symptoms or loss of function and tends to confirm the function of the Swanson arthroplasty as a spacer for the joint. During the initial phases it appears that a fibrous capsule forms around the joint, which then provides sufficient stability if the arthroplasty fractures. Although there is considerable hysteria about the risks of silicone synovitis, this is a very rare complication in Swanson MP replacements and rarely requires surgical intervention.

THE PROXIMAL INTERPHALANGEAL JOINTS

The proximal interphalangeal joints are also commonly affected in rheumatoid arthritis, though it is not unusual to find that if the PIP joints are affected, then the MP joints are spared, and vice versa. This may be caused by a tendency for remission of synovitis in the PIP joints, something that rarely occurs in the MP joints. Kay, who followed-up 33 rheumatoid patients for 2.5 years, showed that MP joint synovitis persisted, while there was a 63% remission rate of synovitis of the PIP joint.

In the PIP joint, the volar plate appears to protect the front of the joint from major problems, and particularly protects the flexor tendons. Unfortunately the rather complex extensor tendon mechanism on the back of the PIP joint is extremely vulnerable. The problems associated with the PIP joints can effectively be divided into three principal conditions:

1. swan-neck deformity
2. boutonnière deformity
3. articular damage.

It is not unusual for tendon and joint surface involvement to co-exist and the treatments for these inevitably overlap.

Symptoms

When presenting with PIP joint involvement in isolation, it is more common to see the effects of tendon involvement, such as the swan-neck or boutonnière deformities rather than purely arthritic change in the joints.

Although pain can be a problem at the PIP joint, it is more common that loss of movement is the major complaint: either loss of extension in the boutonnière deformity, or loss of flexion in the swan-neck deformity.

In some of the other arthritides which are more erosive and less likely to involve the tendons, instability of the joint can be the reason for presentation. This is particularly the case in SLE, where the joint surfaces are often unaffected, or in psoriasis where the joints may be completely destroyed without significant tendon involvement.

Examination

Examination of the PIP joint is similar to examination of any joints in the rheumatoid hand and obviously cannot be examined in isolation from other joints as well as the tendons. However, particular facets of the PIP joints again should be examined for in systematic fashion.

Look

It is often relatively simple to see synovitic proliferation in the PIP joint as this tends to present dorsally. Any redness around the joint is also readily apparent. It is important to observe the posture of the fingers, both in flexion and extension, which may give a guide as to whether any tendon imbalance is flexible or stiff.

Feel

Palpation of the PIP joint confirms the synovitic presence. The presence of localised tenderness is often of limited usefulness in helping to diagnose the cause of PIP joint problems.

Move

Assessing the movement of the PIP joint is quite complex and should be done in quite a careful fashion.

As in other joints, it is worthwhile looking at active flexion and extension prior to looking at passive movement. It must also be remembered that both the extensor and flexor mechanisms have effectively two functions as they cross the PIP joint, one being to move the PIP joint itself, and the other being to move the more distal joint. Assessing the integrity of these tendons at the distal joint is as important as assessing the function of the PIP joint itself.

Therefore, having seen the active movement that the patient can achieve, it is important to examine both the flexion and extension of the PIP joint in isolation. Passive movement of the joint will tell you how much of the loss of active movement is caused by articular involvement (in which case the passive and active movements are going to be similar), or by tendon involvement (in which case the passive and active movements will be different).

It is important to ensure that deformity or loss of function in the PIP joint is not caused by flexor tenosynovitis. This can cause not only lack of active flexion and passive extension, but may also prevent passive flexion in severe situations, particularly when secondary joint contractures occur due to long-term loss of active flexion. Therefore, the presence of flexor tenosynovitis should be actively sought, particularly in the fingers at the level of the A2 pulley and also in the palm proximal to the A1 pulley. If there is any uncertainty, then the flexor tendons should be explored at the time of surgery.

Investigation

Radiographs should be obtained. If the joint surfaces are significantly damaged this alters the management, as tendon reconstruction in the presence of articular damage is doomed to failure.

Swan-neck deformity

The swan-neck deformity (*Figure 4C.10*) does not occur exclusively in rheumatoid disease. Moreover, unlike the boutonnière deformity, it can be secondary to problems either at the MP joint or the DIP joint.

In essence it can be divided into three main types:

1. Long extensor overactivity due to:
   (a) more proximal joint contracture, particularly at the MP joints

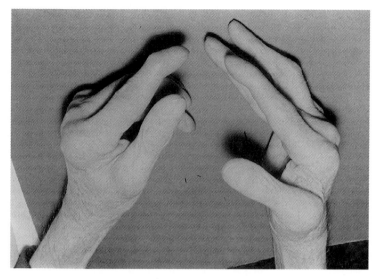

Figure 4C.10 Mild swan-neck deformities.

(b) mallet deformity of the DIP joint

(c) extrinsic spasticity.

2. Intrinsic muscle overactivity which can be caused by:
   (a) primary contracture of the intrinsics
   (b) intrinsic tightness secondary to MP joint disease.

3. Failure of the palmar stabilising structures of the PIP joint which can be:
   (a) volar plate insufficiency
   (b) FDS insufficiency
   (c) generalised joint laxity, usually due to synovitis.

Although this classification gives an idea of the primary cause, it does not tell you how to treat swan-neck deformities. Nalebuff classified them into four types of increasing severity and requiring different levels of treatment. They are:

Type 1 – PIP joint totally flexible

Type 2 – PIP joint flexion limited in certain positions of the MP joint (intrinsic contracture)

Type 3 – PIP joint flexion limited in all positions of the MP joint, but PIP joint preserved

Type 4 – PIP joint stiff and with joint changes.

Type 1 – joint totally flexible

The swan-neck deformity can start in either of the IP joints. In the DIP joint it is caused by stretching or rupture of the extensor mechanism (mallet finger). This

sometimes occurs in rheumatoid arthritis. If the PIP joint is the initiating cause, it is due to synovitis within the joint causing weakening of the volar plate, although occasionally isolated rupture of the superficialis tendon may cause this deformity; in this situation the mallet finger still occurs but this is a secondary deformity and on examination can be differentiated by the ability of the DIP joint to extend if the PIP joint is passively flexed.

In general, in this situation the major complaint is inability to extend the DIP joint rather than the PIP joint problem, although the cosmetic appearance can be a factor here. If the PIP joint is the primary problem then the simple application of an extension restriction splint, which effectively prevents the hyperextension, will usually be sufficient as it allows full flexion. However, as long as the PIP joint remains flexible, the application of the splint may be more of a problem than the deformity itself.

If the DIP joint is the primary site of pathology, then fusion of the DIP joint is usually sufficient to deal with the presenting complaint. However, this joint is not often affected in rheumatoid arthritis.

Although some authors might recommend some form of tenodesis to prevent the hyperextension of the PIP joint, this seems to me to be a purely cosmetic procedure and the extent of the operation does not really justify the presenting complaint. This method of treatment is discussed in later sections.

Type 2 – PIP joint flexion limited when MP joint extended

In this situation the primary problem is intrinsic tightness. However, secondary to this, the volar plate is often stretched and pure release of the intrinsic muscles may be insufficient to allow the deformity to correct itself. This may cause the so-called 'locked swan-neck deformity'. Here the patient is unable to initiate flexion in the PIP joint unless the PIP joint hyperextension is overcome. Once flexion is initiated, full flexion of the PIP joint is then possible.

As the primary problem is intrinsic tightness, treatment should be addressed to this. This involves excision of the intrinsics on either side of the long extensor tendon distal to the MP joint; it is important that the fibres joining the extensor mechanism to the palmar plate at the MP joint level are preserved. A triangle of tissue is excised from each side of the long extensor tendon distal to the MP joint. This includes the lateral bands and the tissues connecting this to the long extensor tendon. Theoretically this could result in inability to extend the DIP joint, but in practice the fibres related to the long extensor will take up the slack and start to act on the DIP joint as well as the PIP joint.

Although often in MP joint disease it is the ulnar lateral band that is particularly tight, the radial lateral band can also be involved and failure to release this also may result in persistence of the deformity.

For many years surgeons only performed an intrinsic release in this situation, but we have become aware that this does not address the laxity of the volar plate that has often occurred secondarily, so the patient is still unable to overcome the locked hyperextended position. Therefore, we usually combine this treatment with some form of tenodesis on the volar aspect of the PIP joint. There are two main operations described to achieve this.

Oblique retinacular ligament reconstruction. This involves taking one of the lateral bands, dividing it proximally and, instead of excising it, re-routing it below Cleland's ligaments which are the palmar fascia ligaments extending laterally from the PIP joint area. This band of tissue is then reefed into the flexor sheath or the bone. The object of the exercise is to place this band of tissue volar to the axis of the rotation of the PIP joint so that it acts as a tether to prevent hyperextension of the PIP joint.

This is a tidy solution in that it uses a segment of tendon that would otherwise be discarded as part of the intrinsic contracture release.

FDS tenodesis. This is a relatively straightforward procedure but obviously is not appropriate in FDS rupture unless this rupture has occurred more proximally. This is also particularly useful if several fingers are being operated on, as it involves a less extensive procedure. Through a volar incision, one limb of the FDS tendon is divided proximally, passed around the proximal end of the A2 pulley and sutured back onto itself to effectively provide a volar tether to hyperextension. Some authors recommend passing this through the bone, as the A2 pulley can be stretched by the synovitic process.

In both these procedures, at the end of the operation the PIP joint should be in approximately 30° of fixed flexion as it is likely that these repairs will stretch, ending up with a slight flexion contracture of between 10 and 15°. If the tether is performed with insufficient flexion, the deformity may recur with time. Postoperatively I maintain flexion for approximately four weeks with K wires and then start mobilisation with a dorsal block splint to prevent hyperextension of the PIP joints. After 6–8 weeks the splintage can be removed, but often it takes a considerable period of time for full flexion to be achieved.

Type 3 – limitation of flexion in all positions of MP joint, but PIP joint preserved

Loss of flexion of the PIP joint is a significant disability. There is disagreement as to whether these patients are best treated by attempting to regain movement by some sort of soft-tissue procedure, or whether arthrodesis should be performed. Usually when such a loss of movement occurs, there is joint damage, which precludes a purely soft-tissue procedure. The treatment programme suggested below takes a considerable period of time and in rheumatoid patients where often other joints are significantly affected, it may not actually be in the patient's interests to try and achieve this improved range of flexion when extensive damage to other joints has also occurred.

Manipulation under anaesthetic. It is essential to obtain full flexion of the PIP joint before doing any soft-tissue reconstruction. It should first be manipulated gently, preferably under regional or general anaesthesia, as complete relaxation of the long extensor muscles is essential. It is important to remember that osteoporosis is a feature of rheumatoid arthritis and, however gentle you are, fractures can occur. If there is long-standing deformity, the soft tissues may be contracted. If the skin on the dorsum of the PIP joint blanches during full flexion, it may be necessary to do oblique tension-relieving incisions distal to the PIP joint.

Having achieved a full range of movement, the PIP joint can be treated very much as described in the previous section, by intrinsic release if appropriate and some form of tenodesis to prevent recurrence of the hyperextension.

If manipulation under anaesthetic fails to correct the deformity, it will be necessary to perform a soft-tissue release of the dorsal structures of the PIP joint to achieve flexion. Again it must be stressed that skin over the dorsum of the PIP joint is often tight and this may need to be dealt with by skin-relieving incisions. It is said that adherence of the lateral bands is the predominant cause of the inability to correct the extension deformity. This can be corrected through a dorsal incision. The lateral bands are separated from the sides of the middle slip of the extensor tendon so that they can move in their normal way down the side of the joint during flexion. In some situations it is necessary to lengthen the long extensor tendon.

Type 4 – joint stiffness with joint surface damage radiologically

In this situation, achieving improvement in joint motion by soft-tissue procedures only is doomed to failure. As in all joint surface arthritis, the options here are either arthrodesis or arthroplasty. I have always found arthroplasty in the presence of significant tendon contractures to be a difficult procedure to achieve any lasting functional advantage. This is particularly so in the presence of an arthroplasty at the MP joint, which is not an unusual requirement in such patients. However, in the ulnar two fingers certain authors have recommended arthroplasty as having a better functional result than arthrodesis, as the degree of lateral instability of the arthroplasty is less important in these fingers. I feel however, that arthrodesis is a more reliable and predictable procedure in this situation. The techniques of arthrodesis are discussed in the next section.

Boutonnière deformity

The boutonnière deformity is the reverse of the swan-neck deformity in rheumatoid disease and is a direct result of synovitis in the PIP joint. Boutonnière is the French word for button-hole, used because the PIP joint button-holes through the extensor hood secondary to rupture of the central slip (*Figure 4C.11*). Curiously, the French call this deformity 'le button-hole'. I always thought it was called boutonnière because that was the position that your finger went into when you pushed hard down on a button, which may help to remember the appearance of the deformity though not the pathology.

The functional loss as a result of the boutonnière deformity is a lot less than with the swan-neck deformity and therefore, although early identification is important, it may in the end be inappropriate to match this early diagnosis with early surgical treatment.

Pathology

The pathology of boutonnière deformity is at the PIP joint only: expanding synovium in the PIP joint weakens the terminal portion of the central slip of the extrinsic extensor tendon, causing a lag to extension. It also weakens the fibres that connect from this central slip to the lateral bands from the intrinsics. The weakening of these fibres allows the lateral bands to dislocate in a palmar direction. Once the lateral bands have dislocated past the axis of the joint, they change from being extensors to flexors of the joint so it is now

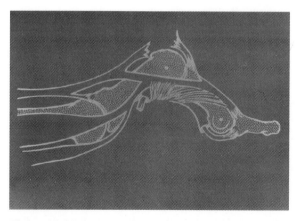

Figure 4C.11 Diagrammatic representation of boutonnière deformity.

impossible for the deformity to correct itself. Due to the change in direction of pull, the lateral bands are also able to act more strongly at their insertion which produces the classical hyperextension deformity at the DIP joint. The strength of this flexion also stretches the central slip even further and may in the end produce rupture. With the tendency to contracture of the PIP joint with prolonged flexion, this often results in a stiff joint in which correction becomes impossible. The synovitis may also affect the PIP joint, resulting in destruction of the cartilaginous surface.

Classification

Nalebuff and Millender have classified boutonnière deformity into mild, moderate and severe, and this is based on the degree of deformity, the presence of passive correctability and the state of the joint surfaces.

Mild deformity. There is only a slight lag of 10°–15° in extension. This can be corrected passively but, when that is done, there is limited flexion of the DIP joint. There may be active synovitis in the PIP joint and the DIP joint may or may not be slightly hyperextended. The MP joint, which often becomes hyperextended later, is normal at this stage.

At this stage the majority of the patient's functional loss is related the lack of full DIP joint flexion rather than the lack of extension at the PIP joint.

Moderate deformity. As the PIP joint flexion contracture reaches 30°–40°, the functional loss of the finger becomes more significant. Hyperextending the MP joint usually compensates for this. However, at this stage the deformity is still correctable passively. The main complaint is now inability to straighten the digit. In the little finger the potential for MP hyperextension is greater and this often prevents presentation until a more severe or fixed deformity has occurred. However, restoring PIP extension without attending to the problems associated with the DIP joint may actually make the functional result unhelpful to the patient.

Severe deformity. In long-standing boutonnière deformity, the PIP joint becomes fixed in a flexed position with little or no passive extension possible. In the more ulnar fingers the MP joint is usually fixed in hyperextension, as is the DIP joint. Despite radiographic changes often not being severe there is usually intra-articular cartilage destruction together with flattening of the anterior aspect of the articular surface on the head of the proximal phalanx. This means that even if the soft-tissue deformity is corrected, the joint is no longer congruous and range of movement cannot be restored.

Treatment

In general, non-surgical treatment is of little benefit and tends to merely reduce the function more than the disease has.

Mild deformity. Trying to correct the PIP joint deformity is probably of little benefit to the patient and is liable to result in more stiffness of flexion of the PIP joint, making function worse. At this stage, it has been recommended that the lack of flexion of the DIP joint should be corrected by an extensor tenotomy. This is performed over the centre of the middle phalanx and the whole extensor tendon is divided. Although theoretically this should cause a mallet finger, the oblique retinacular ligaments, which lie more volar, remain intact and, as they extend into the extensor mechanism at the DIP joint a complete mallet deformity is prevented. Following tenotomy, there is less hyperextension stress on the DIP joint and the flexion of the PIP joint is lessened. With dynamic splinting to extend the DIP joint postoperatively it may be possible to regain PIP joint extension, although the primary function should be to regain the DIP joint flexion.

It must be remembered that seeing patients with these early boutonnière deformities is unusual in British rheumatoid practice and that, if they are seen, rarely a cause of significant problems to the patients to the extent that they request surgical treatment.

Moderate deformity. Again non-operative treatment is rarely of any use to the patient. There have been many operations recommended for the treatment of this type of deformity. As is common in orthopaedics, multiple solutions to a problem imply that none of them is very satisfactory, and the results are unpredictable.

These techniques include:

- resection of part of the elongated central slip and relocation of the lateral bands into a more dorsal position;
- using one of the lateral bands as a form of reconstruction of the central slip;

- side-to-side suture of the lateral band over the top of the central slip;
- crossing over of the lateral bands.

There are a number of criticisms of these techniques.

1. Placing the lateral bands in a more dorsal position than they normally occupy is likely to be doomed to failure because the natural muscle pull will tend to pull the lateral bands back into their normal position.
2. Repairing the central slip does involve using what is often attenuated tissue, over the top of a joint that is already synovitic. Often, despite full synovectomy, recurrent synovitis makes the benefit short-lived.
3. Trying to recreate the anatomy by repair of the central slip often does not correct the loss of DIP joint flexion and, to deal with this, most authors recommend also dividing the extensor mechanism over the middle phalanx, as described in the last section.

After most of these reconstructive techniques it is recommended that a K wire is placed across the joint for between three and four weeks followed by protected mobilisation using some form of Capener-type sprung splint for a further three to four weeks.

As Kiefhaber and Strickland reported in 1993, the results of the different techniques described above are highly variable and unpredictable. There appears to be reasonable evidence that, even in the absence of radiological changes, joint damage is already present in many of these cases and, if this is found, I would have a low threshold for converting such patients to some form of arthrodesis.

Severe deformity. Some surgeons have tried using arthroplasty in this situation. Most readers will be familiar with the results of knee replacement after patellar tendon rupture and the finger, if anything, is less forgiving. The results are usually either rupture of the tendon repair or severe stiffness because of the prolonged splintage necessary to protect the tendon reconstruction.

In general, the more radial the finger the better it copes with arthrodesis and, as arthroplasty in the PIP joint is at best of unpredictable functional benefit, I would usually recommend fusion in these cases and this is likely to be the majority view.

PIP arthrodesis should be performed in varying degrees of flexion depending on which finger is being fused, ranging from approximately 20° in the index finger to about 45° in the little finger.

The bone ends should be either squared off to produce two flat surfaces at the appropriate angle or shaped into a cup and dome which is more forgiving in maintaining good bone-to-bone contact, while allowing changes in position of the flexion of the finger. Usually the DIP joint should also be released by an extensor tenotomy. Fixation is usually with K wires or tension band wiring. Some surgeons have used Herbert screws but often the bone stock is not sufficient to provide an adequate hold.

PIP joint synovitis and articular damage

Symptoms

Patients may present with pain or loss of range of movement, but more commonly a combination of the two. Presentation without some form of tendon imbalance can occur, although in a patient with boutonnière or swan-neck deformity the treatment is governed by the management of the tendon problem.

Examination

Examination of the PIP joint in the absence of a boutonnière or swan-neck deformity is reasonably straightforward. Assessment should be made in the usual way of look, feel and move; particularly feeling for the presence of swelling and synovitis and looking for the passive as well as active range of movement. Do not be misled by the presence of crepitation, which may be emanating from the flexor tendons rather than from the joint itself. Assessment of the stability of the joint is also important, particularly in relation to the collateral ligaments. The most important factor in examination of the PIP joints is differentiation of PIP joint pathology from flexor tendon pathology, as the treatment for the two is completely different. There may be synovitis in both sites and it is not always clear whence the symptoms are emanating.

Investigation

Radiographs of the PIP joint are essential in staging the degree of arthritis in the joint and therefore planning its management.

Treatment

Conservative. Conservative treatment is aimed at relieving pain and reducing synovitis. In general, medication in the form of anti-inflammatory tablets or intra-articular injections is the mainstay of treatment in the absence of radiological signs. Splintage of the PIP joint usually worsens function rather than improves it and it is better to proceed to surgical treatment if medical treatment fails.

Surgery. Surgical treatment depends to a great extent on the degree of articular surface damage. For treatment of the PIP joint in the presence of a boutonnière or swan-neck deformity see the section above.

Synovectomy. Synovectomy of the PIP joint is less rewarding than at the MP joint, as the joint is smaller and access to the volar part is extremely difficult. The results of synovectomy are mixed and it is not uncommon to develop a boutonnière deformity following the procedure. It is also common to lose range of motion following surgery and synovitis can recur. In a carefully controlled study by Raunio in 1977, relief of pain was complete in 60% of the joints but more than 50% of the joints eventually showed a recurrent synovitis. However, the synovectomy patients certainly did better than those treated by other means.

In Ellison's series in 1971, the mean loss of movement was 22° and, surprisingly, the MP joint also lost movement of about 10° following surgery.

Despite all this, it is sometimes possible to prevent further joint damage and possibly tendon damage in patients with extensive synovitis which does not respond to medical treatment.

The procedure is performed through a longitudinal incision, splitting one or both lateral bands away from the central slip of the tendon. Care must be taken to ensure that synovium is removed from around the insertion of the collateral ligaments and as much as possible from around the volar aspect of the joint. Finding early signs of articular cartilage damage is also not uncommon during this procedure; if this is significant, a bony operation is required.

Arthrodesis. Arthrodesis of the PIP joint has for a long time been the mainstay of treatment when there is disabling pain from these joints. The loss of motion does have a significant effect on hand function but, in an already poorly functioning hand, the relief of pain produced by PIP arthrodesis makes it a reliable, predictable and useful method.

The indications for arthrodesis are:

- malposition of the finger making grip and pinch impossible;
- a flail uncontrolled joint that is affecting the function of the hand;
- painful destruction of the joint.

Arthrodesis is particularly useful in the more radial fingers, where lateral stability is crucial to the function of the finger. It may be possible to perform arthroplasty in the more ulnar fingers although the results of this are variable. The angle of arthrodesis depends upon the finger: about 20° in the index finger and increasing to about 40° in the little finger. In patients with severe erosive disease and particularly in those with psoriasis the results of fusion are less certain, but in general are better than the results of arthroplasty (*Figure 4C.12*).

Arthroplasty. Arthroplasty of the PIP joints is a controversial topic. In general if all the PIP joints are involved, then it is better to arthrodese at least the index and middle fingers which are predominantly subjected to lateral forces and possibly consider arthroplasty in the smaller fingers, though this will not restore a full range of movement. If only one PIP joint is affected (though this is uncommon in rheumatoid disease), then to have it stiffened may interfere with the use of the other fingers.

There are several different approaches and to some extent they can be varied dependent on any underlying

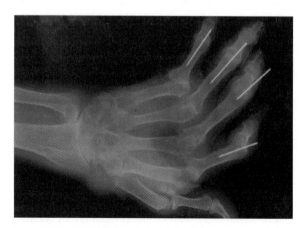

Figure 4C.12 PIP arthrodesis using K wires.

tendon abnormality. In a swan-neck deformity the central slip is divided proximally and then sutured in a slacker position. Similarly in a boutonnière deformity a segment of the central slip may be excised leaving a distally-placed portion to reattach the tendon.

Although the Swanson arthroplasty is again the gold standard here, recent more anatomical replacements have been introduced, but the results of these are limited.

As in all arthroplasty, soft-tissue balancing is essential particularly in the PIP joint where lateral stability is crucial. Approaches from the ulnar side have also been performed, dividing the ulnar collateral ligament and then reattaching it. This avoids the problem of disrupting the extensor mechanism although in published series there seems to be little major advantage in this approach. Others recommend a volar approach, retracting the flexor tendons.

THE RHEUMATOID THUMB

The thumb has been described as functionally half of the hand, and more than two-thirds of rheumatoid patients have some involvement of the thumb. It is therefore worth considering in some detail. In a study by Polkey, 35% of the patients with some involvement showed limited opposition because of restricted rotation; 45% had instability of the MP joint and 10% instability of the interphalangeal joint. Probably about one in three have significant disease of the carpo-metacarpal joint.

As in the fingers there is usually one joint that initiates deformity and the other joints in the thumb collapse into a particular instability pattern dependent on the primary joint deformity. However, the secondary joint involvement often becomes fixed and therefore also requires treatment.

For this reason, it is impossible to consider one joint in the thumb in isolation and the effect of treatment on one joint must be considered in relationship to its effect on the other joints. As in the fingers, the thumb collapses into varying zig-zag patterns which are not only in the flexion/extension plane, but also in the abduction/adduction plane.

It is important to remember that instability in the thumb, particularly at the MP and IP joints, is more disabling than loss of flexion and extension.

The most important functions of the thumb are:

- adduction to allow the hand to be placed flat on a surface;
- palmar abduction so that the fingers can be used for gripping and to allow pinch grip between thumb and index finger for fine manipulations;
- opposition, the rotation which comes after abduction to bring the pulp of the thumb opposite that of the fingers;
- extension ('radial abduction') in order to remove the thumb from the palm of the hand.

All treatment should be aimed towards ensuring that these functions are maintained or at least not significantly reduced.

Classification

Nalebuff has classified thumb deformities into five major groups, although only types one, three and four are commonly seen. It is important to realise that this classification is not sequential, i.e. type five is not worse than type three and so on, but only describe different patterns of deformity.

1. boutonnière-like deformity (MP flexion with IP hyperextension) (*Figure 4C.13*)
2. probably not a type at all but type 1 with carpo-metacarpal subluxation
3. swan-neck-like deformity (CM subluxation with MP-hyperextension)
4. 'gamekeeper's thumb'
5. MP hyperextension only
6. arthritis mutilans

Treatment

In general, treatment of thumb deformities involves surgery. Although medical treatment is useful for its anti-synovitic effect and its analgesic effect, it will rarely affect the outcome of an already deformed thumb and is unlikely to improve its function greatly. Similarly splintage is usually more of a hindrance to thumb function.

Boutonnière-like deformity

Pathology

This is the most common pattern of deformity in the rheumatoid thumb. It is initiated by proliferative MP

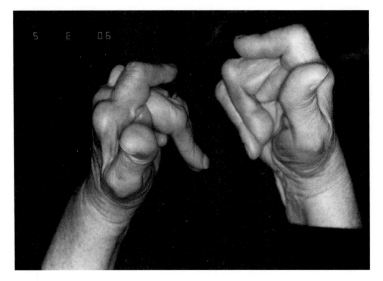

Figure 4C.13 Boutonnière (Type 1) thumb deformity.

joint synovitis bulging dorsally and causing attenuation of the extensor pollicis brevis tendon insertion. The extensor pollicis longus tendon, which is to the ulnar side, gradually subluxes more ulnarly, rather like the long extensors to the fingers in ulnar drift at the MP joints. As a result, extension of the MP joint becomes weak and the extensor pollicis longus over a period of time starts to act as a flexor of the MP joint rather than an extensor, somewhat like the boutonnière deformity in the fingers.

As in the fingers the IP joint gradually hyperextends because all the muscles (including the intrinsics) now extend the IP joint. In the early stages both the MP flexion and IP hyperextension are passively correctable. Relatively rapidly, fixed deformities develop: initially of the MP joint and later of the IP joint as well. It is important before deciding on treatment to assess the correctability of these deformities.

Treatment

Correctable MP joint and IP joint. Treatment here is designed to rebalance the tendon mechanism and maintain function of the joint. As in the early boutonnière deformity of the fingers, some authors have recommended merely reconstruction of the extensor mechanism, but here too the results are unpredictable because the tissues being dealt with are of already poor quality. Nalebuff has described a method of re-routing the

extensor pollicis longus tendon to help this deformity. In this operation the extensor pollicis longus (EPL) and brevis (EPB) tendons are separated proximal and distal to the joint. The EPL tendon is divided over the proximal third of the proximal phalanx. Both the EPB and EPL are elevated off the joint capsule and a transverse incision made in the joint capsule at its proximal insertion, preserving the more thickened distal capsule intact and attached to the base of the proximal phalanx. The EPL tendon is then passed through the dorsal capsule and then turned back onto itself and sutured, thus converting it from an IP joint extensor to an MP joint extensor. Synovectomy of the joint should be performed prior to re-routing the tendon.

In the initial description of this, Nalebuff left the EPB tendon as reinforcement to this manoeuvre, but he found that IP joint extension was too weak. He therefore modified his technique and now attaches the EPB tendon to the stump of the EPL tendon distally, thus providing EPB as an extensor of the IP joint in addition to the intrinsics. After operation, the MP joint requires splintage for four weeks with a K wire followed by external splintage for two more weeks.

An alternative technique, described by Harrison, is to pass the EPL tendon through the base of the proximal phalanx and suture it back onto itself.

MP joint fixed but IP joint correctable passively. The treatment of the MP joint is either by arthrodesis or by arthroplasty. In the thumb, stability is probably more important than movement, especially at the MP joint. Lateral stability of the thumb is as important as dorso-palmar stability and functionally MP arthrodeses seem to perform very well.

The best position of fusion is in about 15° of flexion; if there is concern about involvement of the CM joint then approximately 15° of abduction and 15° of internal rotation can also be built in to assist in opposition. If the CM joint is unstable, then flexion should be increased to about 25°.

The bone ends can be cut flat to ensure the correct angle of flexion. I prefer the cup-and-dome technique that allows correction of the flexion/extension position after fashioning of the bone ends. This method also allows a little bit of variation in abduction/adduction and rotation of the thumb without losing significant bone-to-bone contact.

Methods of fixation include Herbert screws, crossed K wires or the tension band wire technique, the latter being the one that I would favour. Ensure that the K wires are placed laterally in the metacarpal so that when bent and rotated round they sit flat against the side of the metacarpal rather than on the dorsal surface.

After fusion of the MP joint, the IP joint should correct itself as the balance of the thumb has now been corrected. Occasionally the assessment of the IP joint has been incorrect and full passive correction is not possible. In this situation the techniques described in the next section should be applied.

Fixed MP joint flexion and fixed IP joint hyper-extension. It is generally accepted that the only treatment for a badly destroyed IP joint is fusion. However, if the contracture is purely soft tissue and the joint is well preserved, then soft tissue release may actually restore the IP joint's ability to flex. Obviously, what surgery is performed at the MP joint depends to a great extent on the state of the IP joint, so in this situation it is usually advisable to explore the IP joint first and check on its joint surfaces.

If the IP joint is preserved, then a joint release can be performed. One of the major problems with this joint is that the dorsal skin is usually contracted, which limits the amount of flexion that can be obtained.

There are two ways of dealing with this.

1. Approach the joint from the lateral side and perform a tenolysis of the extensor mechanism.

The dorsal capsule of the joint can be incised by sliding the blade volar to the extensor mechanism and rotating it 90°; the dorsal portion of the collateral ligament can be released in the same way. The joint can then be manipulated into flexion and usually it can be held in 25°–30° of flexion without unduly affecting the dorsal skin.

2. A longitudinal incision is made over the dorsum of the joint and a Z-plasty then performed to lengthen the skin.

In both situations the joint needs to be pinned with a K wire in its flexed position for a couple of weeks. If it proves impossible to release the joint, or if there is significant joint destruction, then an arthrodesis needs to be performed, using K wires, tension band wire or Herbert screw. The ideal position for the IP joint in the thumb is straight, although a little bit of flexion can be built in.

Having dealt with the IP joint, it is then necessary to do something to the MP joint. It is often recommended that if the IP joint has required fusion, then the MP joint should be replaced. However I feel that the lateral stability provided by an arthroplasty is insufficient and I prefer to fuse both joints, provided that there is reasonable movement at the carpometacarpal joint to avoid the thumb being fixed into an adducted position and unable to move away from the plane of the hand.

Type 2 thumb

This is extremely rare and is probably a combination of the type 1 boutonnière-type deformity with subluxation or dislocation of the carpometacarpal joint and is to a great extent considered above.

Swan-neck-like deformity

Pathology

The type 3 thumb is the reverse of the boutonnière-type deformity (type 1). It occurs when disease of the CM joint allows dorsal and radial subluxation at that joint. This also happens in osteoarthritis, and in both diseases makes it impossible to get the thumb out of the palm without hyper-extending the MP joint, as a consequence of which the IP joint flexes. It is important to be aware that the CM joint is the precipitating factor, so correction of this deformity must start with correction of the CM joint.

Clinical assessment

Assessment of whether the CM joint is reducible is crucial. If there is hyperextension of the MP joint, it must be shown whether this too is correctable passively. It is worthwhile checking that with flexion of the MP joint, the IP joint then will extend passively.

Treatment

CM joint painful but MP joint normal. Primary treatment here is conservative with splintage and intra-articular injections or systemic medication. If symptoms worsen despite this treatment, then surgery to the CM joint is necessary before hyperextension of the MP joint occurs. Theoretically synovectomy should help this situation but this is rarely successful and it is usually better to perform some form of arthroplasty, as described below under the CM joint in osteoarthritis.

Subluxed CM joint with MP hyperextension. The CM joint has progressed and the MP joint now has a hyperextension deformity but this is passively correctable. Again the best treatment here is arthroplasty of the CM joint. It is important to realise that all the soft tissues are abnormal in rheumatoid arthritis and reconstruction of the ligament, such as with FCR tendon, is not always possible as the tendons themselves are often of poor quality.

After treatment of the CM joint, it is necessary to correct the hyperextension of the MP joint by a flexor tenodesis.

Fixed adduction of CM joint and fixed hyperextension of MP joint. In this advanced stage, the adduction of the metacarpal becomes fixed; there is fixed hyperextension of the MP joint and usually complete dislocation of the CM joint. As in the more moderate cases, some form of arthroplasty procedure should be performed at the CM joint, but at this stage the MP joint usually requires fusion. Sometimes there is a significant web-space contracture and, if there is any doubt that adequate abduction will be achieved, a Z-plasty should be performed of the thumb web.

'Gamekeeper's thumb'

Here the disease is confined to the MP joint and is similar to an ulnar collateral ligament rupture. The ligament is usually stretched rather than ruptured (*Figure 4C.14*), as in true gamekeeper's thumb where it was attenuated by breaking the necks of rabbits for many years. This often results in a secondary adduction contracture of the web space, although the CM joint itself is rarely involved. In this situation, obvious ulnar collateral ligament instability will be present but the CM joint is effectively normal as is the IP joint.

Treatment

Surgical treatment is aimed at the stabilisation of the MP joint. This may be achieved in the early stages by some form of reconstruction of the collateral ligament along with synovectomy of the joint. It may also be necessary to release the fascia over the web-space to allow correction of the adduction of the CM joint. In

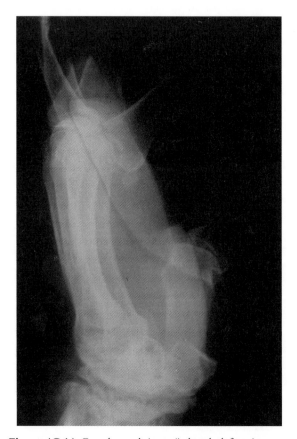

Figure 4C.14 Gamekeeper's (type 4) thumb deformity.

more advanced cases where joint destruction is present, then arthrodesis of the MP joint, again with or without a web-space release, provides a stable thumb.

Hyperextension of MP joint

This is a rare type of thumb deformity and is caused by isolated hyperextension of the MP joint due to slackening and lengthening of the volar plate. There is no adduction of the metacarpal, which distinguishes it from the type 3 deformity. As this hyperextension increases, there will be compensatory flexion of the IP joint due to the FPL tightness. As this is purely an instability problem, the deformity is always correctable.

Treatment

Treatment is relatively simple with some form of capsulodesis or tenodesis, or, if necessary, arthrodesis. The object is to provide the necessary stability to the MP joint in extension.

Arthritis mutilans

In thumbs in which there is severe joint disruption of all joints, there is gross instability and shortening of the thumb. It is very difficult to provide an effective and functional splint in this situation, so treatment is usually by fusion. Because of the destruction, it is often necessary to use bone grafting. This sort of surgery is very difficult and should not be undertaken without careful thought.

OSTEOARTHRITIS

Osteoarthritis can affect single or multiple joints. Although synovitis may occur in this condition, it is not the primary feature and therefore the soft tissues are reasonably well preserved. The commonest sites for osteoarthritis in the hand are in the first carpometacarpal joint at the base of the thumb and the DIP joints of the fingers; less frequently, the PIP joints and the IP joint of the thumb are affected. Although radiological changes in osteoarthritis are common in the hand, they often cause no symptoms. Clinical assessment and diagnosis are in general simpler than in

rheumatoid disease so these patients are often used as short cases in the FRCS Orth exam.

As in osteoarthritic joints in the rest of the body, the presentation in the hand is with pain and loss of function. In the fingers *pain* is the main indication for treatment as loss of movement is difficult to restore following surgical or medical intervention. In the thumb, however, *loss of function* (particularly inability to abduct the thumb and later the fixed adduction) are indications for surgery, although pain usually mirrors the lack of motion.

CARPOMETACARPAL JOINT OF THE THUMB

Anatomy

The carpometacarpal (or trapeziometacarpal) joint is the key joint of the thumb. The movement that makes the thumb such a useful addition to the human hand is its ability to oppose to the fingers, requiring a combination of rotation, flexion, adduction and extension. The joint is saddle-shaped with axes a dorso-palmar direction (which is the direction of abduction and adduction of the CM joint) and the radio-ulnar (in the plane of flexion–extension of the thumb). This shape of the joint allows the wide range of movements described above.

Three main ligaments support the joint:

1. lateral ligament: a broad band running from the lateral surface of the trapezium to the radial side of the base of the first metacarpal;
2. dorsal ligament: this is thin and is reinforced by the expanded insertion of the abductor pollicis longus;
3. volar (palmar) or beak ligament: this is the most important of the three ligaments and attaches into the beak of the first metacarpal where it abuts on the second metacarpal. It is immensely strong. It is thought that problems related to this ligament are the cause of the osteoarthritic process in this joint.

Symptoms

Patients usually complain of poorly localised pain around the base of the thumb. They may also be troubled by inability to abduct the thumb, due to subluxation of the joint caused by a large volar osteophyte.

It is important to differentiate several other conditions affecting the thumb before being certain osteoarthritis is the cause of the patient's symptoms. At least a third of postmenopausal women have radiological evidence of osteoarthritis in this joint, but only between a third and a half of these actually complain of any pain around the base of the thumb. De Quervain's tenovaginitis, non-union of a scaphoid fracture, flexor carpi radialis tendonitis, scaphotrapezial osteoarthritis and referred pain from the carpal tunnel or the MP joint should also be considered as possible causes.

Clinical examination and investigation

Clinical examination should confirm the diagnosis. Two tests are used. One is the grind test, in which the first CM joint is compressed longitudinally and the metacarpal rotated manually; this should produce the pain complained of. The other test for the subluxed joint involves longitudinal traction and pressure over the prominence at the base of the first metacarpal, attempting to reduce the joint. This can also produce pain, as attempts to reduce the subluxed joint push against the medial osteophyte that is invariably present. Uncertainty as to the source of the pain can be helped by injection of local anaesthetic into the first CM joint which should relieve the pain, though it is a difficult joint to inject. Specific radiographs of the first CM, joint, such as Gedda views, should be requested to confirm the diagnosis (see page 103). The joint lies obliquely to the rest of the hand, so the conventional PA and lateral views of the hand will only give you two obliques of the first CM joint.

Staging

It is generally thought that osteoarthritis of the carpometacarpal joint occurs as a result of laxity in the volar beak ligament; subsequently this ligament becomes detached, which allows excessive instability of the joint and gradual degenerative change. Staging of the disease is based on the degree of degenerative change and the degree of subluxation of the joint and was described by Eaton and Littler.

Stage 1. There is a so-called synovitis phase before significant capsule laxity has developed. Radiographs show slight *widening* of the joint space, but normal

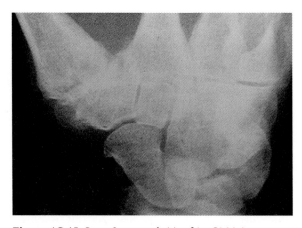

Figure 4C.15 Stage 2 osteoarthritis of 1st CM joint.

articular contours and less than one-third subluxation in any projection.

Stage 2. There is significant capsular laxity and at least one-third subluxation of the joint, which is demonstrated by stress X-ray examination. This is taken with the patient's hands both resting on an X-ray plate, with the thumbs pushing against each other in palmar abduction which particularly stresses the deltoid ligament of the first CM joint. Joint debris in the form of osteophytes or loose bodies not exceeding 2 mm in diameter may have formed. Osteophytes or loose bodies may be present adjacent to the palmar or dorsal facets of the trapezium. The scaphotrapezial-trapezoidal (STT) joint is normal (*Figure 4C.15*).

Stage 3. There is more than one-third subluxation. Osteophytes or loose bodies bigger than 2 mm are present dorsally or palmarly and usually in both places. The joint space is markedly narrow and often there is sclerotic bone and cystic changes (*Figure 4C.16*).

Stage 4. Advanced degenerative change and severe subluxation are present. The joint space is narrow, with cystic and sclerotic subchondral bone changes. There is lipping and osteophyte formation. The STT joint is often also narrowed, sclerotic and may show cystic changes (*Figure 4C.17*).

Treatment

Conservative

As in all osteoarthritic joints rest, alteration in patterns of use and non-steroidal anti-inflammatory drugs can

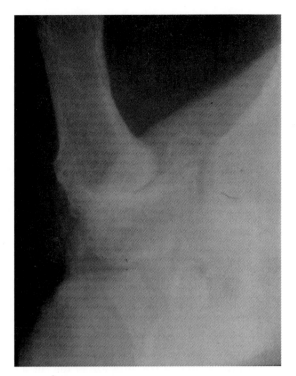

Figure 4C.16 Stage 3 osteoarthritis of 1st CM joint.

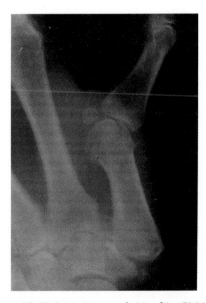

Figure 4C.17 Stage 4 osteoarthritis of 1st CM joint.

control symptoms. These can be coupled with splintage, which is particularly useful in the first CM joint, as applying a protective splint around the base of the thumb reduces the ability to fully abduct. Passive

abduction occurs during pinch grip, which mimics the grind test. Thus avoidance of abduction is useful in controlling symptoms. The joint is also protected from its tendency to sublux.

It is possible to inject steroid into the joint, although this is not easy, particularly when there is significant joint-space narrowing. I usually do this by first stressing the joint palmarly to identify the base of the metacarpal and then put longitudinal traction on the thumb to open up the joint. With an orange needle it should be possible to 'walk' the needle along the bone and into the joint. As with all injections in the hand, 1 ml of fluid containing local anaesthetic and steroid is sufficient.

This may relieve the pain for some time. These procedures tend to be more effective in the earlier stages of disease. In stage 4 disease, steroid injections are rarely helpful, although splintage can often control symptoms and avoid surgery.

Surgery

Stages 1 and 2. Here there is minimal degenerative change in the joint and symptoms are due to instability. Although we seldom see patients at this stage, the general consensus is reasonably consistent as to the best surgical treatment. This is designed to stabilise the joint.

Ligament reconstruction. The most popular ligament reconstruction uses a distally based strip of the flexor carpi radialis (FCR) tendon, passed from its insertion on the base of the second metacarpal from ulnar to radial through the base of the first metacarpal and then looped back round the remaining other half of the FCR tendon and reattached to itself.

Osteotomy. In some small series, abduction-extension osteotomy has been used with good reported results. The theory here is that the operation alters the forces across the joint when the muscles contract, effectively reducing the subluxation. It can also improve the abduction range of the thumb in those who have reduced abduction due to pain. This is not an operation that I have seen or done, but both Wilson in 1973 and Molitor in 1991 reported good results from it, without losing pinch power.

Stage 3 and 4. In stage 3 and 4 disease the degree of degenerative change is such that some form of surgery to the joint itself has to be used. As in other osteoarthritic joints' these are the three classic orthopaedic operations of osteotomy, arthroplasty or arthrodesis.

Osteotomy. Osteotomy similar to that described in stages 1 and 2 has been used in some stage 3 patients under the same rationale, but there are no separate documented results of this procedure in stage 3 patients.

Arthrodesis. Arthrodesis should not be underestimated as a potential procedure (*Figure 4C.18*). As far as the thumb is concerned, stability is more important than movement and certainly power and stability are the main requirements, particularly in the young person and in men. It is particularly useful in those patients with congenital hypermobility of the CM joint. The presence of pre-existing STT arthritis or arthritis of the MP joint of the thumb should be viewed as contraindications to this procedure.

Critics of this type of operation suggest that fusion of the thumb produces an awkward hand that cannot be flattened on a tabletop and is difficult to put into a pocket. However, these criticisms are not borne out by the results in the literature. The position of the fusion is probably the most important aspect and it is generally accepted that 35°–40° of palmar abduction and 20° of radial deviation of the first metacarpal is the best position. In general with the fingers clenched, the thumb should lie on top of the middle phalanx of the index finger, in line with the radius.

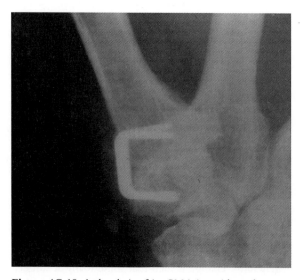

Figure 4C.18 Arthrodesis of 1st CM joint with staple.

Different techniques have been described for performing the fusion, from straightforward parallel resection of the articular surfaces to the cup and dome technique using the trapezium as the dome and the base of the metacarpal as the cup. The latter technique allows some adjustment of position often making the cuts. The fusion is held in most cases by K wires, but the tension band technique is also useful here. Other techniques that have been used include using a Herbert screw, a small T-shaped plate (with its stem on the metacarpal) or power staple fixation. Immobilisation is for six to eight weeks, although with the tension band technique or with a solid screw fixation it is possible to shorten this. Even if non-union does occur, a fibrous ankylosis often functions well for the patient without producing significant pain.

In 1992 Bamerger reviewed CM fusion in 39 non-rheumatoid patients and reported a non-union rate of 8%, which appears to be 3 out of 39 patients. This is quite a high non-union rate for an easily accessible joint but it does indicate the difficulty of obtaining fusion, partly because of the small size of the cut surfaces and also because of the stresses put on the fusion during use of the thumb.

Arthroplasty. As in most joints, excision arthroplasty was the first arthroplastic procedure, described in 1949 by Gurbis, who subsequently had the operation performed on himself. This allowed him to operate again, his rehabilitation being reconstruction of the wooden wheel for his gypsy caravan. *Trapeziectomy* has been widely used since then and there is little doubt that it usually produces very satisfactory pain relief, though patients take several months to get the full benefit. However, concern was soon voiced about the proximal migration of the first metacarpal following such a procedure, as the beak ligament at this stage is usually ineffective. There was considerable weakness of pinch grip and, in a small number of cases, late recurrence of pain due to articulation of the base of the first metacarpal with the head of the scaphoid. However, the majority of criticisms of this technique have been on the basis of radiographic loss of joint space between the scaphoid and the metacarpal rather than on the prevalence of pain related to direct articulation of the metacarpal against the scaphoid. Varley in 1994 published the long-term results of trapeziectomy, which tended to suggest that the long-term results were as good as those reported for any other technique. In 1997 Davis published the results of a randomised comparison between trapeziectomy with and without ligament reconstruction, with functional results in the early stages that were equal in both groups.

Several techniques have been introduced to try and avoid the problems of weakness of pinch grip and proximal migration of the first metacarpal base.

These can be divided into:

- hemi-arthroplasty and interposition with tendon or silicone;
- trapeziectomy and interposition with tendon or silicone;
- trapeziectomy and ligament reconstruction;
- complete joint replacement.

Hemi-arthroplasty. This involves resecting the base of the first metacarpal and trimming the osteophytes off the trapezium. Various forms of silicone interposition have been tried, but these tend to fragment because of their thin nature. The best results are of tendon interposition using a slip of FCR, which is also used for ligament reconstruction. This can be used in stage 3 disease without scaphotrapezial osteoarthritis. The early results seem good, although proximal migration may be a problem in the future.

Trapeziectomy with interposition. In practice many patients presenting with arthritis at the trapeziometacarpal joint also have arthritis in the joints between the scaphoid, trapezium and trapezoid. In this situation, the trapezium must be excised. Although palmaris longus and the FCR tendon have been used as interposition materials, the best results appear to be following silicone interposition using a stemmed implant, the stem being inserted into the metacarpal. Swanson's report of 147 out of 150 cases with an average 3.5 years follow-up, indicated subluxation in 14.5%, dislocation in 6% and a re-operation rate of 3.3%.

However, it appears that development of carpal and metacarpal erosion due to silicone wear products is an increasing problem with longer follow-up. As many as 25% of cases appear to have some cyst formation and bone resorption, but some studies have shown no correlation between the occurrence of pain, swelling or tenderness and the presence of interosseous cysts. Improvement of the wear characteristics of this arthroplasty are said to occur if some form of

tendinous reconstruction is performed with the silicone arthroplasty.

Although subluxation is common, pain only seems to occur with complete dislocation of the arthroplasty. Nevertheless, subluxation of the arthroplasty certainly does result in loss of pinch strength.

Trapeziectomy with ligament reconstruction. Procedures of this nature have become the most popular techniques of treating osteoarthritis of the first CM joint. The resection arthroplasty is to relieve pain and the ligament reconstruction is to prevent proximal migration of the first metacarpal.

The most commonly used method is that described by Burton and Pelligrini, using a strip consisting of half the width of the FCR tendon, which is passed through the first metacarpal to try and reconstruct the volar beak ligament. The remainder of this strip of FCR is then used rolled up and interposed in the trapezial space as a cushion.

A similar procedure has been described using the abductor pollicis longus (APL), also a distally-based strip, wrapped round the FCR tendon to pull the two tendons together; the remainder of the slip of tendon being again rolled up in the space. This technique is criticised as it de-functions the APL and thus may reduce abduction power, the problem that the operation is designed to help. Whether this occurs in practice is difficult to ascertain from the literature.

In general the results following ligament reconstruction and resection arthroplasty are very similar to those of trapeziectomy, in that the pain relief is almost universal but there is persistent loss of pinch strength, although this is claimed to be less following ligament reconstruction than simple trapeziectomy.

Burton and Pelligrini, following patients for a mean of nine years, have noticed that pinch strength improved by 20% from preoperative levels, and this continued to improve for up to six years. By nine years there was a 50% improvement in preoperative pinch strength. It does appear that loss of the arthroplasty space is reduced by ligament reconstruction, a loss of 50% being described in the simple spacer technique compared with only 13% in the ligament reconstruction group. However, there is no correlation between revision dates and loss of arthroplasty space.

Total joint replacement. Several total joint replacements have been produced, but have been used on a limited basis. The main ones are those used by Braun and by de la Caffinière, but these have significant loosening rates relatively early on and the results of most other surgeons with these prostheses have not been as favourable as those of the original designers. There remains a continuing problem of fixation of the trapezial replacement, although de la Caffinière also had problems with the metacarpal stem and had to redesign his implant. Both joints were intended to remove the necessity for ligament reconstruction, but how supplementation by ligament reconstruction might add to the stability and longevity of these prostheses is unknown.

Summary of operative methods. There is considerable variation in the results reported with the same technique by different surgeons. Much of this may be caused by patient selection; certainly the more elderly female patients with less demands on their hands and for whom the main indication is pain relief have excellent functional results from all the techniques described above. There is now one randomised trial (by Davis *et al.*) comparing trapeziectomy and ligament reconstruction as described by Burton and Pelligrini, with simple trapeziectomy which, in the short-term at least, showed no benefit from the difficult and time-consuming ligament reconstruction. Although theoretically the advantage of ligament reconstruction in addition to trapeziectomy appears considerable, there is some doubt whether pinch strength is actually much better with this technique and whether this actually matters to the patients anyway.

The almost hysterical reaction to cyst formation following silicone arthroplasty in the USA is not really borne out by the need for revision surgery. Whether silicone arthroplasty is actually in any way better than over simple trapeziectomy is, however, in some doubt as the results vary from centre to centre. Silicone arthroplasties are now difficult to obtain and the majority of them have been replaced by titanium implants, although it is still possible to get the silicone implants if required. There are no long-term results available from the titanium implants.

In younger patients with isolated trapeziometacarpal arthritis, there is considerable merit in considering osteotomy for the early disease and fusion of the first CM joint in advanced cases.

PROXIMAL INTERPHALANGEAL JOINTS

In osteoarthritis the proximal interphalangeal joints are affected much less commonly than the DIP joints. They may develop arthritis as a result of intra-articular fractures or fracture–dislocations, but even this is not common. The major complaints are pain and loss of function.

Examination

The usual findings are a swollen thickened joint that may be deformed. Movement is often restricted and this may be the main reason for presentation. Crepitus is often felt on passive movement. Although differentiation from tendon damage or tenosynovitis is usually easy, tendon function should be checked. Radiographs show the classical osteoarthritic changes of joint-space narrowing and osteophyte formation.

Treatment

In general, the PIP joints respond poorly to conservative treatment, as splintage is often more disabling than the pain and slight stiffness. Thus the options of treatment are either analgesia or surgery. Arthrodesis and, more recently, arthroplasty have both been used to treat arthritis in this joint.

Unfortunately the loss of motion arthrodesis causes has a significant effect on hand function, especially in the more ulnar digits. However, it is reliable in relieving pain and non-union is unusual. The angle of fusion of these joints is crucial in optimising function following surgery. The angle should vary from 20° in the index finger to 40° in the little finger, although some texts recommend more flexion in osteoarthritic patients as they do not lack the MP extension often present in rheumatoid patients. Techniques vary from the cup-and-dome method to cutting the bone transversely at the appropriate angle. Fixation also varies from crossed K wires or tension band wiring to plate fixation.

The lowest non-union rates have been described using the tension band, interosseous wiring, plate fixation, and Herbert screw fixation, all publishing rates of less than 2%. The functional results are less easy to quantify, although solid fusion is usually associated with good pain relief.

Because of the perceived functional deficit from arthrodesis many surgeons have tried arthroplasty, but the difficulty in replacing the PIP joints is that the stresses on the joint occur in both coronal and sagittal planes. The most commonly used prosthesis has been the Swanson silicone implant, which has poor stability in both planes. Thus in osteoarthritis, where the surrounding joints are often normal, the stresses on the replaced joint are such that early failure occurs. Recently more anatomical prostheses have been used with better effects but long-term results are unavailable in sufficient size-groups to make conclusions valid.

DISTAL INTERPHALANGEAL JOINTS

The distal interphalangeal joints are most commonly affected by osteoarthritis (*Figure 4C.19*). There is pain and swelling in the joints and there may be a so-called mucous cyst, which is a ganglion arising from the DIP

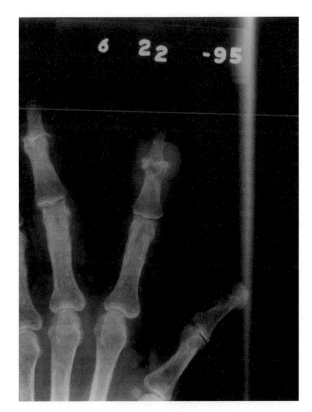

Figure 4C.19 Osteoarthritis of DIP joints.

joint (see pages 125–6). This can often deform the nail. Female patients often complain about the deformity of the nail or the joint rather than pain. Psoriasis and gout are the only inflammatory arthritides which commonly affect the DIP joint; psoriasis usually causes bone loss resulting in instability rather than significant pain.

Examination

Clinical findings are usually swelling, deformity and pain on active and passive movement of the joint. It is important to elicit pain on movement, as often pain can arise from a mucous cyst rather than arthritis in the joint. The deformity in the nail is characteristic and should indicate the presence of a cyst. Multiple joint involvement should assist in the diagnosis.

Treatment

Treatment is seldom necessary. Mucous cysts can be removed both for pain and for cosmetic appearance, but recurrence is common because the underlying joint remains abnormal. They may be reduced by removing osteophytes, or by replacing the thinned-out skin over the cyst by a rotation-advancement flap.

Surgery to the DIP joint itself is very rarely called for. Although DIP joint flexion is important in power grip, this flexion is only useful with stability. Thus the best surgical solution in a painful DIP joint is arthrodesis. This is an excellent procedure which provides a pain-free and stable finger (*Figure 4C.20*).

The surgical approach to the DIP joint can be a problem because mucous cysts often cause significant thinning of the skin that can be difficult to dissect off the cyst. Therefore, it is sometimes necessary to rotate skin from proximally to cover a skin defect. I have found that a trap-door type incision, which is radially or ulnar-based like an incision for a cross-finger flap but more distal, is particularly good in that the incision line avoids the dorsum of the joint.

In psoriatics achieving a satisfactory arthrodesis is difficult. There is often significant loss of bone stock and bone grafting may be necessary. Infection is not an uncommon sequel and the circulation never seems very good. Amputation is a recognised complication. There is said to be an erosive form of osteoarthritis producing a very similar pattern to psoriatic arthritis with instability.

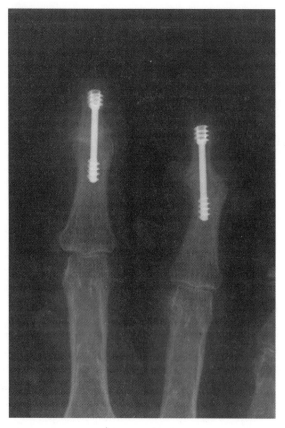

Figure 4C.20 Arthrodesis of DIP joints with Herbert screw.

FURTHER READING

Burton RI, Pelligrini VD. Surgical management of basal joint arthritis of the thumb. Part II. Ligament reconstruction with tendon interposition arthroplasty. *J. Hand Surg* 1986; **11A:** 324–332.

Davis TRC, Brady O, Barton NJ, Lunn PG, Burke FD. Trapeziectomy alone, with tendon interposition or with ligament reconstruction: a randomised prospective study. *J. Hand Surg* 1997; **22B:** 689–694.

Eaton RG, Glickel SZ. Trapeziometacarpal osteoarthritis staging as a rationale for treatment. *Hand Clin* 1987; **3:** 455–471.

Ellison MR, Kelly KJ, Flatt AE. The results of surgical synovectomy of the digital joints in rheumatoid disease. *J Bone Joint Surg* 1971; **53A:** 1041–1060.

Flatt AE. *The Care of the Arthritic Hand*, 5th edn, St Louis: Quality Medical Publishing, 1995.

Kiefhaber TR, Strickland JW. Soft tissue reconstruction for rheumatoid swan neck and boutonnière deformities: long term results. *J Hand Surg* 1993; **18A:** 984–989.

Nalebuff EA. The rheumatoid thumb. *Rheum Dis Clin North Am* 1984; **10:** 589–595.

Oster LH, Blair WF, Steyers CM, Flatt AE. Crossed intrinsic transfer. *J Hand Surg* 1989; **14A:** 963–971.

Souter WA. Planning treatment for the rheumatoid hand. *Hand* 1979; **11:** 3–16.

Swanson AB. Flexible implant arthroplasty for arthritic finger joints. *J Bone Joint Surg* 1969; **54A:** 435–455.

4D

Miscellaneous

Colin Dent

INFECTIONS OF THE HAND

Despite the availability of antimicrobial chemotherapy, a significant number of hand infections require surgical treatment. The sequelae of improper treatment of infections are stiffness, contractures, osteomyelitis and destructive arthritis leading to functional impairment and pain.

Infections of the hand are usually described by their anatomical location and are divided into recognisable named conditions. Alternatively, infections can be classified on the basis of the infective organism. The majority of surgically important infections are caused by bacteria and *Staphylococcus aureus* is the most commonly isolated organism, although multiple organisms are often found. Many other organisms including viruses and fungi have been reported to be responsible for hand infections and some of these have been associated with specific predispositions which often involve occupation (*Table 4D.1*).

Most bacterial infections affecting the soft tissue of the hand will result from a penetrating injury through the skin. Osteomyelitis is not common in the hand, but may be secondary to an open fracture or blood-borne infection. A group of hand infections can be considered to be iatrogenic, having commenced as a complication of a surgical procedure. There are well-recognised groups of patients who are susceptible to postoperative infection, including those with rheumatoid arthritis who may be taking corticosteroids and immunocompromised patients; in these cases the infecting opportunist organisms are often atypical and are less likely to be bacterial.

A typical bacterial infection will commence as a cellulitis and at this stage presents with pain, red skin discolouration and may be associated with localised and proximal tender lymphadenopathy. Treatment is by antibiotic therapy, the choice of which is based on the history of any precipitating injury and taking into account occupation and other activities. Subsequent identification of the infecting agent can occasionally be obtained from wound swabs or blood cultures taken prior to instigation of antibiotic therapy. There is no indication for surgical incision and drainage at the stage of cellulitis, so there is rarely any opportunity to culture infected matter. Elevation of the affected limb is essential to minimise swelling and stiffness and will help by preventing use of the hand at this time. It is also important to splint the hand with the joints in the appropriate positions to prevent development of any contractures. Early treatment in this manner may prevent the progression to a localised anatomically defined infection within the hand.

There are many anatomical spaces and compartments in the hand within which infections can become established and inaccessible to antibiotics. The production of pus causes increased pressure within the tissues

Table 4D.1 Infective agents in specific occupational groups

Agent	Occupational group
Erisipelothrix rhusiopathiae	Slaughterhouse workers
Mycobacterium marinum	Fishkeepers
Herpes simplex	Health workers
Sporothrix schenckii	Gardeners
Vibrio vulnificus	Fishermen
Pox virus (Orf, Cowpox)	Animal handlers
Mycobacterium tuberculosis	Anatomists

which leads to swelling and abscess formation in superficial areas, but in deeper compartments causes significant tissue destruction. Surgical incision and drainage is necessary when infections are seen later than the earliest cellulitis phase or when non-operative treatment has not led to resolution of symptoms. At this stage the patient will complain of marked pain in the hand and will be reluctant to use the affected part or the whole hand. There will typically be signs of infection with pyrexia, tachycardia and lymphadenopathy. The classical presentation of a suppurative infection is less commonly encountered in hospital practice. The majority of hand infections are seen when patients have already commenced on antibiotic therapy prior to referral to the hand surgeon, and the clinical picture will not correspond to either a classical cellulitis or abscess. In these cases it may be difficult to determine whether a longer period of conservative treatment alone will effect resolution. Any infections which have not markedly improved within 24 hours of effective antibiotic therapy should be treated surgically, not least to obtain specimens for bacteriological examination.

There are few contraindications to surgery if the principles for carrying out incision and drainage are adhered to. It is advisable to use a tourniquet to maximise visualisation of the anatomy of the hand and avoid damage to the neurovascular structures. Exsanguination of the limb should not be carried out as there is a risk of disseminating infection, but elevation prior to inflating the tourniquet is helpful.

The accepted principles for planning of incisions for the surgical treatment of hand infections are shown in *Table 4D.2*.

Table 4D.2 Principles of siting of incisions in surgical management of hand infections

---

Incision must allow direct access to the abscess

Incision should permit easy extension in either direction

No incision should cross any flexion crease at a right angle

Incision should avoid injuring nerves, vessels, or tendons

The approach should avoid compromising blood supply to any skin-flaps created

If possible, scars should be sited away from sensitive tactile areas on the volar surface of the hand and digits

---

The specific incision used will clearly depend on which anatomical compartment of the hand is suspected to be the site of infection. It is not always apparent before exploration which part of the hand is affected, in particular which of the palmar spaces, though the position of any entry site for infection may indicate this. At the time of drainage specimens for microbiological examination are collected. When an atypical organism is suspected different forms of biopsy material and specimens may be required and special culture media used.

The management of wounds following incision and drainage is an area of controversy. Open management of wounds is a well-established technique in which the wounds are packed for a period of 48 hours and then allowed to heal by secondary intention. Some authors advocate primary closure of wounds when complete drainage of pus and debridement of dead tissue has been achieved. It is claimed that there is little risk of increased morbidity using this technique which produces cosmetically better scars. A combination of these two methods involves closing the wound around two drains which allow wound lavage and free drainage. Postoperative treatment, regardless of wound management, should include antibiotic therapy and splintage of the affected part in the safe position and in elevation to minimise swelling.

Paronychia

A paronychium or whitlow is an infection of the nail-fold. The causative organism is usually *Staphylococcus aureus* introduced into the soft tissue area by a minor injury. These simple infections are straightforward to treat when they present early; at this stage the infection is superficial and can be drained by opening the abscess with a scalpel blade. The wound is left open and regular soaks and dressing changes are instigated to complete the drainage of pus. More extensive, so called 'run-around abscesses', occur when the pus tracks round the eponychial fold deep to the nail sulcus, reaching the other side of the nail, and may accumulate deep to the nail itself. This requires a more extensive surgical drainage procedure.

These surgical procedures are best performed under ring block anaesthesia. Damage to the nail-bed and germinal matrix can cause scarring which may result in deformity of the nail, which is the main late complication of these infections. The aim of surgery is to obtain decompression and drainage of pus through as conservative an approach as possible. For a typical one-sided abscess, the paronychial fold may be incised; if the pus is deep to the nail itself, the nail-fold is bluntly elevated and a one-quarter sized sliver of the adjacent nail is removed. Deeper and run-around infections are treated by removal of a portion of the base of the nail after bluntly elevating the nail-fold at each side. Alternatively, the eponychial fold can be elevated and turned back on itself to remove the base of the nail. In removing the nail, care must be exercised to not damage the germinal matrix.

Chronic paronychia occur especially in people whose hands are constantly moist through occupation or other activities. *Candida albicans* is present in the majority of these chronic infections but Gram-negative bacteria have also been isolated. It has been suggested that there must also be a degree of obstruction to the nail-fold for a chronic infection to occur. Non-operative treatment utilises concomitant topical steroids and antifungal chemotherapy, but is unsuccessful in a high proportion of cases. Surgical treatment has been described and reported to give an effective cure in up to 90% of cases. The method has been termed eponychial marsupialisation. An area of skin is excised from the dorsal surface of the finger proximal to the nail. The skin is excised to the full width and depth to the germinal matrix but the surgeon avoids damaging this structure. This allows drainage of the germinal matrix prior to epithelialisation. The other surgical method described is to remove the entire nail and apply topical agents to the exposed nail-bed.

Felon

Felons are volar closed-space infections in the distal pulp of the finger. A felon is situated in one of the small compartments of the finger pulp formed by the vertical fibrous septa. The dorsal aspect of the compartment is the rigid bone of the terminal phalanx. Felons are usually the result of a penetrating injury to the pulp and contamination with Staphylococcus *aureus*. Pain in the fingertip is often intense as the abscess forms within the unyielding compartment. As the pressure builds, the septa of the fingertip may break down and necrosis and osteomyelitis of the terminal phalanx may occur. The diaphysis receives its blood supply from the digital

arteries within the pulp compartment and pressure may lead to nutrient artery thrombosis.

The majority of felons at the time of presentation will need surgical incision and drainage. The choice of incision is contentious. The classical technique is a fish-mouth incision around the end of the finger tip; however complications of this incision have been reported, including painful scar formation in the tactile area. Many other approaches have been described, but a unilateral longitudinal incision is most favoured. This is placed on the side of the fingertip, dorsal and distal to the distal interphalangeal joint crease, but not crossing the tip. The incision is deepened to gain access to the pulp compartment. If there is a sinus, the incision should be modified to incorporate the sinus track. Following drainage, the abscess is held open with a pack to ensure drainage for three days.

Infective tenosynovitis

Infection of the flexor tendon sheath necessitates prompt diagnosis and rapid treatment. A *pyogenic* infection in the sheath creates adhesions between the tendons and the sheath itself, causing loss of the normal sliding motion of the tendon. Infections of the tenosynovium almost exclusively affect the flexor tendon sheaths and the radial and ulnar bursae. The ring, middle and index fingers are most commonly affected. The infection follows an injury which penetrates the flexor tendon sheath. The usual infective organism is *Staphylococcus aureus*.

Kanavel described the four cardinal signs of pyogenic flexor tenosynovitis (*Table 4D.3*).

Table 4D.3 Kanavel' cardinal signs

1. Flexed or semi-flexed position of the finger
2. Uniform symmetrical swelling of the finger
3. Excessive tenderness along the sheath, limited to the sheath
4. Excruciating pain on passively extending the finger, most marked at the proximal end

Operative treatment is required in the large majority of cases. A protocol for non-operative treatment of early cases has been described. These early cases of less than 48 hours duration are splinted in a compressive dressing and elevated. Intravenous broad-spectrum antibiotic therapy is commenced and the hand is observed for signs of improvement. There is less risk of inappropriate treatment if all suspected cases are dealt with operatively, to achieve drainage of pus and obtain bacteriological specimens. The surgical approaches to the finger are variable and include techniques for both open drainage and closed irrigation through small incisions in the skin.

A Bruner incision placed on the volar surface of the finger is suitable for gaining good access to the entire flexor tendon sheath. An alternative approach for open drainage is a mid-lateral incision extending from the web space to the distal interphalangeal joint. The neurovascular bundle is elevated with the volar flap and the sheath is visualised between the annular pulleys. From this point the sheath is irrigated and drained through a small transverse incision at its proximal end. Other less invasive methods of surgical drainage utilise through-irrigation with a catheter inserted into the flexor sheath proximally and draining through a distal portal. Thorough lavage is essential to remove the pus and prevent the development of adhesions within the flexor sheath.

Early mobilisation of the infected finger following surgical incision and drainage is the preferred form of rehabilitation. The hand is elevated and immobilised for 24 houirs and at this stage the dressings are changed and made less bulky. Active mobilisation is commenced up to four times a day. This requires the patient to remain in hospital. The rehabilitation must be supervised by a hand therapist, with attention to regaining the sliding movement between the profundus and superficialis tendons.

A less common form of tenosynovitis occurs which is caused by *mycobacterial* infections. Many atypical mycobacterial infections have been described and often relate to occupational risks of exposure to specific organisms. Presentation is usually in the form of pain and swelling in a single digit. The diagnosis is usually made following laboratory testing of operative biopsy material. The laboratory should be warned of the possibility of atypical mycobacteria, which require special culture media. This takes a few weeks and antituberculous therapy should be commenced on clinical suspicion. When the diagnosis is confirmed, the treatment should be continued for six months. At operation there is an obvious chronic proliferative synovitis. Surgical synovectomy is essential in order to preserve the ten-

dons, but efforts are made to preserve the pulley structures of the fibrous flexor sheath.

Web-space infection

The subfascial web-space is situated on the palmar surface of the hand and interdigital area. The limits of the web-space are the natatory ligaments distally, the deep attachment of the palmar fascia proximally and its attachment to the tendon sheaths laterally. The deep transverse metacarpal ligament is the floor of the space.

The infection arises from a wound to the skin between the fingers. The infection presents within a few days of the injury, and the swelling and pain are localised to the web-space and distal palm. The fingers adjacent to the infected web-space adopt a characteristic abducted posture.

Web-space infections with swelling always require incision and drainage. The planning and siting of the incision should follow the basic surgical principles (*Table 4D.2*). A transverse incision is avoided as it would lead to contraction of the web-space and reduced finger abduction. Suitable incisions can be sited on either the palmar or dorsal surface and may incorporate both approaches. Web-space infections may lead to a collar-stud abscess. This occurs when a narrow sinus through the space connects a superficial collection of pus to a deeper collection in the looser connective tissue of the palm. This must be considered at the time of surgical exploration to ensure complete drainage of pus.

Palmar space infections

The mid-palmar and thenar spaces are potential fascial spaces in the palm. These two spaces are situated deep to the flexor tendons and lumbrical muscles in zone 3, and superficial to the interossei and adductor pollicis. Both spaces are limited proximally by fascia at the carpal tunnel and distally by vertical septa of the palmar fascia at the web-space.

The two spaces are separated by a vertical septum in line with the middle finger (*Figure 4D.1*). The thenar space is radial to this septum and its lateral border is the thenar septum which is attached to the palmar aponeurosis and the first metacarpal. The thenar eminence muscles are radial to the thenar space.

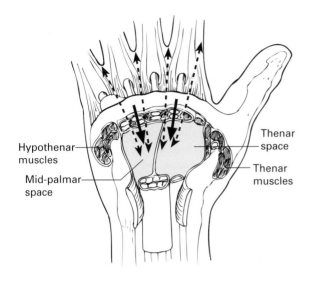

Figure 4D.1 Surgical approach to thenar and mid-palmar spaces. Broken arrows, propagation of infection from the web-spaces; solid arrows, direction of surgical approach to drain the thenar and mid-palmar spaces. Redrawn from Tubiana R, McCullough CJ, Masquelet AC. *An Atlas of Surgical Exposures of the Upper Extremity*, London: Martin Dunitz, 1990.

The mid-palmar space is medial to the vertical septum and bordered on the medial side by the hypothenar septum.

Infections of the palmar spaces can arise from a penetrating wound, propagation from a web-space infection, or rupture of the fibrous flexor sheath in infective tenosynovitis. Pain and loss of function appear within a few days of injury, and the hand presents with marked swelling of the dorsal surface, loss of palmar concavity and fixed finger posture. Passive movement of the fingers is possible, in contrast to infective tenosynovitis.

Palmar space infections always require incision and drainage. The preferred approach to the thenar space is a longitudinal incision in the mid-palm overlying the third metacarpal. The neurovascular bundle and the flexor tendons are retracted and the tense thenar space is exposed. The mid-palmar space is best approached by using a longitudinal incision placed obliquely across the palm. The adjacent neurovascular bundles and tendons are retracted in opposite directions to gain access to the underlying mid-palmar space. Postoperative management may involve simple drainage or the use of indwelling catheters for continuous lavage to ensure complete evacuation of infected material.

Septic arthritis

Infections occur due to an overlying infected wound, or from a direct injury involving penetration of the joint or articular surfaces. The metacarpophalangeal (MP) joints are most commonly affected, and the typical mechanism is a blow to someone else's mouth using a clenched fist with the MPs fully flexed. This often results in a tooth producing an open fracture of the metacarpal head. Adequate treatment of a bite injury requires surgical excision of the wound margins from the skin, tendon and capsule supported by broad-spectrum antimicrobial chemotherapy.

All forms of suspected septic arthritis must be aspirated for laboratory examination. Confirmed septic arthritis is treated by a wide surgical arthrotomy with lavage and debridement of all infected material. Postoperatively the joint should be both passively and actively mobilised, which is beneficial to the preservation of the articular hyaline cartilage. A late consequence of septic arthritis, despite prompt treatment, may be the onset of osteoarthritis in the affected joint.

Fungal infections

The majority of fungal infections of the hand are cutaneous or subcutaneous. Deep and systemic infections can arise from direct inoculation of fungus into the deep tissues of the hand, but these systemic infections are usually restricted to immunosuppressed individuals.

Cutaneous infections are caused by dermatophytes which colonise dead superficial layers of the skin and lead to distinct types of clinical infections in different areas of the body. Tinea manum is an infection of the interdigital areas and palms of the hands. Tinea nigra also affects the palmar surfaces and causes variably-sized macular black lesions which can be mistaken for a melanoma. Onychomycosis refers to any fungal infection of the fingernails. The majority of cutaneous infections can be diagnosed by examination of skin specimens and treated by topical chemotherapy. It is common for secondary bacterial infection to occur which can bring about a delay in diagnosis.

Spirotrichosis is the most common subcutaneous infection and is caused by *Sporothrix schenckii*. This presents with ulcerated lesions on the hands and regional lymphadenopathy. This is often an occupational infection from the habitat of this organism in soil and plants. The treatment of choice, which usually successfully eradicates the infection, is a six-week course of oral potassium iodide.

Mycobacterial infections

Mycobacterium tuberculosis presents in the hand in three forms: a tenosynovial infection, infection of the wrist joint, and an osteomyelitis of the fingers known as dactylitis. Atypical mycobacteria have been identified and recognised as a cause of infections in the hand: tenosynovitis affecting the flexor tendons is the most common form, although osteomyelitis has been reported. *Mycobacterium marinum* is found in warm water and is introduced through skin lesions. *Mycobacterium kansasii* is a cause of lung disease but can lead to hand infection through haematogenous spread. The diagnosis of these atypical organisms is based on a history of possible exposure in the face of a characteristic clinical presentation. Confirmation requires special culture of biopsy specimens, which can lead to appropriate chemotherapy.

JOINT INJURIES

We shall consider first the fingers then the thumb.

The carpometacarpal joints of the fingers

Acute dislocations of the carpometacarpal (CM) joints of the fingers are uncommon. These joints are intrinsically stable and there is no clinically detectable movement at the second and third CM joints. There is a small degree of flexion and extension at the fourth CM joint. The fifth CM joint has the greatest mobility: the shape of the articulating surfaces of the metacarpal base and the hamate provides up to 20° of flexion and extension, and the slight obliquity allows supination which is demonstrable when the little finger is opposed to the thumb. The great stability of these joints is a consequence of the strong dorsal, volar and interosseous ligaments and adjacent muscular insertions. The shape of the articular surfaces contributes little to stability.

The fifth is the most commonly injured CM joint, reflecting its greater mobility and position of relative vulnerability. In the majority of cases, the base of the metacarpal is dorsal to the carpus although volar dislocations have been described. Multiple dislocation of all four joints has been reported usually as a component of major upper limb injuries.

These injuries are often overlooked in the presence of more obvious injuries. The history is of significant trauma causing compression and flexion along the line of the metacarpal shaft. Examination reveals marked swelling and ecchymosis of the dorsum of the hand. The swelling may obscure the visible deformity of the displaced metacarpal base and diagnosis is confirmed from radiographs. Standard posteroanterior and lateral radiographs should be supplemented by a 30° pronated film to give better visualisation of the CM joints. Key points in not missing these injuries are to consider the diagnosis and perform a thorough examination, supplemented by an adequate number of radiographs (which must include a lateral) to establish congruity of all CM joints.

Closed reduction of an *acute dislocation* can be achieved in the majority of cases by longitudinal traction, flexion and direct pressure over the metacarpal base. Interposition of soft tissue and failure to achieve a congruent reduction will necessitate open reduction. The approach to the joint is from a direct dorsally-placed longitudinal incision. Stability, which is dependent on the ligamentous structures, is compromised following dislocation and percutaneous Kirschner wiring of the joint maintains reduction (whether closed or open) during the period of soft tissue healing. The wires should be left in place for a period of four weeks. It is difficult to maintain the reduction with plaster immobilisation alone; as the swelling lessens, movement occurs within the plaster which allows re-dislocation. These dislocations are often associated with other hand fractures which may preclude the use of plaster splintage with the need for functional splintage of the fingers. Some authors advocate open insertion of the Kirschner wires in order to avoid tethering of the extensor tendons. My experience is that small stab incisions and the use of an artery forceps to spread the soft tissues is a satisfactory technique. Fluoroscopy is useful to check wire placement.

Late-presenting dislocations are rarely amenable to closed reduction and are difficult to reduce even at open arthrotomy. In these cases it is often necessary to excise the joint surfaces in a manner similar to that used in a chronic dislocation.

Chronic dislocations and *instability* present with pain associated on gripping and a subjective feeling of reduced grip strength, most commonly in individuals undertaking heavy handling work, or using hand-held machinery. On examination, the dorsally dislocated or subluxing metacarpal base becomes more apparent if the patient is asked to grip strongly. Radiographs will confirm the diagnosis and dynamic screening is useful in difficult cases. These late injuries always require open reduction and stabilisation. The ligaments are incised and the articular surfaces always need to be excised to obtain a reduction. Subsequently arthrodesis of the joint is essential to prevent continuing pain and instability. This is achieved by inserting a bone graft and postoperative immobilisation with percutaneous Kirschner wires. This seemingly straightforward arthrodesis has a reputation for forming a pseudarthrosis and great care and attention to detail of operative technique is needed to obtain solid bony union. A period of immobilisation of the hand is helpful to discourage premature return to activity.

The metacarpophalangeal joints of the fingers

The metacarpophalangeal joints of the fingers permit flexion and extension, with a lesser degree of abduction and adduction and a small amount of rotation. The metacarpal head is much larger than the base of the proximal phalanx in the anteroposterior dimension, but has a smaller transverse axis. The volar plate forms a significant part of the anterior articular surface for the metacarpal head, facilitating the large range of motion in flexion and extension. The shape of the articulating surfaces means they contribute little to joint stability, which is provided by the capsule and ligaments.

The soft tissues of the MP joint form a box-shaped structure, the volar surface of which is formed by the thick volar plate, which is thick and fibrocartilaginous at its distal attachment: an adaptation to its function as part of the articular surface for the metacarpal head. Each volar plate is continuous on its radial and ulnar sides with the deep transverse metacarpal ligament, forming a continuous fibrous structure in the palm of the hand. At the sides of each joint the capsule is strengthened by the collateral ligaments, which arise on the side of the metacarpal head where it is most

narrow; the distal attachment is to the volar part of the base of the proximal phalanx. Some authors describe an accessory collateral ligament, which is a proximal portion of the collateral ligament. The collateral ligaments are tight in flexion because the ligaments diverge to pass across the wider anterior projection of the metacarpal head, in contrast to the position in extension when the ligaments cross the narrower dorsal part of the metacarpal head. Consequently the MP joint is at its most stable in the position of flexion, whereas in extension there is a significant degree of abduction and adduction as a result of the lesser tension in the ligaments.

Injuries to the collateral ligaments in isolation are extremely rare because the ligaments are lax when the fingers are extended at the MP joint which is the position of vulnerability to injury. If an injury does occur, the radial collateral ligament is more commonly affected. To test for stability to an adduction or abduction force the MP joint must be fully flexed, at which position the collateral ligaments are tight and there is no movement. These injuries, when there is no dislocation or volar plate disruption, are treated nonoperatively, with the MP joints of the fingers splinted at a minimum of 50° flexion. If the MP joint is splinted in extension, the collateral ligaments will contract and form a block to subsequent flexion. This is important if there is an acute joint injury, when an effusion or haemarthrosis will tend to extend the joint as this is the position of greatest joint capacity.

Dislocations of the finger MP joints are rare injuries, the usual form is a *dorsal dislocation* with the metacarpal head coming to lie volar to the proximal phalanx. The index and little fingers are most commonly affected because they are in the more vulnerable positions on the hand. The mechanism of dislocation is forceful hyperextension at the MP joint and requires a considerable force. Two forms of injury have been described. In both, the volar plate is detached proximally but its subsequent position is important in selecting the appropriate treatment.

The less significant injury is termed a *simple subluxation*. The MP joint has been forcibly extended and the finger shows considerable hyperextension at the MP joint. The volar plate remains attached distally and remains in its normal position volar to the metacarpal head. Therefore, although the articulating surfaces have subluxed, the volar plate retains its position relative to the joint and is not interposed between the two surfaces. In contrast, a *complex irreducible dislocation* occurs when the proximally detached volar plate becomes displaced between the articulating surfaces, with its proximal margin dorsal to the metacarpal head. The flexor tendons within the fibrous flexor sheath remain attached to the volar plate and consequently lie dorsal and to one side of the metacarpal head, which comes through like the button through a buttonhole. In the index finger the metacarpal head is then encircled by the flexor tendons to the ulnar side and the lumbrical muscle radially; the little finger metacarpal head has the flexor superficialis and profundus tendons and lumbrical muscle on its radial side, and the tendon of flexor digiti minimi and abductor digiti quinti to the ulnar side.

Diagnostic differentiation between the two types of injury is clinical and radiological. A simple subluxation will show marked hyperextension at the MP joint. A complete dislocation will show a much lesser degree of extension as the two dislocated articular surfaces overlap and effectively shorten. There will be an associated lack of flexion due to the interposed volar plate and tendons and the metacarpal head will be palpable in the palm. Radiographs are essential to exclude any fracture. A lateral radiograph of a complete dislocation will show a widened joint space due the soft tissue interposition.

Treatment of a simple subluxation is by closed reduction and splintage with a block extension splint (*Figure 4D.2*) and early movement followed by a period of neighbour strapping to an adjacent finger. The reduction requires flexion at the wrist joint to reduce

tension in the flexor tendons, and dorsally applied pressure to the base of the proximal phalanx. Inappropriate hyperextension will convert the injury into a complete dislocation with the interposition of the volar plate.

Complete dislocations always require operative reduction. Protagonists of the volar approach describe the advantages of direct visualisation of the displaced neurovascular bundles, and direct access to the volar plate and tendons interposed between the articulating surfaces. Division of the A1 pulley to partially mobilise the flexor tendons is readily carried out through this approach. The dorsal approach is claimed to produce less iatrogenic neurovascular damage by avoiding these structures, but is restricted in access to the interposed soft tissues. Following open reduction the joint is immobilised in flexion with an extension block splint.

Late sequelae of dorsal dislocations include osteoarthritis from cartilage injury at the time of injury or operation, and loss of movement often secondary to prolonged splintage.

Volar MP joint dislocations are exceedingly rare injuries. The literature contains reports of successful management by closed reduction, but operative reduction is usually required to remove the dorsal capsule from the joint space where it forms a block to a congruent reduction.

The proximal interphalangeal joints of the fingers

The proximal interphalangeal joints of the fingers together with the metacarpophalangeal joint of the thumb, are the most commonly injured joints in the hands.

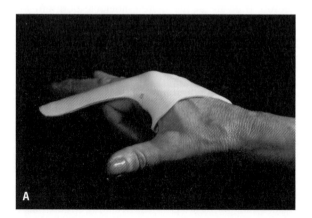 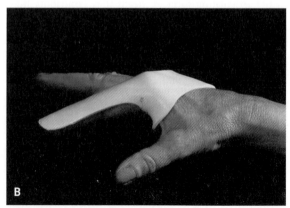

Figure 4D.2 Extension block splint applied to MP joint showing finger in (a) limited extension and (b) flexion.

The mobility of the fingers requires that the PIP joints are stable in all positions of hand function. The two joint surfaces form a true hinge with two articular facets on each bone. There are two condyles on the proximal phalanx and two shallow reciprocal facets on the middle phalanx. Little stability of the joint is derived from the constraints of the articulating joint surfaces, although between the two condyles is an intercondylar notch which provides some rotational stability. Significant stability is derived from soft tissue structures: the collateral ligaments, the volar plate and the fibrous flexor sheath. The collateral ligament on each side is subdivided into the true and accessory collateral. The origin of these ligaments is a recess on the lateral side of the condyle of the proximal phalanx. The origin of the accessory collateral is slightly proximal and volar to that of the true ligament. In contrast to the collateral ligaments of the metacarpophalangeal joint, these ligaments remain taut throughout the complete range of flexion and extension, providing stability to abduction and adduction forces. This is a result of the more volar origin of the collateral ligament at the PIP joint and the absence of an increased transverse diameter on the volar aspect of the proximal phalanx. The volar or palmar plate of the PIP joint is a complex structure forming the volar aspect or floor of the joint. The distal part of the volar plate is formed from thick fibrocartilaginous connective tissue which provides tensile strength, and sufficient strength in compression to allow the volar plate to function as part of the articular surface for the proximal phalanx. The volar plate attaches distally to the volar base of the middle phalanx where it blends with the periosteum. The accessory ligament inserts onto the lateral margins of the volar plate, lying both proximal and volar to the true ligament. The strongest points of attachment are at the lateral margins of the base of the middle phalanx where the volar plate is attached to the true collateral ligament. The proximal attachments of the volar plate are through check-rein or volar check ligaments which are proximal lateral extensions of the fibrous volar plate. The check-rein ligaments originate from the volar surface of the proximal phalanx at the level of insertion of the second annular pulley. The accessory collateral ligaments are joined to the check-rein ligaments effectively forming the side walls of the joint. Between the check-rein ligaments is the membranous part of the volar plate, which is thinner and weaker and does not form part of the articulating surface. The inherent strength of the soft tissues of the PIP joint is its box type structure, which requires disruption in two planes to produce instability.

There is a spectrum of ligamentous injuries affecting the PIP joint. Incomplete ruptures do not produce instability, but complete ruptures can lead to dorsal, lateral and volar dislocation. The description refers to the position of the middle phalanx relative to the proximal phalanx.

Diagnosis of these injuries is usually straightforward, although many dislocations will have been reduced by the patient immediately after injury. These injuries are often sustained while undertaking sporting activities involving physical contact, or ball-handling games.

Dorsal dislocations which are the commonest, are typically caused by hyperextension of the finger with a simultaneous force transmitted along the length of the finger. This can be caused by a forceful blow to the end of the finger from a ball, or direct contact whilst the finger is extended. The volar plate is damaged by the hyperextension, being ruptured at its distal attachment to the middle phalanx. Tears in the membranous part of the volar plate are rare. The collateral ligaments are disrupted, as a split develops between the true and accessory ligaments; the true ligament remains attached to the volar aspect of the base of the middle phalanx. The middle phalanx comes to lie dorsal to the head of the proximal phalanx, roughly parallel to the proximal phalanx, and the true collateral ligament now passes dorsally from its intact origins on the proximal phalanx. The accessory ligament remains attached to the check-rein ligaments on the lateral margins of the volar plate. As the volar plate shortens the accessory ligament is sited in a more proximal position on the proximal phalanx. The attachment of the extensor tendon to the middle phalanx acts as a dislocating force, because it pulls the middle phalanx both proximally and dorsally.

Fracture–dislocation is the most serious type of injury to the PIP joint and is the most difficult to treat successfully. The volar aspect of the middle phalanx is fractured in association with the dorsal dislocation. The volar plate may remain intact but pull off a small fragment of bone from the middle phalanx. Small fractures are effectively similar to simple dislocations with volar plate detachment; however, fractures involving more than 30% of the base of the middle phalanx are inherently unstable. The loss of the volar articular surface results in alteration of the action of the extensor mechanism of the finger. The central slip of the extensor tendon imparts a dorsal dislocating force through its attachment to the middle phalanx.

Lesser *dorsal hyperextension* (*subluxation*) injuries occur in which the PIP joint does not dislocate but the volar plate is detached distally and there is a split between the edges of the true and accessory collateral ligaments. The middle phalanx still articulates with the most dorsal surface of the condyles of the proximal phalanx and the volar plate is not interspersed between the articulating surfaces.

The appearance of the unreduced injury can give some indication of the type of injury sustained. With a hyperextension injury the finger is often hyperextended at the PIP joint and examination reveals no loss of length at the joint and the head of the proximal phalanx is not palpable on the volar aspect of the finger. Dorsal dislocations and fracture–dislocations have less hyperextension at the PIP joint, as the finger shortens. The proximal phalanx is palpable on the volar surface of the finger, and the base of the middle phalanx is palpable dorsally.

Both PA and lateral radiographs are essential to ascertain the presence of a fracture; oblique views may also be required. Assessment of the injured finger itself is necessary to determine skin loss, tendon damage or neurovascular injury. If the painful joint is stable to lateral stressing with a full range of active and passive movement, the injury is limited to partial rupture of the soft tissues. Testing stability in all directions by passive stress is the final part of assessment.

The aim of treatment of all PIP joint injuries is to achieve a stable joint with a minimal restriction in the range of movement. Any restriction usually takes the form of a loss of extension resulting in a fixed flexion deformity. Early mobilisation of the joint is essential in all forms of treatment, in contrast to most joints which require immobilisation after injury. Dynamic extension splints are useful in the later stage of mobilisation and rehabilitation. These allow active flexion but also promote healing of the extensor mechanism without elongation. Continuing instability is uncommon. Fracture–dislocations with significant damage to the articular cartilage of the middle phalanx can predispose to the development of osteoarthritis.

Treatment of hyperextended and dorsally dislocated PIP joints is straightforward. Hyperextended joints readily reduce, with anaesthesia if necessary, and are found to be stable on examination, despite the detached volar plate. Appropriate treatment would be active movement protected by neighbour strapping to an adjacent finger for three weeks. Dorsal dislocations in the absence of a fracture are also usually stable to both passive and active stressing, and can be treated in a similar manner.

Fracture–dislocations are difficult to treat satisfactorily and a number of different methods have been described. Fractures forming less than 30% of the joint surface should be examined to confirm stability and treated as stable dislocations. When the extent of the fracture is greater than 30% and there is a single fragment, open reduction and internal fixation through a volar incision has been advised using both pull-out wire and screw fixation. The restoration of the joint congruity and the effective reattachment of the volar plate restores stability and early active movement is instigated. An extension block splint restricting 20° of movement is utilised for three weeks to protect the fixation. Smaller and comminuted fracture fragments are less amenable to this method of treatment. An alternative technique is a distal volar plate advancement. At open reduction the bone fragment is excised and the volar plate is advanced and attached to the site of the fracture at the base of the middle phalanx restoring stability in extension. This is termed a volar plate arthroplasty, as the volar plate covers the area of articular cartilage deficit on the middle phalanx. Following surgery, the finger is splinted in a similar manner to that described for internal fixation.

Non-operative treatment methods have been described utilising splintage alone. This was traditionally carried out with the PIP joint in flexion to prevent chronic hyperextension, but this often leads to a significant degree of fixed flexion. The technique used should prevent full extension, in which position the joint may redisplace. *Extension block splintage* alone has been described. This has the advantage of providing stable splintage and a protected range of active motion. This splint is cumbersome to wear and requires expertise to manufacture and fit to the patient, although it is possible to make a device from metal splints in the fracture clinic. This treatment relies on a compliant patient who will actively flex the PIP joint through a range of motion limited by the splint to prevent recurrent dislocation. The same effect can be achieved by using *extension block pinning*. A single Kirschner wire is inserted percutaneously into the dorsal surface of the head of the proximal phalanx in a position to block the final 30° of extension. The wire remains in place for a period of three weeks. Care is required at the time of insertion of the wire so as not to tether the extensor tendon which would lead to restricted tendon excursion. *Dynamic traction devices* utilising wires and springs have been described. These provide traction across the joint which restores the alignment of the fracture fragments. At the same time the splint is designed to provide an extension block to prevent dislocation whilst allowing active flexion. Proponents of the various techniques have all described satisfactory results; however it is clear that treating these most difficult injuries demands attention to technical detail and close supervision. I prefer extension block pinning which is simple to do and is less dependent on patient co-operation than extension block splinting.

Hyperextension injuries without dorsal dislocation may be undiagnosed and untreated at the time of injury, resulting in a chronic detachment of the distal margin of the volar plate from the middle phalanx. The *late presentation* is of pain in the PIP joint associated with persistent hyperextension and swan-neck deformity. There is often a complaint of a snapping finger, which is caused by the lateral bands of the extensor tendon passing from the dorsal to the volar aspect of the PIP joint as the joint is flexed from the position of hyperextension. The situation differs from a genuine swan-neck deformity in that the function of the distal interphalangeal joint is normal. Treatment, if required, is directed at strengthening the volar structures of the PIP joint by reattachment of the volar plate or a tenodesis using one half of the distal part of flexor digitorum superficialis.

Volar dislocations of the PIP joint occur much less commonly from a twisting force to the flexed finger. The collateral ligament complex on one side of the joint is disrupted and the ipsilateral condyle of the head of the proximal phalanx may buttonhole the central slip and lateral band of the extensor tendon. This usually results in an irreducible dislocation which requires open reduction and repair of the collateral ligament. A number of volar dislocations can be treated by closed reduction by traction with flexion of both the MP and PIP joint. Splintage in extension for three weeks is required to prevent repeat instability. Following closed reduction radiographs are required to assess the congruity of the reduction, and active extension is tested to confirm function of the extensor mechanism. When there is any concern regarding closed reduction, a mid-lateral incision is utilised to affect an open reduction with direct visualisation of the joint surfaces and the lateral bands.

Lateral PIP joint dislocation occurs from direct stress to one side of the joint causing rupture of both the true and accessory collateral ligaments and the adjacent volar plate. The dislocation spontaneously reduces, and instability is detected on stress testing of the joint. The vast majority of unstable injuries to the collateral ligaments will heal well with non-operative treatment. There is no equivalent displaced lesion similar to the Stener lesion of the MP joint of the thumb. Splintage is similar to that used in the treatment of dorsal dislocations.

The distal interphalangeal joints

The distal interphalangeal joints of the fingers are similar to the PIP joints but are less commonly injured. Dislocations are usually caused by a force to the fingertip whilst the finger is extended. The terminal phalanx is displaced dorsally and there is a higher incidence of open injuries as a consequence of the small amount of soft tissue at the level of the DIP joint.

The aim of treatment of DIP joint injuries is to regain pain-free stability of the joint in order to maintain a stable pinch grip. Unlike the PIP joint, stiffness at the DIP joint is not a significant disability if the terminal phalanx is in correct alignment. The majority of dislocations can be managed by closed reduction followed by a short period of immobilisation in the position of function of slight flexion. Open reduction is required when there is soft tissue interposition within the joint, and there are reports of tendons and the volar plate blocking reduction. Fracture–dislocations usually involve detachment of the extensor tendon resulting in a mallet finger. These injuries are treated on the basis of the more significant loss of extension.

Dislocations of the thumb

The most commonly dislocated joint of the thumb is the MP joint. This is a two-axis joint allowing predominantly flexion and extension but also a small degree of abduction and adduction. The articular surfaces contribute little to stability, which is provided by the strong collateral ligaments and volar plate. Dorsal dislocation is the usual pattern of injury, resulting in the proximal phalanx lying dorsal to and slightly overlying the metacarpal. The mechanism is hyperextension, often occurring in physical contact sports. The dislocation is always associated with a rupture of the volar plate and part of the collateral ligaments. The diagnosis can usually be made clinically but radiographs are mandatory to determine the presence of any associated fracture.

Treatment of these injuries is straightforward. Closed reduction is possible in most cases and is followed by four weeks immobilisation in a spica cast or a form of extension block splinting. Open reduction is required when closed reduction fails; this usually results from interposition of the volar plate or the tendon of flexor pollicis longus between the articular surfaces. Open reduction is best achieved through a volar approach, which allows direct visualisation of the joint space. The neurovascular bundles may be sited in a more anterior position until the dislocation is reduced, and are vulnerable to injury through this approach. Following reduction, a Kirschner wire may be required to maintain the position of the joint if the MP joint feels particularly unstable. Instability with recurrent dorsal dislocation or subluxation is an uncommon complication. The volar plate remains detached distally and is unable to provide stability and resistance to hyperextension. Reattachment of the volar plate at the time of open reduction is indicated, using either a pull-out suture on the dorsum of the thumb or a small tissue-anchor device.

Chronic dorsal instability is occasionally seen in rheumatoid arthritis, although it is not the most typical deformity seen at this joint in this disease.

Volar dislocation at the MP joint is less common and usually requires open reduction.

Traumatic dislocations and instability of the CM joint of the thumb are uncommon. The articulation between the trapezium and the first metacarpal is a saddle joint, with a slight concavity on the metacarpal surface, and a reciprocal convexity on the trapezium. Consequently there is little inherent joint stability from the shape of the articular surfaces. Stability is provided by ligaments and it is injury to these ligaments which leads to dislocation or instability.

An acute CM joint dislocation does not usually present a diagnostic difficulty, although these are rarely encountered injuries. Reports usually describe significant trauma associated with sporting activities or motorcycle accidents. In such cases it is important to consider the possibility of CM joint dislocation, as examination of the thumb may be overlooked in the presence of other injuries. Partial ligament tears lead to varying degrees of instability which are difficult to detect. Post-traumatic pain should be investigated by plain and stress radiography aided by comparison with the contralateral thumb.

Treatment of these injuries has not been described in any large series of published results. Open injuries require operative wound lavage and operative reduction. Most reported cases of dislocation suggest open reduction and ligament repair to prevent late instability. Other authors suggest closed reduction assessed by post-reduction radiographs to confirm joint congruity; in the absence of clinical instability at this stage non-surgical treatment produces a satisfactory result. If the reduction is not congruent, operative treatment is indicated. In all cases immobilisation in a cast for between four and six weeks is essential. Kirschner wire fixation of the CM joint is utilised to further protect the reduction following operative treatment. The position of immobilisation of the thumb in the cast is pronation and extension to allow approximation of the volar anterior oblique and intermetacarpal ligaments.

Chronic painful instability of the CM joint is commonly encountered but is rarely a consequence of any significant trauma. Instability is associated with both osteoarthritis and rheumatoid arthritis, which frequently affect the thumb CM joint. Various surgical methods have been described to treat this instability, including reconstruction of the volar surface ligaments and the fashioning of tendon sling for the base of the first metacarpal. If chronic instability is associated with osteoarthritis there are many forms of treatment including excision arthroplasty, hemi- and total arthroplasty and arthrodesis.

The *interphalangeal joint* of the thumb is less often injured than the MP joint. Dislocation occurs in a similar dorsal direction, and is treated by closed reduction and splintage in slight flexion. Instability is a rare sequel to this injury and stiffness causes little disability if the joint is in a functional position for pinch grip. Open reduction for interposed soft tissue may occasionally be necessary.

Chronic instability at this joint is most often a feature of rheumatoid arthritis.

Ulnar collateral ligament injury of the thumb

Lateral stability of the MP joint is provided by the collateral ligaments, which arise on the metacarpal and pass to a more volar insertion on the proximal phalanx. The medially–sited ulnar collateral ligament provides stability to an abduction force. The laterally–sited radial collateral ligament resists adduction force. Volar stability is provided by the volar plate which merges at its edges with the collateral ligaments and attaches distally to the volar margin of the proximal phalanx. Further dynamic volar stability to the joint comes from the intrinsic thenar muscles.

Injuries of the ulnar collateral ligament of the MP joint of the thumb are common. A tear of this ligament is better termed a gamekeeper's thumb, although this more correctly refers to instability secondary to chronic attenuation of the ligament. An acute traumatic ligament injury is often referred to as skier's thumb reflecting a more typical cause of injury, resulting in a fall onto the thumb or entrapment with a ski pole. However, disruption of this ligament can occur in many forms of athletic pursuits involving contact or ball–handling and from a fall onto the out-stretched hand. The force applied to the thumb results in radial deviation or abduction at the MP joint. The ulnar collateral ligament is avulsed from the base of the proximal phalanx and may include a fragment of bone. The dorsal capsule, volar plate and accessory collateral ligament are torn in more severe injuries. An important feature of this pattern of injury is that described by Stener: the avulsed ulnar collateral ligament is usually displaced and comes to lie superficial to the adductor expansion which normally covers it. As the realignment of the joint occurs, when the deforming force ceases, the adductor expansion may displace the distal end of the ligament in a proximal direction, away from its site of insertion. Consequently the ligament is separated from its point of attachment on the proximal phalanx by the interposed extensor expansion.

Management of these injuries is dependent on the differentiation of a partial from a complete rupture of the ulnar collateral ligament, and a complete undisplaced from a complete displaced rupture or Stener lesion.

Many methods have been described to differentiate the types of ligament injury.

The most simple test is palpation of the ulnar side of the joint; if you can feel a torn ligament that implies that it is displaced. My own experience is that this is a difficult assessment to make with any degree of confidence, due to the considerable swelling associated with this injury. An anatomical study has been reported showing that radial stress testing can be highly predictive of a Stener lesion. Division of the collateral ligament in isolation produced laxity on stressing at a position of 30° flexion, but the laxity was significantly less when tested in extension. When, in addition, the accessory collateral ligament and volar plate were divided, testing produced instability of greater than 35° in full extension. In the clinical study, greater than 35° of instability with radial stressing indicated disruption of the three structures and was associated with a Stener lesion confirmed at operation. Clinical testing may require local anaesthesia or nerve block to overcome pain and guarding.

Radiographs are essential to establish the presence or absence of a fracture of the proximal phalanx at the point of ligament attachment. The majority of fractures will not involve a significant part of the articular surface. An undisplaced avulsion fracture is difficult to detect on a radiograph and will suggest a complete undisplaced ligament rupture. Displacement of the fracture indicates a complete displaced lesion. A lateral radiograph may reveal volar subluxation of the proximal phalanx showing significant disruption to the dorsal capsule and a more severe type of injury.

Stress radiographs may be helpful in assessing the degree of laxity, although this information can usually be obtained without the addition of radiography. Any stress radiographs should be conducted by the surgeon to assess the end-point of the laxity. Abnormal stress radiography is always associated with a Stener lesion.

The effectiveness of ultrasound scanning in recognising a Stener lesion has been discussed in a number of studies. All authors report that ultrasound is sensitive in detecting displacement of the ligament, although there is an incidence of false positives in most studies. The value of ultrasound is that it is a non-invasive and inexpensive investigation. A disadvantage of ultrasonography is the difficulty in the diagnosis of less acute injuries.

Magnetic resonance imaging has become popular in the investigation of these injuries. MRI is both highly sensitive and specific in the diagnosis of displacement of the ulnar collateral ligament. There have been reports of misdiagnosis of normal cases as undisplaced tears; however the value of any investigation is in the detection of the displaced lesion.

An approach to diagnosis in a patient with an appropriate history of injury is first to make a clinical examination, which may demonstrate tenderness and swelling at the site of the ulnar collateral ligament. A radiograph should always be carried out, which may reveal a fracture and degree of displacement of the fracture fragment. Next, stress testing may suggest a displaced Stener lesion but, if doubt remains, it may be valuable to proceed to either ultrasonography or MRI scanning. In a number of cases doubt regarding the extent of the ligament injury may persist, which can only be resolved by surgical exploration.

The goal of treatment is the restoration of a pain-free thumb which is stable at the MP joint, with an unrestricted range of movement. The choice of treatment for these acute injuries is dependent on an accurate diagnosis. *Incomplete* and *undisplaced* complete ligament injuries can be treated non-surgically with the expectation of an excellent result; immobilisation in a thumb spica for a period of four weeks is an appropriate conservative treatment. Care should be taken to inspect the cast when the swelling goes down, to make sure the thumb MP joint is immobilised in slight flexion and ulnar deviation. The use of cast-braces has been reported to produce as good a result as a traditional spica. A percutaneous Kirschner wire across the MP joint can be utilised to maintain this position if a complete rupture is particularly unstable.

Displaced ligament injuries require surgical treatment as there is no hope of the displaced ligament healing in a proper anatomical position, and persistent instability is inevitable. A curved incision is sited on the ulnar side of the joint in the mid-lateral line. Following separation of the soft tissues the aponeurosis of adductor pollicis (usually termed the extensor expansion is reached). The collateral ligament may be apparent on the surface, or may be folded back proximally. This extensor expansion is incised longitudinally. If there is a fragment of bone displaced from the distal

articular surface, it may be feasible to reduce the fragment and the attached ligament to its correct position. Many techniques have been described to provide stable fixation of the fracture fragment following reduction. A reliable method utilises pull-out sutures and wires tied over a button on the radial side of the thumb. Small soft–tissue anchors in the proximal phalanx are an alternative method. Small interfragmentary screws are a popular technique; a single screw is usually adequate. My experience is that the bone fragment is often found to be larger at the time of surgery than was suspected from the preoperative radiographs and screw fixation is feasible. However, many fragments of bone are too small to fix successfully; in these cases it is best to excise the fragment and treat the injury as a soft tissue repair.

Displaced soft–tissue ligament ruptures are confirmed at the time of surgery when the ligament is identified prior to incision of the adductor aponeurosis. The ligament is replaced and fixed at its point of avulsion. It is important to suture the ligament back to the edge of the volar plate. Suture of the the extensor expansion is not essential; some authors state that this leads to restriction in movement at the IP joint.

A period of immobilisation following surgery is required following fixation of the bony fragment. It is advisable to immobilise the MP joint with both a Kirschner wire inserted percutaneously at the time of surgery and a plaster spica for four weeks. Review of the many reported series suggests that there is little loss of motion or recurrent instability following surgical repair. The most significant morbidity following this injury is when a displaced complete ligament rupture has not been diagnosed accurately and consequently inappropriately treated non-surgically.

Reattachment of an acute ulnar collateral ligament rupture is difficult if diagnosed after an interval of six weeks since injury. At this stage the injury can be considered chronic. The ligament is usually attenuated and it is not possible to reattach its distal end to the phalanx with a strong fixation. The disability associated with a chronic lesion is usually of a functional incapacity secondary to instability at the MP joint. This affects span grasp, as used when lifting a glass, and power grasp when gripping. Pain is a variable symptom and may be of little significance, although a long-standing instability may lead to the development of osteoarthritis in the joint. A few patients can be managed conservatively with the provision of a removable polypropylene thumb-splint, but this course of action is usually only feasible in elderly or very low demand patients. In my experience the splint needs to be made for each patient individually, to ensure close fitting and maximum benefit. The majority of patients will require surgical treatment to restore stability and eliminate pain; however, the majority of surgical techniques will result in some restriction in motion at the MP joint.

Assessment of the thumb should be carried out to confirm the degree of instability and radiographic views are required to ascertain the presence of any osteoarthritic change affecting the joint, particularly in long-standing chronic injuries. Treatment falls into three groups: reconstruction of the ulnar collateral ligament, tendon transfers and arthrodesis. Reconstruction of the ligament from the existing tissues is difficult and a free tendon graft, preferably palmaris longus, is required. A figure-of-eight technique using two holes in both the metacarpal and phalanx or using a V-shaped pattern passed through holes in the bone have been described. Postoperatively, immobilisation with a Kirschner wire and spica is required for six weeks. Hand therapy is necessary following mobilisation to minimise the loss of flexion and extension. The best published results show preservation of 85% of full motion. Dynamic tendon transfers have been described using adductor pollicis, the insertion of which is transferred to the ulnar side of the base of the proximal phalanx. Arthrodesis of the MP joint is the treatment of choice where there is osteoarthritis affecting the joint and is a cause of symptoms. It is clear that tendon reconstruction or transfer will not alleviate osteoarthritic pain. Arthrodesis results in a stable pain-free thumb and in most individuals who do not have widespread arthritis a full range of motion at the carpometacarpal and interphalangeal joints permits good function of the thumb as a whole. In heavy manual workers the reconstructed ulnar collateral ligament may fail to provide adequate stability, and arthrodesis may be the preferred surgical option to provide a strong stable thumb. Arthrodesis also serves as a salvage procedure for failed ligament reconstruction. I favour the chevron arthrodesis, using immobilisation with two percutaneous Kirschner wires and a spica; this technique results in slight shortening but allows the thumb to be fused in a functional position.

Radial collateral ligament injury of the thumb

The radial collateral is less commonly injured than the ulnar collateral ligament, but can also lead to a significant degree of pain and instability if inadequately treated.

The mechanism of this injury is an adduction or varus force to the thumb at the level of the MP joint. In contrast to the ulnar side, the site of rupture is variable and often occurs at the proximal origin on the metacarpal head. Diagnosis requires radiography to detect the presence of an avulsion fracture. A useful sign is volar subluxation at the MP joint, apparent on a lateral radiograph, which is suggestive of an extensive radial collateral ligament injury. There is no equivalent Stener lesion on the radial side of the MC joint, so displaced ruptures of the ligament are less common. Ultrasound scanning is also useful in ascertaining the degree of ligament disruption.

There is no consensus in the literature on the best means of treating these injuries. Similar good results have been reported with both conservative treatment by immobilisation in plaster or splints and following surgical repair. It has also been reported that results are not compromised by a delay in treatment in the same way as with ulnar collateral ligament injuries. Incomplete lesions without volar subluxation and less than 30° of instability on varus stressing are immobilised in pronation and extension for a period of four to six weeks. Extensive and complete lesions are probably best treated by an operative procedure aiming to reattach or repair the ruptured ligament. When there is volar subluxation, surgery is indicated; if not conservative.

Chronic lesions are managed in a similar manner to chronic ulnar collateral ligament instability.

VIBRATION WHITE FINGER

Vibration white finger is a form of secondary Raynaud's phenomenon associated with the use of hand-held vibrating tools and has been a prescribed occupational disorder in the UK since 1985. The earliest descriptions of the condition were in limestone-cutters and quarrymen; more recent reports describe this syndrome in lumberjacks, riveters and other occupations. Vibration white finger is the most commonly recognised and used name for this condition, although some authors prefer hand–arm vibration syndrome. Manifestations of occupational vibration in the upper limb include Raynaud's phenomenon, peripheral neuropathies, muscle injury, joint pain and stiffness and bone changes. Many factors affect the development of symptoms: the type of machinery used, the duration of exposure, the temporal pattern of exposure and environmental factors including noise and temperature. Vibration is a vector quantity, meaning that the direction and amplitude of the movement is important. The degree of physical stress associated with occupation is affected by the frequency, displacement, velocity and acceleration of the vibration. The latent period between exposure and onset of symptoms may be many years.

Many theories have been put forward to explain the mechanism of decreased blood flow in vibration white finger. A number of authors have stated that the cause is an abnormally high sensitivity and responsiveness to normal vasoconstrictive stimuli. The sensory vibration receptors (Pacinian corpuscles) may become over-excited by vibration and produce reflex vasoconstriction, supporting the theory of vibration-induced hyperactivity in the central sympathetic system causing vasoconstriction in predisposed individuals. Proponents of this theory have reported increased catecholamine excretion in sufferers of vibration white finger.

The other group of theories of pathogenesis emphasise the local effects of vibration leading to a defect in the vessel and increased peripheral resistance. A study has shown that smooth muscles of the blood vessels are directly affected by vibration and respond more strongly to noradrenaline causing reversible vasospasm. The effect of alteration in the composition of blood is not clear; there are reports of both normal and increased plasma and whole blood viscosity.

The pathophysiology is probably multifactorial, with a local effect in the digital artery wall, hyper-responsiveness of the peripheral arteries, and central sympathetic hyperactivity induced by cold, vibration and noise. A low temperature in the working environment is known to exacerbate the effect of any physical stressor. The effect of cold has been demonstrated on both sensory and motor performance, although the mechanism of this effect on tissue tolerance to a physical stressor is not known. The association of vibration white finger with peripheral nerve compression is recognised, and it has been suggested that the nerve

compression is a primary event in the subsequent development of vibration white finger.

Typical symptoms of vibration white fingers are blanching of the fingers associated with tingling and numbness. Initially the symptoms are often precipitated by cold but, if the condition becomes more marked the blanching occurs in warmer temperatures. The characteristic changes of Raynaud's phenomenon usually ensue: pain associated with blue and finally red coloration. Both hands are usually affected. The index, middle and ring fingers are most frequently involved and the thumbs seldom. Two classification systems are commonly used. Both the Taylor–Palmear and the 'two-tier' Stockholm hand–arm vibration syndrome classifications quantify the symptoms of blanching, numbness and tingling in relation to disruption of work and home activities. In the later stages symptoms affect all the fingers in summer and winter, leading to a change in occupation. These classifications are based solely on a subjective assessment.

The diagnosis is from a history of exposure to vibration and the absence of a systemic disease as a cause for secondary Raynaud's phenomenon. It can be difficult to distinguish the early symptoms from peripheral nerve compression, which also may be associated with the use of vibrating machinery. Neuropathy affecting the median nerve in the carpal tunnel, the ulnar nerve and the brachial plexus have all been described as consequences of exposure to vibration. Intraneural and extraneural compression and demyelination have been reported from nerve biopsies in vibration white finger.

Nerve conduction studies are useful to determine median nerve function at the carpal tunnel and surgical decompression, if indicated, sometimes relieves the symptoms of blanching as well as numbness and tingling.

A number of tests specifically for vibration white fingers have been described, of which none are considered diagnostic. The cold provocation test relies on inducing blanching by immersion in cold water, typically ten minutes immersion at 10°C. Finger systolic pressure, thermography, finger skin temperature and finger re-warming times have also been reported as useful. Grip–strength measurement has been claimed to detect muscle weakness. Bone cysts in the carpal and metacarpal bones on radiographs, distinct from osteoarthritis, have been reported. However, it has also been stated by other authors that these changes do represent osteoarthritis which has developed as a direct consequence of exposure to vibration.

There is no specific treatment for vibration white finger. Preventive measures to remove the exposure to vibration in cold, noisy conditions and good maintenance of machinery to minimise the physical stress to the hands are clearly important. Most patients get better when occupational exposure is eliminated. Drug therapies and sympathetic blockade treatment have shown little success in alleviating symptoms, and are not recommended.

PRESSURE GUN INJURIES

High-pressure injection injuries of the hand can cause severe damage to the soft tissues. These injuries often appear insignificant on examination, so the examiner may not realise the degree of underlying tissue damage.

Many different materials can be injected including paint, grease, diesel fuel and hydraulic fluid. More recently the injection of water from high pressure water–sprayers has also been described. Victims are usually employed in industry or agriculture.

The initial tissue damage and extent of spread of material depends on the pressure within the injection system. Less viscous liquids injected at high pressure will disseminate furthest from the point of injury and consequently will cause the greatest degree of physical injury to the soft tissues.

The injected material may have a direct toxic effect on contact with the tissues which is additional to any direct physical damage. The degree of damage is dependent on the relative toxicity to living cells and connective tissues of the injected material. The length of time the toxic material remains in contact with the tissues will also have a direct effect on the amount of cellular and connective tissue damage. This is a factor where therapeutic intervention and appropriate treatment can significantly alter the natural history of these injuries, by limiting the contact time between tissue and the toxic material. High-pressure paint-gun and airless-paint sprayers are the most damaging and dangerous injuries. Other oil-based solvents also cause serious damage. In contrast, water-sprayer injuries are considered more benign.

Once a diagnosis has been made from the history of the mechanism of injury, urgent surgical exploration is needed. Initial inspection may only reveal a deceptively small skin lesion, although there is typically oedema and marked tenderness in the affected digit. It is most important to ascertain the degree of spread proximally into the limb by careful inspection and palpation and, with some radio paque materials, a radiograph can be helpful.

High-pressure injection injuries are very painful and first-line treatment should include analgesia, elevation and immobilisation of the limb. Broad-spectrum antimicrobial therapy is commenced and the need for anti–tetanus treatment must be considered. There is little evidence that corticosteroid therapy or any other form of pharmacological intervention improves the outcome from this type of injury.

Surgical treatment is always required and it has been shown that a delay in removal of the foreign material leads to a poor outcome. The aim of surgery is to *remove all the injected material*, necessitating wide exposure of the digit with proximal extension until the full extent of tissue contamination is seen. The best approach is through zig-zag incisions, usually sited on the volar surface of the limb; this will need to be modified in the rare case in which the point of entry is on the dorsal surface of the arm. A tourniquet will minimise bleeding which would obscure the contaminating material. Devitalised and dead tissue is excised and thorough lavage of the entire wound is essential. After all the material has been removed, the wounds can either be loosely opposed or left open. Repeat surgery for further lavage and wound closure may be required. It is essential that the patient receives intensive physiotherapy to the hand to minimise swelling and retain movement in the affected digit and hand; in particular it is most important to obtain active mobilisation of the flexor tendons within the fibrous flexor sheaths as early as possible.

Reported series describe an incidence of amputation varying from 16% to 48%. Poor prognostic factors which can not be influenced by treatment are the type and quantity of injected material. A most important factor which can be modified by effective surgical treatment is the length of time injected material is in contact with the tissues.

Outcome is based on the presence of pain and stiffness of the fingers. The fingers typically stiffen in a partially flexed posture, and the lack of active flexion and extension leads to a very significant level of functional impairment.

REFLEX SYMPATHETIC DYSTROPHY

The clinical condition of disproportionate burning pain associated with swelling and discoloration of the hand and upper limb has long been recognised. Many terms have been used to describe this condition including causalgia, shoulder–hand syndrome, complex regional pain syndrome and pain-dysfunction syndrome. In its extreme form it used to be called Sudek's atrophy. Reflex Sympathetic Dystrophy (RSD) is the term currently in common usage for this characteristic condition, which has a great deal of variation in its clinical manifestations. Reflex describes an involuntary response to an initiating stimulus, the term sympathetic refers to the neurological pathways subserving the syndrome, and dystrophy describes the trophic changes resulting from the persistent sympathetic stimulation. A definition of RSD has been proposed by Prithvi Raj as 'continuous pain in a portion of an extremity after trauma which may include fracture but does not involve a major nerve, associated with sympathetic hyperactivity'.

The pathogenesis of RSD is not fully elucidated. A sympathetic response is normal following injury. Afferent sensory fibres carry a painful stimulus to the spinal cord and synapse in the dorsal horn. The impulses enter ascending pathways to the brain, connect to the anterior horn cell initiating a motor reflex and the sympathetic nerve cell bodies. The sympathetic reflex efferent travels in the peripheral nerve to the extremity, causing vasoconstriction. This normal sympathetic response is temporary and as healing progresses the reflex ceases, leading to gradual vasodilatation and repair of the injured tissues. In the condition of RSD it is hypothesised that the sympathetic response is abnormal, leading to continuing and subsequently inappropriate vasoconstriction resulting in tissue ischaemia and pain. This subsequently leads to more afferent pain impulses, causing further stimulation through the reflex pathway. It is not known why the normal reflex sympathetic response to an injury continues beyond the length of time of a normal physiological response and produces what has been described as a hyperdynamic sympathetic state. A recent study has demonstrated elevation of bradykinin and calcitonin gene-related peptide levels in RSD patients compared to a normal control group, which suggests an inflammatory mechanism for the symptoms and signs of RSD.

An RSD diathesis has been described; these individuals normally show increased sympathetic activity in the limbs in the form of cold hands and hyperhidrosis. It has also been demonstrated that individuals affected by RSD show personality traits towards depression and anxiety. Smoking has been implicated as a risk factor.

In practice, the stimulus leading to the onset of RSD is usually traumatic, infective or following surgery. Relatively minor injuries to regions rich in nerve endings are more likely to result in RSD than major trauma involving direct injury to nerves and vessels. Minimising the risk of the development of RSD is important. A previous history of RSD following injury or surgery is a most significant risk factor. Elevation of the limb and good pain control are probably beneficial. Some authors have utilised sympathetic blockade of the limb at the time of surgery, although there is no clear reduction in subsequent RSD from this treatment.

Clinical features

The most significant feature of RSD is pain which is greater than expected from the underlying stimulus alone. There is no single characteristic pattern to the pain although it is often described as burning or cutting. The pain is usually continuous and is made worse by both active and passive movements of the joints of the affected part. The pain is rarely localised, tending to affect the whole hand with radiation into the proximal part of the arm, and does not correspond to any anatomical distribution of peripheral nerves, dermatomes or myotomes. Hyperaesthesia of the hand is a typical complaint, sometimes resulting in protective behaviour towards the limb. The other features of RSD are less constant, which has led to the course of the condition being divided into three stages with distinct features (*Table 4D.4*).

Stage 1 is termed the *acute or hyperaemic stage*. This commences at the time of injury. The duration of stage 1 is variable, but most authors describe a period of between three and six months. In common with the two later stages, the principal symptom is pain. The hand is invariably oedematous and swollen, more marked than the usual post–operative swelling. Stiffness is characteristic and involves all the joints of the affected hand; the muscles appear to be in spasm and are tender to palpation. The skin condition is more variable; in the earliest period the hand may be cyanotic, but the

Table 4D.4 Stages and characteristics of RSD

Characteristic	Stage		
	1: Acute	2: Dystrophic	3: Atrophic
Pain	Burning/neuralgia +++	Burning/throbbing +++	Burning/throbbing ++
Dysaesthesia	++	+++	+
Function	Minimal impairment	Restricted	Severely restricted
Autonomic dysfunction	Increased blood flow	Normal or decreased flow	Decreased blood flow
Temperature	Increased	Decreased	Decreased
Discoloration	Erythematous	Mottled/dusky	Cyanotic
Sudomotor dysfunction	Minimal	++	+++
Oedema	++	+++	+
Trophic changes	−	++	++++
3-phase bone scan	Increased activity, all images	Normal uptake all phases except increased static phase	Decreased activity all phases
Osteoporosis	−	+	+++

+ − Feature is present.
+ + − Feature is present to greater degree.
+ + + − Feature is present at grade (level) 3.
+ + + + − Feature is present at grade (level) 4.

usual finding in stage 1 is of warm red skin. Towards the end of this stage the skin appears smooth and tight, with the loss of skin patterns and wrinkles.

Stage 2 is called the *subacute, dystrophic* or *ischaemic stage*, and follows if there is no therapeutic intervention during stage 1. It lasts for three to six months. Pain is maximal at this stage and is more closely linked to motion and use of the hand. The swelling is more pronounced and firmer, often with thickenings in the palmar fascia; consequently stiffness and functional disability are more marked. The skin is cyanosed and cold and in the later stages is dry. The fingernails show atrophic changes and become brittle.

Stage 3 is the *atrophic* or *chronic stage*. Pain is less troublesome and the predominant features are of atrophy and stiffness. The skin is thin, dry, cyanosed and cold with absence of normal creases. Muscle wasting is marked and, with the marked stiffness, leads to profound weakness and functional limitation. Many of the trophic changes of stage 3 are irreversible, and therefore some authors consider the third stage to be a permanent state.

Diagnosis

It is important to consider RSD in any individual who has an unexpectedly high level of pain following a recent injury or surgical procedure; the additional features of stiffness, swelling and discoloration would represent a classical case of RSD presenting no diagnostic difficulty. Many cases will differ from the typical features described in the three stages. There is no single feature or investigation diagnostic of RSD in less classical cases. There are a number of scoring systems which have been devised to attribute diagnostic value to a number of criteria which are both signs and special investigations (*Table 4D.5*).

Investigations

Plain radiographs show diffuse osteopenia which can be attributed to a combination of increased blood flow and consequent bone turnover. The patchy bone loss is typically in the periarticular regions of all the joints in the hand. This is usually more marked than the effect of disuse alone. The bone loss persists longer in RSD and has been seen at twelve months after onset.

Three-phase scanning is carried out after intravenous administration of technetium-labelled diphosphonate. The first phase, recorded immediately after injection, consists of angiographic images. The second-phase scans show regional blood pool distribution, recorded 1–5 minutes after injection. The third-phase scans,

Table 4D.5 Putative diagnostic criteria for RSD

Clinical symptoms and signs
  Burning pain
  Hyperpathia/allodynia
  Temperature/colour changes
  Oedema
  Hair/nail growth changes

Laboratory results
  Thermography/thermometry
  Bone radiograph
  3-phase bone scan
  Quantitative sweat test
  Response to sympathetic blockade

Interpretation based on number of criteria present
  > 6=probable RSD
  3–5=possible RSD
  $3 <$ unlikely RSD

recorded at 2–4 hours after injection, demonstrate uptake within bone. The third-phase images, which are considered to be the most reliable in the diagnosis of RSD, show diffusely increased uptake and increased periarticular uptake involving multiple joints of the hand. Critical review of the reported series of three phase bone scanning in RSD shows that the assessment of the images is very subjective and difficult to quantify. Specificity is poor, as similar findings occur in vascular occlusion and cellulitis. The best correlation between RSD and scanning is with patients in the initial stages at a time up to 20 weeks after onset. However, in the best reports the sensitivity in diagnosing RSD from these typical appearances is only 50%. The increased uptake into bone in the third phase of the scan has been related to the increased blood flow in the first phase. This is consistent with a similar length of time when blood flow is known to be increased in the initial stage of RSD prior to the onset of vasoconstriction. Three-phase bone scanning following sympathetic blockade shows increased blood flow and uptake in the first and third phases of the scan. Sympathetic blockade in the second stage of RSD had little effect on scanning results.

Thermography has been suggested as a means of quantifying temperature difference in an affected extremity. It is common for the affected hand to be warmer in the early stages of RSD and colder in the later stages. There is no consensus in the literature on the interpretation of these results, an obvious difficulty arising when the findings vary from time to time during the natural history of the condition. Other conditions affecting vascularity to the hand will also have a significant effect on the skin temperature independent of sympathetic activity. It is possible that this non-invasive but expensive investigation may have a more useful role in monitoring progress and response to treatment than in diagnosis.

Treatment

One should avoid tight dressings and plasters, ensure elevation of the limb to avoid swelling and provide adequate analgesia. Attention to these details in the management of both post–operative and injured patients is good surgical practice, but there is no evidence that RSD is preventable.

Early diagnosis is important in order to instigate early treatment in stage 1 in the hope of preventing progression to stages 2 and 3. The basis is to eliminate the painful stimulus and interrupt the overactivity in the sympathetic nerve supply. Interruption of the sympathetic reflex can be achieved using pharmacological and surgical techniques. Physiotherapy is important to try to maintain function in the affected hand if this can be accomplished without significant pain and discomfort.

Nerve blocks are the favoured method of producing sympathetic blockade. In the upper limb the usual sites are at the stellate ganglion, the brachial plexus or utilising an intravenous regional block. The best results are achieved using repeated blocks in combination with therapy until pain has resolved. The most widely used approach is a guanethidine block. Guanethidine acts at the ganglionic level to block the autonomic reflex. A modified Bier's block with 20 mg of guanethidine in 40 ml of 0.5% prilocaine for a period of 30 min is appropriate for most adults. The patient can benefit from physiotherapy to the hand which is carried out whilst the Bier's block provides analgesia; this is an opportunity for the therapist to passively mobilise the joints. The number of treatments an individual patient will require is very variable, and in some cases there is no response to the treatment. Reports of results are difficult to assess due to the variability in expressing outcomes. In general, most patients experience improvement or complete resolution of symptoms with repetitive sympathetic blocks, although there is a significant rate of relapse following cessation of treatment. Similar results are described using continuous blockade at the stellate ganglion and brachial plexus using indwelling catheters.

Chemical or surgical sympathectomy are not commonly practised for upper limb RSD because the close proximity of the cervical roots to the sympathetic chain precludes chemical neurolysis and surgical techniques are difficult, involving a transaxillary or posterior approach.

Many other treatments including systemic corticosteroids, adrenergic blockers, calcium channel blockers and oral guanethidine have been described. All have predictable and significant side–effects and none are in common usage.

Physiotherapy is a vital adjunct in the treatment of RSD, best carried out when sympathetic blockade has shown good effect. The role of therapy in the painful acute stage 1 is not clear: some reports suggest that therapy may exacerbate the RSD by increasing the intensity of painful stimuli. There is no doubt over the value of therapy in the later atrophic stage when mobilisation of contractures and exercises to counter muscle wasting are essential.

FURTHER READING

Boyle JC, Smith NJ, Burke FD. Vibration white finger. *J Hand Surg* (1988), **13B**: 171–176.

Dray GJ, Eaton RB. Dislocations and ligament injuries in the digits. In: Green DP (ed.) *Operative Hand Surgery*, 3rd edn. Edinburgh: Churchill Livingstone, 1993.

Fowler JR. Infections. *Hand Clin* (United States) Nov. 1989, **5:** 613–627.

Green DP. Carpal dislocations and instabilities. In: Green DP (ed.) *Operative Hand Surgery*, 3rd edn. Edinburgh: Churchill Livingstone, 1993.

Kasdan ML. Occupational hand and upper extremity injuries and diseases. Philadelphia: Hanley and Belfus 1991.

Lankford LL. Reflex sympathetic dystrophy. In: Green DP (ed.) *Operative Hand Surgery*, 3rd edn. Edinburgh: Churchill Livingstone, 1993.

Lee GW, Weeks PM. The role of bone scintigraphy in diagnosing reflex sympathetic dystrophy. *J Hand Surg* 1995; **20A:** 458–463.

Mackinnon S, Holder LE. The use of three-phase radionuclide bone scanning in the diagnosis of reflex sympathetic dystrophy. *J Hand Surg* 1984; **9A:** 556–563.

Nevaiser R. Infections. In: Green DP (ed.) *Operative Hand Surgery*, 3rd edn. Edinburgh: Churchill Livingstone, 1993.

Phipps AR, Blanshard J. A review of in-patient hand infections. *Arch Emerg Med* 1992; **9:** 229–305.

Prithvi Raj P. Reflex sympathetic dystrophy. In: Prithvi Raj P (ed.) *Pain Medicine a Comprehensive Review.* St Louis: Mosby, 1996.

5

Compartment Syndrome and Ischaemic Contracture

Colin Dent and Michael Waldram

COMPARTMENT SYNDROME

Compartment syndrome is a clinical situation resulting from increased pressure in a fascial compartment. This can lead to muscle ischaemia when the compartment pressure is greater than the perfusion pressure in the arterial vessels supplying the muscle. The ischaemia causes severe pain, exacerbated by passive stretching of the muscle. If not treated increased compartment pressure will lead to development of irreversible muscle necrosis; the final consequence is Volkmann's ischaemic contracture. Raised pressure may also affect any nerve within the compartment, causing first parasthaesiae and then paralysis of the muscles supplied by the affected nerve. Occlusion of the arterial vessels as a result of increased compartment pressures is not common: it will only arise as a late complication of an undiagnosed or poorly managed case. The pressure required to occlude the main artery within a compartment is significantly higher than the pressure that will cause muscle necrosis.

In the upper limb, compartment syndrome can occur in the flexor, extensor or radial compartments of the forearm, the intrinsic muscle compartments of the hand, and the digits.

The syndrome results from trauma to the limb, most notably closed compression injuries with extensive soft tissue damage, and can occur in the absence of any fracture. The features of raised compartment pressure are similar to those seen in the lower limb, where the patient experiences severe rest pain which is exacerbated by passive stretching of the muscles in the affected compartment. The presence of peripheral arterial pulses does not exclude the diagnosis, which is based on a history of severe unremitting pain in the injured limb. Examination usually reveals swelling of

the affected compartment, and the worst pain on passive stretching (*Figure 5.2(a)*). In the face of equivocal findings, the surgeon should proceed to carry out fasciotomy and decompress the compartments. Fasciotomy using an appropriate technique has a low morbidity, in contrast to an untreated case. The two most widely used methods of measuring compartment pressure are the infusion technique and the indwelling recording catheter. Most authors recommend surgical decompression when the pressure is 40 mmHg or higher. Normal pressure recordings should not preclude surgical decompression in the presence of unequivocal clinical signs. The value of pressure measurements is in a case where signs are equivocal, and the decision to operate is based on sequential pressure recordings showing a sustained rise in pressure.

The three compartments of the forearm are the flexor, extensor (dorsal) and radial compartments (*Figure 5.1*).

The flexor compartment contains both the wrist and finger flexor muscles and the median and ulnar nerves. The incision to decompress the flexor compartment is sited on the volar aspect of the forearm, commencing at the palm and continuing proximally in a curve as far as the elbow. The median nerve is identified in the carpal tunnel and is followed proximally on the deep surface of the flexor digitorum superficialis. The forearm fascia is divided as part of this extension of the incision. Alternative incisions can follow a zig-zag line along the volar aspect of the forearm or along the volar–ulnar border. The three compartments are interconnected, so release of the flexor may also decompress the extensor and radial compartments; however I always use a separate approach to these.

The extensor compartment contains the finger and thumb extensors and the radial compartment contains

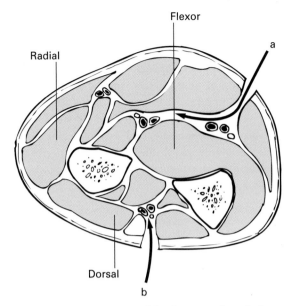

Figure 5.1 Compartments of the forearm and surgical approaches. a, Approach for release of flexor compartment; b, approach for release of dorsal compartment. Redrawn from Tubiana *et al.* (1990).

brachioradialis and the wrist extensors. These two compartments can be decompressed through a single midline incision on the extensor surface of the forearm extending distally to the extensor retinaculum.

The intrinsic muscles of the hand are decompressed through two incisions on the dorsum of the hand. One incision is sited between the index and middle finger metacarpals and the second between the ring and little finger metacarpals. The incisions are deepened each side of each metacarpal bone.

Fingers are decompressed through incisions sited along each mid-lateral line.

Skin incisions are always left open following fasciotomy and decompression. Closure is attempted about 5 days later, with a secondary procedure at 10 days which may require the application of split skin grafts to any remaining wound.

VOLKMANN'S ISCHAEMIC CONTRACTURE

Volkmann's contracture is the end result of untreated compartment syndrome. Pressure within a fascial compartment builds up to a level high enough to occlude capillary circulation. Muscle ischaemia and necrosis then result in an *ellipsoid infarct*, where circulation is most severely impaired in the centre of the muscle belly. This occurs when the extracapillary pressure rises above 40 mmHg. Holden divided Volkman's ischaemic contracture into two types based on aetiology.

The first is the result of a major vessel occlusion proximal to the elbow, resulting in secondary ischaemia distal to the injury. It usually occurs in young children (e.g. after a supracondylar fracture of the elbow) and the extent of degree of the ischaemia is severe.

The second is caused by direct trauma when the ischaemia develops at the site of the injury. The common causes are external pressure from a tight cast placed on a fresh fracture, or direct pressure on a limb in an unconscious patient. Such patients, with overdose or collapse, are often admitted under physicians as a medical rather than a surgical emergency and the diagnosis is made too late.

Nerves passing through ischaemic muscle degenerate and become thin and cord-like. Initially sensory symptoms are present but, if the ischaemia is severe, then motor signs ensue. The degree of damage and paralysis depends on the size of the ellipsoid infarct. Naturally the median nerve, which passes through the centre of the forearm, is most commonly affected.

Muscle regeneration can occur to a variable amount, depending on the degree of damage. New fibres grow longitudinally along existing sarcolemmal tubes, but there is only partial recovery towards the centre of the infarct, where intense fibrosis develops. In extreme cases complete necrosis results in a yellow pulpy mass which can be scooped out with a spoon.

Treatment

The best treatment is to avoid the problem in the first place. If ever in doubt whether you should decompress a compartment acutely, you should do it without delay. Late decompression (after 48 hours from onset) will not restore circulation to frankly ischaemic muscle and may result in infection of necrotic tissue, especially if there is skin blistering. This could end up with an amputation. Remember to talk in an exam about compartmental pressure monitoring in the acute situation (Whiteside technique).

Classification according to severity (after Tsuge)

Another classification, perhaps more practical, is according to the severity of the damage. Three types are described, with suitable surgery for each type.

Mild

This is localised to part of the profundus muscles; there are flexion contractures of two or three fingers (usually the middle and ring fingers). There is usually no sensory disturbance, but if present it is slight. A tenodesis effect can be demonstrated; on wrist extension the finger flexion increases, and on wrist flexion it relaxes. A common example is after a forearm fracture or supracondylar fracture in children. Surgery can consist of a muscle slide operation as described by Scaggliati. This consists of detaching the common flexor origin, and deeper muscles if they are involved, from the medial epicondyle, anterior aspects of the ulna and the interosseous membrane, with careful preservation of the ulnar nerve and all its branches. The muscle slides 2–3 cm.

Moderate

This is also known as the classic or typical type. The muscle involvement involves the flexor digitorum profundus and flexor pollicis longus, but can also involve the superficial flexors and wrist flexors. Flexion contractures of all the fingers and thumb develop and the wrist adopts a flexed posture. There is sensory disturbance of the median and the ulnar nerves and intrinsic

paralysis results in a claw hand. Surgery consists of a more radical release of the flexor muscles, including detaching flexor pollicis longus from the radius (take care of the superficial branch of the radial nerve) and the insertion of pronator teres from the radius. Great attention must be given to the nerves and vessels passing through the flexor mass. Tendon transfers can be used, taking brachioradialis and extensor carpi radialis longus around the radial side of the distal forearm and attaching them to the distal flexor digitorum profundus stumps and flexor pollicis stumps, respectively.

Severe

This involves both the flexor and extensor compartments. There is severe neurological involvement and marked contracture (*Figure 5.2(b)*).

This may be seen after untreated supracondylar fractures or complicated forearm fractures with cicatrisation of the skin and also after overdoses and prolonged unconsciousness during which the patient is lying on the arm. Surgery can consist of early excision of necrotic muscle and neurolysis. The reason for early muscle excision is to try to preserve nerve function, as muscle fibrosis strangles a nerve of its blood supply. Tendon transfers can also be used, as in the moderate type. Free muscle microvascular transplantation using sartorius or semitendinosis attached to the medial epicondyle proximally and the flexor tendons distally, with anastomosis to the anterior interosseous nerve and artery, was first described in China in 1976. Slight muscle contraction can be felt three months after the transfer. Skin can also be incorporated with the transfer if there is a deficiency.

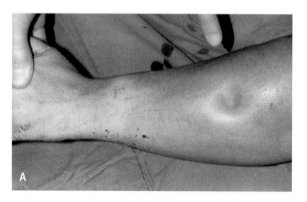 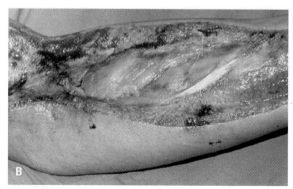

Figure 5.2 (a) Extensor compartment oedema from severe compartment syndrome. (b) Irreversible necrosis of the flexor compartment muscles; severe Volkmann's ischaemia.

FURTHER READING

Rowland SR. Fasciotomy: The treatment of compartment syndrome. In: Green DP (ed.) *Operative Hand Surgery*, 3rd edn. Edinburgh: Churchill Livingstone, 1993.

Tubiana R, McCullough CJ, Masquelet AC. *An Atlas of Surgical Exposures of the Upper Extremity*. London: Martin Dunitz, 1990.

Whitesides TE Jr, Haney TC, Morimoto K, Hirada H. Tissue pressure measurements as a determinant for the need of fasciotomy. *Clin Orthop* 1975; **113:** 43–51.

6

Tendons

Ian A Trail

The anatomy, biology, healing and function of normal and diseased tendons has fascinated hand surgeons for decades. Much has been written and in certain areas great strides have been made in the understanding and treatment of tendon-related conditions. Despite this there is still much to do and our understanding of tendon healing and tenosynovitis remains incomplete.

The aim of this chapter is to prepare the reader for his/her final examination of training. As such, it is assumed that the reader will have a reasonable knowledge of tendon anatomy, although certain key areas will still be described in detail. In addition certain topics which the author considers controversial, e.g. tendon healing, rehabilitation, tenosynovitis and repetitive strain injury (RSI) will be considered in greater detail.

CLINICAL EXAMINATION

For a detailed discussion of examination of tendons in the hand the reader is referred to *The Hand, Examination and Diagnosis*, published on behalf of the American Society for Surgery of the Hand by Churchill Livingstone (2nd edn, 1983).

However, of particular importance for the fingers is that the flexor digitorum profundus usually has a common belly to the ulnar three digits, such that flexion of the distal phalangeal joints with the others restrained can only occur in the presence of an intact flexor digitorum superficialis. The examiner should also be aware that 30–40% of normal individuals have a very attenuated or absent flexor digitorum superficialis to the little finger. Finally flexor digitorum profundus and flexor pollicis longus are the only tendons that can actively flex the distal joints.

With regard to the extensor tendons, the abductor pollicis longus and extensor pollicis brevis are evaluated by asking the patient to bring the thumb out to the radial side, i.e. to extend the thumb away from the fingers. For extensor pollicis longus integrity, the best manoeuvre is to ask the patient to pull the thumb backwards behind the plane of the other digits (*Figure 6.1*). With regard to the long extensor tendons to the fingers, these are the only structures that actively extend the metacarpophalangeal joint, either as a unit or independently in the case of the index and little fingers. The wrist extensors and flexors are tested by asking the patient to move the wrist in the appropriate direction while simultaneously palpating.

Secondly, consideration should be given to the tightness of the long flexor/extensor tendons, due either to muscle shortening or adhesion formation. Identification of both depends on the fixed length phenomenon of tendon; more specifically if the extensors are stuck

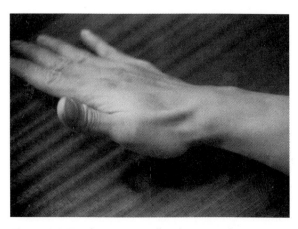

Figure 6.1 Test for extensor pollicis longus tendon integrity.

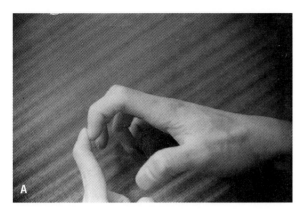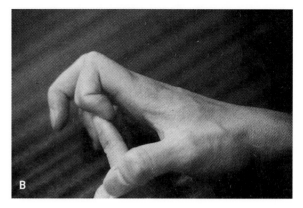

Figure 6.2 Intrinsic tightness preventing PIP flexion with MP's extended (a) abnormal impaired (b) normal.

down or shortened, the proximal interphalangeal (PIP) joint will not passively flex when the metacarpophalangeal (MP) joint is also flexed, but will do so when it is extended. Conversely, for flexor tendon tightness the PIP will not extend with the MP joint extended, but will if they are flexed. In short, one joint can be flexed or extended but not both simultaneously

Thirdly, intrinsic function should be considered. Much of this is outside the scope of this chapter although it is important to remember that an inability to flex the proximal interphalangeal joint, with the MP joint extended, is more often caused by intrinsic tightness (*Figure 6.2*). This is the reverse of extrinsic tightness.

Finally the reader is reminded that certain neurological conditions can mimic the findings of divided or ruptured tendons. For example, anterior interosseous nerve palsy will present as weakness of the flexor pollicis longus and often flexor digitorum profundus to the index. Similarly a posterior interosseous nerve palsy can result in loss of extension at the metacarpophalangeal joints.

CUT FLEXOR TENDON

The healing process

Human flexor tendons are composed of three structures: collagen, mucopolysaccharides and cells (tenocytes). The high intrinsic strength of tendons is derived from the fact that most of the structure is composed of closely packed collagen fibres. These fibres can be as long as the tendon and have numerous cross-linkages. Essentially,

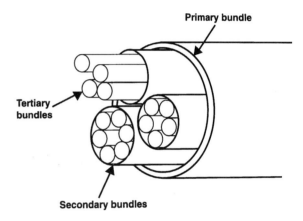

Figure 6.3 Diagrammatic representation of the cross-section of a tendon.

collagen fibres are grouped together in primary bundles separated by mucopolysaccharides (*Figure 6.3*). These primary bundles are in turn assembled into larger secondary bundles or fasicles. These in turn form tertiary bundles which together comprise the tendon. The loose connective tissue lying between these bundles is referred to as endotenon. It is in this layer that the blood supply, lymphatics and nerves of the tendons run. This layer is also continuous with a fine connective tissue sheath surrounding the tendons. This latter structure is known as the peritenon or epitenon. Further, surrounding this is a loose fatty areolar layer known as the paratenon; this latter structure is replaced in the flexor sheaths by a synovial lining.

Flexor tendons in the hand have been divided into zones. Of particular importance to the surgeon are injuries in zones 1 and 2 where the tendons pass through the flexor sheath (*Figure 6.4*). It is in these particular zones that the results of surgery are often disappointing. The surface anatomy of zone 2 lies from the volar crease at the level of the PIP joint down to the transverse palmar creases.

Contrary to earlier views, flexor tendon is not an avascular structure, but does contain living cells. It is known to possess respiratory activity, although this is extremely low: 0.1 μl/unit weight/h. It has also been demonstrated that there is a small but definite turnover of amino acids and collagen within adult tendons.

Controversy still surrounds the exact mechanisms involved in tendon healing. Considerable research has been undertaken and most authors now all fall into one of three schools of thought. These are as follows.

1. The healing process is due to proliferation of tissues surrounding the tendon, i.e. extrinsic mechanisms.
2. The healing process is due to proliferation at the divided tendon ends, i.e. intrinsic mechanisms.
3. Both mechanisms are important.

As can be seen from the above, the main area of contention centres on the origin of the various cells participating in and responsible for healing of the injured tendon. Further confusion occurs as a result of the ability of tendons at various anatomical sites to heal

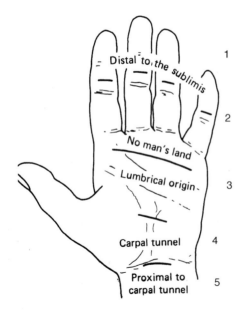

Figure 6.4 Zones of flexor tendons.

differently. This is well demonstrated by the Achilles tendon of rats where lacerations will heal spontaneously under any circumstances, even if a large section is excised. However, when the intrasynovial flexor profundus tendon in the same animal is severed, it shows much less propensity for spontaneous healing. This should be remembered when evaluating the results of animal experiments and extrapolating them to humans. The role of surrounding tissues (extrinsic mechanisms) was principally championed by Potenza who, following extensive work using the flexor tendon of the dog, found that healing resulted from proliferation of the tissue surrounding the tendon and throughout this process the tendon itself remained inert. Indeed he also concluded that tendons do not contain cells naturally able to synthesise collagen. The contrary view was taken by Lundborg who concluded, following an ingenious series of experiments, that rabbit flexor tendon has the ability to heal within a synovial environment. Indeed explanted flexor tendons from various animals were shown to have an intrinsic capacity to heal.

Most surgeons now believe that both the extrinsic and intrinsic mechanisms are at work in tendon healing. Obviously the surgical ideal is the latter, particularly in zones 1 and 2, because this will allow healing yet prevent excessive adhesion formation. A factor of particular importance appears to be the gap between the sutured tendon ends, as experimental evidence has shown that if this gap is not too great (i.e. less than 2 mm) it can be bridged by the tendon itself. For a gap greater than this, however, the extrinsic mechanism seems to be more important. Mobilisation has been shown to have a beneficial effect in that it stimulates the intrinsic healing mechanisms.

More recent work has raised the possibility of there being several types of cell within tendon (*Figure 6.5*). In fact there are even variations within the flexor sheath as in 'areas of compression' (overlying the joints) healing processes are more dependent on diffusion, whereas in 'tension areas' (overlying the bones) the intrinsic blood supply is of more importance.

There are many other factors involved in healing of which, unfortunately, few can be altered by the surgeon. These range from:

1. material and technique of suture;
2. the opening or excision of the flexor sheath;

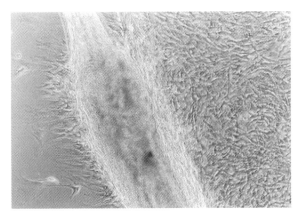

Figure 6.5 Human flexor tendon tenocytes as a monolayer (× 20 magnification).

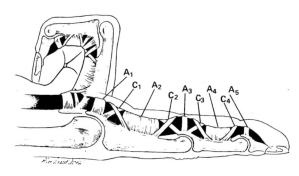

Figure 6.6 Flexor sheath pulley system.

3. the excision or preservation of the flexor digitorum superficialis tendon and the vincular blood supply;
4. the immobilisation or mobilisation of the tendon whilst healing takes place;
5. surrounding materials applied to isolate the repair site;
6. pharmacological manipulation of adhesions;
7. other factors.

A number of these will be discussed later, particularly the material and technique of suture and the immobilisation or mobilisation of the tendon.

With regard to the flexor sheath, experimental evidence remains confusing in that some authors believe that it is important to restore the integrity of the sheath because this encourages tendon healing and reduces adhesion formation. Others, however, have found no difference if the sheath is left unrepaired or indeed excised. On a more practical level, most surgeons believe it is important that the pulleys (particularly the A2 and A4) are preserved (*Figure 6.6*). Rispler *et al.* found that the division of one of the major pulleys, either the A2 or A4, resulted in significant changes in the efficiency of finger flexion, whereas division of the minor pulleys A1, A3, A5, led to a smaller reduction. With regard to the rest of the sheath, however, repair is often difficult. It is the author's view that pulleys should be preserved at all costs and that any division of the sheath to facilitate exposure and repair should be kept to an absolute minimum.

If there is an additional injury to the flexor digitorum superficialis so that the vincular blood supply is compromised, it is generally held to be preferable to repair both tendons as this potentially restores the intrinsic blood supply through the vincula. Again, however, experimental evidence does not give a clear answer in that some investigators have shown that excision of the superficialis tendon at its insertion has no effect on healing of the profundus, whereas others have demonstrated an increased number of adhesions and reduced function. Clinically, however, most surgeons believe that it is important to repair both tendons and that this produces superior results.

Finally various investigators have looked at the possibility of isolating the repair site by inserting materials around the repair. These have ranged from allantoic membrane through to polyethylene, fibrin, silicone fluid and hyaluronic acid. Unfortunately, despite some initial success these materials have not found widespread use. Similarly, pharmacological manipulation of adhesions has been tried: drugs used include steroids, either topically or orally, antihistamines and lathrogenic agents. Again, although these have found favour in certain centres, they are not generally in widespread use. The area of concern is that although they undoubtedly reduce adhesion formation, they also have an effect on normal tendon healing. Finally a number of other modalities have been used to promote tendon healing, including electromagnetic stimulation, ultrasonographic treatment, as well as direct electrical stimulation; again none are in widespread use.

Techniques of repair and rehabilitation

There are several factors affecting the outcome of tendon repair many of which are outside the control of the surgeon, the most important of these being the site and extent of trauma to the tendon. However, some can be influenced and of particular importance are the techniques of repair and subsequent therapy.

With regard to suture materials, there now seems little doubt that some of the earlier materials used, such as silk, produced an intense tissue reaction. However, it is now possible to use materials that are relatively inert, such as nylon, polypropylene or coated polyester. Experimental evidence has confirmed the minimal inflammatory response produced by these materials. More recently biodegradable materials, such as monofilament polyglyconate, have also become popular; although research indicates that these may stimulate an increase in inflammatory response whilst remaining *in situ* long enough to allow satisfactory healing of the tendon. At this time the author's preferred suture material is polypropylene, as it is easy to use and relatively atraumatic as it is passed through tendon. Care, however, should be taken when knotting.

With regard to techniques of tendon repair, over the years every conceivable configuration of suture insertion has been described (*Figure 6.7*). Traditionally, a Bunnell criss-cross suture was used, although later research indicated that this caused an increase in the amount of adhesion formation, and necrosis at the tendon ends, due to strangulation of the blood supply

to the tendon. As a consequence this was modified initially by Kessler and later by Kleinert. These techniques or variations thereof are the most commonly used at this time. In 1985 Savage described a new technique where six instead of two strands of suture material joined the cut ends. This has been shown to increase the strength of the tendon repair, both *in vitro* and *in vivo*. Concern, however, remains with regard to the considerable volume of suture material used and the potential for this material on the surface of a tendon to stimulate an inflammatory response. At this time the author's preferred suture technique is that described by Kleinert (1973) using a 4/0 suture material with an additional superficial 'running' suture using a 6/0 material.

Experimental evidence in the area of mobilisation is also conflicting. Initially many investigators found that tendons that were mobilised early tended to retract, giving a gap between the sutured ends: the wider the gap, the more scar tissue formed and as a result the poorer the result.

Contrary work found that mobilisation *reduced* the number of adhesions formed. Following on from this, it was concluded that not only did tendons have the intrinsic ability to heal themselves but that early controlled passive motion stimulated this response. Based on this work, a number of surgeons have advocated early mobilisation of tendon repairs. Experience has been reported with the 'Kleinert regime' which is effectively a passive flexion with active limited extension technique of mobilisation. In this technique, extension is resisted by tensioning a rubber band, theoretically reducing the force transmitted along the

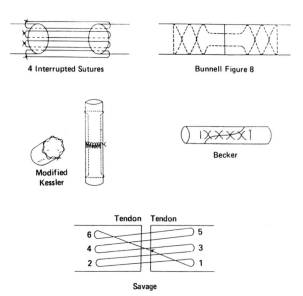

Figure 6.7 Various commonly used suture techniques.

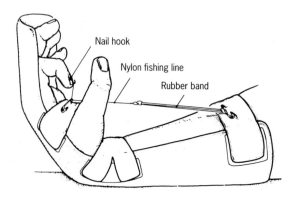

Figure 6.8 Kleinert mobilisation technique.

flexor tendons (*Figure 6.8*). Surgeons from Belfast have demonstrated that controlled early active mobilisation is even more beneficial. An independent evaluation of this in a comparative study, found that a controlled active motion regime conferred significant benefit on the final range of motion following flexor tendon repair. However, concern has been expressed that in certain cases this type of mobilisation technique can lead to an increased re-rupture rate and careful monitoring is essential. In the author's unit the preferred method of mobilisation at this time is one of active flexion within a controlled range and resisted extension as described by Kleinert. If, however, the patient is well motivated and shows satisfactory progress, rapid progression to a more active mobilisation programme is encouraged.

Results

Prior to assessing the outcome of any tendon repair technique, it is important to understand the various methods of assessing outcome. The simplest technique measures the distance between the tip of the actively flexed finger and the distal palmar crease. Less than half an inch was an excellent result; between 0.5 and 1 inch was good; between 1 and 1.5 inch was fair, and greater than 1.5 inches was poor. Other authors recommend measuring absolute angles, particularly of the proximal and distal interphalangeal joints. At this time, probably the most widely used classification is that adopted by the American Society for Surgery of the Hand where the sum of the inactive PIP and DIP joint flexion is subtracted from the sum of the active PIP and DIP joint flexion. This is then divided by 175° (a normal value) × 100 to give a percentage, greater than 75% being good, 50–75% fair, and less than 50% poor. The second most commonly used system is a complex scoring system including active flexion, extension deficit and finger pulp distal crease distance. Interestingly all these techniques ignore functional outcome. Given this and the fact that there are a large number of variables with each case (such as severity of injury, number of tendons involved, additional nerve and vascular damage), any meaningful interpretation is difficult. Analysis of early papers, however, indicates that with standard core suture techniques, usually that of Bunnell, after which the finger was splinted for three weeks prior to mobilisation, good to excellent results occurred in 45–65%. With the advent of improved suture techniques, and, more importantly, early mobilisation, results appear

to have improved: Kleinert *et al.* (1973) reported good to excellent results in 80%. Further evidence for the importance of mobilisation was given by Strickland and Glogovac who assessed digital function following flexor tendon repair in zone 2, comparing a three-week period of immobilisation against a controlled passive motion technique. The former gave fair to excellent results in 40%, the latter 72%. Other factors to consider are the number of digits and tendons involved, as well as the delay before repair. For the latter a review of literature would indicate that repair within the first three weeks after the injury probably has little detrimental effect although most surgeons agree that where possible it is better to repair within the first 24–48 hours. More recently several authors have indicated that it is not total mobilisation of the finger postoperatively that is important but that of the proximal interphalangeal joint in particular. Indeed it has been noted that the active range of motion of the PIP joint three weeks after surgery is a good indicator of the eventual outcome.

With regard to the flexor pollicis longus tendon, the same criteria as with the fingers apply, although given the peculiarities of the anatomy there is more likely to be associated digital nerve damage. Otherwise techniques and therapy proceed along similar lines with the results comparing favourably.

In children, the particular difficulty lies with postoperative therapy; indeed many authors believe that in the very young rigid immobilisation in plaster is the only safe technique, as these children are unable to co-operate with complex mobilisation programmes. Interestingly, however, from published results mobilisation does not appear to have a significant deleterious effect, in that generally the outcome in children seems to be markedly superior to that in adults. One should also note that the scope for improvement still exists whilst skeletal maturity continues.

What happens if the primary repair fails to give satisfactory results? This can be due to a number of reasons: principally adhesions around the tendon; usually from the surrounding sheath or underlying bone or separation of the tendon ends. In the first instance, most surgeons would consider tenolysis to be the procedure of choice. During this procedure the tendon repair is explored and the adhesions freed, often by sharp dissection. Of crucial importance, however, is mobilisation which should be started either during the procedure, if it is undertaken under local anaesthesia, or immediately afterwards. Given the exposed scar tissue, the tendency for the adhesions to form again is great. Indeed the importance of therapy following this procedure is even greater than after primary repair. It is also important for the surgeon to be aware that all the joints in the finger must have a full passive range of motion prior to the procedure being undertaken. Published literature indicates a wide variation in outcome, probably related to the timing of the procedure. There seems little doubt that if tenolysis is performed at three months the chances of success are greater than if it is undertaken at twelve months or more, but it should not be done before then as the repair process may not be complete and risk of rupture would be increased.

Should tenolysis fail or at exploration the findings are unsatisfactory with excessive scarring of the flexor sheath and tendon bed, then tendon grafting should be considered. At one time it was generally held that, given the poor results of direct tendon repair, it was the procedure of choice. However, with the increasing success of direct repair it is now being undertaken less frequently. Prior to undertaking the procedure, it is again important to check for a full passive range of motion in the finger joints, satisfactory soft tissue coverage, and adequate vascular perfusion of the finger. Tendon grafting can be undertaken in either one or two stages. For the latter the introduction of a silicone rod (*Figure 6.9*) for a three-month period allows a membrane to condense, providing a tunnel for improved gliding; subsequent to this a donor tendon, either palmaris longus or a spare toe extensor tendon, can be

used for reconstruction. It is important to realise, however, that these tendons used as grafts do not normally run in a sheath and, as a consequence, have a completely different metabolism. Unfortunately, however, there is no other suitable alternative. Of particular importance with this procedure is that the graft should be securely anchored distally into bone and proximally by a weave onto the appropriate tendon. This should allow a more aggressive postoperative mobilisation programme. For the tendon graft to function satisfactorily it is also important that the pulley system of the flexor sheath is intact. If the A2 and A4 pulleys are deficient a number of procedures have been described for reconstruction, but it is generally held that the results of tendon graft with pulley reconstruction are poor.

Finally, in the extreme circumstance where, after several operations, the patient is left with a flexed rigid digit which may also be insensate, one should consider either arthrodesis of a contracted PIP joint in a functional position, or even amputation of the ray.

For the thumb an alternative to tendon grafting would be a tendon transfer, particularly flexor digitorum superficialis of the ring finger, or alternatively arthrodesis of the interphalangeal joint which is a simple and satisfactory procedure.

Extensor tendons

Injuries to the extensor tendons are more common than those of their flexor cousins. Although the extensor tendons generally do not suffer from the unique biology of the intrasynovial flexor tendons, the anatomy on the dorsum of the wrist and hand is complex which can lead to difficulty in diagnosis, and indeed, failure to diagnose various injuries.

Lacerations on the dorsum of the hand and wrist can occur at any level and involve variable numbers of tendons. In diagnosis, it is important to remember which tendons extend the wrist only and which extend the fingers, the latter acting only at the metacarpophalangeal joint. Distal to this, extension is principally a factor of both the interossei and the long extensor tendons. Diagnosis of an extensor pollicis longus laceration or rupture can be difficult as patients will often retain some extension by way of the extensor pollicis brevis and abductor pollicis longus tendons. In the author's experience, the best test for integrity of the extensor pollicis longus tendon is to ask the patient to

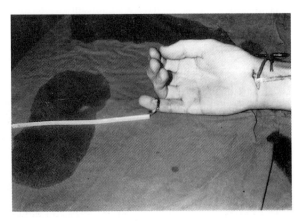

Figure 6.9 Second stage flexor tendon grafting showing silicone rod being removed from tip of the finger.

adduct the thumb back in the plane of the other four digits. When this is undertaken, the pollicis longus tendon can be both visualised and palpated.

Acute extensor tendon injuries have been classified, as with the flexor tendons, into zones (*Figure 6.10*). Effectively injuries in zones 1 and 2 produce a mallet finger deformity, which is discussed later. Similarly injuries in zones 3 and 4 produce a boutonnière deformity, which is discussed in the next section. Zone 5 lies over the metacarpophalangeal joint, the standard treatment being open repair of the divided tendons. The technique of repair, given the flat shape of the tendon at this site, takes the form of simple or mattress sutures. After repair the tendons are immobilised, with the wrist and fingers in extension, for a period of three to four weeks. For zone 6 (overlying the metacarpal), the treatment is identical although many now recommend early mobilisation using wrist extension splints and dynamic out-riggers on the fingers. Initial MP flexion may be restricted to 30° but this can be removed at two to three weeks. A number of authors have shown improved results using this technique, in particular a lower incidence of adhesions between the extensor

tendon and the underlying metacarpal bone. For lacerations over the wrist and carpus, that is zones 7 and 8, exploration and repair are again recommended with splintage of the wrist in extension for a period of four to six weeks.

With the extensor pollicis longus, diagnosis can be difficult. However, many of the principles that apply to the extensor tendons at other sites also apply in the thumb, where acute repair is recommended particularly for divisions in zones T3, T4 and T5. Splintage generally involves a thumb spica cast for between four and six weeks, with the MP and IP joints in extension and the first carpometacarpal joint adducted and extended.

Fortunately, complications of extensor tendon injuries are few and the results of surgery often satisfactory. If not, this is more often due to limitation of flexion than loss of extension. However, with complex injuries involving skin and soft tissue loss with additional associated fractures, adhesions around the extensor tendon are not uncommon and will result in loss of flexion at the metacarpophalangeal joint. Treatment for this involves extensor tenolysis with dorsal capsulotomy of the MP joint if appropriate, after which immediate mobilisation is instigated. Should this fail there are a number of surgical alternatives including side-to-side suture or 'piggy-backing' tendons on the dorsum of the hand; more specifically, the extensor tendon to the little finger can be sutured to that of the ring and even the middle finger. Otherwise tendon transfers are possible as well as extensor tendon grafting, the latter often being used in severe cases when the whole of the extensor apparatus on the back of the hand is involved in the trauma.

Boutonnière deformity

Injury to the extensor mechanism at the proximal interphalangeal joint can result in a boutonnière deformity, in which there is loss of active extension at the PIP joint. The particular structure damaged is the central slip of the extensor tendon which inserts into the base of the middle phalanx. This can be damaged by trauma, either open or closed, as well as in various inflammatory conditions particularly rheumatoid arthritis. As can be seen from *Figure 6.11*, the extensor mechanism over the dorsum of the fingers is a complex structure. Effectively the long extensor

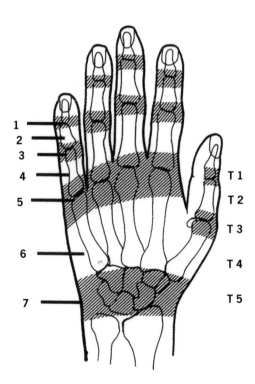

Figure 6.10 Zones for extensor tendons.

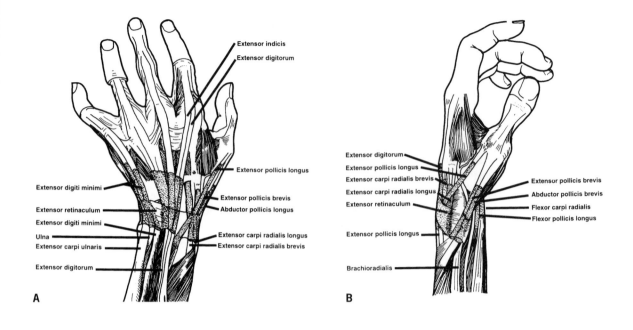

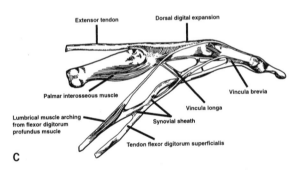

Figure 6.11 Extensor mechanism overlying the wrist (a and b) and fingers (c).

progresses to form the majority of the central slip. However, it also forms two lateral slips that merge with contributions from the intrinsic muscle to form lateral bands; these proceed distally, becoming more dorsal over the middle phalanx, join together and insert into the base of the distal phalanx. Surrounding these bands are various ligaments which maintain balance of the tendon during active extension. Should the central slip be damaged, this allows the head of the proximal phalanx to gradually push dorsally between the lateral bands, resulting in their displacement more laterally and volarwards. As a consequence of this, their axis of rotation passes volar to the PIP joint, resulting in an inability to extend fully that joint. The pull of the

intrinsic muscles is then directed exclusively at the distal joint, that is the DIP joint, which progressively hyperextends. Finally the MP joint may also hyper-extend through the action of the long extensor tendon.

Acute damage to the central slip can be difficult to diagnose, as patients often retain the ability to extend the middle phalanx. Various tests have been described, the best known being that described by Boyes who noted that by holding the PIP joint in full extension the amount of flexion of the distal joint is decreased. However, this test only becomes positive later when the lateral slips are displaced. In the acute injury the reader is referred to the test described by Elson; here the patient has an inability or weakness of extension of the PIP joint from a position of 90° of flexion with the DIP joint fixed in extension (e.g. flexed over the end of a book or table).

Treatment of the acute injury remains controversial. In lacerations it would seem sensible to repair the central slip and splint the PIP joint in full extension for a period of six weeks. Indeed a number of surgeons advocate K wire fixation in this position. For closed injuries, however, if the diagnosis is made early and a full passive range of motion maintained, closed treatment (again by immobilisation in the extended position) would seem to be the treatment of choice. This can be achieved by a number of means, ranging from plaster of Paris to simple thermoplastic splints. Again, a period of K wire fixation may be advisable, the joint being splinted for a period of six weeks. Finally, if there has been a large fragment of bone avulsed from the dorsum of the middle phalanx, then internal fixation would be appropriate.

For the chronic deformity with loss of passive extension, initial treatment should be to restore a full range of motion by correcting contracture. Again this can be undertaken by using serial plaster of Paris casts or a dynamic extension splint, e.g. Capener. Once full passive extension is achieved this should be followed by a period of immobilisation to allow tendon repair. Should this fail, then one may wish to consider operative intervention. However, care must be taken when deciding to operate on the PIP joint, as although extension may be regained it is so easy to lose flexion, a situation that is functionally worse than the original boutonnière deformity. There are a number of techniques available. These include a direct anatomical repair or reinsertion of the central slip, reconstruction of the central slip with a tendon graft, mobilisation and restoration of the dorsal location of the lateral slips, or tendon transfer utilising the ulnar lateral band. A number of authors recommend additional tenotomy of the distal extensor tendon over the middle phalanx; this procedure allows correction of any DIP joint extension contracture whilst improving flexion of that joint. The author's personal preference would be mobilisation of the lateral slip with a transfer of the ulnar lateral band into the central slip.

For fixed deformities of the PIP joint that have failed to respond to conservative methods of correction, surgical exploration may be indicated; the release of various tight structures, including the transverse retinacular ligament, and mobilisation of the lateral bands may be of benefit. In addition, the accessory collateral ligaments or even the volar plate may have to be released. Usually, however, the more surgery required for mobilisation the poorer the prognosis. In cases with advanced articular stiffness, where it is found from radiographs or at surgery that there is severe articular cartilage damage, then surgical options range from arthrodesis in a functional position or arthroplasty.

Mallet finger

Mallet finger is a term used to describe a flexion deformity of the DIP joint which has occurred as a result of detachment of the extensor tendon at the base of the distal phalanx. The injury often occurs as a closed injury although obviously can also be caused by a traumatic laceration. There may be an avulsed fragment of bone from the dorsum of the distal phalanx and, if this involves a significant portion of the articular surface, this may lead to volar subluxation of the distal phalanx. If this is the case then treatment should take the form of surgery, either with internal fixation of the articular fragment, if it is large enough, or K–wire immobilisation of the DIP joint in the reduced position. For the pure tendon avulsion injuries, most clinicians treat the condition by conservative means, that is by splinting the distal phalanx in a position of full extension for a period of six to eight weeks. Various splints are available for this purpose; in the UK the most commonly used being the plastic one designed by Stack. Patient compliance, however, can be a problem as it is important that the joint remains hyperextended uninterruptedly for the full period of six to eight weeks. Despite this, however, most authors report a success rate for this type of treatment of 75–90%, success being judged by a return of most, if not all, extension of the joint. If, however, there is concern about the reliability of the patient, K wire fixation of the DIP joint may be more sensible. Finally, for the open laceration (as with the boutonnière deformity) direct tendon repair is appropriate, followed by splintage.

For the patient in whom conservative treatment has failed, the choice lies between accepting the deformity, which generally causes little functional disturbance, or surgery. Options range from secondary suture, tenodermadesis, tendon graft or if all else fails arthrodesis. The results of all these procedures are less than optimum, the author's preference being secondary suture or reconstruction of the extensor tendon using local tissues.

TENOSYNOVITIS AND TENOVAGINITIS

Where tendons pass through sheaths lined with synovium, the latter can become inflamed, resulting in the condition known as tenosynovitis. This condition can be caused by a number of factors ranging from trauma, usually repetitive, through to inflammatory conditions such as rheumatoid arthritis. In a number of cases no obvious aetiological factor can be identified. Thickening of the fibrous sheath (tenovaginitis) is commonly seen in three locations; in the first extensor compartment overlying the radial styloid, and in the flexor sheath of the fingers or thumb. These are discussed in more detail later. Finally, it should be noted that inflammation in and around tendons outside a synovial sheath should not be called tenosynovitis, a better terms being tendonitis or peritendonitis.

de Quervain's disease

This was probably first described by Tillaux in 1892 and more specifically by de Quervain in 1895. Indeed it was de Quervain who first described the surgical management. In 1930 Finkelstein reported a number of cases and also described the well-known Finkelstein test. By this manoeuvre the extensor pollicis brevis and abductor pollicis longus (APL) tendons are caused to move within their sheath of the first dorsal compartment whilst under load. More specifically, on grasping the patient's thumb and quickly abducting the hand ulnawards, the pain over the styloid tip is excruciating.

The aetiology of de Quervain's disease is unknown, although like all forms of tenovaginitis it appears to be more common in females. Its relationship to repetitive resisted extension and abduction movements of the thumb is disputed and the author knows of no conclusive evidence one way or the other. However, there is no doubt that inflammation around tendons can be associated with movement particularly if undertaken repetitively and under load. Many authors over the years have found this condition more common among persons performing manual work; indeed at one time it was known as 'washer-woman's' thumb.

Diagnosis is made from the history together with localized pain overlying the first dorsal compartment. There may be swelling in this area with crepitus on movement of the thumb. Finkelstein's test should be positive.

Treatment in the first instance should take the form of rest, often with the aid of a thumb spica splint, physiotherapy to reduce inflammation, or an injection of local anaesthetic and steroid around the tendon but in the sheath may be beneficial. If these fail, however, surgery in the form of release of the first dorsal compartment is indicated. Essentially this is a straightforward procedure, although care must be taken to protect the superficial branch of the radial nerve as this lies in close proximity. In addition although APL usually has two tendons, it is not unusual to find accessory tendons: often three and occasionally four. Because of this it is important to check that all sheaths for both tendons have been released.

Flexor tenovaginitis/trigger digits

The most common form of flexor tenovaginitis in the hand is trigger finger. Although this condition is quite common, there is still considerable controversy regarding its relation to activities at work. The condition has a spectrum of presentations ranging from pain overlying the flexor sheath, through swelling, crepitus, clicking or, triggering to a fixed contracture of the finger. Although the exact aetiology is unknown, something is known about the pathophysiology which is dependent on the peculiar anatomy of the region; more specifically the passage of flexor digitorum profundus and flexor digitorum superficialis through the closed compartment of the flexor sheath. Whether the tightness of the fibrous sheath results in inflammation or conversely tendon degeneration results in enlargment and nodule formation remains unclear. Indeed it may well be that both occur as a response to inflammation. In any event, trigger finger and thumb occurs most commonly in postmenopausal women without any history of trauma, either acute or repetitive. In some cases there are associated conditions such as diabetes mellitus, haemodialysis, carpal tunnel syndrome or amyloid deposition. It is also seen in generalised inflammatory conditions, particularly rheumatoid arthritis where there may be a lump of tenosynovitis producing the difficulty in gliding.

It should also be noted that there is also a so-called congenital variety which more often than not affects the thumb. Whether this is truly a congenital abnormality is unclear, as it does not appear to present in newborn babies, but is generally noticed several months after birth. If it does not resolve spontaneously, or indeed presents with a fixed flexion deformity, operative release is indicated.

Examination of a patient with trigger finger will demonstrate pain on both passive and active movements of the digit. The patient can often voluntarily demonstrate triggering. Again crepitus may be felt. It should also be remembered that in some patients the finger can be locked in flexion and the patient cannot actively extend the digit. With regard to the latter it is obviously important to exclude other conditions that can lead to flexor contracture, e.g. infection, arthritis, Dupuytren's contracture.

Treatment as with many of these inflammatory conditions, may be either conservative or operative. In most cases, conservative treatment is tried first unless it has failed previously or in the presence of fixed contracture. Conservative treatment takes the form of splintage, with the MP joint in extension. This, combined with the avoidance of any repetitive activity, should be in place for a period of anywhere between three and six weeks. In the author's experience, although a number of patients report a temporary improvement, the splint is often poorly tolerated and the problem recurs. A more common form of conservative treatment is to inject a small amount of local anaesthetic and steroid into the sheath either at the site of the nodule or distally; the author favours the former. The reported success ranges from 60–70%. This figure is lower if the triggering is secondary to an inflammatory condition, such as rheumatoid arthritis or diabetes. It has also been reported that an injection of local anaesthetic alone can cause resolution. A second modality of treatment is physiotherapy which again is often successful although more time-consuming. Finally, it has been noted that in a number of patients the condition can spontaneously resolve with time.

In patients whose triggering has failed to respond or indeed recurred after a satisfactory course of conservative treatment, or if they present with a fixed contracture, most surgeons proceed directly to open release. The procedure is best performed as a day-case under local anaesthesia using a small transverse incision over the distal palmar flexor crease. Using this approach the entrance to the flexor sheath can be identified and the first centimetre of the A1 pulley is released; some authors recommend a V-shaped excision of the sheath to prevent recurrence. In any event the release should be sufficient to allow free movement of the nodule as the finger fully flexes and extends. If the operation is being performed under local anaesthesia this can be confirmed by asking the patient to actively move the digit. It goes without saying that the A2 pulley should not be involved in the release as this results in bow-stringing across the MP joint with a resultant contracture.

In surgical release of trigger thumb the digital nerves are more at risk because they lie anterior to the sheath rather than laterally. As a consequence it is recommended that the skin incision alone is undertaken by sharp dissection, that the digital nerves are then identified by blunt dissection and protected whilst the proximal A1 pulley is again released.

The reader should be aware that the condition can recur even after surgery although this is uncommon, occurring in less than 10% in most reported series.

Finally, mention should be made of the use of a percutaneous release using a small tenotome or even the sharp edge of a large needle. Enthusiasts of this technique claim 80–90% success rate with little morbidity. Obviously, however, the procedure is undertaken without visualisation of the sheath and as a consequence tendon and neurovascular damage is possible. It is the author's opinion that this procedure should only be undertaken in the fingers when the physician or surgeon involved is fully experienced with the technique.

Tenosynovitis and tendonitis at other sites

Tenosynovitis can occur and has been described in and around all flexor and extensor tendons in the hand. It can be caused by infection, often after a penetrating injury; common organisms are *Staphylococcus aureus* or *Streptococcus* or more rarely *Mycobacterium marinum* from tropical fish (see also pages 171–2). Another cause is rheumatoid arthritis where multiple tendon involvement is the rule; however, this is outside the remit of this chapter. Thirdly, the problem can arise spontaneously and fourthly, be related to over–use, more specifically repetitive actions involving movement of the tendon under load.

In the infected case the finger or wrist is extremely painful with little or no movement. In addition an external wound can often be seen and the patient is often systemically unwell. Although the diagnosis is often easy to make, the condition is unfortunately difficult to treat successfully. An early intravenous course of high-dose antibiotics may be effective, but generally the preferred treatment is exploration and decompression followed by continuous intravenous and then oral antibiotics. As an alternative, a number of surgeons recommend continuous irrigation of the wound with antibiotic-laden saline. In any event the results can often be poor and the patient may be left with a stiff digit.

With regard to idiopathic and work-related forms of tenosynovitis, the only difference between the two is the clear history of ove—ruse. They are known by their specific anatomical locations. Symptoms and signs, however, are often similar in that the tenderness is quite localised, the pain being made worse by specific movement of the tendon involved, either passive or active. Less frequently, swelling and crepitus are seen and palpated at the site of tenderness. Further investigation can be undertaken and a number of authors recommend either ultrasonography or indeed magnetic resonance scanning.

Of the particular locations, inflammation around the extensor pollicis longus tendon as it passes close to Lister's tubercle was originally described in Prussian drummer-boys.

Another tendon often involved in an inflammatory condition is flexor carpi radialis. Here there is acute localised tenderness over the tendon just proximal to the scaphoid tubercle. The condition is sometimes seen in patients suffering from degenerative change of the scaphotrapezial joint. Similarly extensor and flexor carpi ulnaris tendonitis can occur. These conditions form part of the differential diagnosis of ulnar-sided wrist pain.

Finally 'intersection syndrome' or peritendonitis crepitans occurs at the intersection of the extensor carpi radialis longus and brevis with the abductor pollicis longus and extensor pollicis brevis tendons on the radial side of the distal forearm, just proximal and dorsal to the site of de Quervain's tenovaginitis. This is said to occur in patients who undergo rapid flexion/extension of the wrist whilst gripping, e.g. oarsmen.

Over–use syndrome: repetitive strain injury

No other condition arouses such controversy within hand surgery at this present time. Opinion ranges from those who believe the problem is common and often caused by activities at work to those who believe this never occurs. As in all such situations the truth probably lies somewhere in between. At this time, apart from one or two notable exceptions, there is nothing in the way of hard evidence either one way or the other. There does, however, appear to be some consensus in that symptoms and signs tend to fall into two categories. The first is where a definite diagnosis, e.g. tennis elbow or trigger finger, can be made and the second where the symptoms and signs do not fit into a recognised medical pattern. Although most clinicians would accept that symptoms from tennis elbow and trigger finger can be aggravated if not caused by activities, particularly if repetitive and stressful, it is the latter group that is particularly contentious. This has resulted in many theories being postulated. One such is that each individual has a constitutional ability to perform various activities with their upper limbs. If one particular action is undertaken repetitively and with increasing force, then at some stage it does not seem unreasonable that a patient may develop pain and discomfort in the tendons and muscles producing that activity for the duration of the task and sometime thereafter. This can initially take the form of muscle fatigue and later, if the activity continues, to more prolonged symptomatology. Key factors are the movements undertaken and the patient's exposure to a new work practice or the alteration of an existing process.

Although little headway has been made with regard to pathogenesis, a number of researchers have shown that the introduction of sensible and sympathetic modifications to the work–place can reduce the number of upper limb disorders.

CLINICAL PROBLEM

A closed flexor digitorum profundus avulsion injury is a particularly difficult injury for hand surgeons to manage. The condition can occur often after quite trivial trauma but is relatively common in contact sport, e.g. rugby. It commonly occurs in the ring finger, the reason for this being the comparitively weaker insertion of the tendon in this digit. The diagnosis is made from the history and clinical examination. Here the patient loses the ability to independently flex the DIP joint. In addition to this, there will be localised tenderness overlying the volar aspect of the finger and occasionally down into the palm if the tendon has retracted that far. Indeed, the retracted tendon may be felt as a lump in the palm. If, however, the diagnosis is unclear then further investigation by ultrasonography or MRI may be appropriate.

If the clinician is aware of the possibility of this type of injury, then the diagnosis is usually easily made. Unfortunately, this does not apply to treatment. Undoubtedly if the diagnosis is made early then it is worthwhile exploring the finger and reinserting the tendon. By far and away the best method of insertion is by passing the suture through the bone onto the dorsum of the distal phalanx. This particularly strong repair allows a more aggressive mobilisation pro-gramme. On occasion a fragment of bone may also be avulsed with the tendon; if this is the case then reduc-tion and internal fixation is the best option.

Unfortunately, if the diagnosis is made long after the injury the results of surgery are very dependent on the level at which the tendon has arrested proximally. If there is no contracture and the avulsed end is at the level of the A4 pulley, reinsertion is possible. If, however, the avulsed segment is at the level of the A2 pulley or indeed in the palm, then reinsertion may lead to a flexion contracture of the finger, the reason for this being the contracted nature of the tendon and its devascularisation due to vincular damage. Options here are to allow a flexion contracture to develop at the DIP joint or to undertake a formal arthrodesis of this joint.

FURTHER READING

Amadio PC, Hunter JM, Jaeger SH, Wehbe MA, Schneider LH. The effect of vincular injury on the results of flexor tendon surgery in zone 2. *J Hand Surg* 1985; **10A:** 626–632.

Bainbridge LC, Robertson C, Gillies D, Elliot D. Comparison of post-operative mobilisation of flexor tendon repairs with 'Passive flexion – active extension' and 'controlled active motion technique'. *J Hand Surg* 1994; **19B:** 517–521.

Bunnell S. Repair of nerves and tendons of the hand. *J Joint Bone Surg* 1928; **10:** 1–26.

Gelberman RH, Menon J, Gonsalves M, Akeson WH. The effects of mobilisation on the vascularisation of healing flexor tendons in dogs. *Clin Orthop* 1980; **153:** 283–289.

Kleinert HE, Kutz JE, Atasoy E, Stormo A. Primary repair of flexor tendons. *Orthop Clin North Am* 1973; **4:** 865–876.

Lundborg G. Experimental flexor tendon healing without adhesion formation; a new concept of tendon nutrition and intrinsic healing mechanisms. *The Hand* 1976; **8:** 235–238.

Potenza AD. Tendon healing within the flexor digital sheath in the dock. *J Bone Joint Surg* 1962; **44A:** 49–64.

Rispler D, Greenwald D, Shumway S, Allan C, Mass D. Efficiency of the flexor tendon pulley system in human cadaver hands. *J Hand Surg* 1996; **21A:** 444–450.

Savage R. In-vitro studies of a new method of flexor tendon repair. *J Hand Surg* 1985; **10B:** 135–141.

Strickland JB, Glovac SV. Digital function following tendon repair in zone two. A comparison of immobilisation and controlled passive motion techniques. *J Hand Surg* 1980; **5:** 537–543.

The Hand, Examination and Diagnosis, 2nd edn. American Society for Surgery of the Hand. Edinburgh: Churchill Livingstone, 1983.

ACKNOWLEDGEMENT

The author would like to acknowledge the Department of Medical Illustration at the Royal Manchester Children's Hospital for the preparation of figures and Mavis Luya for typing the manuscript.

7

Nerves

James Crossan

Nerve damage, in one form or another, is a common and important part of orthopaedic practice. Such injuries may vary enormously in severity from intermittent tingling experienced in mild compression syndrome to complete paralysis of the upper limb in brachial plexus lesions. One of the main purposes of taking a history in a patient with a nerve problem is to establish the type of lesion and whether its management should be conservative or operative. In many cases, it should be possible even at this very early stage to have a confident idea of the prognosis. The prognosis is related very closely to the pathological changes which occur within the substance of the nerve as a result of the damage. These changes often correlate well with the history of compression lesion of nerve and the symptoms of which the patient complains.

PATHOLOGY

Intermittent ischaemia

The mildest form of nerve compression occurs when the tissue pressure around the segments of nerve rises even a few millimetres. This type of pathology is characteristic of the nerve compression syndromes within tunnels and an elevation of venous blood pressure to as little as 20 mmHg will cause cellular ischaemia. The ischaemic cells will no longer be able to operate the Na/K pumps and nerve conduction will be impaired. The symptoms which the patient experiences are of intermittent tingling in sensory nerves or mild paralysis in motor nerves.

Intermittent sustained ischaemia

This type of ischaemia occurs when the venous pressure rises to more than 30 mmHg. In addition to cellular ischaemia the pressure within the endoneurial fluid rises and axonal transport of 'building bricks' and the return of used products is compromised. This type of pathology causes the more prolonged periods of numbness and tingling in the fingers which a patient with carpal tunnel syndrome may experience overnight. The symptoms may last for 30 min or more but will settle eventually, often when the patient gets up and moves the hand about. This level of compression will also produce neurophysiological changes characterised by slowing of nerve conduction.

When venous pressure rises above 50 mmHg, epineurial oedema ensues and this will induce motor and sensory changes for longer periods of time. Complete intraneural ischaemia occurs with pressures greater than 60 mmHg and we know, from experience with the use of tourniquets, that these pressures can be tolerated for between two and three hours without producing permanent motor or sensory changes. Beyond three hours there is great risk of tourniquet palsy developing and this can lead to motor and sensory changes which take some considerable time to recover.

Localised loss of myelin sheath

If intraneural ischaemia lasts more than three hours or so, an inflammatory reaction ensues and the increased capillary permeability leads to invasion of the tissues by macrophages which attack the myelin sheath in the affected area. This leads to demyelination of the local segment of the nerve (neurapraxia*). This is the primary pathology in lesions such as the 'Saturday night palsy'. It is important to appreciate that with this injury the myelin sheath in the nerve remains intact, not only proximally but also distal to the site of the lesion. This means that electrical stimulation of the distal segment, as might be undertaken during the course of electrophysiological testing, will result in transmission of the electrical impulse distally. The conduction velocity will, however, be slowed over the damaged demyelinated segment and this forms the basis of electrophysiological testing for nerve compression syndrome. When pressure is removed from the nerve, the body is capable of regenerating the myelin sheath and a good recovery can be anticipated.

Combination of local demyelination and some axonal loss

This type of injury is characterised by traction lesions which are most commonly seen within the brachial plexus. The stretching and intraneural bleeding which these injuries induce can cause demyelination over segments of the brachial plexus. In addition, if the traction is sufficiently severe, a variable number of axons within the substance of the nerve can be disrupted (axonotmesis). In those fibres which have simply become demyelinated, the distal axons will retain their myelin sheath and recovery will be similar to that observed in the previous group of patients. In those axons which have been disrupted, the myelin sheath will disappear from the distal segment in the process of Wallerian degeneration.

Complete disruption of nerve substance

This is the type of injury which we see most commonly as orthopaedic surgeons. Although it can occur in a partial form in traction injuries, it is complete in injuries involving transection of nerves (neurotmesis). When a nerve is transected, the proximal part of the nerve retains its myelin sheath. The distal part retains its myelin sheath for only a few days before Wallerian degeneration occurs. Injuries of this nature require accurate repair of the nerve to permit the process of regeneration which will take place slowly, at the rate of 1 mm per day. The prognosis of this type of injury varies considerably and is affected by a number of fac-

tors. The most influential factor is the age of the patient, recovery being much more complete in young patients than old patients. The second factor which affects recovery is the degree of scarring which occurs after the injury. If very little scar tissue forms and nerve repair has achieved good alignment of the fascicles, particularly the matching of motor and sensory fibres proximally and distally, a good recovery can be anticipated if the lesion lies reasonably close to the muscles which the nerve supplies. On the other hand, if a great deal of scarring occurs, the young nerve sprouts will be unable to migrate across the scar and, if they do, are likely to be matched much less well with their distal motor and sensory tubes. This will produce a poor result. It is, therefore, possible to make a fairly accurate assessment of the pathological nature of the injury and its subsequent prognosis from the very earliest stage.

Although we deal with nerve compression syndromes and nerve injuries as orthopaedic surgeons, we must remember that other pathologies occur within nerve. A number of pain syndromes occur, such as brachial neuritis, and this can mislead the unwary orthopaedic surgeon into misdiagnosing the problem as a surgical one rather than a medical one. It must also be remembered that a number of patients will present with peripheral neuropathies. Such neuropathies include disorders of motor and sensory neurones, such as motor neurone disease and carcinomatous neuropathy. Demyelinating conditions such as the Guillain–Barré syndrome, neuropathies from toxic substances such as alcohol or heavy metals and finally lesions caused by disturbance of the blood supply to nerves such as occurs in the collagen diseases, diabetes, leprosy and amyloidosis. One must always beware of the ulnar neuritis caused by a Pancoast tumour in the apex of the lung which can present in similar fashion to cubital tunnel syndrome, although severe pain is usually associated with the carcinomatous lesion.

CLINICAL ASSESSMENT

Sensory examination

One can be alerted to the presence of sensory disturbances in the upper limb by a variety of skin changes which characterise sensory damage. The skin in the affected area loses its capacity to sweat and becomes smooth and dry. At times it almost looks as if it has been polished. This is sometimes accompanied by

---

*Neur-a-praxia = nerve not working.

colour changes in the affected area due to circulatory changes induced by loss of sympathetic nerve control. This can cause the skin to become red and shiny. If the sensory loss has been present for some time there may be evidence of ulcerated skin lesions, particularly at the finger-tips or in areas in which the patient has bruised the hand accidentally.

The distribution of these changes can be described in terms of *dermatomes* or cutaneous nerve distribution (*Fig. 4A.1*, p. 99). The dermatomes are as follows:

C5   over the deltoid muscle
C6   thenar eminence
C7   indeterminate
C8   ulnar border of hand
T1   ulnar border of elbow
T2   inner aspect of upper arm.

Proximal to the wrist, the *cutaneous branches* of these nerve roots reach the skin through a variety of cutaneous nerves. There is considerable overlap in the areas supplied by these nerves so that testing of the forearm and upper arm is generally unreliable if one is attempting to localise the site of the lesion, apart from axillary nerve injury which commonly causes loss of sensation over a small patch of the deltoid mass. The two cutaneous nerves supplying the upper arm are the lateral inferior cutaneous nerve of arm and the intercostobrachial nerve which supplies the inner aspect of the upper arm and which can be a useful nerve for nerve grafting. The area over the front of the elbow is supplied by the medial cutaneous nerve of arm. The forearm is supplied by the lateral cutaneous and medial cutaneous nerves of the forearm. Localisation can be much more accurate in the hand where the ulnar, radial and median nerves have characteristic autonomous zones. For the median nerve the autonomous zone is the palmar aspect of the index finger and for the ulnar nerve the palmar aspect of the little finger. The autonomous zone of the radial nerve lies on the dorsum of the hand in the web between the thumb and index finger.

Simple observations may localise an area of sensory loss and one may be able to deduce the site of nerve damage. However, in order to achieve an accurate index of sensory loss, more sophisticated tests must be undertaken. The suitability of these tests varies according to the underlying pathology. Two sensory tests are particularly valuable when assessing nerve compression lesions (see below), whereas other tests may be of more

value when assessing nerve injury or when monitoring the patient during the process of nerve regeneration. There are many different types of sensory receptors in the skin which can detect changes in different forms of energy and translate them into nerve action potentials. In the skin we can test light touch receptors, crude touch receptors, receptors for heat and cold, and pain receptors. When, for instance, we test for light touch, the transduced signals are transmitted along the afferent nerves to the primary sensory neurone, the cell body of which lies in the dorsal root ganglion outwith the spinal cord. Such a primary sensory neurone with its fibres and its branches constitutes a sensory unit. The receptive unit is the area of skin supplied by a sensory unit and is circular in shape. These receptive units overlap to varying degrees. In the fingers, there are large numbers of receptive units which greatly overlap. In less sensitive areas, such as the upper arm, there is much less overlap and reduced tactile discrimination.

In the course of sensory testing, you should test for two types of tactile discrimination: intensity or threshold discrimination and innervation density. We find that threshold tests are particularly useful when testing for compression syndromes whereas innervation density tests are much more useful for monitoring nerve regeneration. It must also be remembered that complex cortical integration takes place during nerve regeneration and this can be taken into account by undertaking Moberg's picking-up test (picking up a paper-clip or pin from a flat surface).

In assessing the results of nerve repair, the difficulty is that we have no reliable and quantitative method of measuring sensory recovery. One reason for this is that patients do not regain 30% to 70% of normal sensation; they develop a different *quality* of sensation, which may be unpleasant.

Testing for innervation density

Two-point discrimination is determined by the density of receptor fields and their degree of overlap. In the finger-tips there are many small receptive fields with large overlap and this permits a two-point discrimination of as little as 1–2 mm. Proximally, however (for instance at the elbow) the two-point discrimination may be as much as 6 mm. *Static* two-point discrimination is assessed by holding two points against the skin for a number of seconds and determining whether the patient feels one or two prongs. This test is repeated on three occasions and the critical distance noted in millimetres. The static test is mediated through slowly-adapting nerve fibres, whereas moving two-point discrimination is assessed through rapidly-adapting receptor fibres. *Moving* two-point discrimination is conducted by moving the two prongs longitudinally from the tip of the finger proximally and assessing whether one or two prongs are felt by the patient. Critical distances are recorded in millimetres. The value of two-point discrimination tests in nerve regeneration is that the tests measure not only the peripheral parameters of nerve function but also the central interpretation of these events in the cerebral cortex. Following nerve division, the perceived pattern of the affected area is altered in the cerebral cortex. As part of the recovery of sensation, a certain degree of plasticity is required within the cerebral cortex to allow the patient once more to interpret external stimuli accurately. This plasticity is much greater in the child than it is in the adult and may account in large measure for the much better levels of recovery following nerve injury in children.

Threshold testing

In compression syndromes, cortical organisation is unimpaired. Two-point discrimination may remain intact even if only a few sensory fibres are left in the skin. The results of sensory testing can therefore be misleading. It is much better in nerve compression syndromes to undertake threshold tests. A popular method of measuring pressure thresholds is the use of *Semmes–Weinstein monofilaments*. These are nylon monofilaments of different diameter and degrees of stiffness. The test is performed by applying the monofilament perpendicularly to the area of skin to be tested and increasing the pressure until bending of the monofilament takes place. The method can be tedious and it is sometimes difficult to achieve full co-operation from the patient. Nevertheless, it is a test which can be reproduced and which can permit reasonably accurate assessment of nerve recovery. A more sensitive test of receptor function is *vibrometry*. This measures the threshold of quickly-adapting fibres. The test is conducted by placing the vibrometer against the skin and measuring the smallest vibrating stimulus which can be detected by the patient. This is measured in micrometres

and, although it is tedious to conduct, it does give a very accurate measurement of this particular sensory modality.

Motor examination

Inspection of the upper limb can often give a clear indication of the type of motor loss which has been sustained by a patient. In the acute situation paralysis of certain groups of muscles may lead to an abnormal posture of the arm or the hand, whereas in longer-standing lesions muscle wasting becomes obvious and gives some clues as to the site of the underlying injury. Postural abnormalities include the porter's tip position from an Erb's palsy in which the arm hangs by the patient's side internally rotated, fully extended and with a pronated forearm. The drop-wrist and drop-fingers are characteristic of a radial nerve palsy. Ulnar nerve palsy is manifested by varying degrees of clawing of the fingers, usually the ring and little fingers. A simian posture of the thumb, adducted against the side of the hand, can be characteristic of a median nerve palsy. The distribution of the changes can be recorded in a variety of ways. The myotomes are as follows:

C5   deltoid and infraspinatus
C6   pectoralis major, biceps, brachialis, coracobrachialis
C7   triceps, wrist and finger extensors, pronator teres
C8   wrist flexors, flexors to fingers and thumb
T1   intrinsic muscles. (See also *Table 4A.1*, p. 99).

A number of key muscles could be tested in the course of examining the upper limb. A full description of the tests can be found in the MRC publication on examination of peripheral nerve injuries. This is a well-illustrated booklet which cannot be bettered. In the following paragraphs some of the anomalies encountered during peripheral muscle testing will be described.

Axillary nerve (C5/6)

It is important to look for muscle contraction in the deltoid when testing this nerve and to palpate muscle contraction. A number of patients learn trick movements involving the long head of the biceps, coracobrachialis or trapezius and use these to initiate shoulder abduction.

Radial nerve (C5–T1)

Triceps. When testing triceps, hold the arm horizontally and fully abducted at the shoulder so that one eliminates the effects of gravity, which can deceive the unwary examiner.

Brachioradialis. It is important to ensure that the forearm is in neutral rotation before undertaking this test so that the brachioradialis muscle stands out when the elbow is flexed against resistance.

Extensor carpi radialis longus and brevis. These muscles can be tested easily with the wrist in extension. A further refinement is that testing of grip strength in patients with paralysis of these muscles will be reduced, as the wrist tends to flop into flexion when this test is performed. As recovery takes place in these muscles, the strength of extension increases to the point where the patient can hold the wrist in extension actively and the grip strength will thereby increase.

Extensor digitorum. Remember to test these muscles by examining active extension at the *metacarpophalangeal joints* and noting resisted extension against the proximal phalanges. Extension of the fingers at the proximal interphalangeal joints is brought about largely by the activity of the intrinsic muscles.

Extensor pollicis longus. If this muscle is tested for with the palms together, it will avoid the inadvertent palmar abduction of the thumbs which some patients are prone to exhibit when asked to test in other positions. If this muscle appears weak, make sure that the extension is not being induced by abductor pollicis brevis or adductor pollicis brevis, both of which have some attachments to the extensor mechanism distal to the metacarpophalangeal joint.

It is also wise to be aware that loss of extension of the wrist, fingers or thumb can be brought about by other pathologies such as attrition rupture of extensor tendons in rheumatoid arthritis or following Colles' fracture. Some viral neuropathies can cause wrist-drop.

Musculocutaneous nerve (C5/6)

This nerve supplies the biceps and brachialis and can sometimes be injured in the course of shoulder surgery for recurrent dislocation or replacement. When testing these muscles, it is wise to supinate the forearm and thereby eliminate the action of brachioradialis and pronator teres, both of which can in some patients contribute to elbow flexion.

Ulnar nerve (C8–T1)

It is important to test contraction in the muscle belly of flexor carpi ulnaris with the wrist flexed and ulnar deviated. In some patients, often those with combined ulnar and median nerve lesions, gradual migration of the abductor pollicis longus tendon towards the volar aspect of the wrist joint can produce movement which can be misinterpreted as coming from flexor carpi ulnaris.

Flexor digitorum profundus of the ring and little fingers. Although this test is simple to perform, it can sometimes be misleading if there has been a severe injury in the mid-forearm which has caused fibrous adhesions between the muscle bellies of the flexor muscles.

Abductor digiti quinti. Make sure that the common extensor tendon to the little finger has not subluxed in an ulnar direction, as this can produce a misleading result.

Interosseii.
First dorsal interosseous muscle. Make sure that ulnar abduction of the index finger is not being induced by extensor indicis proprius. While examining this and the other interosseii muscles it is worth testing for intrinsic contracture. This is determined with the metacarpophalangeal joint in full extension; if the proximal interphalangeal joint can be flexed fully, there is no intrinsic contracture.

Adductor pollicis. Testing for this muscle is the reverse of testing for abductor pollicis brevis. The thumb should be laid in the line of the second metacarpal and in so doing the thumb-nail will lie in a vertical position.

Median nerve (C5–T1)

Pronator teres. The pronator quadratus also takes part in forearm pronation and is also supplied by the median nerve.

Flexor carpi radialis. Beware that the abductor pollicis longus can sometimes act as a wrist flexor when the flexor carpi ulnaris is paralysed.

Flexor digitorum superficialis of the fingers. Make sure that the fingers which are not being tested are fully extended by holding them beyond the distal interphalangeal joints. This locks the flexor digitorum profundis muscle mass in the forearm and the examiner can then test for flexion at the proximal interphalangeal joint, as described by Apley. Note that some patients cannot co-ordinate separate movements of superficialis and profundus tendons in the little finger.

Flexor pollicis longus.

Flexor digitorum profundus to the index and middle fingers.

Abductor pollicis brevis. Place the thumb in the line of the second metacarpal so that the nail of the thumb lies at right angles to the nails of the digits. The thumb should be lifted vertically from this position and the abductor pollicis brevis muscle palpated as the thumb is being tested.

Opponens pollicis. The simplest way to test this muscle is to ask the patient to flex the index finger to the thumb to form a figure O. The examiner attempts to break the circle by pulling his finger through the it.

One should be aware that inability to flex the flexor digitorum profundus tendons in the fingers may be due to non-neurological causes such as rupture from rheumatoid synovitis and isolated paralysis of flexor pollicis longus and flexor digitorum profundus to the index finger is caused by an anterior interosseous nerve palsy.

Anomalous innervation in the upper limb

Anomalies of nerve innervation can occur at any level. Those which occur most commonly and which cause most confusion to orthopaedic surgeons are the anomalies involving the muscles of the forearm and the hand. These anomalies involve interconnections between the median and ulnar nerves and comprise the following.

1. *A connection between the anterior interosseous branch of the median nerve and the motor branch of the ulnar nerve.* This interconnection occurs within the substance of the muscle belly of flexor digitorum profundus in the proximal forearm. In the presence of this anomaly, the flexor digitorum profundi to the index and middle fingers (which are usually innervated by the median nerve) will be supplied by the ulnar nerve. The opposite situation can also arise, in which the median nerve supplies all of the profundus group.

2. *The Martin–Gruber 'anastomosis'*★ is a communicating branch between the median nerve in the proximal forearm and the ulnar nerve. It occurs in 15% of the population and its presence produces a similar clinical picture to that described above.

3. *The ulnar nerve can communicate with the median nerve in the distal forearm.* This anomaly occurs much less commonly than the Martin–Gruber anastomosis.

4. *The Riche–Cannieu* anomaly is formed by a neural connection between the recurrent branch of the median nerve in the thenar eminence and the deep branch of the ulnar nerve. Usually it involves only motor fibres. This anomaly is much more common than the Martin–Gruber anastomosis and has been recorded in one series as occurring in as many as four out of five people.

The significance of these anomalous nerve distributions is that if a main nerve trunk has been divided distal to the origin of one of these anomalies, significant function of the damaged nerve can still exist and is mediated through the nerve fibres within the anomalous loop.

Electromyography and nerve conduction tests

Although an accurate assessment of the neurological status of a patient can usually be determined from a careful history and clinical examination, situations arise in which further information is necessary to establish a diagnosis or to assess the degree of recovery following nerve injury. Electrophysiological testing has a valuable role in assessing compression lesions of nerves, in determining the nature of a traction injury to nerve and in assessing the recovery of nerve function before clinical signs become apparent.

★This is a misnomer: strictly speaking an anastomosis is a connection between two hollow tubes.

Nerve stimulation

The simplest test which can be performed on a nerve is to deliver a pulse of current to the nerve via cutaneous electrodes and to see and feel contracting muscles. For instance stimulation of the median nerve at the elbow should, under normal circumstances, produce contraction of the flexor muscles to the thumb, index and middle fingers. Variable effects may be noticed in relation to the ring and little fingers, depending on the presence or absence of anomalous nerve distribution. By using this simple test one can detect the presence of, for instance, a Martin–Gruber anastomosis in a particular patient.

Nerve stimulation will cause contraction in the muscles supplied by that nerve if the nerve remains myelinated. Thus abnormalities caused by intermittent ischaemia or by local areas of demyelination will still permit an electrical stimulus over the nerve to produce contraction in the muscles which it supplies. Over a segment of demyelinated nerve, however, the conduction velocities are reduced. When a nerve is transected it takes a number of days for the myelin sheath distal to the level of the injury to degenerate and therefore nerve stimulation will continue to activate the innervated muscles for a few days following a transection of the nerve. Within ten days, however, Wallerian degeneration will have taken place and stimulation of the demyelinated component of the nerve will no longer induce muscle contraction.

Nerve conduction studies

Nerve compression lesions such as carpal tunnel syndrome or cubital tunnel syndrome will eventually produce an area of loss of myelin in the segment of nerve which is being compressed. When nerve conduction tests are performed on myelinated nerves, the conduction velocity within the nerve is fast as the nerve impulse jumps between the nodes of Ranvier (sultatory conduction). This process proceeds at a velocity of about 50 m/s or 120 miles/h; that is to say, the speed at which a racing car might travel. When a segment of nerve is denuded of its myelin, the conduction velocity is no longer determined by the impulse jumping between the nodes of Ranvier but is conducted down the cable and is known as cable conduction. This proceeds at a rate of 10 m/s which is the equivalent to about 25 miles/h; that is the speed of a world-class 100 m sprinter. In all but the most severe cases of nerve compression syndrome, axonal loss has not occurred at the area of damage and therefore Wallerian degeneration has not occurred distal to the lesion. It is therefore possible to measure conduction above, below and across the damaged segment of nerve to establish the site of nerve compression. For instance, motor conduction at the wrist in carpal tunnel syndrome can be measured by stimulating the median nerve proximal to the wrist and measuring the time it takes for the potential to reach abductor pollicis brevis. Under normal circumstances, the time taken between stimulation and recording in the muscle (that is, the distal motor latency) measures less than 3 ms. The equivalent value for the ulnar nerve at the wrist is 2.2 ms. Prolongation of this latency indicates slowing of conduction across a demyelinated segment of nerve and is a good indication of nerve compression at that site. Similarly, distal sensory latencies can be measured by applying stimulating electrodes to the appropriate finger and measuring the nerve action potential at the wrist. The appropriate values for median and ulnar nerves at the wrist are 3 and 1.8 ms respectively. Increase in this distal latency is caused by a local conduction block due to demyelination and indicates the presence of a compression syndrome.

Electromyography

Normal muscle is electrically silent. In other words, if a needle is placed in abductor pollicis brevis, one cannot (apart from a slight blip as the needle goes into the muscle) record electrical activity within the muscle at rest. A muscle which has been denervated reverts to its embryonic state and exhibits spontaneous fibrillation. This becomes apparent some three weeks after a denervation injury and the fibrillations which are seen on the oscilloscope can be demonstrated graphically by a high-pitched clicking sound. If a nerve has been transected and repaired, re-innervation will eventually occur and this can be detected by electromyography in the form of reduced levels of fibrillation. In addition, when the patient is asked to undertake voluntary movement of the muscle, the unit action potentials are all of small amplitude. These changes only become normal when the myelin sheath has regenerated fully. The intermediate stage of partial denervation is characterised by giant units on the oscilloscope and these can sometimes be seen clinically in the form of fasciculations.

Not only does electromyography give some indication of the type of injury sustained by the nerve and the degree to which recovery has taken place, but it also differentiates traumatic nerve lesions from medical problems such as neuropathies.

DIVIDED NERVES

Before considering the role of the surgeon in repairing divided nerves, it is worth reviewing briefly what happens to the nerve following injury and, in general terms, what the surgeon can do to gain maximum benefit from this process. When a nerve is transected by a sharp instrument (neurotmesis), the nerve distal to the transection undergoes Wallerian degeneration, followed by regeneration. Initially, almost all the cellular material in the distal segment of the nerve is phagocytosed to leave a skeleton of axonal tubes composed of residual basement membrane containing Schwann cells. Regeneration then proceeds by proliferation of Schwann cells, which manufacture new axons. These become functional only when motor axons regenerate into distal axonal motor tubes and reach motor end-organs. Sensory fibres, likewise, must reach sensory end-organs. Regeneration proceeds at the rate of 1 mm/day. During this time the pattern of representation of function in the cerebral cortex becomes altered and, as re-innervation takes place, this pattern can be manipulated by intensive motor and sensory rehabilitation to produce the best possible result. It is never possible to restore completely normal function, either motor or sensory.

Loss of continuity of nerves also occurs in avulsion injuries caused by traction. When a nerve is avulsed in mid-substance, there is considerable axonal disruption distally. Repair is by Wallerian degeneration and regeneration, but results are generally poor because of severe disorganisation of the tissues and subsequent severe scar formation. It must be remembered that traction injuries in which the nerve remains in continuity can also contain areas in which axons are disrupted (axonotmesis) and repair of these segments will again take place by Wallerian degeneration followed by regeneration. In these circumstances, axon matching is usually poor and severe intraneural scarring generally produces a poor outcome.

Principles of treatment
Primary repair

This should be performed in all uncontaminated nerve divisions. Tension-free repair can be obtained and orientation of the nerve established by matching epineural blood vessels and fascicles using magnification with loupes or a microscope. Epineural repair with fine nylon sutures (no larger than 8/0) is favoured. Individual fascicular repair can be performed but the outcome is no better than that following epineural repair. The repaired nerve should be protected by plaster immobilisation in a position which reduces tension for up to two weeks. Unprotected joints should be kept mobile by intensive physiotherapy and later a sensory re-education programme should be undertaken.

Secondary repair

This procedure is reserved for contaminated wounds and is generally undertaken six weeks or more after injury. There is good supportive evidence that the quality of result obtained in secondary repairs undertaken three months or more after the injury is less good than repairs performed in the first three months. In undertaking this procedure the surgeon trims the scarred proximal and distal ends of the nerve. It may be possible in some circumstances to suture the ends of the nerve without tension or flexing adjacent joints but usually nerve graft is required.

Nerve grafting

This is used for secondary repair and failed primary repair where tension-free repair of the trimmed nerve ends is not possible. Nerve graft is usually obtained from the sural nerve, but may also be obtained from other sources such as the intercostobrachial nerves or the medial cutaneous nerve of forearm. Parallel strands of nerve graft are sutured across the defect. Alternative sources of graft are now available and these include vascularised nerve graft, freeze-thawed muscle conduits, allografts and biodegradable tubes. None of these latter techniques is superior to standard sural nerve grafting but may be appropriate in unusual circumstances.

The older method of 'cable grafting', where the strands of nerve graft were glued together to produce a structure of similar diameter to the nerve trunk to be grafted and then sutured or glued in place at each end, is seldom used today.

Tendon transfers

These are used following failed nerve repair. A muscle whose function is duplicated by another muscle or muscles is mobilised and redirected to produce the desired function. For example the tendon of flexor carpi ulnaris can be mobilised from the flexor aspect of the forearm to its dorsal aspect and sutured into paralysed extensor units to provide extension of the fingers in a radial nerve palsy. Meanwhile, wrist flexion is maintained by flexor carpi radialis and palmaris longus.

Technical factors

The best results of nerve repair are invariably obtained in youngsters. This may be a reflection of an increased capacity of the younger patient to regenerate nerve tissue. It is more likely, however, that these patients exhibit a greater degree of cerebral plasticity, so that the sensory and motor cortices of the brain can create more efficient patterns of reconfiguration than is the case in adults.

Across all age groups, the next most critical factor is likely to be the development of scar tissue at the site of the repair, whether one has undertaken a primary or secondary nerve suture. The surgeon can play an important role in reducing the development of scar tissue following nerve repair. It is important to resect obviously damaged and fibrosed segments of nerve, particularly at secondary repair. One must find a clean, healthy and well-vascularised area of tissue in which to undertake the nerve repair. Particular care should be taken where the nerve repair is conducted in a subcutaneous situation such as the median nerve at the wrist. One must ensure that there is no risk of adherence of the cutaneous scar to the nerve repair. One should equally ensure that contiguous nerve and tendon repairs are separated by healthy tissue and, at the level of the wrist, this is often possible by mobilising flaps of flexor synovial tissue to isolate a median nerve repair from the surrounding tissues and thus minimise the amount of perineural and intraneural scarring.

Absolutely critical to the surgical repair of a nerve is the reduction of tension at the repair site. Nerves have a degree of elasticity and a gap will always appear

following clean division of a nerve; therefore a small degree of tension is inevitable even when there is no tissue loss. If the laceration is not clean-cut and there is significant damage to the ends of the divided nerve requiring trimming of the nerve stumps, one must be very careful in one's assessment of the degree of tension created by trimming the nerve stumps. This is particularly crucial in areas where there is little gliding or excursion of the nerve, as in the digital nerves. Where there is more mobility, for instance in the median nerve at the level of the wrist, slightly larger gaps can be tolerated. If in doubt, one should consider filling the defect with a nerve graft. Although tension in nerve repairs can be reduced by flexing joints on either side of the injured nerve at the time of the repair, this release of tension will only occur during the period of plaster immobilisation and tension will develop once more when the joints are mobilised. The increased tension which develops during mobilisation will promote the formation of dense scar tissue within the substance of the nerve and in its immediate environment. Such procedures are no longer recommended.

In complex injuries which are not amenable to primary repair, the surgeon should make sure that reconstruction takes place within three months and certainly less than six months. This is particularly important with regard to return of motor function. If the muscle end-organ is deprived of trophic stimuli from its nerve, it will undergo interstitial fibrosis and atrophy from about 18 months onwards. Thus if early re-innervation of a muscle cannot be obtained within a year of injury, the prospect of successful re-innervation is low. This is best illustrated by the natural history of an ulnar nerve repair in the upper arm. With nerves regenerating at the rate of 1 mm a day, it will take almost two years for any potential re-innervation to reach the intrinsic muscles in the hand. Thus in adults, recovery of intrinsic muscle function in the hand following this type of injury has not been recorded. There is more latitude in the return of sensory function, no matter how long the interval between the injury and repair. In addition, although nerve grafting over distances of more than 3 cms, can be disappointing with regard to return of motor function, return of sensory function may be anticipated using grafts of up to 15 cms.

Finally, a vigorous rehabilitation programme following nerve repair is mandatory if one wishes to achieve the best possible result. Traditionally, great emphasis has been laid on the return of muscle function. The first step is to ensure that the joints distal to the injury are not allowed to stiffen. This often requires intensive physiotherapy, particularly for proximal nerve lesions where active movement in a large number of joints is not possible. Although the physiotherapist should concentrate on this aspect of rehabilitation in the early stages, efforts should be directed to increasing muscle strength and function in the later stages of recovery. In recent years it has become apparent that an intensive sensory re-education programme can improve the clinical results of nerve repair substantially. This phase of re-education starts when nerve regeneration reaches its end-organ. It has the benefit of improving the patient's perception of his environment by touch and it can also correct any hypersensitivity, which is a common feature in areas which have lost their sensory supply. As more nerve fibres reach their end-organs in the later phases of sensory re-education, the physiotherapist concentrates on improving the patient's tactile ability to recognise objects.

The surgeon often encounters patients in whom primary or secondary nerve repair has produced little or relatively little benefit. The question then arises as to whether the repair should be explored further. Indications for so doing include the absence of a progressing Tinel's sign and electrophysiological data which reveal no evidence of motor or sensory re-innervation. At the time of such late explorations, the nerve is often found to lie in a mass of scar tissue and external neurolysis of the nerve can be effective in promoting further regeneration in a number of patients. There is good evidence now that intraneural neurolysis (separating out the individual fasciculi within the scarred nerve, which was favoured some years ago, is not worthwhile and may create even more scarring in an already damaged nerve.

Median nerve

Upper arm

Complete division of the median nerve in the upper arm causes extensive motor and sensory deficits. The pattern of involvement may vary to some degree from patient to patient, depending on whether or not they have cross-over fibres between the median and the ulnar nerves in the forearm. Generally one would expect loss of function in pronator teres, the superficial and deep flexors to the index and middle fingers and flexor pollicis longus. In addition, a number of the small muscles in the hand will be paralysed: these include abductor pollicis brevis and the lumbrical muscles to the index and middle fingers. The distribution of sensory loss may vary also from patient to patient depending on median/ulnar crossover in the forearm, but classically the thumb, index and half of the ring fingers will be affected. The median nerve can be located easily in the upper arm as it usually overlies the brachial artery at this level. Although one might anticipate varying degrees of recovery in the forearm muscles, lesions of the median nerve at this level are generally too far removed from the thenar muscles and lumbricals to permit their re-innervation. Recovery of modest sensory function can be anticipated but this rarely approaches normal levels of tactile sensation.

Elbow

The neurological deficit in divisions of the median nerve at this level is closely similar to those in the upper arm, except that pronator teres is usually spared as its nerve-supply originates proximal to the elbow joint. It should be remembered that other forms of nerve injury are more common than laceration at this level. A number of iatrogenic injuries are induced these days by injection injuries, secondary to cannulation of a brachial artery or vein, and others from self-administered opiates or other drugs. The latter cases can also be associated with the rapid development of a Volkmann's ischaemic contracture, which in itself can directly injure the median nerve which becomes firmly entrapped beneath the unyielding lacertus fibrosus and the proximal arcade of the deep flexor muscles of the forearm. Similar problems can arise in association with supracondylar fractures of the humerus.

Wrist

Most median nerve injuries at this level are caused by sharp divisions which may be accidental or self-inflicted. At this level the median nerve's most important function is to provide sensation to the radial half of the palm of the hand and to the palmar surfaces of the thumb, index and middle fingers. A majority of patients with complete division of the median nerve at this level experience no functional problems from loss of innervation of the thenar muscles, because the ulnar nerve may also innervate the thenar muscles (other than abductor pollicis brevis). In clean lacerations of the nerve at this level, functional recovery of sensation can be expected in two out of three patients.

Ulnar nerve

The ulnar nerve, like the median nerve, carries motor and sensory fibres. It is vulnerable to injury as it runs inferior to the proximal brachial artery and then courses obliquely towards the elbow. In the distal third of the upper arm it gives off its branch to flexor carpi ulnaris and thereafter it supplies flexor digitorum profundus to the little finger and often to the ring finger. Its main function is to supply the many intrinsic muscles within the hand and repair of the nerve in the upper arm is often disappointing because nerve regeneration cannot proceed at a pace which will permit re-innervation of these intrinsic muscles prior to their atrophy and fibrosis. The nerve also supplies sensation to the little finger and the ulnar half of the ring finger and, by its dorsal branch, to the dorsal skin on the ulnar half of the hand. If a patient experiences weakness and clumsiness in the hand from this type of injury, one should consider early tendon transfers to restore satisfactory levels of hand function.

Elbow

The ulnar nerve is at its most superficial as it passes beside the olecranon notch and behind the medial epicondyle. It is vulnerable to laceration at this site. Because flexor digitorum profundus function to the little and ring fingers is compromised with this type of lesion, it is less likely to be associated with clawing of the fingers than an injury at the level of the wrist where profundus function is not compromised. If a delayed repair of a transected ulnar nerve at this level is undertaken, it is often worthwhile performing a subcutaneous anterior transposition prior to repair and this can avoid the use of nerve grafts.

Wrist

The ulnar nerve is deeper than the median nerve at this level and lies on the radial side of the flexor carpi ulnaris tendon. It subsequently divides into its motor

and sensory branches within Guyon's canal. The examiner can often be misled into thinking that there may be a partial lesion of the ulnar nerve if there are cross-over fibres from the median nerve in patients with connections such as the Martin–Gruber anastomosis. Almost invariably, however, abductor digiti quinti and opponens digiti quinti function will be severely compromised. Adduction of the thumb is also generally weak. At this site, as with the median nerve, industrial accidents can cause division of the nerve with marked damage to the divided ends and to the surrounding tissues: resection of nerve tissue is then necessary and it should be emphasised that, in these circumstances, one should not be tempted to suture the trimmed nerve ends under tension or with the wrist in any significant degree of flexion. It is preferable to undertake nerve grafting with the sural nerve. This is particularly gratifying at this level, as the motor and sensory branches of the ulnar nerve can often be identified quite readily and accurate matching of motor and sensory fibres thereby obtained. It is particularly important when repairing the ulnar nerve at this site to interpose some synovial tissue between the nerve repair and the tendon of flexor carpi ulnaris, which is almost invariably also divided, to prevent perineural and intraneural fibrosis occurring. Although clinical results show that both motor and sensory function can be restored to some degree, the return of high levels of manual dexterity following this injury is rare. Thus patients in occupations which require swift and skilful use of the hands (such as car mechanics or musicians) will rarely achieve their former level of expertise.

Radial nerve

The radial nerve is quite different from the median and ulnar nerve in a number of respects. Firstly it is primarily a motor nerve and loss of its sensory function which supplies a small area of skin on the dorsal web between the thumb and index finger is not a problem to most patients. Injuries to the radial nerve also occur quite close to the insertion of the branches into the muscle of the triceps and the extensor muscles of the forearm. A good motor recovery following primary nerve repair can therefore be anticipated. However, injuries caused by sharp division of the radial nerve are rare. More often the radial nerve is injured as a result of fractures of the humerus or in association with high-velocity gun-shot wounds. In the former situation the nerve remains in continuity and the injury occurs as a result of neurapraxia of some of the large motor fibres and sensory fibres within the nerve. These lesions can be expected to recover within a few days if they have been caused by oedema or within a few weeks if they have been caused by disturbance of the myelin sheath around the nerve. There is also commonly an element of axonotmesis, where bundles of axons have been interrupted at multiple levels within otherwise intact epineural sheaths. The degree of recovery anticipated in these lesions is related to the amount of intraneural scarring and this is commonly greater in high-velocity injuries such as gun-shot wounds in which the bullet has passed through the adjacent tissues without actually interrupting the continuity of the nerve. If there are no signs of recovery in the predicted timescale, electromyography may give some indication of the prognosis if performed 6–12 weeks after the injury. In the presence of a severe injury with a considerable degree of axonotmesis, fibrillation and de-innervation potentials will be present within muscles such as brachioradialis and muscle action potentials will also be absent. If the injury has produced neurapraxia, stimulation of the nerve proximal to the injury will not produce muscle contraction, whereas distal stimulation will cause the muscle to contract as the myelin sheaths distal to the injury remain intact. Thus electromyography may prevent an unnecessary exploration although the surgeon must always appreciate that this technique provides only qualitative evidence for regeneration and one cannot be certain that functional levels of recovery will ensue.

BRACHIAL PLEXUS AND THORACIC OUTLET SYNDROME

The brachial plexus provides the nerve supply for most of the shoulder girdle and the entire upper extremity. It extends from the intervertebral foramina of the spinal column to the axilla, across a distance of some 15 cm in the adult. It is therefore one of the largest structures of the peripheral nervous system and is vulnerable to injury.

Anatomy

The roots comprise the anterior primary rami of the five mixed spinal roots C5, C6, C7, C8 and T1 (*Table 7.1,* p. 220). These lie between the scalenus anterior and scalenus medius muscles and pass across the phrenic nerve as it travels down towards the chest in this area. The three trunks of the brachial plexus are derived from the roots. The anterior primary rami of the C5 and C6 roots converge to form the superior trunk whereas those of C8 and T1 form the inferior trunk. The anterior primary ramus of C7 continues as the intermediate trunk. Each trunk then splits into an anterior and posterior division, producing six elements in total. The anterior divisions of the upper and middle trunks unite to form the lateral cord, whereas the anterior division of the lower trunk continues as the medial cord. The posterior divisions of all three trunks converge to become the posterior cord. The cords are infraclavicular and lie in the axilla. They are the longest parts of the brachial plexus and their names reflect their positions in relation to the second portion of the axillary artery which they surround.

It is important to remember that three significant peripheral nerves originate from the brachial plexus above the clavicle. The dorsal scapular nerve arises from the C5 nerve root and innervates the rhomboid muscles. The long thoracic nerve derives from C5, C6 and C7 to innervate serratus anterior. The suprascapular nerve arises from the upper trunk and supplies supraspinatus and infraspinatus.

The remaining peripheral nerves derive from the cords in the inferior part of the brachial plexus. The lateral cord supplies the musculocutaneous, the lateral head of the median and the lateral pectoral nerves. The medial cord supplies the medial pectoral, the medial cutaneous nerves of the arm and forearm, and the ulnar and medial heads of the median nerve. Finally the posterior cord supplies the subscapular, thoracodorsal nerve to latissimus dorsi, axillary nerve to the deltoid, and radial nerves.

Finally, it is important to remember that the first thoracic anterior primary ramus contributes its preganglionic sympathetic fibres to the stellate ganglion. Injury to those fibres produces Horner's syndrome consisting of miosis, ptosis, enophthalmos and loss of sweating around the eye on the affected side.

Classification

Various classifications of brachial plexus injury have evolved. These often focus on parameters such as the affected population, the specific causes, the nature of the injury, the anatomical location of the injury or the mechanism of injury. This reflects the difficulty in classifying an injury such as that of a motorcyclist who has sustained a closed supraclavicular preganglionic traction lesion of the plexus. The anatomical classification which will be used in this chapter is shown in *Table 7.1*. Most *injuries* are closed ones producing traction or avulsion lesions of the brachial plexus. Less commonly we see contusion, compression, neurovascular or orthopaedic injuries. Open injuries are much less common but are usually gun-shot wounds or lacerations. In addition, open neurovascular injuries can be sustained and the brachial plexus can be damaged in the course of operative interventions or surgery around the neck. An increasingly common cause of problems is the insertion of needles and cannulae for therapeutic or diagnostic purposes.

The second major group of injuries is *non-traumatic lesions* of the brachial plexus and these include primary and secondary tumours, the most common of which is the Pancoast lesion at the apex of the lung which can irritate the lower roots of the brachial plexus and cause a severe painful ulnar neuropathy. Neuralgic amyotrophy (sometimes known as brachial neuritis) is also a common cause of non-traumatic brachial plexus dysfunction characterised by severe pain from its outset. Radiation-induced brachial neuritis often occurs many years after the primary treatment with deep X-ray therapy, so that patients who received intense treatment 20 or 30 years ago for breast cancer may present with unremitting painful brachial neuropathy. Thoracic outlet syndrome will be considered in its own right.

Incidence

A common type of brachial plexus lesion seen by orthopaedic surgeons is the high-velocity injury. In the past, young motorcyclists were the predominantly affected group but the recent introduction in the United Kingdom of high insurance premiums together with alterations in motorcycle design, particularly tyres and brakes, have led to a progressive fall in the incidence of motorcyclists in this group. Other causes include high-velocity car accidents and pedestrian accidents. Much of what we have learned about peripheral nerve lesions in general and brachial plexus injuries in particular, has been as a result of injuries sustained during war-time. For instance, out of the 25,000 peripheral nerve injuries seen in the United States Military Hospitals at the end of World War II, there were approximately 1200 brachial plexus injuries.

Mechanism of injury

Before going into detail regarding the various pathological mechanisms involved in brachial plexus injury, it is worthwhile taking a broad view of these injuries by arbitrarily dividing them into supraclavicular and infraclavicular plexus lesions. These differ significantly in incidence, severity and prognosis. Within the group of supraclavicular injuries, we have preganglionic and postganglionic lesions, which can occur either in the upper plexus or lower plexus depending on whether the C5/6 roots or the C8/T1 roots are involved.

Injuries may also occur behind the clavicle at the level of the divisions of the brachial plexus as a result of clavicular fractures. Finally, the injuries can occur in the infraclavicular part of the plexus and involve the cords or the peripheral nerves which derive from these cords.

The lesions may be complete or incomplete, otherwise known as total or partial. In incomplete lesions, there is usually evidence of some recovery within two or three months of injury. In most series, complete

Table 7.1

Roots	Trunks	Divisions	Cords	Nerves
C5★	Upper★★	Anterior	Lateral†	Musculocutaneous Median (50%)
C6★		Posterior		
C7★	Middle	Anterior	Posterior	Axillary Radial Subscapular Thoracodorsal
		Posterior		
C8	Lower	Posterior	Medial	Median (50%) Ulnar
T1		Anterior		

★Peripheral nerve derived from C5, 6, 7 roots – long thoracic
★★Peripheral nerves derived from upper trunk – dorsal scapular
                                    suprascapular
                                    nerve to subclavius
†Peripheral nerve derived from lateral cord – anterior thoracic

involvement of the affected root has been found more often than partial involvement, no matter which roots were involved. In addition, complete plexus involvement can be found in 45–70% of patients. The most severe type of injury, the avulsion injury, is becoming more common.

Transient ischaemia of the plexus can occur as a result of carrying heavy rucksacks and most people have been aware at one time or another of a slight weakness in the arm with tingling, radiating usually into the thumb. The changes are reversible and cause inconvenience rather than disability.

Other than transient ischaemia, the mildest clinical disorders are caused by conduction block. In this situation, nerve impulses cannot be transmitted across the site of the lesion, although axonal continuity remains intact. The nerve segment distal to the lesion does not undergo Wallerian degeneration and will continue to transmit electrical impulses which can be demonstrated by electrophysiology.

This type of lesion is caused by mild traction and/or compression. Weakness due to conduction block is clinically indistinguishable from that due to axonal loss in the early stages, but within a few days or weeks the conduction block will resolve leaving persistent deficits only in those areas in which elements of the plexus have undergone loss of axons.

The majority of brachial plexus lesions, however, have a significant element of axon loss and degeneration. The milder degrees of this disorder occur most often within infraclavicular lesions. Usually the regenerating axons encounter no major barrier when traversing the site of the lesion, because their endoneural tubes are intact. Motor recovery is often quite good if there is a short distance between the lesion and the affected muscles. On the other hand, if the T1 nerve roots have been damaged in the axilla, their regenerating fibres will be unable to reach the intrinsic muscles in the hand within the 18 months during which the muscle fibres will survive. In adults, therefore, the 'time-distance' factor is extremely important. The more severe grades of axon loss occur usually in supraclavicular lesions due to a mixture of stretch and contusion but, although many of the nerve elements may remain in continuity, the amount of destruction caused by haematoma formation and the later deposition of fibrous scar will lead to a poor return of function. The milder lesions cannot be distinguished from the more severe lesions

clinically or by electrophysiology and the only opportunity for assessing the extent of axon loss is to perform intraoperative nerve conduction studies in the course of dissecting out fascicles of a lesion in continuity. The most severe injury involves separation of axons, either by avulsion of the root from the spinal cord or from rupture of nerve in a specific portion of the plexus. In surgical series, 80% of patients are likely to have complete disruption of one or more elements of the brachial plexus. Upper plexus traction lesions are more common than lower lesions and rupture is more common than avulsion. This is because the fibres of C5 and C6, unlike those of C8 and T1, are firmly anchored by fascia close to the intervertebral foramina. On the other hand lower plexus lesions, although less common, are more likely to take the form of preganglionic avulsion injuries and therefore are not amenable to surgical correction. In a typical surgical series involving C5 and C6 nerve roots, 40% were avulsions and 60% ruptures. In contrast, similar injuries to C8 and T1 produced 85% avulsions and only 15% ruptures.

Clinical presentation

In broad terms, supraclavicular lesions generally produce motor and sensory deficits in the distribution of one or more myotomes and dermatomes. In contrast, infraclavicular plexus lesions more commonly present clinically as proximal peripheral nerve lesions.

Upper plexus

Injuries involving the C5 and C6 nerve roots or the upper trunk of the plexus are the commonest type of supraclavicular lesion. The shoulder-girdle muscles and the biceps are generally involved. When the lesion is severe, the upper limb hangs by the side of the body, extended at the elbow and adducted and internally rotated at the shoulder so that the palm of the hand may be visible from the rear (waiter's tip position). When the lesion is at the level of the nerve roots the affected muscles will include serratus anterior, the rhomboids, supraspinatus, infraspinatus, deltoid, biceps, brachialis and brachoradialis. If the lesion is more distal in the trunk, the serratus anterior and rhomboids may be spared as their nerve supply rises quite proximally. Sensory loss is usually present over the deltoid and the outer aspect of the arm and forearm.

Intermediate plexus

This type of isolated injury is rare and usually co-exists with elements of upper or lower plexus lesions. It has been found that the overlap of neural function is such that this type of lesion may cause little functional disability, although one would expect impairment of the elbow, wrist and finger extension.

Lower plexus

Severe lesions of the C8 and T1 nerve roots or the lower trunk cause the well-recognised Klumpke paralysis. Muscle weakness occurs in areas supplied by the ulnar nerve in the hand and forearm together with some median-innervated hand intrinsic muscles and muscles supplied by the anterior interosseous nerve. In addition, muscles such as extensor indicis proprius and extensor pollicis brevis may also be paralysed. The classical sensory loss is found along the medial aspect of the forearm and the ring and little fingers. If the T1 nerve root has been avulsed, a Horner's syndrome will be present. Surgery has no functional value in this type of injury, other than perhaps reducing the amount of pain experienced by the patient.

Assessment

Evaluation of a brachial plexus injury requires a very detailed clinical examination. Unless surgery is undertaken immediately, this examination will need to be repeated over a number of weeks and months. If the patient has a non-traumatic brachial plexus lesion, one will require to undertake electrophysiological testing to eliminate the possibility of other neuromuscular disorders which can be confused with plexus lesions. These include motor neurone disease, C5 and C6 cervical radiculopathies, mononeuropathies of nerves such as the suprascapular, axillary and musculocutaneous nerves. In addition, one must remember that some forms of shoulder pseudo-paralysis are due to large rotator cuff tears. With C8 and T1 radiculopathies it is also imperative to exclude an underlying apical lung tumour by radiography.

Neurophysiology

Nerve conduction studies have a useful place to play in assessment of brachial plexus lesions. Using surface electrodes, the amplitudes of the motor responses provide a semiquantitative measure of the number of viable nerve fibres innervating the recorded muscle. For instance, if one stimulates the ulnar nerve at the wrist while recording from the hypothenar muscles, normal amplitude responses will be elicited if the weakness is due to neurapraxia or is non-organic, but will produce low amplitude or unelicitable responses when axon loss has occurred. Thus these amplitudes become reliable indicators of axon loss once Wallerian degeneration has occurred seven days or more after injury.

Sensory nerve conduction tests are extremely valuable and are probably the most sensitive indicators of axon loss. One has to wait two or three weeks before undertaking these tests, to allow Wallerian degeneration to take place. Sensory nerve conduction studies are extremely valuable in differentiating between nerve root avulsion and disruption of the peripheral sensory fibres of the nerve. With nerve root avulsions, the peripheral sensory fibre cell bodies located in the dorsal root ganglia are still in continuity so that normal sensory responses will be obtained. Thus avulsion of a root will be characterised by a combination of normal sensory responses and unelicitable motor responses.

Electromyography can be of value in a number of ways. It can demonstrate residual levels of muscle innervation and can also detect re-innervation of muscles many weeks before this becomes apparent clinically. In patients with nerve root avulsions, fibrillation potentials are often found in the cervical paraspinal muscles. Although fibrillation potentials are the most sensitive indicator of motor axon loss, they will take three weeks or so to develop in denervated muscle.

Somatosensory evoked potentials

Somatosensory evoked potentials (SEP) are obtained by stimulating a variety of peripheral nerves while recording over the supraclavicular region and the contralateral somatosensory cortex. SEPs can also be obtained intraoperatively by stimulating above or below a brachial plexus lesion exposed during surgery. The initial hopes that SEPs would offer a reliable means of preoperative assessment have not been fulfilled and they have not proven to be of use in evaluating the C5 nerve root. Intraoperative SEPs, however, remain a valuable procedure and can assess C5 nerve root fibres.

Intraoperative nerve action potentials

This is probably the most valuable technique for assessing the state of a brachial plexus injury. By stimulating and recording across the element of the lesion, the presence or absence of conduction through the affected region can be determined. If a distal nerve action potential can be recorded, normal or regenerating fibres are traversing the lesion which should therefore be left undisturbed. If an action potential cannot be elicited, the abnormal segment can be resected and a nerve graft inserted.

Histamine test

This is rarely used now that the nerve conduction studies can be used to assess the status of a lesion. The test is performed by injecting a small quantity of histamine intradermally in the distal forearm. A normal response causes a weal and flare and indicates the presence of intact peripheral sensory fibres. With a preganglionic lesion a normal flare is seen because the peripheral sensory fibres remain in continuity with the cell bodies in the dorsal root ganglion. A negative result will be obtained in the presence of peripheral rupture of nerve.

Neuro-imaging

Radiography. Radiography can be of value in excluding the presence of cervical spine injuries. Fractures of the lower cervical transverse processes, along with first rib fractures, commonly occur in association with avulsion injuries. Proximal humeral injuries or clavicular injuries can also be detected. In non-traumatic cases, malignant neoplasms may be detected both in the apex of the lung and in other bone structures.

Computed axial tomography. This is probably the most valuable imaging procedure for assessing the condition of the nerve roots. It is best combined with contrast material and may detect nerve root avulsions.

Magnetic resonance imaging. To date this procedure cannot provide sufficient definition to demonstrate clear-cut nerve lesions in the brachial plexus, but may be of value in the later stages in detecting affected muscles involved in the injury.

Typical feature of a patient with nerve root avulsion

Typical patients have a history of violent trauma and present with a complete brachial plexus palsy. They often have a severe burning pain in their anaesthetic limb and a Horner's syndrome. Because of the high level of the lesion, paralysis of the serratus anterior, rhomboids and spinatii is present and sensory loss extends proximal to the clavicle. Tinel's sign will be negative in the supraclavicular fossa and some patients with a particularly severe injury may have some long tract signs. Radiographs may show the presence of fractures of the transverse processes of the lower cervical vertebra together with traumatic meningocoeles. Electrophysiological examination will show reduced sensory nerve conduction with absent motor nerve conduction. Somatosensory evoked potentials will be negative to the opposite cortex and the patient will have a positive or normal histamine test.

TENDON TRANSFERS

In the context of failed nerve repairs, tendon transfer is a useful procedure to restore some motor function in many areas in the upper limb. The object of the exercise is to identify the muscles whose function has been lost and to seek to duplicate this function by using one or more normal muscles, which have to be mobilised and redirected to produce the desired function. If many muscle units are paralysed as in combined nerve palsies, one may have to be selective in choosing which functions to restore, concentrating on functions which are most important to enable the patient to undertake the normal activities of daily living. The surgeon must identify the appropriate tendon or tendons for transfer and thereafter create a smooth gliding pathway with minimal adhesion formation between the transferred tendon and the surrounding tissues. The patient will have to re-educate himself to gain voluntary control to use the transferred muscles in the context of a new pattern of co-ordination in the upper limb.

General principles

1. One must ascertain that the transferred muscle tendon unit can be used without creating a

functional deficit for the patient. For example, there are three wrist extensors: namely extensors carpi radialis (ECRL), longus and brevis, together with extensor carpi ulnaris. ECRL is used commonly for tendon transfer and the normal patient will experience no great loss of wrist extension, as this is maintained by the remaining two muscles. In contrast, a muscle such as flexor pollicis longus should never be used for a tendon transfer as its function is not duplicated by any other muscle tendon unit.

2. One must ascertain that the transferred muscle is sufficiently strong to perform the task required of it. For instance, ECRL has a large strong muscle belly and is a good muscle for transfer, but palmaris longus with its vestigial muscle cannot be expected to act as a functional tendon transfer in most situations. Although palmaris longus is used in reconstruction following failed nerve repair, it tends to exert its effect through a tenodesis action rather than by providing active movement across any joint.

3. One must ascertain that the transferred muscle-tendon unit has sufficient amplitude to produce the movement required. For example brachioradialis has very little excursion and it cannot be expected that it would produce sufficient movement to flex the fingers as the flexor tendons glide over a distance of some 7 cms at the level of the wrist.

4. The muscle must be under good voluntary control and it is best that the selected muscle is synergistic with its desired action or that the patient can be re-trained to use it in this fashion. A good example of this phenomenon occurs when ECRL is used to produce finger flexion, as it often is in patients with quadriplegia. When one attempts to grasp an object with one's fingers, the brain induces co-ordinated extension of the wrist at the same time; in addition there is a natural tenodesis effect which induces flexion of the fingers when the wrist is extended. It is clear, therefore, that transfer of ECRL into the combined flexor tendons produces a synergistic effect which makes it easy for the patient to learn how to control the new transfer.

5. Under most circumstances one should design a tendon transfer so that the tendon runs in a straight line. This permits it to exert its maximum effect. There are some exceptions to this rule, such as the use of extensor indicis proprius as an opposition transfer for the thumb. It may be that this transfer works so well because a large element of tenodesis effect is induced.

6. One must avoid areas which are scarred by previous injury and tendons should not be passed through sheets of fascia or across raw bone.

7. One should not consider undertaking a tendon transfer unless the joints which the transfer is designed to move have retained full or almost-full passive movements. Surgeons should therefore ensure that patients suffering from nerve injuries maintain such movements by their own volition or, more commonly, by supervision in physiotherapy.

8. One should ensure that there is no potential area where infection can develop; for instance, one would be reluctant to consider tendon transfer in the presence of a chronic post-traumatic osteitis.

9. The muscle which is to be transferred should be of normal power. If the patient has had a previous extensive injury involving more than one nerve, one must ensure that any muscle used for tendon transfer has not been significantly weakened for longer than two weeks, because it is likely that the muscle would then be too weak to effect a satisfactory degree of function.

10. Finally patients must be fully aware that the purpose of tendon transfer surgery is to restore a degree of function to the hand and that the return of normal function cannot be anticipated. In addition they must be made aware that the surgery will have no effect on the sensory aspects of their deficit.

Operative techniques

Scarring must be reduced to a minimum and it is best that tendons for transfer are mobilised through a series of small transverse incisions rather than through a longitudinal incision along the line of the tendon. For instance one can mobilise ECRL through three incisions: at the wrist, in the distal third of the forearm and in the mid-forearm. Through a proximal incision, the muscle belly of ECRL should be mobilised by dissecting proximally up to a point about 12 cms, distal to the elbow. One must not mobilise the muscle belly too far proximally lest one interfere with its nerve supply.

One should not consider resecting the muscle belly of the paralysed motor tendon unit as this would simply create a further area for potential haematoma formation and scarring. Often tunnels for the tendon transfer can be created in the subcutaneous tissues of the forearm using a blunt tunneller. Areas of pre-existing scarring should be avoided and, if necessary, the tendon may have to be passed beneath skin-flaps which are free of subcutaneous scar. One must ensure that the tendon transfer passes across only one joint. If it passes over two or more joints, its function is dissipated across these joints and it will be much less effective in achieving the desired goal because the unwanted movement may use up most of its amplitude.

Tendon transfers for median nerve palsy

Low median nerve palsy

The only motor branch given off from the median nerve distal to the wrist is the one to the thenar muscles. In about one-third of patients who fail to re-innervate this branch of median nerve, considerable dysfunction of the thenar muscles ensues. This produces the clinical deformity of the simian (monkey-like) hand in which the thumb lies down alongside the second metacarpal and cannot be abducted to produce useful function with the finger-tips. This function can be replaced in a variety of ways, the commonest being transfer of extensor indicis proprius (EIP) around the ulnar border of the wrist and across the base of the palm of the hand in a subcutaneous tunnel. The transferred tendon must be brought into this subcutaneous tunnel through multiple small stab incisions to ensure that the transferred tendon does not impinge on the flexor tendons or median nerve crossing the front of the wrist. It can then be inserted into the tendinous insertion of abductor pollicis brevis and the radial border of the extensor tendon. In undertaking this transfer, one must use the full length of EIP; otherwise it is not long enough. The capsular defect which is produced in taking the distal end of EIP must be carefully repaired to prevent later radial subluxation of the common extensor tendon to the index finger. The transfer must be immobilised in plaster with the thumb in abduction and opposition for four weeks before graduated mobilisation. A good result can generally be anticipated with this transfer. Other motor units such as palmaris longus can be used but are generally less effective.

High median nerve palsy

In addition to loss of thenar muscle function, a high median nerve palsy will produce paralysis of the long flexors to the thumb, index and middle fingers. Index and middle finger flexion can be restored by suturing their profundus tendons to the adjacent profundus tendons serving the ring and little fingers, in the form of a tenodesis. Thumb flexion can be restored by transferring brachioradialis across to the flexor pollicis longus tendon proximal to the wrist joint.

Tendon transfers for ulnar nerve palsy

Low ulnar nerve palsy

Failed recovery of an ulnar nerve divided at the level of the wrist has profound effects on hand function, in that the patient loses a stable pinch between his thumb and index finger and develops hyperextension deformities at the metacarpophalangeal joints and a compensatory flexion deformity of the interphalangeal joints, causing clawing.

Thumb adduction is generally restored using the split insertion of flexor digitorum superficialis (FDS) to the middle finger. This tendon is mobilised and brought through a defect created in the palmar aponeurosis. In order to reach the tendon of adductor pollicis, the FDS tendon has to pass across the palm at 90° to its normal line of action but, despite breaking the rules which have been previously laid down for tendon transfer, it appears to work rather well.

Restoration of adduction of the thumb is one element of producing a stable pinch grip between thumb and index finger. The second element is to restore function to the first dorsal interosseous muscle and this is best done by a simple transfer of extensor indicis proprius into the insertion of the first dorsal interosseous. These two transfers in combination can be very effective. They can make the difference between a workman being unable to use a hammer without it flying out of his hand and retaining his ability to perform this function to a reasonable level.

The correction of clawing presents a more difficult problem and various techniques have been designed to reverse this problem. The best procedures appear to be those with a dynamic element to them, of which the most commonly used are the transfer of extensor carpi radialis longus elongated by a tendon graft into the intrinsic mechanisms in the fingers. To some extent this has been superseded in certain centres by the use of the Zancolli lasso technique, in which a transverse incision is made between the A1 and A2 pulleys to isolate the superficialis tendon; this is then looped volar to the A1 pulley and sutured through itself in such a manner as to produce 20° of flexion at the metacarpophalangeal joints. This procedure requires much less soft tissue dissection and tunnelling and is of proven worth.

High ulnar nerve palsy

It is rarely necessary to restore function of flexor carpi ulnaris following failed repair of the ulnar nerve proximal to the elbow. These patients are unable to flex the distal interphalangeal joints of the little and ring fingers and, under those circumstances, a simple tenodesis of the affected profundus tendons to the normally functioning profundus tendons of the middle and ring fingers will achieve adequate function.

Tendon transfers for radial nerve palsy

A patient with radial nerve palsy which has failed to recover will experience functional problems because of his inability to extend the wrist, fingers and thumb. Wrist extension is restored by transfer of pronator teres to extensor carpi radialis brevis. Restoration of extension in the fingers and thumb is most commonly achieved by transferring flexor carpi ulnaris from the volar surface of the forearm to its distal aspect obliquely. In so doing, it can be woven into and sutured to each of the common extensor tendons to the finger and extensor pollicis longus.

Occasionally in patients with radial nerve palsy proximal thumb instability occurs as a result of loss of function in abductor pollicis longus. If this is a problem, it can be corrected by a tenodesis in which palmaris longus is sutured to extensor pollicis brevis.

Tendon transfers for combined nerve palsies

Combined nerve palsies, such as a high median and ulnar nerve palsy, provide a formidable challenge to reconstruction as there are generally fewer motor units which can be used for tendon transfer and more functions which have to be restored. Having discussed the situation with the patient, an attempt should be made to restore the most important basic functions for the individual patient rather than trying to restore every function which has been lost.

NERVE COMPRESSION SYNDROMES

Compression neuropathy in the upper limb can take place at a variety of specific sites between the intervertebral foramina of the cervical spine and the wrist. In most instances it is thought that increased pressure within a tight canal induces pathological changes in the nerve. This can be caused by the development of bony protuberances, such as an exostosis, growing from the walls of the canal. In other cases, it may be due to increase in the volume of associated structures which run within the canal, such as the presence of hypertrophic synovium in the carpal tunnel. Inflammatory conditions producing synovial swelling can also be a potent cause of compression neuropathy. General medical disorders such as the neuropathies associated with diabetes or alcoholism can render the peripheral nerves more sensitive to the effects of relatively small increases in pressure and can precipitate a clinical syndrome. Occasionally deposits of abnormal tissue occupy the canal, as in the mucopolysaccharidosis and in amyloidosis which is often seen in patients on renal dialysis.

The phenomenon of double-crush syndrome can play a potent role in precipitating compression neuropathies, particularly carpal tunnel syndrome. In this situation a compression lesion at one point in a peripheral nerve, say in the intervertebral foramen of the cervical spine, may occur in association with very mild increase in carpal tunnel pressure. In this situation, minimal compression of the median nerve in the carpal tunnel can lead to clinically prominent symptoms. It is thought that this increased sensitivity to pressure is brought about by restriction of transport mechanisms within the axon.

A further phenomenon has been recognised in recent times. It is known that nerves have considerable ability to glide throughout the tissues: for instance, the median nerve may glide as much as 1 cm when the wrist is brought from full extension into full flexion. After an injury, adhesions may tether the nerve to the surrounding tissues and it is now recognised that repeated episodes of traction can produce an electrical conduction block within the nerve.

The clinical presentation of these disorders may be acute or chronic. Most acute cases are due to trauma, such as severely displaced Colles, fractures or perilunar dislocations, and these must be dealt with immediately. By far the majority of cases, however, are chronic in onset. They are characterised by a gradual onset of symptoms and signs in part or all of the distribution of a specific peripheral nerve. In most instances, an accurate diagnosis can be made by taking a careful history and undertaking a careful physical examination. It is particularly important to employ the relevant sensory tests when examining a patient with a suspected compression neuropathy. These are threshold sensory tests, which can detect changes in nerve function related to the loss of large numbers of nerve fibres. The threshold tests which should be used are the Semmes–Weinstein monofilament test, which is simple to perform, and/or vibration testing which is more time-consuming and probably no more reliable or sensitive. It is worthwhile reiterating that testing innervation density using static and moving two-point discrimination is not sensitive to the changes produced by compression neuropathy and should be reserved for examining patients in whom one is following the course of nerve regeneration after injury.

Confirmation of the presumed diagnosis can be made using electrophysiological testing. The characteristic changes found in compression neuropathies are that the conduction velocities over the compressed segment of the nerve are decreased and the latencies are increased. On occasions, however, particularly in relation to carpal tunnel syndrome, patients with classical symptoms and signs of a compression disorder but with normal electrophysiology can benefit from decompression of the nerve. This indicates that a small group of patients may be symptomatic in the presence of normal nerve conduction. These patients may have a dynamic situation in which the pressures within the tunnel fall to relatively normal levels at rest and increase only with prolonged use of the limb, or, alternatively, during sleep though the reason for this is not clear.

One of the most important aspects of electrophysiological testing is that it permits the examiner to predict the probable clinical outcome following surgical decompression. Rapid and full recovery following surgical decompression can be predicted in those patients with mildly impaired electrophysiological testing. These patients almost certainly experience minor intermittent episodes of ischaemia induced by increased pressure and this is often a dynamic situation in which the pressure decreases at rest and increases with the use of the limb. Patients who exhibit severe slowing of conduction within increased latencies have developed abnormalities in the myelin sheath at the site of the compression. Recovery in such patients is likely to take a number of weeks or months, during which the oedema within and around the nerve will settle and a normal myelin sheath will be reconstituted by the Schwann cells. Finally, if electromyography demonstrates the presence of significant denervation of the target muscles it can be presumed that axonal loss has taken place by the process of Wallerian degeneration and that regeneration might be incomplete or may fail to occur. These patients often have obvious perineural fibrosis and intraneural fibrosis may cause an hour-glass deformation in the nerve at the level of compression. Patients with significant intraneural fibrosis will fail to recover function despite surgical decompression, although their pain may be decreased.

Carpal tunnel syndrome

The classical clinical features of carpal tunnel syndrome are well known to readers of this book: nocturnal pain in the hand, associated with paraesthesiae in part or all of the median nerve distribution and in the later stages, wasting of the thenar muscles. It should be noted that due to anomalous nerve supply with various abnormal connections between the ulnar nerve, a small proportion of patients with carpal tunnel syndrome may present with pain, numbness and tingling in the ulnar-innervated fingers. This variant form of carpal tunnel syndrome can be diagnosed electrophysiologically. However, even when you have pins-and-needles, it can be difficult to decide their exact distribution: many patients just notice symptoms in the hand and assume the little finger is involved, but are cured by standard carpal tunnel decompression.

Anatomy of carpal canal

Boundaries
Radial wall: scaphoid and trapezium.
Ulnar wall: triquetrum, pisiform and hamate.

Floor: lunate, capitate and proximal metacarpals.

Roof: flexor retinaculum ('transverse carpal ligament').

Contents. The carpal canal contains flexor digitorum superficialis and profundus tendons to all fingers, flexor pollicis longus, synovial sheaths around the tendons and the median nerve.

The most consistent abnormality associated with carpal tunnel syndrome is the presence of changes in the flexor tenosynovium. Pathological features in most cases of idiopathic carpal tunnel syndrome show that the tenosynovium is subject to fibrous hypertrophy associated with oedema and vascular sclerosis. Relatively few inflammatory cells are present with the synovial tissues. These findings have been found in 98% of patients with idiopathic carpal tunnel syndrome.

Branches. Although the branch of the median nerve to the thenar muscles usually leaves the nerve on its radial aspect towards the end of the tunnel, this branch may lie immediately beneath the Flexar retinaculum or even pass through it. When it takes this unusual course it is more likely to be injured in the course of surgery, particularly endoscopic surgery. A number of variations occur, including the presence of accessory branches in the distal carpal canal and the high division of the median nerve in the forearm. It is also worthwhile remembering the presence of a persistent median artery which can lie within the median nerve in the canal; thrombosis of such an artery can cause an acute onset of carpal tunnel syndrome.

Treatment

Conservative. Many women experience symptoms of night pain and tingling which can be relieved if they shake their hand about or if they begin to use it during the day. These patients undoubtedly experience intermittent ischaemic symptoms which are readily reversible and a considerable proportion of patients at this stage of the disorder will respond well to the use of a night splint designed to hold the wrist in a neutral position. Studies have shown that injection of cortico-steroids into the canal in patients of this nature will produce relief in four out of five, but only one patient out of five will remain asymptomatic one year later.

Operative treatment

Open. Open carpal tunnel decompression remains the mainstay of treatment in most hospitals. The reliability of this approach has been established over many years and allows good visualisation of the median nerve and the contents of the carpal tunnel. It allows one to identify anomalies within the nerve and to protect anomalous branches from damage. It also may enable one to draw some conclusions about the physiological state of the nerve: should an hour-glass deformation be present beneath the carpal tunnel, this would indicate that intraneural fibrosis is present and has progressed to a concentric contracture. The prognosis for such patients is not good. In addition, one may be able to identify perineural adhesions binding the nerve to the undersurface of the flexor retinaculum or the side walls of the canal. Many investigators believe that some of the symptoms attributable to carpal tunnel syndrome are due to intermittent traction of adherent nerves. A recent study demonstrated, however, that the results obtained from simple carpal tunnel release without extraneural neurolysis were no different from those in which an external neurolysis had been performed.

Open operation may be complicated by damage to the palmar cutaneous branch of the median nerve or entrapment of this nerve in the associated scar tissue. In addition, a number of patients develop 'pillar' pain at the base of the hand following carpal tunnel release. The aetiology of pillar pain is not understood clearly. Some authors have attributed this pain to gradual stretching of the intercarpal ligaments which are no longer de-tensioned by the flexor retinaculum. Other authors believe that division of the flexor retinaculum disturbs the alignment of the pisotriquetral joint and that this is the source of pillar pain. They have sup-ported their theory by demonstrating that an injection of local anaesthetic into this area relieves the symptoms of pillar pain and they have even used this test as a basis for excising the pisiform, which they consider to be a useful procedure.

Endoscopic carpal tunnel release. Endoscopic release of the carpal tunnel has gained popularity in recent times on the basis that it might promote an earlier return to work for patients and that it may reduce the perceived complications of open release, namely damage to the palmar cutaneous branch of the median nerve and pillar pain. The advantages of a small scar have been outweighed by the reported incidence of damage to the median nerve and other nerves (including the ulnar nerve) in the course of endoscopic release. The hopes that palmar tenderness caused by damage to the palmar cutaneous branch of the median nerve would be eliminated, have not been confirmed and pillar pain has not been reduced. The only objective measure of improvement using endoscopic release as opposed to open release has been the demonstration that grip strength, which returns to preoperative levels three months after open release, returns by six weeks in patients undergoing endoscopic carpal tunnel release. Most British surgeons believe that the potential risk of iatrogenic injury to the neural structures within the canal outweighs the small advantage in earlier return of grip strength, especially if the operation is likely to be performed by a junior surgeon.

In the course of MRI investigations of carpal tunnel syndrome, it has become apparent that division of the flexor retinaculum allows the contents of the carpal canal to bulge in a volar direction by $\geq$ 2 mm. However, fears that carpal tunnel release would produce bow-stringing of the flexor tendons across the front of the wrist have not been confirmed and this appears to be a theoretical complication rather than one which happens in clinical practice. It is also of interest that the MRI evidence has demonstrated that release of the carpal tunnel alone also produces increase in the cross-sectional area of Guyon's canal and will thus also decompress the ulnar nerve at the wrist.

Complications of carpal tunnel syndrome

Tenderness. It is normal for the scar to be tender for a month or two, probably due to division of the very fine terminal branches of the palmar cutaneous nerve in the fat beneath the skin. All patients should be warned of this beforehand. One of the main arguments for arthroscopic decompression is to avoid this, but it does not necessarily do so.

Rarely, there is great and very troublesome tenderness, perhaps due to damage to the main palmar cutaneous nerve. Since this nerve (which is about the size of a digital nerve) always lies radial to the mid-line (usually close to the tendon of FCR), the incision should be in the mid-line or slightly ulnar to the mid-line.

Unfortunately, this unpleasant complication is very difficult to treat. Even division of the palmar cutaneous nerve more proximally and diathermy of its proximal

end to prevent a new neuroma from forming does not always solve the problem.

Bleeding. If haemostasis has been inadequate, there may be oozing of blood out of the wound, but this will stop with elevation and pressure. Some bruising ensues but clears fairly soon. Careless division of the superficial transverse arterial palmar arch in the distal end of the wound produces a spectacular haematoma which requires re-exploration.

Infection. This is uncommon, but it can happen. Sometimes the usual tenderness is wrongly diagnosed by the GP as infection.

Dehiscence. This usually only affects the superficial epidermal layers of the skin and does not matter if the deeper layers are healed. It is best always to leave the suture in place for at least two weeks.

Damage to nerves. See below.

Reflex sympathetic dystrophy. Fortunately this distressing complication occurs very rarely after carpal tunnel syndrome.

Recurrence. This is uncommon, but possible. However, if, for any reason, you have to re-explore a carpal tunnel you will find that the flexor retinaculum has reconstituted and looks almost normal, even if it is only a few weeks after the first operation which you did yourself and know you did adequately!

Many cases of 'recurrence' prove, on close questioning, to have symptoms in the hand which are not quite the same as before operation (see below).

Carpal tunnel syndrome in the other hand. This is generally said to occur in 25% of cases, but it may be more common.

Failed carpal tunnel decompression

When any operation fails to achieve its aim, one must consider two explanations: the diagnosis was wrong or the operation was carried out incorrectly. One must go back to the beginning and take a careful history all over again.

Symptoms unchanged.

Wrong diagnosis. The most common differential diagnosis is a cervical disc lesion. This, like carpal tunnel syndrome, is a common condition, so both may be present. Other levels of compression, such as in the thoracic outlet and forearm, must be considered.

Inadequate operation. The flexor retinaculum measures at least 3 cm from proximal to distal and the surgeon may have failed to divide either end, especially if the skin incision was too small. However, there is no need for the skin incision to cross either of the transverse wrist skin creases: the flexor retinaculum is essentially in the hand.

New symptoms.

Normal structures damaged at operation
- Palmar cutaneous branch of median nerve (see above).
- Digital branches of median nerve.
- Motor (thenar) branch of median nerve.
- Ulnar nerve (it has been reported!).

The last three are more likely to be damaged during endoscopic decompression of the carpal tunnel, but can also be injured during open operation.

New diagnosis. Here again the most likely explanation is that the patient has now developed a cervical disc lesion, but all possibilities must be considered, including general medical causes of neuropathy.

Median nerve compression around the elbow

The median nerve is also said to be vulnerable to compression at a variety of sites around the elbow. These have been grouped together under the heading 'pronator syndrome' as they share a common clinical presentation. They are very uncommon. The patient typically complains of an ache or discomfort in the forearm associated with weakness or clumsiness of the hand and numbness in all or part of the median nerve distribution. The clinical presentation differs in a number of respects from carpal tunnel syndrome, in that night pain is not a common feature and certain movements around the elbow can provoke pain. In addition, tests such as Tinel's sign and Phalen's test are negative. It is often difficult to demonstrate any electrophysiological abnormality in this syndrome. Systematic clinical examination in these patients may indicate the precise site at which the nerve is being compressed.

Struther's ligament. This is a fibrous band which extends inferiorly from an anterior supracondylar spur

in the distal shaft of the humerus. This congenital abnormality occurs in less then 1% of the population. The bony spur can be visualised on a lateral radiograph of the distal humerus.

The bicipital aponeurosis. When there is a high origin of pronator teres, the lacertus fibrosus may compress the median nerve. Resisted elbow flexion with the forearm in supination may provoke symptoms in such patients.

The pronator teres. Resisted forearm pronation with the elbow in full extension may provoke symptoms in these patients when the median nerve becomes compressed between the two heads of pronator teres.

Proximal fibrous arch of the flexor digitorum superficialis. Resisted flexion of the proximal interphalangeal joint of the middle finger may produce paraesthesiae in the median nerve distribution in patients in whom that nerve is trapped beneath the fibrous arch of origin of flexor digitorum superficialis.

In most instances of pronator syndrome it is wise to explore the median nerve as it passes beneath the bicipital aponeurosis, the pronator teres and the flexor digitorum superficialis and to perform release of these structures as indicated by the surgical findings. Not infrequently blood-vessels are seen to cross the median nerve at a variety of sites within this area and some authors consider that these are potent factors in precipitating median nerve compression. It is recommended that such vessels should be ligated and divided to decompress the nerve fully.

Anterior interosseous syndrome. This syndrome is a variant of the so-called pronator syndrome but tends to arise in a different manner. Not infrequently the symptoms occur acutely with a sudden onset of dull pain in the forearm. This is associated with weakness of flexion in the distal interphalangeal joint of the index finger and the interphalangeal joint of the thumb. Sensory disturbances do not occur in this syndrome. Occasionally the syndrome can occur bilaterally and a number of cases have been shown to be caused by a viral neuropathy affecting the anterior interosseous nerve. On other occasions there is a history of unaccustomed overactivity involving the use of these muscles.

Treatment

Treatment of the pronator syndrome and the anterior interosseous syndrome should initially be conservative. In many patients symptoms and signs will gradually resolve over a period of a few weeks. In those who exhibit no resolution of symptoms and whose symptoms remain severe, surgical exploration may be indicated as described above. Recovery following such surgery is unpredictable.

Ulnar nerve compression syndromes

Ulnar nerve compression at the elbow

Entrapment of the ulnar nerve at the elbow is the second commonest nerve entrapment syndrome in the upper limb, after carpal tunnel syndrome. The patient usually presents with numbness involving the little finger and the ulnar half of the ring finger and this may be accompanied by weakness and clumsiness in the use of the hand. The motor symptoms may cause difficulty in doing up buttons and many manual workers find that they can no longer use tools such as screwdrivers.

Physical examination generally reveals tenderness over the ulnar nerve at the elbow, often with a positive Tinel's sign on percussion of the nerve close to the cubital tunnel. The presence of sensory involvement on the dorso-ulnar aspect of the hand also suggests that the lesion is a proximal one occurring at the elbow rather than at the wrist. Paradoxically entrapment of the ulnar nerve at the elbow generally produces less clawing of the fingers than distal entrapment of the ulnar nerve at the wrist. This phenomenon is accounted for by the fact that dysfunction of the ulnar nerve at the elbow or the wrist produces weakness of the intrinsic muscles. The intrinsic muscles in the hand act as flexors at the metacarpophalangeal joints and extensors of the proximal interphalangeal joints. When ulnar nerve entrapment occurs at the elbow, paralysis of the flexor digitorum profundus muscles to the ring and little fingers occurs so that the weakness of extension of the proximal interphalangeal joints is counterbalanced by weakness of flexion in the finger, resulting in relatively little tendency to clawing. However, if the ulnar nerve compression occurs at the level of the wrist, the function of the flexor digitorum profundus muscles to the ring and little fingers is not compromised and the action of these flexor tendons is not counteracted by the intrinsic muscles as it would be under normal circumstances. Hence, clawing is exaggerated in patients with distal ulnar nerve entrapment in Guyon's canal.

Anatomy. Potentially the ulnar nerve can be trapped in several areas around the elbow.

The arcade of Struthers.★ This structure, which is present in 70% of the population, is formed by superficial muscle fibres of the medial head of the triceps attaching to the medial epicondylar ridge by a thickened condensation of fascia. This structure lies up to 10 cm proximal to the cubital tunnel and care must be taken to decompress this area at the time of surgery.

The olecranon groove. At the level of the elbow the nerve lies within the groove on the dorsal aspect of the medial epicondyle and the canal is completed superficially by a fibrous aponeurotic arch.

The cubital tunnel. This tunnel is formed by a fibrous arch connecting the two heads of flexor carpi ulnaris and lies just distal to the medial epicondyle. Within this canal, the nerve gives off its motor branches to flexor carpi ulnaris and these must be protected at the time of decompression.

The deep flexor pronator aponeurosis. Just beyond the cubital tunnel and about 5 cm distal to the medial epicondyle, the nerve passes through the deep flexor pronator aponeurosis which can also produce entrapment of the nerve in some patients.

Causes of entrapment. The nerve may be compressed by constricting fascial bands such as the arcade of Struthers or bands of scar tissue running across the medial epicondylar groove. This area lies close to the elbow joint, from which hypertrophied synovium and synovial cysts may compromise the passage of the nerve. An accessory muscle called anconeus epitrochlearis may also compromise the canal. Bony abnormalities around the elbow, such as osteophytic spurs or cubitus valgus following previous supracondylar fracture may cause tardy ulnar nerve palsy. In some patients the ulnar nerve dislocates forwards from the groove during flexion. This can be detected both clinically and at the time of surgery.

Treatment.
Conservative. It has been shown repeatedly that conservative treatment may relieve symptoms of ulnar nerve

---

★Not to be confused with his ligament, which arises from a supracondylar spur and may compress the median nerve.

dysfunction at the elbow in as many as 50% of patients. They should be given general instructions to avoid leaning on the elbow when it is flexed and can be provided with night splints to maintain the elbow at an angle of 45° of flexion.

Operative treatment. The principles of operative treatment for ulnar nerve entrapment at the elbow are to identify the ulnar nerve a good 10 cm proximal to the elbow and to free Struther's arcade if it is present. One should then proceed distally until one locates the nerve as it passes under the deep flexor-pronator aponeurosis. Having decompressed the nerve thoroughly, a wide variety of options is available to the surgeon. In an extensive review of reports published over the last 100 years, Dellon demonstrated that there was little difference in outcome in most straightforward cases whether the nerve was treated by simple decompression, by medial epicondylectomy, by subcutaneous transposition or by submuscular transposition. A satisfactory outcome was achieved in more than four out of five patients using any of these techniques and function returned in these patients within six months.

There are certain exceptions to this rule of thumb. If there is a bony deformity in the groove behind the medial epicondyle or if the nerve exhibits a tendency to sublux or dislocate, it is best to perform an anterior transposition of the nerve, either subcutaneously or submuscularly (beneath the muscles arising from the common flexor origin). If the patient's symptoms have been prolonged and if there is constant numbness in the fingers with marked wasting of the ulnar intrinsic muscles, anterior submuscular transposition has been shown to produce the best results with the lowest recurrence rate.

Those patients who fail to respond to surgical decompression may do so either because of the presence of severe intraneural fibrosis or to inadequate decompression. It is, therefore, very important to ensure that the nerve is mobilised and decompressed fully for some distance proximal and distal to the elbow joint.

From time to time a surgeon is confronted with a patient who has undergone failed surgery for ulnar nerve entrapment at the elbow. In most cases the nerve will have been simply decompressed or transposed subcutaneously. There is evidence to suggest that anterior submuscular transposition of the nerve in such instances may result in improvement in symptoms and function in as many as three out of four patients.

Ulnar nerve compression at the wrist

The ulnar tunnel syndrome occurs when the ulnar nerve is compressed as it passes through Guyon's canal in the wrist. It is much less common than entrapment of the ulnar nerve at the elbow. Patients who present with this lesion have less pain than their counterparts with ulnar nerve compression at the elbow. Most commonly compression occurs as a result of a ganglion originating from one of the carpal joints, usually the triquetrohamate joint, and impinging on the nerve within the canal.

Anatomy. The ulnar nerve enters Guyon's canal accompanied by the ulnar artery and vein. Guyon's canal lies in the space between the flexor retinalulum and volar carpal ligaments.

The proximal part of Guyon's canal is bounded by the pisiform medially, the proximal edge of the flexor retinaculum on its floor and the edge of the volar carpal ligaments superficially. Its floor is formed by the pisohamate and pisometacarpal ligaments. The roof is formed by palmaris brevis muscle merging with the volar carpal ligament. Guyon's canal ends at the hook of the hamate where a fibrous arcade is formed by the pisohamate ligament. This is the level at which the deep branches of the nerve pass through the pisohamate hiatus. The ulnar nerve bifurcates at the distal part of Guyon's canal.

Clinical presentation. Compression of the ulnar nerve within the canal produces motor and sensory deficits and the commonest causes of compression are ganglia and fractures of the hook of the hamate. Deep ganglia often cannot be detected by palpation. Distal to Guyon's canal, these may cause compression of the deep motor branch of the ulnar nerve with no compromise of the sensory branch. Alternatively, the sensory branch can be compromised in isolation; this usually occurs as a result of thrombosis or an aneurysm of the ulnar artery. Lesions within and beyond Guyon's canal can be detected by magnetic resonance imaging. In the case of thrombosis or aneurysms of the ulnar artery, Doppler testing may help confirm the diagnosis.

Treatment. Surgical treatment of lesions with Guyon's canal is usually straightforward. Most patients make a good recovery and, because the lesion occurs close to the motor units supplied by the nerve and close to the sensory units, a good and rapid recovery can be anticipated in most patients.

Radial nerve

Ulnar nerve compression at the elbow

This is unusual but has been reported and may be associated with compression beneath the fibrous arch originating from the lateral head of the triceps muscle. Clinical examination will demonstrate weakness of extension of the wrist and digits. Some patients will have impairment of sensation in the dorsal web of skin between the thumb and index finger. Electromyography can establish the diagnosis in certain cases and surgical decompression is rarely indicated as the condition, which often occurs following strenuous exercise, often settles spontaneously.

Posterior interosseous nerve

Just as the median nerve may be compressed at a variety of sites close to the elbow, the posterior interosseous nerve can be equally vulnerable to entrapment. In the case of the posterior interosseous nerve, entrapment generally occurs as it passes between the two heads of the supinator muscle in the radial tunnel. The boundaries of this tunnel are:

Medial: biceps tendon
Lateral: brachioradialis and extensor carpi radialus longus and brevis tendons
Roof: brachioradialis
Floor: deep head of the supinator muscle.

The posterior interosseous nerve then enters the arcade of Frohse formed by the proximal edge of the superficial head of the supinator muscle. Within the tunnel, a transverse leash of vessels crosses the nerve and these may compromise its function.

Presentation. The onset of this syndrome is often insidious. Initially the patient may be aware of a dull ache in the proximal forearm but later becomes alarmed when he or she encounters difficulty in extending the fingers and thumb. Wrist extension is not affected, as the branch of the radial nerve to extensor carpi radialis longus is not involved. Extensor carpi radialis brevis is affected, however, and when the patient attempts to extend the wrist he or she does so with an element of radial deviation. On occasions electrophysiology is required to confirm the diagnosis. This is often the case in patients suffering from rheumatoid arthritis. However, the inability of these patients to extend their fingers may also be due to rupture of the extensor tendons at the level of the wrist or indeed to pressure exerted on the posterior interosseous nerve by synovium bulging from the elbow joint.

There is some evidence to suggest that a number of patients who develop posterior interosseous nerve palsy do so as a result of a viral infection with a localised peripheral neuropathy of this particular nerve. It is worth observing patients with this diagnosis for a few weeks, as many of then will get better spontaneously. If there is no sign of recovery, full decompression of the nerve should be undertaken with regard to the potential areas of compression. That is to say, one must take care to release the thickened fibrous tissue overlying the elbow joint, to release vessels from the recurrent radial artery (leash of Henry), to release the fibrous edge of extensor carpi radialis brevis and the proximal edge of the supinator (arcade of Frohse). The dissection should be extended to the distal end of the supinator so that the full decompression of the nerve is obtained over some distance.

Radial tunnel syndrome

This condition, unlike many of the problems which have been under review in this chapter, is a pain syndrome. The pain is often acute and can mimic tennis elbow. It is said to co-exist with tennis elbow in 5% of patients. The tenderness in radial tunnel syndrome is more distal than that associated with tennis elbow where the diagnosis can be substantiated when resisted extension of the middle finger reproduces the pain (see also p.52). Electrophysiological studies show no abnormality, which is in contrast to the usual situation with posterior interosseous nerve compression. A number of authors have suggested that this condition is best treated by decompression of the posterior interosseous nerve as it passes through the radial tunnel, but a recent review from the Mayo Clinic has shown that only 50% of patients undergoing surgery obtained satisfactory results. When one considers that a number of these patients may have improved spontaneously had surgery not been undertaken, the place of surgery in the treatment of this condition is not yet established. In particular, it was noted that workers' compensation cases suffering from this condition generally achieved poor outcomes following surgery.

Wartenburg's syndrome

This troublesome syndrome is relatively uncommon and is caused by entrapment of the superficial radial sensory nerve in the distal forearm. The patient experiences pain over the outer aspect of the distal forearm, often associated with a feeling of burning or numbness in part or all of the distribution of the superficial nerve. There is frequently hypersensitivity close to a watch-strap or a shirt-sleeve and the diagnosis can be confirmed by eliciting a positive Tinel's sign over the superficial radial nerve as it passes through the fascia between the brachioradialis tendon and that of the

extensor carpi radialis longus. The symptoms can be further elicited by forceful pronation of the forearm. The diagnosis can be confirmed by a trial injection of local anaesthetic and the presence of abnormalities on sensory testing distinguishes it from a de Quervain's stenosing tenovaginitis. Some patients respond to conservative treatment, which generally takes the form of avoiding watch-straps crossing the area, splinting and the use of anti-inflammatory drugs. About 50% of patients respond to conservative treatment and in those who fail to do so, surgical release of the nerve produces good results in the majority.

FURTHER READING

Angelides AC, Wallace PF. The dorsal ganglion of the wrist: its pathogenesis, gross and microscopic anatomy, and surgical treatment. *J Hand Surg* 1976; **1:** 228–235.

Birch R. Lesions of peripheral nerves: the present position. *J Bone Joint Surg* 1986; **68B:** 2–8

Birch R. Brachial plexus injuries. *J. Bone Joint Surg* 1996; **78B:** 986–92

Bonney G. Iatrogenic injuries of nerves *J. Bone Joint Surg* 1986; **68B:** 9–13

Brain WR, Wright AD, Wilkinson M. Sportaneous compression of both median nerves in the carpal tunnel. Six cases treated surgically *Lancet* 1947; **1:** 277–282

Dellon AL. Review of treatment results for ulnar nerve entrapment at the elbow. *J Hand Surg* 1989; **14A:** 688–700

Jabaley ME, Wallace WH, Heckler FR. Internal topography of major nerves of the forearm and hand: a current view. *J Hand Surg.* 1980; **5:** 1–18

Medical Research Council. Special Report Senes; no. 292: *Peripheral Nerve Lyunes.* London: HMSO 1954

Rowntree T. Anomalous innervallon of the hand muscles. *J. Bone Joint Surg* 1949; **31B:** 505–510.

Seddon HJ. A classification of nerve injuries. *Brit Med J* 1942; **2:** 237–239

8

Amputations

Colin Dent

ELECTIVE AMPUTATIONS

Elective amputations in the upper limb are rarely performed, and consequently few surgeons develop a great experience in carrying out these procedures. Indications include congenital deformities and acquired conditions as diverse as malignant tumours and Dupytren's disease. In contrast to the lower limb, vascular disease is a rare indication for amputation. The majority of elective amputations can be carried out at recognised levels in the upper limb, using well recognised techniques. The aim of surgery is to preserve function by maintaining movement at adjacent joints in the presence of normal sensibility, thus avoiding painful neuromata.

Amputation through the fingers

These distal amputations are most commonly indicated for recurrent Dupytren's disease affecting the little finger. The level is through the proximal phalanx or disarticulation at the MP joint, which preserves the full width of the hand. The incised flexor and extensor tendons must be left unattached. Diathermy is applied to the cut nerve endings, which are allowed to retract proximally.

Ray amputation

Ray amputations are indicated for tumours, infections and failed replantation. In order to preserve the width of the hand disarticulation at the metacarpophalangeal joint might seem a better alternative technique but, with the exception of the little finger, amputation at this level leaves a large gap in the hand which causes

significant functional impairment. Preservation of the index metacarpal leads to a prominence in what is effectively the first web space, whereas ray amputation of the index finger leaves a smooth first web space.

In all distal amputations, it is preferable to use a tourniquet whenever possible. Exsanguination of the limb, however, is contraindicated if the amputation is being performed for a neoplastic or infective condition.

The technique requires planning of skin incisions to ensure adequate coverage and is based on a circumferential incision around the proximal phalanx, extended proximally along the entire dorsal surface of the metacarpal. The extensor tendons are divided at the level of the metacarpal base and the bone is transected at the proximal flare of the shaft. The flexor tendons are divided and released to retract proximally, along with the tendons of the volar and dorsal interossei. The blood vessels are ligated proximally but the digital nerves are transected more distally to ensure that the nerve ends can be placed deep in the interosseous space. After release of the tourniquet, the distal incisions are sutured in a straight line continuing onto the palm of the hand.

Index finger ray

Index ray amputation results in a most acceptable cosmetic appearance, but there is decreased strength of both power grip and key pinch. Hyperaesthesia of the first web-space is a well-documented complication, thought to be a consequence of mobilisation of the radial digital nerve of the index finger, classically appearing eight weeks after surgery. This is usually a permanent complication which is not amenable to any further surgery, so the handling of the digital nerves at the time of amputation is of great importance to ensure the nerve is in a protected position.

Quadriga syndrome is another recognised complication and results from the transected profundus tendon becoming tethered at the level of the amputation. As these tendons originate from a single muscle belly, this can lead to reduced excursion of all the profundus tendons and impairment of finger flexion. This is corrected by releasing the profundus tendon to allow proximal retraction.

Middle finger ray

Middle finger ray amputation requires a modified technique to close the potential space in the hand between the ring and index fingers. (This space is caused by the essential preservation of the base of the third metacarpal.) This can be achieved by an osteotomy to the base of the index finger and transferring this digit to the base of the middle metacarpal after excision of the middle ray. This leaves the base of the index metacarpal deep in the first web-space, in a similar manner to an index ray amputation. Internal fixation is necessary to immobilise the base of the third to the shaft of the index metacarpal. Particular care is needed to ensure there is no rotational deformity, which would result in impaired flexion of the transposed index finger. An alternative technique has been described to prevent a gap forming in the palm, which avoids the need for osteotomy with its potential for further complications. At the time of excision of the middle finger ray, care is taken to preserve the deep transverse metacarpal ligaments from the adjacent ring and index finger metacarpophalangeal joints. These ligament ends are sutured together across the space formed by the base of the third metacarpal. After middle ray amputation utilising either of these techniques, immobilisation of the hand for a period of between six and eight weeks is required, using a temporary Kirschner wire, during which it is essential that the patient is treated by a hand therapist to prevent stiffness occurring in the remaining digits.

Ring finger ray

Ring finger ray amputations can result in a problematic gap in the palm of the hand in a similar manner to middle ray amputation. Osteotomy of the fifth metacarpal and transfer to the base of the fourth metacarpal can be performed. The alternative technique is the suture of the deep transverse metacarpal ligaments across the space; the fourth and fifth metacarpal bases both articulate with the hamate which allows the fifth metacarpal to slide radially following excision of the entire fourth metacarpal including its base, so there is only a small gap between the adjacent bases of the third and fifth metacarpal bases. Suture of the deep transverse metacarpal ligaments serves to maintain the fifth metacarpal in this radially translated position.

Little finger ray

Ray amputation of the little finger does not produce a space within the palm. However, it remains necessary to preserve the base of the fifth metacarpal with the insertions of the tendons of flexor and extensor carpi ulnaris.

Wrist disarticulation

Indications for this are rare, although it has become more favoured with improvements in design of prostheses for what was considered a difficult stump. The advantage of wrist disarticulation over a forearm amputation is in the preservation of a stable distal radio-ulnar joint allowing forearm rotation. The preferred technique utilises a fishmouth type incision with a long palmar and a shorter dorsal flap.

Forearm amputations

Below-elbow amputations are suitable for fitting with prostheses. Forearm rotation is best maintained with the maximum length of stump, though in all cases the rotation will be significantly limited in the absence of the articulation of the distal radio-ulnar joint. More proximal levels provide very little rotation; however, even a very short stump will allow a degree of flexion at the elbow. The skin flaps are sited on the volar and dorsal surfaces of the forearm and are joined at the mid-lateral lines. Muscle bellies are divided marginally distal to the bones to allow a well protected and shaped stump. Nerves should be dissected proximally prior to division to ensure that the nerve ends can be sited deeply in the muscle mass.

The Krukenberg procedure is a specific form of forearm amputation which splits the forearm stump longitudinally to form radial and ulnar components. It is sometimes termed a lobster-claw amputation. Contraction of pronator teres brings together the forearm components giving a functional pincer or pinch grip. This procedure is seldom indicated where there is access to sophisticated and myoelectric prostheses which provide better functional capacity on a standard below-elbow stump. There is a continuing place for this procedure in specific circumstances. The maintenance of proprioception helps blind patients who cannot visualise the position of a prosthetic limb. The other indication for this procedure is in providing grasping ability where sophisticated prostheses are not available.

Above-elbow amputations

A similar design of flaps is employed as for a below-elbow amputation, and the muscles and nerves are divided and allowed to retract in a similar manner. The maximum length of stump possible is preserved, as this will retain the most movement from the gleno-humeral joint.

Shoulder disarticulation

Shoulder disarticulation and above-elbow amputation at the level of the pectoralis major tendon function in a similar manner, but a high above-elbow amputation results in better preservation of the shape and appearance of the shoulder.

For disarticulation the lateral skin incision and flaps are based on the deltoid muscle, extending distally on the arm to the level of the deltoid tubercle. The medial flap is based on a transaxillary approach, with the two incisions joining over the anterior and posterior surfaces of the shoulder joint and extending proximally. The axillary vessels and the thoraco-acromial vessels are ligated through the transaxillary approach in the deltopectoral groove. The main nerves are also divided at this level and allowed to retract proximally deep to pectoralis minor. Following division of the muscle tendons crossing the glenohumeral joint, the rotator cuff and capsule are divided and the joint is disarticulated. The lateral edges of the latissimus dorsi and pectoralis major muscles are attached to the glenoid cavity.

Forequarter amputation

Removal of the entire arm and pectoral girdle of clavicle and scapula produces significant disfigurement and there is no capacity for the fitting of any prosthesis. The principal indication is in the management of malignant tumours of the upper limb. Preoperative planning and staging of disease prior to surgery is performed, usually under the direction of a specialist in musculoskeletal malignancy. There are two recognised surgical techniques.

In the anterior approach, the incisions meet at the attachment of the sternocleidomastoid muscle on the clavicle. The upper incision extends along the clavicle onto the posterior surface of the shoulder region following the spine and vertebral border of the scapula. The lower incision follows the deltopectoral groove through the axilla to meet the upper incision on the posterior surface at the inferior angle of the scapula. The clavicle is divided at a point just lateral to the attachment of sternocleidomastoid, which allows access to ligate the large vessels and divide the brachial plexus. The scapula is mobilised by releasing its many muscular attachments. The upper skin–flap is mobilised distally so the resulting suture line follows the upper border of pectoralis major.

The other technique utilises a posterior approach. The most significant difference from the anterior approach is in the management of the neurovascular structures. These are reached by elevation of the scapula prior to division of any anterior structures or division of the clavicle.

TRAUMATIC AMPUTATIONS
Fingertip injuries

Fingertip injuries are defined as occurring at a level distal to the insertions of the extensor and profundus tendons and are the most common form of amputation affecting the hand. This part of the finger includes the volar pulp, which has a high concentration of afferent nerve endings to function as a sensory organ. The fingertip also functions in grasping and gripping and, in order to provide strength to the fingertip, it is supported by the terminal phalanx and fingernail. The management of these injuries is controversial. The aim is to preserve or restore a fingertip with normal sensory function, adequate padding, and freedom from discomfort. It is desirable to preserve the nail-bed if possible, although in doing so damage to the germinal matrix must be avoided, which could lead to a functional or cosmetic deficit in the fingernail.

These injuries are usually classified and subdivided based on the soft tissue loss and exposure of bone. The shape and position of the excised section is also an important consideration. A volar oblique section will result in a greater loss of pulp tissue. The degree of crush and contamination will also influence the decision on management.

The treatment of choice for these injuries can be generalised into two broad groups: conservative and reconstructive.

Conservative treatment

Conservative treatment is clearly appropriate for injuries with no tissue loss. The majority of simple lacerations can be left open; debridement of non-viable tissue should be minimal. Suturing is generally not required, because the intact septae of the pulp compartment prevent disruption of the shape of the fingertip. Lacerations to the nail-bed should be carefully repaired with small interrupted sutures, to prevent subsequent deformities in nail growth.

In the management of tissue loss from the fingertip in children, conservative treatment is appropriate in the large majority of cases. A number of studies comparing surgical to conservative treatment have been reported. Apart from the advantage of not requiring anaesthesia and time lost from school, two-point discrimination was better in the conservatively managed injuries. These heal by epithelialisation of the wound when the nature of the wound is suitable. However, in cases where the distal phalanx is degloved, shortening of the bone is required to provide a suitable surface for healing. The need for an occlusive dressing when treating injuries conservatively has been stressed by many authors. Many methods have been described, including using non-adhesive dressings and the fingers of surgical gloves.

Dissatisfaction with the results of conservative treatment in adults has led to the description of many surgical techniques of reconstructing the fingertip. However, it is clear that there is a continuing role for conservative treatment of these injuries in adults. Good results have

been reported when the area of defect is relatively small, transversely placed, and the bone is not exposed.

Reconstructive surgery

In all cases where reconstructive surgery is contemplated, the patient's age and general health (including diabetes, arterial disease and a history of cigarette smoking) must be considered. The condition of the peripheral vasculature is of great significance in the potential viability of local and regional flaps. Occupational and other functional requirements may affect the choice of treatment, as well as the patient's ability to comply with a rehabilitation programme.

Surgery to shorten and primarily close the stump, known as *terminalisation*, is not generally recommended. Many patients complain of tenderness and cold intolerance and avoid using the shortened digit. This technique may be indicated in an elderly unfit patient with limited functional requirements who cannot be considered for an alternative form of treatment

Skin grafting is described for small predominantly skin deficits where the bulk of pulp tissue is preserved, leaving a well-vascularised area of soft tissue. Split-skin grafts can be applied to areas on the ulnar side of a digit. The subsequent contraction of the graft will pull skin from the pulp across the defect, providing coverage of the tip, and preserving sensory function. Full-thickness grafts are more appropriate for the radial and volar aspects of the fingertip. The usual donor site is the thenar crease at the MP joint of the thumb. Sensory problems are the principal complication of full-thickness grafts, resulting in poor function which has been described as 'blindfolding the pulp'.

Many *local flaps and regional flaps* have been described, which resurface the fingertip with skin from the injured or an adjacent digit. The advantages include the utilisation of similar skin to cover the deficit and the restoration of normal sensory function. These techniques are technically demanding, and can lead to significant complications, including flap necrosis, if carried out by inexperienced operators.

The two most commonly described local advancement techniques are the lateral advancement flaps and the V–Y advancement flap.

The lateral advancement technique, or Kutler flap, uses two short, wide, laterally–placed flaps based on subcutaneous pedicles incorporating the most distal part of the neurovascular bundle. The flaps are mobilised and advanced distally. The proximal deficits are closed by direct suture, which results in slight tapering or narrowing of the finger. This technique provides good tip coverage and sensory function where a limited degree of advancement is required.

The V–Y flap can be sited laterally on a pedicle in the mid-lateral line, or alternatively on the volar surface if the deficit is transverse or obliquely angled. The V-shaped flap is cut with a proximal apex and mobilised with the neurovascular bundle. The proximal extension of the wound which follows advancement of the flap is closed directly, and forms the longitudinal part of the Y-shaped final wound.

Larger island flaps have also been described involving the entire volar skin from the digit based on both neurovascular bundles, and the step advancement flap based on the mid-lateral pedicle. Failure of these large flaps results in loss of skin cover from the entire digit.

In some situations a local advancement flap is not feasible, and skin needs to be brought in from another part of the hand utilising a regional flap. The cross–finger flap has a donor site on the dorsum of an adjacent finger, requiring a full thickness skin–graft from the groin to cover the donor site on the finger. It is necessary to immobilise both the recipient and donor fingers, and percutaneous Kirschner wires can be used. The risk of developing stiffness in the fingers is apparent and for this reason the flap pedicle is divided at the earliest opportunity i.e. three weeks.

The thenar flap is raised just proximal to the MP joint of the thumb and is restricted to use for the index and middle fingers; the ulnar fingers are unable to reach the donor site. Proximal and distal flaps are raised using an H-shaped incision. The proximal flap is sutured to the fingertip deficit, and the distal flap is sutured to the proximal volar margin of the fingertip wound. The finger is immobilised in flexion for two weeks, at which time the proximal flap is detached at its pedicle and sutured to cover the entire fingertip wound. The distal flap is detached from the finger rather than divided at its pedicle; this allows it to be used to cover the donor site. This flap is less versatile than the cross-finger flap but has less donor site morbidity.

Fingertip injuries are important: think how it would affect you. They require careful assessment of a number of factors before an appropriate choice of treatment can be made. There is a morbidity associated with these injuries which can not be fully prevented by any form of treatment. Review of the many reported series of fingertip injuries reveals that the most significant long-term problems are altered sensation, including hyperaesthesia of the fingertip, and pain in cold conditions.

Replantation

The wider availability of mirosurgical operating skills has led to an increase in reattachment and revascularisation following traumatic amputations. Revascularisation is defined as reconstruction of an incompletely amputated limb in which some soft tissues remain intact. Replantation is the reattachment of a completely amputated part.

The majority of amputated parts can be reattached and vascular viability can be achieved. Crushing and avulsion injuries result in greater damage to the soft tissues of the amputated part and lead to a decreased chance of restoring vascularity. It is now recognised that viability alone does not determine the functional capacity and other factors must be borne in mind when considering replantation. As a general rule, replantation should be attempted in nearly all injuries affecting children, where good recovery and adaptation to give good function is likely.

Amputation of the thumb, multiple digits and the entire hand are strong indications for replantation, although in multiple digit injuries it may only be possible to replant those digits which are the least severely damaged, not necessarily on their original rays. The level of digital amputation is important and replantation is feasible only when veins can be found in the amputated part. In the thumb, restoration of length is more important and replantation can be attempted as far distal as the nail-base. In the fingers, the most distal viable level is 4 mm proximal to the nail-base.

Joint stiffness, cold intolerance and unsatisfactory sensory function produce a poor result. To avoid this a number of contraindications have been defined:

- patients with life-threatening head and chest injuries;
- crush or degloving injury to the amputated part;
- amputations at multiple levels;
- chronic illness precluding surgery;

- disease affecting the peripheral vasculature;
- amputations of a single finger.

The majority of contraindications are relative and the expectation of the patient as well as his functional requirements must be taken into consideration. Single finger amputations proximal to the insertion of the flexor superficialis tendon are rarely indicated. Following successful replantation, the majority of patients avoid using the reattached finger because it has reduced sensitivity and range of motion.

Replantation of a single digit is indicated when the thumb is involved in an attempt to maintain length, though even here good sensation is the most important thing.

Other factors are features of the patient as a whole which may affect the suitability of the vessels to repair. Such relative contraindications are diabetes mellitus, age and cigarette–smoking. Replantation in children has a higher rate of success and in general should always be attempted, as the nerves recover well so restoration of viability leads to restoration of good function.

Ischaemic time is less well–tolerated in proximal amputations because there is more muscle present. The maximum warm ischaemic time for a digit is 12 h and 6 h for a more proximal amputation. Cold ischaemic time can be extended up to 24 h for digits. Amputated parts should be stored in ordinary, not dry, ice, which is not in direct contact with the skin.

There are many technical aspects of the surgical technique of re-implantation. An operating microscope is usually required, as well as specialised instruments and size 10–0 sutures. Perfusion of the reattached part is aided by a warm body temperature and environment. A regional block is the preferred type of anaesthesia, as it provides a degree of sympathetic blockade and vaso-dilatation of the distal vasculature. There is a preferred order of reconstruction, commencing with restoration of skeletal stability. Shortening of the bone is necessary in order to retain adequate length in the nerves and vessels for anastamosis. Internal fixation is essential to provide rigid bone stability. This is achieved using per-cutaneous Kirschner wires or small plates and screws. The next stage is repair of the extensor and flexor tendons, followed by arteries, nerves and finally veins.

Postoperative care of reimplantations has a number of areas of controversy, particularly regarding the role of anticoagulant and vasodilator therapy.

Prosthetics

The role of prostheses following amputation in the upper limb is complex. The majority of patients with a unilateral amputation will manage to function ade-quately with the remaining limb, and will avoid using a heavy complex prosthetic limb.

Many prostheses provide cosmesis alone. These are made from silicone materials and can be designed to provide a good skin–colour match. Functional prostheses are classified as body–powered or externally powered, although most types are a hybrid design.

The most simple form of functional prosthesis is a split hook. The two elements of the hook can provide a basic pinch. These can be either voluntary opening or closing. As the most important function of the hook is in grasping, most are opened voluntarily using a cable-drive system linked to humerus or shoulder motion. The hook itself is fitted with a rubber band mechanism to provide apposition between the two elements of the split hook. These prostheses are heavy and cumbersome and require considerable movement and muscle power in the proximal part of the limb to power the pinch grip at the hook. At the wrist the hook is opened by wrist dorsiflexion and closed with palmar flexion.

The most sophisticated prosthesis available for a distal amputation is the myoelectric hand. The socket of this prosthesis contains electrodes which detect myoelectric potentials from contracting muscle groups in the remaining part of the limb. These potentials are used to activate an electric motor powered by batteries within the prosthesis. The electric motor drives the thumb, index and middle fingers of the prosthesis, providing a three-point pinch grip. The advantages over a split hook are improved cosmetic appearance and the absence of a cable activation system.

With a wrist disarticulation or below–elbow amputation there is a remaining capacity for forearm rotation, so any prosthetic device can be fitted with a sophisticated socket to preserve this movement in addi-tion to the grip provided by the device itself.

In above-elbow amputation, as long a stump as possible should be preserved. This has advantages over a shoulder disarticulation in both cosmetic appearance (with preservation of the shoulder contour) and pros-thetic fitting. With a hinged-elbow prosthesis attached by straps fitting over the shoulder and around the con-tralateral axilla, a number of functions can be achieved.

The elbow can be locked in any one position to allow carrying of a load. A turntable device sited proximal to the elbow hinge can be locked in position; this integral part of the design can allow rotation in the longitudinal axis, and consequently alter the orientation of the flexion and extension motion at the elbow hinge. Active movement of the elbow hinge is achieved using a cable system linked to humeral flexion or by passing around the shoulder from the opposite limb. If the elbow hinge is locked, the cable system can be utilised to move the distal part of the prosthesis.

The socket of a shoulder disarticulation gives a less suitable site for the fitting of a prosthesis. A similar prosthesis to that used for an above-elbow amputation can be fitted, the cable system being activated by the opposite arm.

The only type of prosthesis of any value for a forequarter amputation is cosmetic. This is designed to restore the shoulder contour and allow the use of unmodified garments.

FURTHER READING

Brown PW. Less than ten—surgeons with amputated fingers. *J Hand Surg* 1982; **7**: 31.

Kay SPJ. Fingertip injuries. *Curr Orthop* 1991; **5**: 223–229.

Leclercq C. Management of fingertip injuries. *J Hand Surg* 1993; **18B**: 415.

Lister G. Injury. In: *The Hand: Diagnosis and Indications*, 3rd edn. Edinburgh: Churchill Livingstone, 1993.

Louis DS. Amputations. In: Green DP (ed.) *Operative Hand Surgery*, 3rd edn. Edinburgh: Churchill Livingstone, 1993.

McCarthy JG. *Plastic Surgery*, Vols. 7 and 8. Philadelphia: Saunders, 1990.

Urbaniak JR. Replantation. In: Green DP (ed.) *Operative Hand Surgery*, 3rd edn. Edinburgh: Churchill Livingstone 1993.

Index

Page numbers in *italics* indicate figures and tables.

TRANSURETHRAL
RESECTION

TRANSURETHRAL RESECTION

Fifth Edition

John P Blandy CBE DM MCh FRCS FACS FRSCI
Emeritus Professor of Urology
The Royal London Hospital and Medical College
London
UK

Richard G Notley MS FRCS
Emeritus Consultant Urological Surgeon
The Royal Surrey County Hospital
Guildford
UK

John M Reynard DM MA FRCS Urol
Consultant Urological Surgeon
Department of Urology
The Churchill Hospital
Oxford
UK

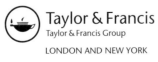

Taylor & Francis
Taylor & Francis Group

LONDON AND NEW YORK

A MARTIN DUNITZ BOOK

© 2005, Taylor & Francis, an imprint of the Taylor & Francis Group

First published in the United Kingdom in 1971 by Pitman Medical Publishing Co Ltd
Second edition in 1978
Third edition in 1993 by Butterworth Heinemann Ltd
Fourth edition in 1998 by Isis Medical Media Ltd
Fifth edition in 2005 by Taylor & Francis, an imprint of the Taylor & Francis Group plc, 2 Park Square, Milton Park, Abingdon, Oxfordshire OX14 4RN.

Tel.:   +44 (0) 1235 828600
Fax.:   +44 (0) 1235 829000
E-mail: info@dunitz.co.uk
Website: http://www.dunitz.co.uk

A CIP record for this book is available from the British Library.

Library of Congress Cataloging-in-Publication Data
Data available on application

ISBN 1 84184 408 X

Distributed in North and South America by
Taylor & Francis
2000 NW Corporate Blvd
Boca Raton, FL 33431, USA

Within Continental USA
Tel.: 800 272 7737; Fax.: 800 374 3401
Outside Continental USA
Tel.: 561 994 0555; Fax.: 561 361 6018
E-mail: orders@crcpress.com

Distributed in the rest of the world by
Thomson Publishing Services
Cheriton House
North Way
Andover, Hampshire SP10 5BE, UK
Tel.: +44 (0)1264 332424
E-mail: salesorder.tandf@thomsonpublishingservices.co.uk

Production Editor: Stephen Nicholls

Composition by EXPO Holdings, Malaysia

Printed and bound in Spain by Grafos S.A. Arte Sobre Papel

Contents

Preface

Thirty-three years ago, when the first edition of this book was written, throughout Europe nearly all prostates were operated on by one of the open methods. Transurethral resection was rarely performed, regarded with suspicion and carried a considerable morbidity. Since those days everything has changed, and there have been many improvements and refinements in the operation and the investigation and preparation of the patient, while a whole new range of alternative methods of management have been introduced. The senior authors welcome the fresh input of their younger colleague John Reynard, who has already made his reputation at the growing edge of urology. One thing has not changed: transurethral resection is difficult to learn and to teach, and this book is aimed at the newcomers to urology who wish to learn how to do it safely.

John P Blandy
Richard G Notley
John M Reynard

Acknowledgements

The authors wish to thank a number of individuals and firms for their invaluable cooperation in the production of this book. The first of these is Alastair Holdoway of Video South Medical Television for his generous help in a number of ways, but especially with the production of the coloured endoscopic photographs. Rimmer Brothers, Karl Storz Endoscopy (UK) and KeyMed have again been generous in their help with the illustrations of the endoscopic equipment.

Chapter 1
History

The ancients, who thought that the bladder was divided by a horizontal septum, knew little about obstruction at its outflow, though Galen must have divided the prostate and bladder neck regularly when performing lateral lithotomy[1]. Oribasius of Pergamum, writing his synopsis at the command of the Emperor Julian in the fourth century AD, proposed to cut through the prostate by a perineal incision in cases of retention of urine where it was impossible to pass a catheter, considering that the risk of fistula after this operation was preferable to death from unrelieved retention. Ambroise Paré seems to have been aware of the entity of bladder neck obstruction, and devised catheters with a sharp cutting cup at the tip with which pieces of the bladder neck could be torn away (Fig. 1.1). Morgagni, Valsalva and Bartholin all wrote on the subject[1–3], but it was John Hunter who demonstrated, in a series of specimens, the progressive effects and complications of prostatic obstruction. One of these was a classic example of obstruction by enlargement of the middle lobe[4] which his brother-in-law Everard Home subsequently published and claimed as his own original observation – plagiary soon denounced by his contemporaries[5] (Fig. 1.2).

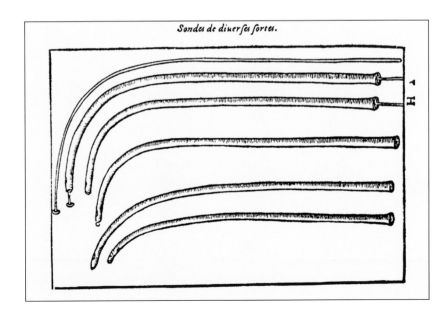

Sondes de diverses sortes.

Figure 1.1
Catheters armed with cups for removing 'carnosities' from the urethra and possibly also the bladder neck. Ambroise Paré 1510–1590.

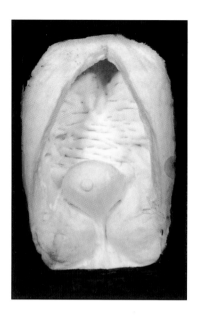

Figure 1.2
John Hunter's specimen showing a large middle lobe. Courtesy of the Trustees of the Hunterian Museum, the Royal College of Surgeons of England.

As for treatment, there was only the catheter and men were admitted to hospital to be 'schooled' in how to pass it. Even at the end of the nineteenth century the mortality of catheterization was still as high as 20% in the first 6 months[6].

Probably the first surgeon to attempt an open division of the bladder neck was Sir William Blizard in about 1806 (Fig. 1.3) who described a patient in the London Hospital who lay with an indwelling catheter and subsequently died with an abscess in each lateral lobe of the prostate[5]. Blizard reflected that:

> This person might have been successfully treated by dividing the prostate with a double gorget cutting on both sides introduced in the usual way on a staff into the bladder. It would have relieved the immediate distress, and might have laid the foundation for a cure. This is not a speculative remark. I have several times performed such an operation in cases of disease of the prostate gland which I have thought within its scope of relief, with complete success.

Of Blizard's contemporaries, Guthrie (Fig. 1.4) at the Westminster Hospital, with an international reputation for the conservative treatment of limb wounds before and after Waterloo, noted the role of the bladder neck in outflow obstruction:

> No greater error has been committed in surgery than that which supposes the third lobe, as it is called, of the prostate to be the common cause of those difficulties in making water which occur so frequently in elderly people and sometimes in young ones. I do not deny that a portion of the prostate does enlarge and project into the bladder, preventing the flow of urine from it; but I mean to affirm that this evil takes place more frequently, and is more

Figure 1.3 (left)
Sir William Blizard.
Courtesy of the President
and Council of the Royal
College of Surgeons of
England.

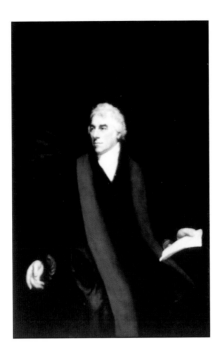

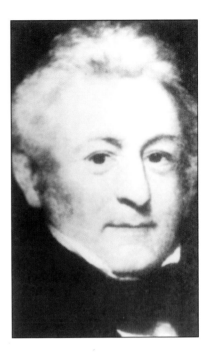

Figure 1.4 (right)
Sir George James Guthrie.
Courtesy of the President
and Council of the Royal
College of Surgeons of
England.

effectually caused by, disease of the neck of the bladder, totally unconnected with the prostate, than by disease of that part[5].

Understanding the nature of the 'bar at the neck of the bladder', Guthrie devised a means of dividing it which would be less traumatic than Blizard's perineal incision. He ordered a sound to be made for him with a concealed knife which could be projected to cut through the 'bar, dam or stricture' without injuring the adjacent parts (Fig. 1.5). It is often said that Guthrie had in mind the kind of bladder neck stenosis which may occur

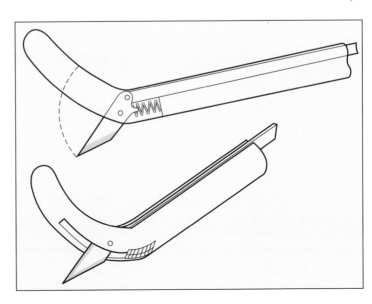

Figure 1.5
Guthrie's concealed knife,
based on his description.

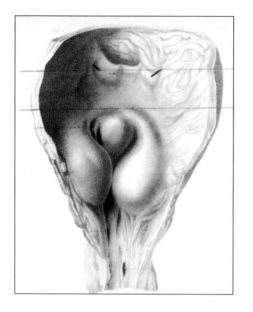

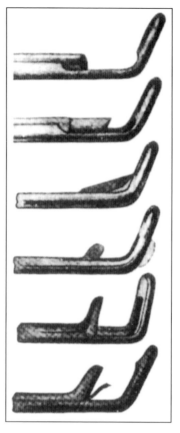

Figure 1.6 (left)
Guthrie's prostate specimen, supplied to him by Goldwyer Andrews of the London Hospital.

Figure 1.7 (right)
Concealed knives devised by Civiale and Mercier.

without enlargement of the prostate, but in his illustration (Fig. 1.6) of a specimen lent to him by Goldwyer Andrews, Blizard's colleague and successor at the London Hospital, it is clear that he was thinking of typical middle lobe enlargement, and the concealed knife was intended to cut the ring of bladder muscle that imprisons and traps the adenoma.

Concealed knives similar to that of Guthrie were later devised by Civiale and Mercier[7] (Fig 1.7). Mercier claimed to have done 300 successful operations – a figure doubted by Guyon[8]. Years later, when Hugh Hampton Young devised his punch, he generously gave credit and priority to Mercier[9].

Inevitably any kind of incision or cold punch resection was more or less blind and bloody: to overcome these defects surgery had to wait for the application of electrical engineering to urology. The first step was taken by Bottini[10], who devised an instrument like a lithotrite whose male blade was heated by direct current to burn a channel through the neck of the bladder (Fig. 1.8). There was no bleeding until the slough came away, but it was still blind, and it was difficult to know exactly which tissues were being burnt. Bottini claimed to have done 57 cases with two deaths and 12 failures[10].

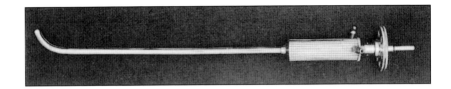

Figure 1.8
Bottini's instrument for heating the prostate. Courtesy of the Institute of Urology.

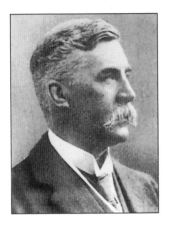

Figure 1.9
Edwin Hurry Fenwick.

Bottini's work was taken up by his contemporaries. Fenwick (Fig. 1.9), Chetwood and Wishard all attempted to improve Bottini's instrument, but the results were unimpressive[11–13]. 'No permanent good ever came of it', wrote Reginald Harrison of St Peter's Hospital[14], who preferred to open the bladder or perform urethrotomy so as to be able to dilate the internal meatus with his finger. If the patient was unfit for either of these procedures, then he was to be given a permanent suprapubic tube of the improved pattern then being introduced by Buckston Browne[14].

At the end of the nineteenth century the standard treatment at St Peter's Hospital was still 'catheter schooling', supplemented by vasectomy (since this was believed to lead to testicular atrophy, and in turn to shrinkage of the prostate[6]). Looking back on these years, Frank Kidd[15] noted that up to 8% of men treated in this way would be dead of uraemia or infection within a month.

It was in this climate that enucleative prostatectomy by the suprapubic or perineal route was introduced[7]. First recorded at St Bartholomew's Hospital in 1884[16] it was independently developed by Goodfellow in Tombstone, Arizona (1885)[17], McGill in Leeds (1887)[18], Mansell-Moullin at the London Hospital (1892)[19], Fuller in New York (1895)[20] and Freyer at St Peter's (1900)[21] (Fig. 1.10). Thanks very largely to Freyer's enthusiasm and energy the transvesical or Freyer operation

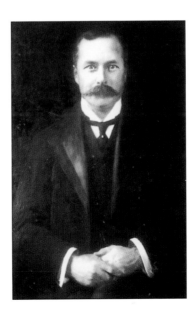

Figure 1.10
Sir Peter Freyer.

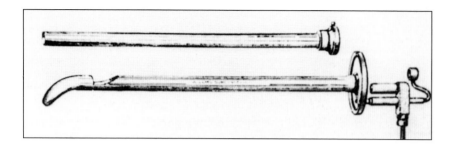

Figure 1.11
Hugh Hampton Young's punch.

soon overtook all other forms of treatment, but even the pioneers in the field were concerned that the amount of tissue removed 'is often so small that it seems ridiculous to have to perform suprapubic operation for its removal'[22].

It was this concern which led Hugh Hampton Young, one of the pioneers of perineal prostatectomy, to look again at Mercier's concept of using a sharp tubular knife, like a cork-borer (Fig. 1.11). 'I called my instrument a prostatic excisor and the operation excision. The internes promptly dubbed the instrument 'the punch'[22]. The first punch was very simple and without any means of haemostasis: this was only possible thanks to the development of diathermy[23].

Soon after the discovery that very high-frequency alternating current did not excite nerve or muscle, the heating effect at the site of contact would be used to cauterize warts on the skin, and by 1910 Beer was using the same current through a cystoscope to cauterize 'warts' in the bladder[24]. The electric cystoscope, pioneered in Germany by Nitze, and introduced to the UK by Fenwick, was now in general use, although it had taken Fenwick a decade to overcome the early prejudice against it. Fenwick was once laughed off the rostrum at the Medical Society of London for suggesting that the electric cystoscope was anything more than a gimmick, since every proper surgeon knew that the right way to explore the bladder was with a finger introduced via the perineum[25].

With the early operating cystoscopes and the early spark-gap diathermy machines one could produce a controlled Bottini burn at the neck of the bladder, although it took a series of sittings before a sufficiently large channel could be burned away. This method was developed in New York by Stevens[26] and Bugbee[27], and in France by Luys[7,28] (Fig. 1.12).

Young's approach was far more bold: he tried to cut away the tissue, and then stop the bleeding with the diathermy (Fig. 1.13). This combination of the cold punch with diathermy haemostasis was rapidly developed by Young, Braasch, Bumpus and Caulk[29] until by 1930 Caulk reported that he could resect 85% of his cases with the punch, and had only one death in 510 cases[30]. The 'cold punch' had arrived. It did, however, have a major

Figure 1.12
'Forage' of the prostate. From Luys (1935)[28].

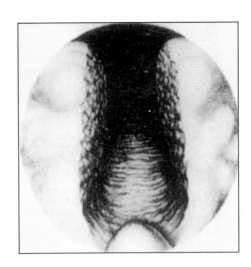

Figure 1.13
Gershom Thomson's combination diathermy and punch. Courtesy of the Institute of Urology.

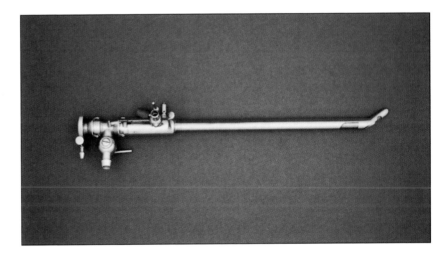

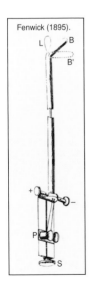

Fenwick (1895).

Figure 1.14
Fenwick's 'galvanic écraseur'.

drawback: the surgeon's view was obscured just as the tissue was being cut off, and this made it difficult and even dangerous to use.

A different principle was being developed at the same time, using a hot wire to cut through the tissue. As early as 1895 Fenwick[11] had designed a 'galvanic écraseur' with a wire snare, heated white hot, to cut through the projecting parts of the middle lobe (Fig. 1.14). In practice it is difficult to cut through the prostate with a hot wire: it drags, sticks and carbonizes. Loop resection was not a practical possibility until 1926 when Maximilian Stern[31] tried out the new powerful radio-frequency valve diathermy machine invented by Wappler. Stern described how this more powerful current would create 'a luminous ring or halo which causes eruption of cells in its path as the loop is advanced, leaving no

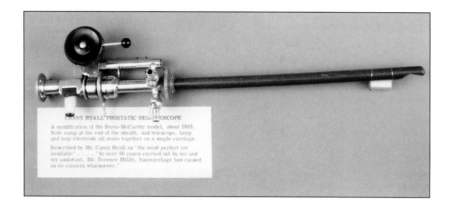

Figure 1.15
The Stern-McCarthy resectoscope. Courtesy of the Institute of Urology.

carbonized tissue either on the loop or the cut surface of the gutter it leaves in the tissues'[31]. It may not have carbonized the tissue, but neither did it stop the bleeding. For a time urologists would use two machines: Wappler's new valve 'endotherm' for cutting, and the old-fashioned spark-gap diathermy for haemostasis. Eventually, enterprising manufacturers supplied both circuits in one box with variable current outputs that allowed the surgeon to cut or coagulate as necessary.

To Stern's diathermy system was soon added the 'foroblique' telescope devised by McCarthy, and the combination became the Stern-McCarthy resectoscope, a sturdy and reliable instrument, which is the prototype of all the present-day instruments (Fig. 1.15).

By 1930 hot-wire or cold-punch instruments were available to any surgeon who would take the trouble to learn how to use them. At first the aim was limited, to cut a groove through the middle lobe, or to excise small glands and little fibrous bladder necks where there were only 5 or 10 g of tissue to be taken away.

It was in the Middle West that transurethral surgery really grew up. By 1936 Thomson and Buchtel of the Mayo Clinic[32] reported 200 cases from whom they had removed more than 20 g of tissue. Five years later in Minneapolis Creevy did not consider a prostate 'large' unless he had removed more than 30 g[33] and it was not long before the concept of transurethral resection had been entirely changed. No longer was it the intention to perform a kind of forage of the gland, but to remove the adenoma right down to the capsule in a way that was no less complete and no less thorough than that of the surgeon's finger at transvesical prostatectomy.

Detailed accounts of how to perform a complete transurethral prostatectomy were published in 1943 by Reed Nesbit of Ann Arbor[34] and Roger Barnes[35] of Los Angeles, but by now the Second World War was raging and at least in Europe there were other matters to occupy the attention of surgeons, and there was a hiatus in the development of transurethral surgery.

Between the two World Wars, transurethral resection using the cold punch had been taken up with enthusiasm by Wardill in Newcastle who, like Lane in Dublin, had been to the Mayo clinic to see for himself[36]. Hot-wire resection had been taken up by Canny Ryall and Terence Millin at All Saints[37,38], Kenneth Walker[39] at St Paul's and Ogier Ward at St Peter's but their efforts were hampered by the unreliability of their diathermy equipment. As Millin was later to confide, 'My personal experiences with TUR commenced in 1930 and by 1949 I had carried out some 2000 TURs. By 1940 my percentage was 80% approximately but with the introduction of safer open prostatectomy the percentage declined to less than 10% in the years before I retired'[40].

One critical factor was that the more powerful diathermy machines were commandeered from hospitals to be used to block enemy radar[41] and even 10 years later few hospitals were equipped with diathermy that would cut under water. The other factor was that, after the Second World War, the returning surgeons were greeted with the news that Millin himself, protagonist of transurethral resection, had almost given it up in favour of the retropubic operation. The new operation was simple, easy to teach, and easy to learn: coupled with the introduction of aseptic measures and the sulphonamides, open prostatectomy became much safer[42]. The fact that it was still nothing like as safe as transurethral resection was ignored[6]. Even as late as 1960, Salvaris[43] pointed out that in 1200 open operations at St Peter's Hospital the mean weight of prostate was only 42 g. His article was turned down by British journals, and eventually only found its way into print in Australia.

With the exception perhaps of those who were fortunate enough to work in Dublin with Lane[36], any young surgeon who wished to learn transurethral resection had to go to North America. There we encountered a whole new world of astonishing urological expertise. Resection of a 50 g prostate was routine: the bleeding was stopped completely, and patients went home within a few days: what a difference from the grisly procedure with which we were familiar back home. On our return Geoffrey Chisholm, Joe Smith and other converts began to practise and preach what we had learned[36]. But change was slow: there was still a shortage of effective diathermy equipment, the telescopes were dim and the lighting unreliable. The operation continued to be very difficult to teach.

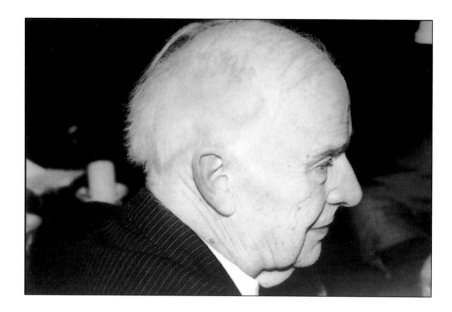

Figure 1.16
Harold Hopkins.

Then came the three inventions of the late Harold Hopkins (Fig. 1.16) which were to change transurethral resection completely. The first was the rod-lens telescope, which owed its development to the imagination and enterprise of Karl Storz (Fig. 1.17). The second was the flexible glass fibre light cable, which provided limitless, unfailing illumination. The third was the coordinated flexible glass cable which made it possible for a pupil to watch the operation.

Thanks to these improvements and to the increasing confidence in transurethral surgery, another equally important development in urology crept in: transurethral resection of bladder tumours. From the early 1930s small papillary tumours were coagulated with cystoscopic electrodes but when they were too large to be 'fulgurated' it was necessary to open the bladder and remove them with a diathermy snare after which the base was sown with radon seeds or tantalum wire[44]. Today these operations have been completely given up.

These changes have come about entirely due to the advances made in urological instruments. When today we sit down to resect a bladder tumour or a prostate we should remember with gratitude those 'grand originals' who struggled so hard to make it possible[45].

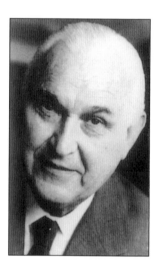

Figure 1.17
Karl Storz.

References

1. Murphy LTJ. *The History of Urology*. Springfield: Thomas, 1972.
2. Paré A. *Oevres Completes avec Figures*. JF Malgaigne (ed.) Paris: Baillière, 1840.
3. Gutierrez R. *History of Urology*, Vol. 2. Bransford Lewis (ed.) Baltimore: Williams and Wilkins, 1933: 137.
4. Palmer JF (ed.) *The Works of John Hunter*. London: Longmans, 1835.

5. Guthrie GJ. *On the Anatomy and Diseases of the Urinary and Sexual Organs*. London: Churchill, 1836.
6. Blandy JP. Surgery of the benign prostate: the first Sir Peter Freyer Memorial Lecture. *J Irish Med Assoc* 1977;70:517.
7. Rognon LM, Raymond G. Historique de l'hyperplasie bénigne de la prostate. *Ann Urol* 1992;26:167.
8. Guyon F. Les prostatiques. *Ann des Mal des Org Génitourin* 1885;3:328.
9. Young HH. A new procedure (punch operation) for small prostatic bars and contractures of the prostatic orifice. *JAMA* 1913;60:253.
10. Bottini E. Die galvanocaustische Diaerese zur Radical-Behandlung der Ischurie bei Hypertrophie der Prostata. *Arch Klin Chir* 1897;54:98.
11. Fenwick EH. *Urinary Surgery*, 2nd edn. Bristol: Wright, 1895.
12. Chetwood CH. Contracture of the neck of the bladder. *Med Rec* 1901;59:767.
13. Wishard WN. Notes on surgery of the prostate. *J Cutan Genitourin Dis* 1925;10:105.
14. Harrison R. *Lectures on the Surgical Disorders of the Urinary Organs*, 4th edn. London: Churchill, 1893.
15. Kidd F. *Urinary Surgery: A Review*. London: Longmans Green, 1910.
16. St Bartholomew's Hospital Reports. *Statistical Tables* 1885;21:79.
17. Goodfellow G. Prostatectomy in general especially by the perineal route. *JAMA* 1904;Nov 12:1448.
18. McGill AF. Suprapubic prostatectomy. *BMJ* 1887;2:1104.
19. Mansell-Moullin CW. *Enlargement of the Prostate: its Treatment and Cure*. London: Lewis, 1894.
20. Fuller E. Six successful and successive cases of prostatectomy. *J Cut Genitourin Dis* 1895;13:229.
21. Freyer PJ. A clinical lecture on total extirpation of the prostate for radical cure of enlargement of that organ. *BMJ* 1901;2:125.
22. Young HH. Discussion after symposium on resection. *J Urol* 1932;28:585.
23. Nation EF. Evolution of knife-punch resectoscope. *Urology* 1976;7:417.
24. Beer E. Removal of neoplasms of the urinary bladder. A new method employing high frequency (Oudin) currents through a catheterising cystoscope. *JAMA* 1910;54:1768.
25. Morson C. Personal communication to JPB. 1969.
26. Stevens AR. Value of cauterisation by high frequency current in certain cases of prostatic obstruction. *N Y Med J* 1913;98:170.
27. Bugbee HG. The relief of vesical obstruction in selected cases: preliminary report. *N Y State Med J* 1913;13:410.
28. Luys G. Traitement de l'hypertrophie de la prostate par la voie endourétrale. *Clinique* 1913;44:693.
29. Collings CW. History of endoscopic surgery. In: Barnes RW (ed.) *Endoscopic Prostatic Surgery*. London: Kimpton, 1943.
30. Caulk JR. Obstructing lesions of the prostate. Influence of the author's cautery punch operation in decreasing the necessity for prostatectomy. *JAMA* 1930;94:375.
31. Stern M. Resections of obstructions at the vesical orifice. *JAMA* 1926;87:1726.
32. Thomson GT, Buchtel H. Transurethral resection of the large prostate: a review of 200 cases in which 25 grams or more of tissue was removed. *J Urol* 1936;36:43.
33. Creevy CD. Resection of the 'large' prostate: technic and results. *J Urol* 1941;45:715.
34. Nesbit RM. *Transurethral Prostatectomy*. Baltimore: Thomas, 1943.
35. Barnes RW. *Endoscopic Prostatic Surgery*. London: Kimpton, 1943.
36. Blandy JP, Williams JP. *The History of the British Association of Urological Surgeons 1945–1995*. London: BAUS, 1995.
37. Ryall C, Millin T. An alternative to prostatectomy. *Lancet* 1932;2:121.
38. Ryall C, Millin T. Endoscopic resection of the prostate—a survey. *Urol Cut Rev* 1933;37:52.
39. Walker KM. Perurethral operations for prostatic obstruction. *BMJ* 1925;1:201.
40. Millin T. Personal communication to JPB. 1969.
41. Jones RV. *Most Secret War*. London: Hamilton, 1978: 126.

42. Wilson Hey H. Asepsis in prostatectomy. *Br J Surg* 1945;33:41.
43. Salvaris M. Retropubic prostatectomy: an evaluation of 1200 operations. *Med J Aust* 1960;47:370.
44. Dix VW, Shanks W, Tresidder GC *et al*. Carcinoma of the bladder: treatment by diathermy snare excision and interstitial irradiation. *Br J Urol* 1970;42:213.
45. Blandy JP. The history of urology in the British Isles. In: Mattelaer JJ (ed.) *De Historia Urologiae Europaeae*, Vol. 2: 11–22. Kortrijk: European Association of Urology, 1995.

Chapter 2

The instruments

When a government purchases a modern missile, it speaks in terms of a 'weapons system', implying not only the rockets but all the complex electronic guidance systems and maintenance arrangements that go with them. So, also, with a resectoscope it is wise to think of the entire weapons system: the light source, the diathermy equipment, and the closed circuit television system.

The resectoscope

Several different instrument systems are available today and the trainee should take the trouble to use as many different resectoscopes as possible. When purchasing one, especially when it comes to equipping a department, it is even more necessary to think in terms of a 'weapons system'. Bear certain points in mind: all these instruments are very expensive, and all resectoscopes can be made to do good work in the hands of an expert. It is humiliating to recall that 50 years ago the master resectionists of the Middle West were removing 100 g an hour with a filament-lit Stern-McCarthy. An expensive tennis racket does not guarantee victory at Wimbledon. If you do have to use an unfamiliar resectoscope it is no more difficult than adjusting to a new car: you do not have to learn to drive all over again.

Interchangeable equipment

The diagnostic flexible cystoscopy, of course, stands by itself, but the indications for using a rigid cystoscope nearly always imply that something else will be done. You may need to catheterize a ureter, biopsy a suspicious lesion, resect a tumour, incise a bladder neck, incise a urethral stricture or crush a stone. You must be able to go ahead and do any of these things without having first to fiddle with different light leads and water connections. The first requirement then is for a complete kit of interchangeable instruments.

Service

The instrument system you finally choose will depend on several factors. First will be the amount of money you or your hospital can afford: but no less important should be the question of after-sales service. You must be able to get rapid and efficient service from a manufacturer's agent who has a representative in your own city, who visits your hospital regularly, knows you and your operating theatre team, and has won a reputation for promptness and reliability. It is no good buying a Rolls-Royce if their nearest agent is in Ruritania.

Spares

Make sure you have an adequate number of spare parts. It is reckless to embark on a resection and be held up because the lamp in the light source has blown and there is no spare; because water has got into the telescope and you can no longer see; because the last loop has broken, the end of the resectoscope sheath has become dangerously worn, or the diathermy machine has broken down. There must always be an adequate number of spares of the things that often go wrong, e.g. light leads, lamps, resectoscope loops and sheaths. Your hospital should always have several spare telescopes and at least one spare diathermy machine.

Telescopes

The story of the invention of the rod-lens telescope by the late Professor Harold Hopkins (Fig. 2.1), and of its development by Karl Storz, is now well known and has been told elsewhere[1]. What is not so well known is the reason why so many resectionists use a 30° rather than a forward-looking or 0° telescope (Fig. 2.2). Sixty years ago, because there was a tiny lamp at the end of the telescope, it was necessary to have a slightly angled line of vision: it was a matter of necessity, not choice. However, it did make it slightly more easy to see the floor of the trough from which a chip of prostate had been taken. Newcomers to the art of transurethral resection will find it easier to use a 0° telescope from the beginning.

Sheaths

The early sheaths were made of bakelite, later of fibreglass and similar plastics which were apt to crack and split. Today sheaths are always made of steel, with an insulated tip made of plastic or ceramic (Fig. 2.3).

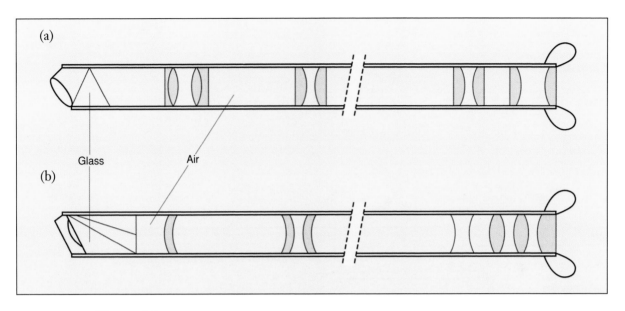

Glass

Air

Figure 2.1
(a) Conventional telescope.
(b) Hopkins' rod lens
telescope.

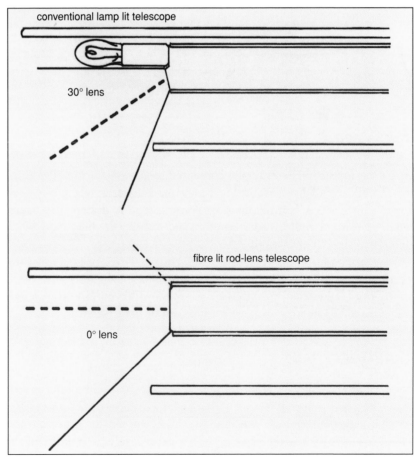

conventional lamp lit telescope

30° lens

fibre lit rod-lens telescope

0° lens

Figure 2.2
The filament lamp at the
end of the telescope
necessitated the use of a 30°
telescope.

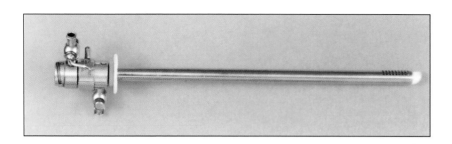

Figure 2.3
Steel sheath with ceramic tip.

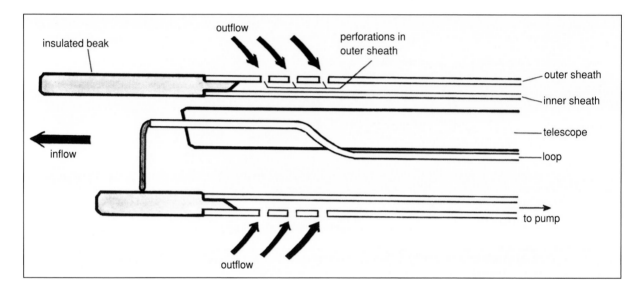

Figure 2.4
Iglesias's continuous irrigation.

Iglesias devised a continuous flow resectoscope[2] which allowed the irrigating fluid to be continually circulated in and out of the bladder to avoid build-up of pressure inside it, and to keep the field clear at all times (Fig. 2.4). A continuous flow resectoscope is particularly useful when resecting larger bladder tumours and to keep the field clear when demonstrating an operation.

From time to time one comes across a patient with a particularly long urethra, such that a normal length resectoscope will only just reach inside the bladder or prostate. In this situation having a long resectoscope (Fig. 2.5) in your armamentarium can be very useful.

Lighting

Modern flexible fibre-lighting is the result of another of Hopkins' inventions. Each glass fibre is coated with glass of a different refractive index, so that light entering at one end is totally internally reflected and emerges at the other. Repeated use of the cable results in fracture of the small glass fibres and gradually the cable transmits less light. Clumsy

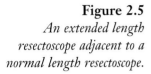

Figure 2.5
An extended length resectoscope adjacent to a normal length resectoscope.

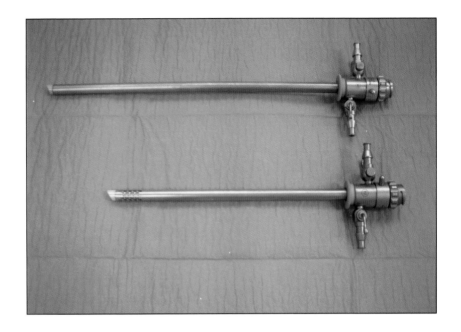

handling accelerates this process of wear and tear, but in time every cable must be replaced and there must always be spares.

Where the light lead is plugged into the source it becomes very hot and must be insulated to prevent staff handling the cable from getting burnt (Fig. 2.6). Absorption of the light at the other end of the cable by dark green drapes may result in local heating and even smouldering of the cloth which may give the patient a burn (Fig. 2.7), so that when

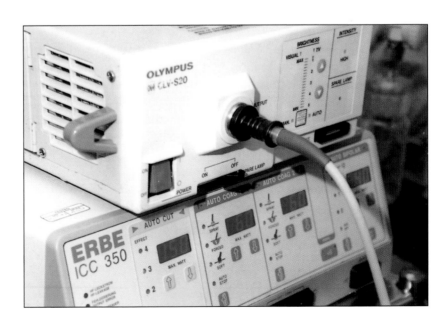

Figure 2.6
Where the light cable joins the light source it gets very hot and must be insulated.

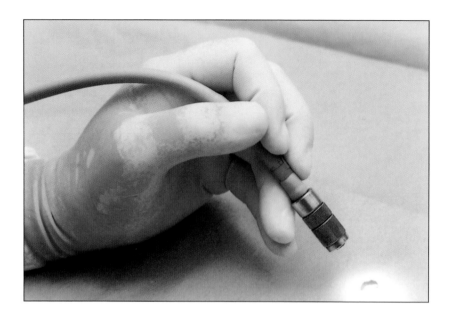

Figure 2.7
If the light cable shines on a dry sterile drape it can smoulder and give the patient a burn.

not in use the end of the cable must always be kept well away from the patient.

It is equally important, when using some of the very bright light sources that are used for television, for the surgeon to safeguard his own retina: only the booby looks at the sun, and one must never allow the full intensity of the light reflected from the bladder to enter one's eye without interposing the teaching attachment or the beam splitter.

The handpiece

Nothing gives rise to more personal fads and fancies than the particular design of the resectoscope handpiece. There are many to choose from, and no one design is outstanding. What you need is a handpiece that is strong, will stand up to wear and tear, and will go on working smoothly in spite of much use. It is irritating and sometimes dangerous when a handpiece sticks or jams in mid-cut.

Many surgeons today work with one finger in the rectum and there is an advantage in a spring action which returns the loop to the starting position without action on the part of the surgeon. There are also advantages in having all the cables on rotating attachments, so that the instrument can be rotated without obstructing or entangling the water pipes, light or diathermy cables.

Light sources

There are many different light sources on the market today. Curiously, they all come with a rheostat to allow the light input to be varied, even

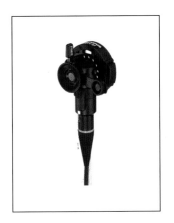

Figure 2.8
Modern, lightweight camera system. Courtesy of Olympus.

though everyone uses the maximum intensity the light can provide. Far more important than a rheostat is that there are plenty of spare lamps, and that everyone in the operating room team knows how to change them. Flash for endoscopic photography is useless.

Teaching equipment

Every surgeon is always a teacher, but to teach endoscopic surgery one must have the right equipment. Teaching attachments have been superseded today by a new generation of lightweight chip cameras that attach directly to the eyepiece of the telescope (Fig. 2.8) (see Chapter 3).

Diathermy

Transurethral resection requires a powerful diathermy machine which can both cut tissue and stop bleeding under water. If your budget is limited, economize on the resectoscope rather than the diathermy. Some of the diathermy machines which are adequate for haemostasis in general surgery will not cut under water.

Many of us take diathermy for granted: there is a big box with two pedals and some dials. When it does not work we ask the nurse to turn up the current. This is often exactly wrong, and diathermy is such an important part of the work of the urologist that he or she must understand its principles. The following account is intended to help the surgeon, even though it may occasionally offend the electrical engineer[3,4].

When an electric current passes between two contacts on the body there is always a certain increase in temperature in the tissues through which the current flows. This increase in temperature depends on the volume of tissue through which the current passes, the resistance of the tissues and the strength of the current. The stronger the current, the greater the rise in temperature.

When a direct current is switched on or off, nerves are stimulated and muscles will twitch. If the switching on and off is rapid enough, as with the Faradic current of a dynamo, there is the sustained contraction familiar to the physiology class as the 'tetanic contraction'.

If the frequency of the alternating current is increased beyond a certain critical level, there is no time for the cell membrane of nerve or muscle to become depolarized and nerves and muscles are no longer stimulated. The critical frequency depends to some extent on the strength of the current; with small currents it is of the order of 10 000 cycles per second (10 kHz). In practice much greater frequencies are used, from 300 kHz to 5 MHz, which today are generated by transistorized valve circuits.

With frequencies as great as this a very large current can be passed through the patient without exciting nerves or muscles, and it is then possible to exploit the heating effect at the points of contact. If one

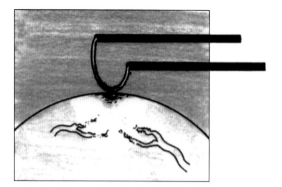

Figure 2.9
The working electrode – the diathermy loop – is thin, so the heating effect is maximum. The coagulating current cooks the tissue for some distance around the loop and congeals the blood vessels.

contact is made large, the heat is dissipated over a wide area and the rise of temperature is insignificant. Such a contact is the earth or neutral electrode under which the rise in temperature is only 1 or 2°C: it is the other end which concerns us, the working electrode or diathermy loop. This is kept deliberately thin so that the heating effect is maximum (Fig. 2.9).

The effect of the diathermy current on the tissues depends on the heat that is generated under the diathermy loop. The effect of heat on tissues is well known to us from everyday experience in the kitchen: when cooking an egg, at first the albumen turns white and shrivels as it coagulates. Then the egg fries, blackens and (in air) may smoke, crackle and eventually catch fire.

These changes are indeed seen in everyday open surgery, though even here it should be noted that good haemostasis depends on poaching, not roasting. It is the drying, coagulation and distortion of small blood vessels and plasma proteins which seals them. This requires only 'white coagulation'. Blackening and smoke are unnecessary and cause needless tissue necrosis.

If the current is increased to raise the temperature still further there is an explosive vaporization of intracellular water in the tissue. In transurethral resection this additional rise in temperature is achieved by a spark, the result of ionization of the water between the electrode and the tissue[3]. The electrode does not actually need to touch the tissue. The sparks explode the cells into steam, but their energy does not reach the deeper layers, so the cut is a clean one, and the blood vessels underneath are not sealed. The cutting current is a pure sine-wave current (Fig. 2.10).

Figure 2.10
*Cutting current: a
continuous sine wave.*

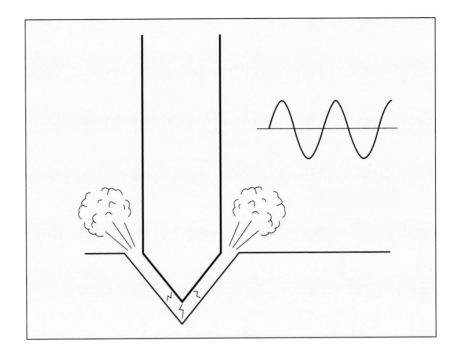

Coagulation is achieved in general with short bursts of sine waves which give longer sparks, but with intervals between them to allow the tissue to cool: the result is sustained heating which leads to poaching rather than explosion of the tissue (Fig. 2.11).

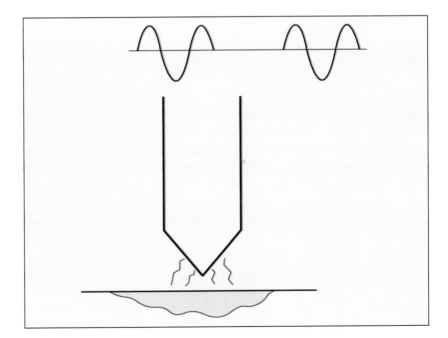

Figure 2.11
*Coagulating current; short
bursts of sine waves produce
local heating and
coagulation.*

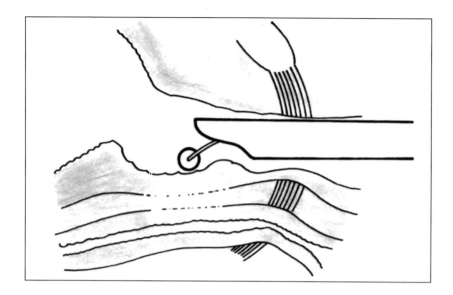

Figure 2.12
Too much coagulation with the roly-ball electrode can cause destruction of deeper tissues, e.g. the sphincter.

By designing the solid-state generator to deliver a mixture of pure sine-wave 'cutting' and interrupted bursts of sine-wave currents for 'coagulation' a current can be designed to allow a combination of cutting and coagulation – the 'blended' current[3].

If a large electrode is used (as with the big roly-ball) there is a danger that the deeper layers of tissue will be cooked, since the heating effect is proportional to the square of the diameter of the contact. This must always be kept in mind when using the coagulating current in the vicinity of the sphincter (Fig. 2.12).

If the current does not seem to be stopping the bleeding, do not make the common mistake of asking for the current to be increased. The problem may be that it is sparking and causing explosion (cutting) of the underlying tissue. Turn it down.

Diathermy burns

If current returns to earth through a small contact rather than the broad area of the earth pad, then the tissues through which the current passes will be heated just like those under the cutting loop. If the pad is making good contact, the current will find it easier to run to earth through the pad and no harm will arise even when there is accidental contact with some metal object.

The real danger arises when the diathermy pad is not making good contact with the patient. It may not be plugged in, its wire may be broken (Fig. 2.13) or, in the older type of earth plate, the conductive jelly may have dried out. Under these circumstances the current must find its way to earth somehow, and any contact may then become the site of a dangerous rise in temperature.

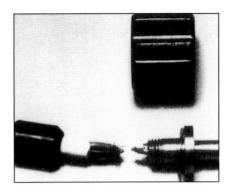

Figure 2.13
The wire may be frayed inside its insulation; always check the circuit from pad to diathermy machine if the loop does not cut.

Figure 2.14
(a) Normal current pathway from loop to earth plate.
(b) If the earth circuit is interrupted, current will find its way via any accidental small metal contact and cause a burn.

It follows that if the diathermy does not seem to be working, the first thing that the surgeon must *not* do is to ask for an increase in current. Instead, check that the diathermy plate is making good contact with the skin of the patient; check that the lead is undamaged; check that the resectoscope loop is securely fixed to the contact (Fig. 2.14). Many modern diathermy machines have a warning circuit which sounds an alarm when there is imperfect contact between the earth plate and the patient (Fig. 2.15). Others have a very low capacitance between the diathermy machine and earth, so that if the earth plate is not attached the current finds it easier to run to earth than through the patient: the surgeon finds the loop does not cut, but the patient cannot be burnt.

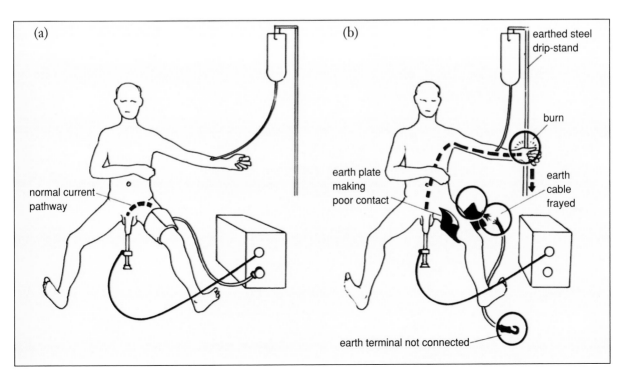

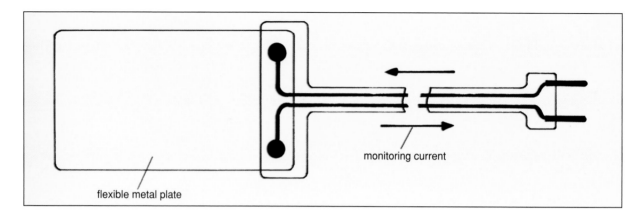

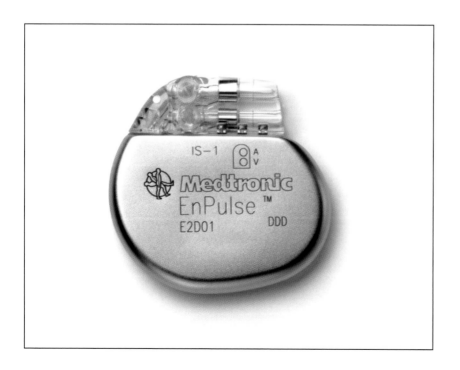

Pacemakers

An increasing number of elderly men come up for prostatectomy with pacemakers (Fig. 2.16). Four types are in common use[5,6]:

1. Fixed-rate pacemakers for patients with permanent heart block: these stimulate the ventricle at a constant rate.

Figure 2.15
Safety circuit incorporated in dry plate; if the circuit is interrupted there is a warning signal, but this does not mean that the plate has been applied to the patient.

Figure 2.16
The Medtronic EnPulse™ pacemaker. Photo courtesy of Medtronic, Inc.

2. Demand pacemakers, which detect ventricular contraction, amplify it, and feed it back to the ventricle. Only if the ventricular impulse is too weak to be detected will the pacemaker deliver its own regular beat.
3. Atrial synchronous pacemakers have one electrode in the atrium which detects a contraction arising there, and a second electrode in the ventricle to supply it with the amplified impulse. If the atrial contractions become too frequent a fixed-rate system takes over.
4. Atrioventricular sequential pacemakers stimulate the atria at a variable but appropriate rate.

The earlier demand pacemakers could sometimes be deceived by the diathermy current into delivering a rate of stimulation that was dangerously high. Several potential problems can occur with the modern devices:

1. Pacemaker inhibition. The high frequency of diathermy current may simulate the electrical activity of myocardial contraction so the pacemaker can be inhibited. If the patient is pacemaker-dependent the heart may stop.
2. Phantom reprogramming. The diathermy current may also simulate the radio-frequency impulse by which the pacemaker can be reprogrammed to different settings, so-called phantom reprogramming. The pacemaker may then start to function in an entirely different mode.
3. Pacemaker damage. The internal mechanism of the pacemaker may be damaged by the diathermy current if this is applied close to the pacemaker.
4. Ventricular fibrillation. If the diathermy current is channelled along the pacemaker lead, ventricular fibrillation may be induced.
5. Myocardial damage. Another potential effect of channelling of the diathermy current along the pacemaker lead is burning of the myocardium at the tip of the pacemaker lead. This can subsequently result in ineffective pacing.

It was formerly recommended that a magnet was placed over the pacemaker to overcome pacemaker inhibition and to make the pacemaker function at a fixed rate. This can, however, result in phantom reprogramming. For demand pacemakers, it is better to programme the pacemaker to a fixed rate (as opposed to demand pacing) for the duration of the operation. Clearly, input from the patient's cardiologist is required for this eventuality.

The other precautions are not difficult (Fig. 2.17):

1. The patient plate should be sited so that the current path does not go right through the pacemaker. Ensure that the indifferent plate is

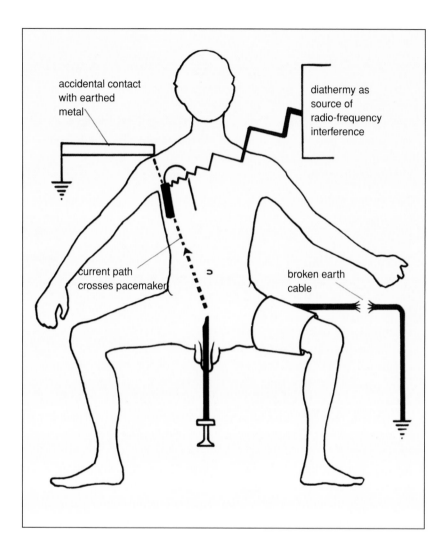

accidental contact
with earthed
metal

diathermy as
source of
radio-frequency
interference

Current path
crosses pacemaker

broken earth
cable

Figure 2.17
*Hazards to be avoided
when using diathermy in a
patient with a pacemaker.*

correctly applied, as an improper connection can cause grounding of the diathermy current through the ECG monitoring leads, and this can affect pacemaker function. The indifferent plate should be placed as close as possible to the prostate, e.g. over the thigh or buttock.

2. The diathermy machine should be placed well away from the pacemaker and should certainly not be used within 15 cm of the pacemaker.

3. The heartbeat should be continually monitored, and a defibrillator and external pacemaker should be at hand.

4. Try to use short bursts of diathermy at the lowest effective output.

5. Give antibiotic prophylaxis (as for patients with artificial heart valves – see Chapter 4).

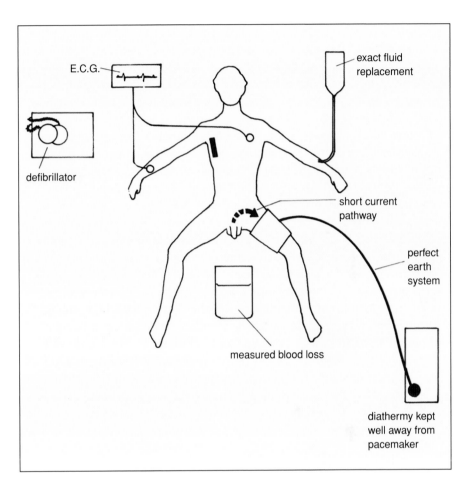

6. Because the pacemaker-driven heart will not respond to fluid overload in the normal way, the resection should be as quick as possible, and fluid overload should be avoided (Fig. 2.18).

Sterilization

The instruments used in urological surgery should, in theory, be no less sterile than those used to operate on the eye or the brain. There is only one way to guarantee the destruction of all known microorganisms, and that is by heat. The ideal method is to put all the instruments through an oven or an autoclave, as is the normal practice for haemostatic forceps and retractors. There are also many parts of the ordinary urological armamentarium, e.g. the metal cystoscope and resectoscope sheath, the taps, obturators, etc., which could and should ideally be sterilized by heat. Modern cystoscopes and resectoscopes including components such as light leads are autoclavable. Standard autoclave regimens heat the instruments to 121°C for 15 minutes or 134°C for 3 minutes. Another commonly used method of sterilization is to soak instruments in formaldehyde solutions. Both methods are entirely acceptable in countries without access to some of the more modern autoclave or liquid sterilization systems.

Theatre autoclaves such as the 'Little Sister' are no longer used in the UK, because they cannot guarantee sterility of the instruments. Central Sterile Supply Units (CSSUs) are used nowadays for sterilizing the majority of urological surgical instruments. The 'turn-around' time of instruments sterilized in CSSUs is inevitably several hours. As a consequence, it is important to have a large enough number of resectoscopes available such that an operating theatre list can be completed without requiring instruments to be sterilized in between cases.

Cameras cannot be autoclaved. Two alternatives are available to prevent transmission of microorganisms between patients. A camera sleeve can be used to prevent contamination of the camera with body fluids. Alternatively, modern cameras can be sterilized between cases in solutions such as Tristel. This is an aqueous solution of chlorine dioxide which is aldehyde-free. There has been a move away from these latter agents (such as formaldehyde) because of health and environmental concerns. Tristel kills bacteria, viruses (including HIV and hepatitis B and C), spores and mycobacteria.

Sterilization and prion diseases

Over the last few years there has been much concern about the potential for transmission of variant Creutzfeldt-Jakob disease (vCJD) between patients via contaminated surgical instruments. vCJD is a neurodegenerative disease caused by an agent known as a prion. Other examples of these neurodegenerative prion diseases include classic CJD, kuru, sheep scrapie and bovine spongiform encephalopathy (BSE). The infectious agent in these diseases is a prion protein (PrP). Variant CJD and BSE are caused by the same prion strain, and represent a classic example of cross-species transmission of a prion disease.

Prions are not readily destroyed by conventional methods of sterilization, using for example, standard autoclave regimens of 121°C for 15 minutes or 134°C for 3 minutes. Similarly, ethylene oxide, formaldehyde and chlorine dioxide are ineffective against prions. There is evidence that classic CJD may be transmitted by neurosurgical and other types of surgical instruments, because normal hospital sterilization procedures do not completely inactivate prions[7]. However, it is not possible at present to quantify the risks of transmission of prion diseases by surgical instruments. In a case–control study of *sporadic* CJD, having had two or more surgical procedures in the past was associated with an increased risk of developing CJD, although there was no association with a particular surgical procedure or anatomic site[8]. This must be put in perspective. Iatrogenic CJD remains rare, with 267 cases reported worldwide up to 2000[9].

The risk of transmission of CJD may be higher with procedures performed on organs containing lymphoreticular tissue such as tonsillectomy and adenoidectomy, because vCJD targets these tissues and is found in high concentrations there. For this reason there was a move towards the use of disposable, once-only use instruments for procedures such as tonsillectomy. However, these instruments have been associated with a higher postoperative haemorrhage rate[10] and as a consequence ENT departments in the UK are no longer obliged to use disposable instruments.

The dilemma then, is how to minimize the risk of transmission of CJD by surgical instruments, while containing costs. Clearly, a policy of disposing of all surgical instruments after only one use is completely impractical, but continuing with current practice may not be regarded as acceptable. In the UK, the Advisory Committee on Dangerous Pathogens and Spongiform Encephalopathy[11] provides advice on appropriate methods of cleaning and sterilization of surgical instruments. This advice stresses that it is not only the process of sterilization that removes infectious agents from surgical instruments, but also the *pre-sterilization process of cleaning* the instruments. Prions are particularly resistant to conventional chemical and thermal decontamination, and it is therefore possible that dried blood or tissue remaining on an instrument could harbour prions that will not then be killed by the sterilisation process. Once proteinaceous material such as blood or tissue has dried on an instrument, it is very difficult subsequently to be sure that the instrument has been sterilized. The chance of leaving such tissue on an instrument can be reduced by prompt cleaning after use, initial low temperature washing (<35°C) with the use of appropriate detergents and an ultrasonic cleaning system to remove and prevent coagulation of prion proteins. This is then followed by a hot wash and air-drying, and only then is thermal sterilization carried out.

The use of ultrasonic cleaning is particularly important for hollow surgical instruments such as resectoscopes, where it can be difficult to remove all the attached debris within the lumen of the instrument. Sonic cleaners essentially 'shake' attached material from the instrument. The latest models of pre-sterilization cleaning devices – automated thermal washer disinfectors – are designed to perform all of these cleaning tasks in one unit.

While prions are not readily destroyed by conventional autoclave regimens, pre-sterilization cleaning followed by longer autoclave cycles at 134–137°C for at least 18 minutes (or six successive cycles with holding times of 3 minutes) or 1 hour at conventional autoclave temperatures may result in a substantial reduction in the level of contamination with prions. There is some evidence that a combination of pre-sterilization cleaning, autoclaving and chemical treatment may be effective in reducing the risk of contamination with prion agents[12]. Enzymatic proteolytic inactivation methods are under development[9].

For urological instruments, such as those used for TURP and TURBT, the risks of transmission of prion diseases are not known and at the present time current sterilization techniques continue to be used. Following good practice by ensuring that the instruments are thoroughly washed and inspected before sterilization should be continued, until it becomes clearer whether iatrogenic prion transmission is a real threat.

References

1. Blandy JP, Fowler CG. Lower tract endoscopy. *Br Med Bull* 1986;42:280.
2. Iglesias JJ, Stams UK. How to prevent the TUR syndrome. *Urologe* 1975;14:287.
3. Fowler CG. Urological technology. In: Blandy JP, Fowler CG (eds) *Urology*, 2nd edn. Oxford: Blackwell Science, 1996:3–17.
4. Mitchell JP, Lumb GN. *A Handbook of Surgical Diathermy*. Bristol: Wright, 1966.
5. Sowton E. Use of cardiac pacemakers in Britain. *BMJ* 1976;2:1182.
6. Spurrell RAJ. Cardiac pacemakers. *Br J Clin Equipment* 1975;1:43.
7. Collinge J. Variant Creutzfeldt-Jakob disease. *Lancet* 1999;354:317–23.
8. Collins S, Law MG, Fletcher A *et al*. Surgical treatment and risk of sporadic Creutzfeldt-Jakob disease: a case-control study. *Lancet* 1999;353:693–7.
9. Collins SJ, Lawson VA, Masters CL. Transmissible spongiform encephalopathies. *Lancet* 2004;363:51–61.
10. Nix P. Prions and disposable surgical instruments. *Int J Clin Pract* 2003;57:678–80.
11. The Advisory Committee on Dangerous Pathogens and Spongiform Encephalopathy. *Transmissible Spongiform Encephalopathy Agents: Safe Working and the Prevention of Infection*. London: HM Stationery Office, 1998.
12. Taylor DM, Fernie K, McConnell I. Inactivation of the 22A strain of scrapie agent by autoclaving in sodium hydroxide. *Vet Microbiol* 1997;58:87–91.

Chapter 3

Closed circuit television for the urologist

Closed circuit colour television (CCTV) is now widely used by urologists in the UK. Few urological surgeons now crane their necks to put an eye to the telescope of their instruments, preferring to sit comfortably looking at the colour monitor conveniently placed in front of them (Fig. 3.1). They thus protect their cervical discs[1] and lessen the risk of facial contamination by blood and irrigant[2].

Urological trainees receive formal training in monitored transurethral resection, as courses are run regularly around the country using CCTV for endoscopy. The improved technology of the miniature chip camera

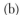
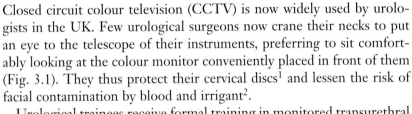
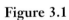

Figure 3.1
(a) KeyMed modern equipment rack. A modern, large monitor allows the surgeon and other theatre staff a clear view of the operation. Courtesy of KeyMed.
(b) One monitor is placed over the patient.
(c) The second monitor is on the wall.

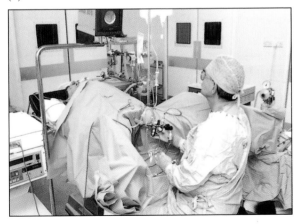
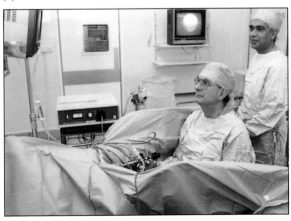

provides such an excellent image that it is now possible to see on the TV screen as much detail – perhaps even more – than one can see by looking directly into the telescope of the instrument. Not only transurethral resection can be done as a 'monitored' procedure, but all varieties of urological endoscopy – urethroscopy, cystoscopy, ureteroscopy and pyeloscopy – are done more easily and effectively using the CCTV camera and working from the monitor.

The urologist who wishes to set up CCTV for use in the operating theatre is faced by a bewildering choice of television equipment. Many manufacturers provide comprehensive packages and it is difficult to choose between them on any grounds other than cost. Ask yourself six basic questions:

1. What do you think you want?
2. What do you think you need?
3. Where will you get it from?
4. Should you buy a package?
5. How much will it cost?
6. What will it cost to run?

What do you think you want?

It is clear that a CCTV set-up in the operating theatre is worthwhile. Apart from saving your neck and helping to protect you from infection by hepatitis and HIV viruses by lessening the risk of facial contamination, CCTV enables you to teach trainees and demonstrate endoscopic technique to theatre personnel. But which parts of the rather expensive system are vital and which are luxuries? You must decide what you want to achieve. The basic wish is to project an image of what the telescope sees onto a TV screen. This may be for a number of reasons. Staff who work in an operating room where almost all the operations are invisible to anyone but the surgeon find it boring. Being able to see what is going on kindles interest. They can see which instrument is going to be needed next and thus anticipate your wishes. There may be students or junior staff to teach. Perhaps you would like to make videotapes, CDs or DVDs for teaching or demonstration purposes[3]. Above all, you may simply want to protect your health. All these are valid reasons to consider the installation of CCTV in the urology operating theatre, but it can be difficult to differentiate between need and luxury.

What do urologists need?

To use CCTV in an operating theatre you need:

1. The usual endoscopic and diathermy equipment.

2. A light source with sufficient output to permit the use of a TV camera; a dim light provides a poor TV image. Your eye can accommodate a dim light because it is an infinitely more efficient optical instrument than the camera.

3. Fibreoptic cables capable of conducting the higher intensity illumination from the light source to the endoscope without suffering heat damage.

4. A good quality telescope. All telescopes deteriorate with use; endoscopic TV needs a really clear telescope. A hazy telescope gives a poor TV image, even if your eye copes adequately.

5. A TV camera.

6. A video monitor or monitors.

7. Some form of constant irrigation system. It is perfectly possible to use CCTV with intermittent irrigation, but constant irrigation enables the watcher to see an uninterrupted operation.

8. Some sort of trolley or cabinet to contain the camera and its ancillary works. This is not essential, but video equipment is expensive and relatively fragile and a trolley is a good way of protecting your investment.

The above list does not include any recording equipment; recording the TV image is not a necessity. It is something to which most urological surgeons will come, but not until they have mastered the general technique of CCTV for endoscopic surgery and have decided what they wish to record and why. This will be discussed later.

Light sources

A suitable general purpose high output light source – high intensity tungsten, metal halide or xenon arc – can be purchased from the urological instrument dealer without difficulty. Tungsten light sources put out between 50 and 150 watts and suit many modern chip TV cameras, but are at the lower end of the spectrum of suitability for CCTV and may not give the best images under adverse operating conditions. Metal halide sources usually operate at 250 watts and xenon arc sources at over 300 watts. Any of these can be used as the standard endoscopic illumination, whether the TV is being used or not, so it is not necessary to have a conventional light source as well. However, a word of caution; high-powered light sources produce light of such intensity that the heat produced can burn holes in surgical drapes, or in patients, if the cable is left unattended (Fig. 3.2).

The lamps are expensive and benefit from a little thought and care; do not turn them off at the end of each operation, as maximum wear on the light source occurs each time it is activated. Lamps will last longer if they are turned on at the start of the list and left on until the last case is

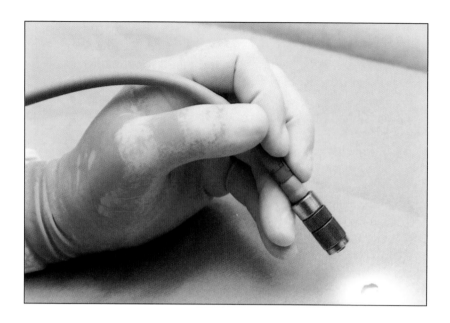

Figure 3.2
If the light cable shines on a dry sterile drape it can smoulder and give the patient a burn.

finished. Always keep a spare lamp and ensure that you know how to change it so that the teaching session does not come to an untimely halt due to a burned out lamp.

As an alternative to a general purpose light source, it is possible to buy a 'dedicated' light source designed to work with a specific TV camera; these come as part of various CCTV 'packages'. The advantage of these dedicated metal halide or xenon arc sources is that they are linked electronically with the camera to produce an image of standard brightness. Feedback from camera to light source gives more light when the field is dark and reduces the light to prevent highlight and flare when the subject matter is over-illuminated. It is a more expensive option than a general purpose light source and it has been the authors' experience that general purpose light sources work well enough, especially if minimizing the capital outlay is important.

Light cables

Armoured, specially insulated, or fluid-filled light cables are widely available. They work just as well with low light intensities, so if CCTV is going to be used one might as well standardize all the cables to be capable of carrying high intensity light, particularly if you plan to use only a high intensity light source. Ensure that the cables are in good condition for TV work; broken fibres and the inevitable melt damage which occurs at the source terminal of the cable are important causes of a poor TV image.

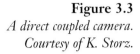

Figure 3.3
A direct coupled camera.
Courtesy of K. Storz.

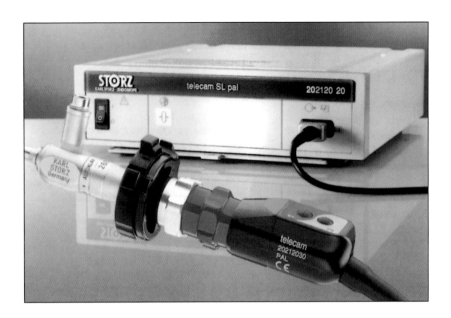

Telescopes

It goes without saying that only rod lens telescopes are suitable for TV work. The slow deterioration of a rod lens telescope from normal regular use is imperceptible to the eye until it is very advanced, as the eye is an altogether superior optical instrument to any TV camera. By the time a telescope looks dim to the eye, it is probably incapable of transmitting an image which the TV camera can visualize at all. You must use a telescope in 'new' condition if CCTV is to be used.

Trolleys

It is essential to house the delicate CCTV equipment safely. This can be in the wall of the operating room, with long cables to the camera, or it can be in a mobile trolley or cabinet, perhaps with an extensible arm to support the 'resecting' monitor (Fig. 3.1). The less it is necessary to manhandle the equipment the less the risk of accidental damage. It is advisable to be able to lock the equipment into its housing, not only to prevent theft, but also to reduce the incidence of malfunction due to knob-twiddling by TV 'experts' or by accidental alteration of switches.

Constant irrigation systems

Constant irrigation with continuous removal of the irrigant during prostatic or bladder tumour resection keeps the TV image constant and makes it easier for an observer to follow. This can be achieved by an irrigating resectoscope sheath (the authors' preference) or a suprapubic cannula system. Intermittent irrigation means that the teaching process has to be interrupted every time the bladder fills and has to be emptied, making the teaching less effective and the operation slower because the surgeon has to find his place again after emptying the bladder.

Cameras

A modern three-element (each element now being a chip, formerly a tube) television camera produces the best image with regard to colour, crispness and resolution, but it is a bulky piece of equipment which does not lend itself to use in an urological operating room without a squad of assistants, cannot be coupled directly to the endoscope because of its size and has to be used through a jointed beam splitter. There is inevitable rotation at the joints with consequent loss of orientation of the TV image.

Modern single-chip cameras are small enough to fit directly onto the endoscope eyepiece without making it too clumsy to manipulate. They produce a remarkably clear image, with excellent depth of focus and colour reproduction. They can also be made waterproof, to allow disinfection by soaking. If the surgeon wants to operate by direct vision, using a beam splitter, this is not jointed and the problems of image orientation are minimal.

Basically only four chips are commercially available for chip cameras, so whatever camera one buys it will have one of them. They all have very similar performance. What else one gets will depend on what the manufacturer has decided to provide. A hand-held camera purchased in the High Street shop has all its working parts in one box – so it is relatively bulky – much too big for the urologist's purposes. In an endoscopic camera the chip has been separated from the works and connected by a cable.

Some camera manufacturers use a 12 volt system to power the camera for reasons of safety. Some put in zoom fitments. Some include colour bar generators. Some have automatic light balance. However, the signal processing is going to be what the chip manufacturer supplies so that, on the whole, modern chip cameras have fairly comparable performance and the urologist must look for what he wants.

Figure 3.4
(a) Modern lightweight camera system with a right-angled beam splitter. Courtesy of KeyMed. (b) Many modern cameras have no eyepiece, so the image can only be viewed on the monitor. Courtesy of Olympus.

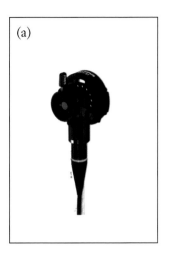

(a)

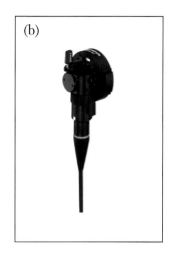

(b)

Cameras may be made to couple directly onto the telescope eyepiece (Fig. 3.3), or may be attached via a right-angled beam splitter (Fig. 3.4a). Many modern cameras have no eyepiece (Fig. 3.4b), so the image can only be viewed on the monitor. A direct coupled camera will rotate with the telescope so that the image will rotate on the monitor. To keep it still the camera must be held steady and not rotated with the endoscope; this needs an extra hand. As most urological surgeons like to use both hands on the endoscope this is inconvenient. A fitted beam splitter is more convenient as it will either swing on the eyepiece or have an inbuilt rotation point that keeps the camera steady in relation to the telescope, so that the image is always kept the right way up.

A camera sleeve should be used to prevent contamination of the camera with body fluids. Alternatively, more modern cameras can be sterilized between cases in solutions such as chlorine dioxide.

Monitors

Video monitors come in all sizes and qualities. As a general principle, the picture will be clearer and sharper if a monitor is purchased rather than a television set. So, if the salesman tells you that the 'monitor' can be used as a television set, you know you will not get the highest quality picture, however convenient it may be to watch the tennis when things get tedious. The size and number of monitors provided in the operating room is a personal (and financial) choice. It is the authors' experience that it is unwise to have a monitor with a screen measuring less than 28 inches. This can easily be suspended above or adjacent to the patient's abdomen for ease of use (Fig. 3.1).

Recording equipment

There is now a wide variety of digital recorders available for saving both still and 'video' footage of endoscopic procedures. The images may be saved in a variety of formats including on Zip discs, CDs and DVDs or as printed images (Fig. 3.5). These images can then be incorporated into lectures or simply saved as a record of what you saw at the time of surgery and what you did. What do you want to record? What will you do with the recordings when you have made them?

If a recording is needed for the records then a still printer is required – for something like a bladder tumour, for instance. But it is difficult to show the whole of a bladder tumour on one print if it is more than 1 cm across. It is necessary to take a long view of a sizeable tumour to keep it in frame. The human eye can cope with the inverse square law, being a better optical instrument, but the video camera cannot, and a large object cannot be illuminated adequately to produce a video image suitable for printing. The still video printer is still an expensive luxury and only one of the new digital recorders will provide prints that are good enough for publication (as in this book) but are mightily expensive as well as being prodigal of computer space.

If the requirement is to keep a tape or CD for a medico-legal record, the tape must be complete and unexpurgated. It will therefore be long (and boring to watch) and a consideration will be the cost of the video-tape or other recording format and the problem of storage. Videotape intended for lectures or teaching requires some method of editing the tape so that it is concise and interesting. That means at least another

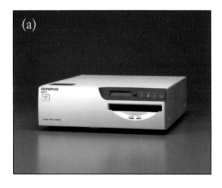

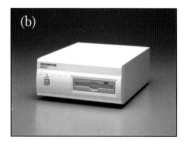

Figure 3.5
Modern recording equipment. Colour video printer and drive for recording images on Zip discs. Courtesy of KeyMed.

video cassette recorder, and it is not possible to get a tidily edited tape simply by cross-recording from one tape to another by using two VCRs. To edit a videotape properly requires an editing suite in which a computer links and controls the two VCRs. Videotape editing involves re-recording the scenes to be kept, in the order that is required, on a second tape (unlike ciné film editing when the film is physically cut with scissors and rejoined). Without computerized coordination of the two VCRs the end result is uneven and the joins between the re-recorded scenes are obtrusive. Such an editing suite is expensive, but you must have access to one because you must do the editing yourself, or supervise it personally, to achieve the result you require. Editing is made considerably easier in this era of digitalized images where sections of the recording can be cut and pasted as required.

The urologist setting up CCTV in the operating room should postpone the purchase of recording equipment until the system is installed and running. You may never want to record. Prints are of no great value. Making a videotape is time-consuming: it takes at least an hour and a half of editing and sound recording time to create 15 minutes of final tape, in addition to the time spent making the original video recording. It is also very expensive.

The best advice for the urologist seeking to put a CCTV system into the operating theatre is to try out all the equipment that is available from all the firms that sell it. See how each performs in your hands in your own operating room; decide what suits your requirements, and purchase as your budget permits. Since the cost of individual items of equipment is comparable wherever they are purchased it is more important to find out which firm will offer service and repair arrangements. Find out if the equipment has to go to Alaska for repair, or if it can be done locally, because one may take longer than the other. And wherever it does go, will the firm provide a loan replacement part to keep the CCTV system in action?

Should the urologist buy a CCTV package?

CCTV for the urological surgeon is provided by specialist suppliers. Most of these suppliers will provide a package which usually consists of their camera and beam splitter, a light source (which may or may not be dedicated) and a VCR. In many cases the package is enclosed in a trolley or cabinet of the supplier's own design, often of a modular pattern that can be varied to accommodate special requirements.

Most suppliers are open to negotiation as to the exact contents of their package. Most offer alternative format VCRs, or will leave it out of the package altogether. Some offer still image recorders. Most will agree to exclude the light source if the surgeon already has a suitable one, although the dedicated light source suppliers make the point that their camera works best with its own dedicated light source.

There are suppliers who will come to see what is required and are then prepared to put together a package to suit your requirements, subject to including their camera in the package. For this it is necessary for you to know what you want and to have had some experience in the use of CCTV, which might perhaps be called 'second generation' CCTV usage. Of course, if you do have experience in the use of CCTV and know all about electronics, go shopping for the necessary components and put together your own package and so save money. However, few surgeons have such expertise and you will find that the suppliers offer a good deal with good performance from most of their packages. The vital thing is to have an extended trial of the package on offer before purchase – if the supplier will not agree to this then go elsewhere.

How much does it all cost?

The cost of CCTV for urology will depend on where you work and whether the equipment is made locally or has to be imported. The most expensive equipment is not necessarily the best for your particular purpose. Look at the equipment that is available in your area; make sure that it is really what you want; compare the costs and try each set of equipment out. Discover the servicing arrangements on offer. You will then be in the best position to purchase a system which works for you and is within your budget.

What are the costs of running a CCTV system?

It is important to have a clear idea of what it will cost to run a CCTV system in the urology operating room or department. Once purchased and installed, electronic equipment is not expensive to run. The consumption of electricity is minimal. Some parts of the system have batteries which need to be replaced from time to time at nominal cost. If recording is to be done the cost of tapes must be added. Apart from these considerations there are no significant revenue implications of running a CCTV system, which is important information for the purchaser, whether this be the urology department, the Supplies Officer of the hospital or a charity providing the equipment. If good equipment is purchased and reasonable care is taken of it, it will cost no more to run than a domestic TV or hi-fi system.

It is essential to plan ahead in order to replace your equipment as time goes by because it will wear out and occasional unexpected breakdowns will occur. So keep spares where possible, particularly a light source lamp, and maintain a reserve of cash so that it is possible to replace parts rapidly and so keep the set-up going. Buy your equipment from someone who will offer a prompt and reliable repair and replacement service: you may wish to take out a service contract, but watch the price and be prepared to bargain.

Equipment with knobs attracts fiddlers like flies to rotten meat, and manufacturers seem impelled to fit multiple knobs on the front of all TV equipment for sales reasons. This lures the fiddler, who is usually a self-professed expert on all matters televisual. When the knob-fiddler has maladjusted everything in sight it can appear that the system has broken down. If the supplier is then called in to rescue the situation it can be expensive for what is actually simple adjustment. So wage war on fiddlers: fit locks, close doors, put up notices and, most important of all, learn how to do the adjustments. Anything which can be locked away after being set up and is thus invisible is an advantage.

Enthusiastic dusters are also a potential problem, changing the setting of a switch at the flick of a wrist. Dust covers and lids help, but take care not to operate electronic equipment under its plastic cover because it may overheat and malfunction. Likewise do not keep electronic equipment in a cold place and expect it to work instantly in a warm room, condensation being a potent cause of malfunction.

Diathermy and other interference

Diathermy interference is a mysterious and troublesome phenomenon which has plagued every urologist who has tried to set up CCTV in the operating theatre. Diathermy machines produce radio-frequency waves which get transmitted around the theatre, the various leads being excellent aerials. Operating rooms have wiring systems producing electrical fields capable of generating interference on CCTV systems, as may electrical equipment in an adjoining room. A surgeon hoping to use CCTV must try out the system in his own operating room. If the interference cannot be eliminated easily, do not buy that system. If interference appears when it was not there before, check that all electrical connections are clean and firm, that no lead is frayed or its insulating cover damaged, and that the various pieces of equipment are properly earthed. This check should be applied to all the electrical equipment in the operating room, and especially to the diathermy. If interference persists after an extensive check of all leads, etc., get the diathermy checked electrically as it may be that a minor circuit malfunction has developed.

References

1. Whitaker RH, Green NA, Notley RG. Is cervical spondylosis an occupational hazard for urologists? *Br J Urol* 1983;55:585–8.
2. McNicholas TA, Jones DJ, Sibley GN. AIDS: the contamination risk in urological surgery. *Br J Urol* 1989;63:565–8.
3. O'Boyle PJ. Video-endoscopy: the remote operating technique. *Br J Urol* 1990;65:557–9.

Chapter 4

Indications and preparations for transurethral resection of the prostate

Indications for TURP and diagnostic tests prior to TURP

The indications for TURP are bothersome lower urinary tract symptoms which fail to respond to changes in lifestyle or medical therapy; recurrent acute urinary retention; renal impairment due to bladder outlet obstruction (so-called high pressure *chronic* urinary retention); recurrent haematuria due to benign prostatic enlargement and bladder stones due to prostatic obstruction.

These indications are all relative. Indeed, one could say that there are no *absolute* indications for TURP. A man with renal impairment due to bladder outlet obstruction can always be managed with a long-term catheter rather than TURP. Some patients, particularly the very elderly and infirm, will find this an acceptable alternative to surgery. For those practising in the UK, one should remember that the British Association of Urological Surgeons (BAUS) Procedure Specific Consent Forms[1] state that alternative management options should be discussed with the patient (see Chapter 13, Medico-legal aspects of transurethral resection), one of which is a long-term catheter. While the surgeon may feel that a TURP is in the patient's best interest, clearly the decision to proceed with surgery rests with the patient. Having said this, most men with urinary retention will not wish to remain with a long-term catheter and will opt for TURP.

TURP for bothersome lower urinary tract symptoms

Changing terminology: 'LUTS' versus 'prostatism'

The 1990s saw a change in the terminology used to describe the symptom complex that we had traditionally associated with obstruction due to benign prostatic hyperplasia (BPH). We came to appreciate that the 'classic' prostatic symptoms of hesitancy, poor flow, frequency, urgency, nocturia and terminal dribbling bore little relationship to prostate size, flow rate, residual urine volume or indeed urodynamic evidence of bladder outlet obstruction[2]. Other studies showed that age-matched men and women had similar levels of urinary symptoms when assessed using the American Urological Association[3] symptom score[4]. Thus, the expression 'lower urinary tract symptoms' (LUTS) came into common use to describe the symptoms hitherto known as prostatism. This is a purely descriptive term which avoids any implication about the possible underlying cause of these symptoms[5].

More recently, one hears the expression 'LUTS/BPH' being used to describe the symptoms of BPH while others still use the term prostatism. In many ways it does not really matter whether one uses 'prostatism' or 'LUTS' to describe these symptoms or 'BPH', 'BPO' (benign prostatic obstruction), 'BPE' (benign prostatic enlargement), or 'BOO' (bladder outlet obstruction) to describe the possible underlying cause. What is important is to remember the non-prostatic causes of hesitancy, poor flow, feeling of incomplete emptying, frequency, urgency and nocturia and therefore to avoid operating on the prostate when the problem lies elsewhere. Knowing this, one can give the patient a realistic idea of how likely it is that his symptoms will respond to treatments 'aimed' at the prostate. He needs to know that prostate operations such as TURP will not always result in resolution of his symptoms. Thus, the new terminology is useful, but only because it reminds the urologist to consider these alternative causes of symptoms, which may have absolutely nothing to do with prostatic obstruction.

Clinical practice guidelines for BPH and LUTS – a word of warning

A number of clinical practice guidelines have been developed to streamline the approach to diagnosis and treatment in men presenting with symptoms suggestive of BPH[6]. While every available guideline for assessing BPH patients agrees that a history and examination should be taken, and that the severity of urinary symptoms should be formally assessed using a symptom score, there is considerable variation between guidelines in terms of the other diagnostic tests that they recommend. This is unfortunate, because clinical practice guidelines were developed to standardize the approach to diagnosis (and treatment) of the man presenting with urinary symptoms thought to be due to BPH. Some recommend that flow rate and residual urine volume should be measured, some state that these tests are optional, while others specifically state that these tests are not recommended. How can such wide variation between guidelines be possible? Surely the 'disease' we are dealing with is the same wherever the patient comes from? The reasons for these varations are complex, but at least part of the answer lies in the way in which guidelines have been designed, i.e. on their 'quality'.

Guideline quality can actually be measured against a set standard, using criteria based on the system used to create the guidelines[7]. Some guidelines make no mention of the search strategy used for obtaining the evidence on which their recommendations are made, while others do not identify the methods used to assess the strength of the evidence they quote. High quality clinical practice guidelines rank this evidence according to whether it is derived from randomized controlied trials or based on descriptive evidence such as case-series or case reports (evidence from randomized controlled trials being regarded as 'stronger'). Low quality guidelines do not do this. Interestingly, higher quality BPH guidelines are *less* likely to recommend lots of diagnostic tests[7]. They seem to keep the diagnostic approach to the man presenting with urinary symptoms fairly simple, measuring symptom scores, analysing the urine, obtaining a voiding diary and doing little else. This should not be taken to mean that a careful history to exclude other non-BPH causes of urinary symptoms is not important (in fact, these additional features of the history and examination, as outlined below, are terribly important). But what it does mean is that there must be good evidence that measuring flow rates or doing pressure-flow studies, for example, really do help in deciding what to do and in predicting the outcome from treatment.

Because there is such variability between the various guidelines, it is not possible to recommend one over the other, and of course what guidelines you use will to a considerable degree depend on what part of the world you practise in[8–15]. However, maintaining a healthy scepticism in such things is no bad thing for the practising urologist.

A history, basic examination and some simple investigations can help to determine whether the cause of the patient's symptoms lies in the prostate, in the urethra or bladder or elsewhere.

History and examination

Baseline symptoms can be 'measured' using a symptoms index and the most widely used is the International Prostate Symptom Score (IPSS), which is a modified version of the AUA symptom index (Fig. 4.1).

A history of macroscopic haematuria or the finding of dipstick or microscopic haematuria is clearly an indication for flexible cystoscopy and upper tract imaging to exclude the presence of, for example, a bladder or renal cancer. Similarly, marked frequency and urgency, particularly when also combined with bladder pain, can occasionally be due to carcinoma in situ

	Not at all	Less than 1 time in 5	Less than half the time	About half the time	More than half the time	Almost always	Score
Incomplete emptying. Over the last month, how often have you had a sensation of not emptying your bladder completely after you finish urinating?	0	1	2	3	4	5	
Frequency. Over the last month, how often have you had to urinate again in less than 2 hours after you finished urinating?	0	1	2	3	4	5	
Intermittency. Over the past month, how often have you found you stopped and started again several times when you urinated?	0	1	2	3	4	5	
Urgency. Over the past month, how often have you found it difficult to postpone urination?	0	1	2	3	4	5	
Weak stream. Over the past month, how often have you had a weak urinary stream?	0	1	2	3	4	5	
Straining. Over the past month, how often have you had to push or strain to begin urination?	0	1	2	3	4	5	
Nocturia. Over the past month, how many times did you most typically get up to urinate from the time you went to bed at night until the time you got up in the morning?	0	1	2	3	4	5	
Total IPSS score							

Quality of life due to symptoms	Delighted	Pleased	Mostly satisfied	Mixed – about equally satisfied and dissatisfied	Mostly dissatisfied	Unhappy	Terrible
If you were to spend the rest of your life with your urinary condition just the way it is now, how would you feel about that?	0	1	2	3	4	5	

Figure 4.1
The International Prostate Symptom Score (IPSS).

of the bladder and one should have a low threshold for obtaining urine for cytology and for performing flexible cystoscopy in such cases.

Recent onset of bedwetting in an elderly man is an important symptom, because it usually allows one to make a diagnosis of high pressure chronic retention. In such cases there is gross distension of the abdomen with high bladder pressures leading to back pressure on the kidneys and impaired renal function[16]. Visual inspection of the patient's abdomen may show marked distension due to a grossly enlarged bladder. The diagnosis of chronic retention can be confirmed by palpation of the enlarged, tense bladder, which is dull to percussion.

Rarely, lower urinary tract symptoms can be due to neurological disease causing spinal cord or cauda equina compression or to pelvic or sacral tumours. There will usually be associated symptoms such as back pain, sciatica, ejaculatory disturbances, and sensory disturbances in the legs, feet and perineum. In these rare cases, loss of pericoccygeal or perineal sensation (sacral nerve roots 2–4) indicates an interruption to the sensory innervation of the bladder and an MRI scan will confirm the clinical suspicion that there is a neurological problem.

Digital rectal examination (DRE)
A discussion of the merits (or otherwise) of prostate cancer screening in men presenting with urinary symptoms is beyond the scope of this book, but it is important to know that the UK National Institute for Clinical Excellence (NICE) Guidelines[17] and the European Association of Urology (EAU) Guidelines[18] on diagnosis of BPH recommend that a digital rectal examination should be done to detect nodules which may indicate an underlying prostate cancer. Most current 'BPH' guidelines recommend a discussion with the patient about the pros and cons of PSA (prostate-specific antigen) testing.

Assessment of prostate size
Apart from being recommended to determine whether the patient has prostate cancer or not, a digital rectal examination (DRE) is also used to give an indication of prostate size. While the size of the prostate does not correlate with severity of symptoms and prostatic enlargement is not in itself an indication for treatment, it is useful to have an idea of prostate size before embarking upon surgical treatment. DRE gives a *rough* estimate of prostate size and if one suspects that the prostate is markedly enlarged, a transrectal ultrasound can be performed to provide a more accurate assessment of its volume. A large prostate could be an indication for an open prostatectomy. It is better for the surgeon to know in advance that an open prostatectomy may be necessary. An accurate assessment of prostate size prior to operation can avoid unexpected conversion from TURP to open prostatectomy. In the National

Prostatectomy Audit[19] there was a need to convert from TURP to open prostatectomy in 10 of 4226 TURPs (0.2%).

The larger the prostate, the more challenging TURP is likely to be and the more inclined the surgeon is to recommend open prostatectomy. Precisely what constitutes 'large' is a matter of opinion. Some surgeons are happy to resect 75 g of prostate, while others will struggle to remove this volume of tissue transurethrally. Many surgeons, however, will give serious consideration to open prostatectomy for glands estimated to be greater than 75g in size. Apart from detecting prostate cancer, this is the principal reason for palpating the prostate by rectal examination when you are thinking about performing a TURP. Prostate size can also have a bearing on drug treatment of prostate symptoms. Treatment with prostate-shrinking 5-alpha reductase inhibitors tends to be confined to the larger prostate.

There may be other factors present which incline one towards open prostatectomy and these can usually be established from the history and examination. Some patients have orthopaedic problems which prevent abduction or flexion of their hip joints, such that the surgeon simply cannot get between their legs to perform a TURP. The presence of bladder stones which are too large for endoscopic cystolitholapaxy, combined with marked enlargement of the prostate is an indication for open prostatectomy. Rarely the patient may have such a long urethra that even a long resectoscope may not allow transurethal access to the entire length of the prostate, and in this situation one has no choice but to remove the prostate by an open technique. This finding usually only becomes apparent at the time of surgery (although a particularly large prostate on DRE may alert you to this possibility), so it is as well to mention the occasional need to resort to open prostatectomy to all patients prior to TURP. However, it is uncommon nowadays not to know in advance that you are likely to have to perform an open prostatectomy.

Tests

Urine culture
The urine should be cultured to determine whether there is infection. This may be the cause of the patient's symptoms, although if this is so, it will usually be obvious from the presence of suprapubic discomfort and pain or 'scalding' in the urethra on voiding. In patients with a positive urine culture, a short course of antibiotics for a few days before TURP will reduce the likelihood of postoperative septicaemia.

Frequency-volume chart
Patients with nocturia should be asked to estimate the volume of urine they void at night. Elderly men and women lose the diurnal rhythm of

urine production, whereby daytime urine output is greater than that at night. Production of large night-time volumes of urine – nocturnal polyuria – can be confirmed by getting the patient to complete a frequency-volume chart or voiding diary, where urine volume is recorded along with the time of each void (Fig. 4.2). It is not surprising that nocturnal polyuria, a fluid balance disorder rather than a prostate problem, does not improve following TURP. Failure to appreciate that nocturia could be due to nocturnal polyuria might account, at least historically, for nocturia being one of the least likely symptoms to improve following TURP. Many men treated with TURP for nocturia probably had nocturnal polyuria.

Serum creatinine
Serum creatinine should be measured to detect renal failure secondary to high pressure urinary retention[18,20,21]. An elevated creatinine may obviously also be due to primary renal disease, which by impairing renal

Figure 4.2
Frequency volume chart.

Monday	Tuesday	Wednesday	Thursday	Friday	Saturday	Sunday
7am 100 ml	7.30am 250 ml	8am 200 ml	7.30am 250 ml	7am 250 ml	7am 100 ml	7.30am 250 ml
10 am 300 ml	9am 200 ml	9.45am 200 ml	10 am 300 ml	10.15am 175 ml	9am 200 ml	10 am 300 ml
1pm 250 ml	11am 200 ml	11am 250 ml	1pm 250 ml	12.00 150 ml	1pm 250 ml	1pm 250 ml
4pm 200 ml	1.30pm 150 ml	1.30pm 150 ml	4.15pm 150 ml	2pm 150 ml	8.30pm 300 ml	2pm 150 ml
8.30pm 300 ml	4.30pm 150 ml	5pm 350 ml	6.30pm 200 ml	5pm 250 ml	10pm 250 ml	6.30pm 200 ml
11pm 200 ml	7pm 150 ml	8pm 200 ml	10pm 200 ml	7.30pm 150 ml	2am 250 ml	7.30pm 150 ml
1am 150 ml	10pm 250 ml	11.30pm 200 ml	2am 250 ml	11pm 200 ml	4am 200 ml	11pm 250 ml
4am 200 ml	2am 250 ml	2.30am 150 ml	4.30am 150 ml	3am 200 ml		2.30am 150 ml
	4.30am 150 ml	5am 200 ml				5am 250 ml
	6am 200 ml					

concentrating ability can lead to high day and night-time voided volumes and hence daytime frequency and nocturia. One should consider other causes for polyuria, such as poorly controlled diabetes, the resulting glycosuria causing an osmotic induced diuresis, with consequent frequency and nocturia. A simple urine dipstick test for glucose can make the diagnosis.

Post-void residual urine volume
Post-void residual urine (PVR) volume measurement – the volume remaining in the bladder at the end of micturition – is recommended by the 4th International Consultation on BPH[21], but is regarded as an optional test by the AUA[20] (Fig. 4.3).

Residual urine volume measurement is useful (along with measurement of serum creatinine) as a safety measure. It gives an indication about the likelihood of the patient experiencing back pressure on his kidneys and thus it tells the urologist whether it is safe to offer watchful waiting rather than TURP. The Veterans Administration Cooperative Study on Transurethral Resection of the Prostate has shown that in men with moderate urinary symptoms it is safe *not* to operate where the post-void residual volume is <350 ml[22]. In this study over 500 men with residual urine volume <350 ml were randomized to watchful waiting or TURP. Most patients in the watchful waiting arm did not progress to requiring a TURP nor did they show a rise in creatinine or in residual urine volume. At 3 years of follow-up in the watchful waiting group, average residual urine volume had actually decreased by 40 ml from baseline.

Bates *et al* have recently shown that when one observes men with large residual urine volumes over several years (rather than proceeding with

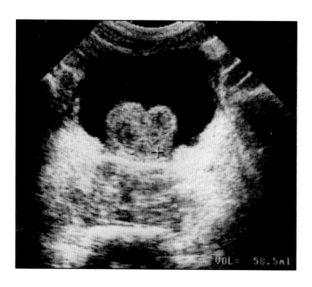

Figure 4.3
Abdominal ultrasound scan showing a small volume of residual urine in the bladder (approximately 58 ml) and a large middle lobe impression.

TURP) complications such as renal failure, acute retention and urinary tract infection are uncommon[23]. In this study, 93 men with residual urine volumes averaging 363 ml and ranging from 250 to 700 ml were observed for an average of 5 years. Over this time period residual urine volume remained stable in 50%, fell in 30% and increased in 20%. A third of men went on to have a TURP for serum creatinine elevation, acute retention, increasing residual urine volume or for worsening symptoms. Thus, one can 'get away' without the need for TURP in men with relatively high residual urine volumes, but as the study authors recommended, out-patient surveillance in this group of patients is a sensible idea.

One of the problems of using residual urine as an indication for TURP is its day to day variability. In a substantial proportion of patients there is considerable variation in residual volumes measured either on the same or on different days[24,25]. In two-thirds of men Birch et al[24] found wide variations in residual volumes on at least two measurements on the same day. Bruskewitz et al repeated residual volume measurements between two and five times on the same day by in and out catheterization and found wide variation within individual patients between repeat measurements[25]. Dunsmuir et al[26] measured residual volume in 42 men with 'BPH symptoms' on *different* days over a 3-month period and found that in two-thirds the volume varied between 150 and 670 ml! This represented an average variation within a single individual of 42% between repeated measures. Thus, a patient may have a high residual urine volume on one day and a low one on another. Which volume measurement does one then believe?

The second problem with residual urine volume measurement is that it cannot predict symptomatic outcome from TURP[27,28]. For these reasons, residual urine volume measurement is regarded as an optional test in the AUA guidelines.

It has been suggested – indeed it seems intuitive – that an elevated residual urine volume predisposes to urinary infection. There is surprisingly little evidence that this is the case. In fact, what evidence there is relating residual volume to urine infection suggests that an elevated residual urine may not, at least in the neurologically normal adult, pre-dispose to urine infection. Riehmann et al[29] found that the presence of bacteriuria in 30 of 99 institutionalized men was *not* associated with residual urine volume, nor with age, previous diagnosis of 'BPH' or presence of urinary symptoms. Hampson et al[30] studied the presence of pyuria and active urinary infection in a large group of adult male and female patients, measuring residual urine volumes by ultrasound or during urodynamic studies. Pyuria and active urinary tract infection (UTI) were present in 18% and 10% of patients with a residual urine volume of <100 ml and in 26% and 18%, respectively, of patients with a residual volume >100 ml. There were no significant differences in the chances of pyuria or UTI between any of these groups and it was concluded that an elevated residual urine volume did not predispose to infection in neurologically normal adults.

Flow rate measurement

Measurement of flow rate (Fig. 4.4) is regarded as an *optional* test by the AUA[20], *recommended* by the 4th International Consultation on BPH[21], and the EAU BPH Guidelines state that it 'is *obligatory* prior to undertaking surgical treatment'[18].

   In men with 'prostatic' symptoms, flow rate varies substantially on a given day[31] by an average of 2 ml/s between first and second voids, by 4 ml/s between the first and third void and by as much as 5 ml/s if a fourth flow is done. These changes occur in the absence of any change in voided volumes between repeated flow tests. Rather as with residual urine volume estimation, which flow rate should you base your decision on treatment on?

   Uroflowmetry alone cannot distinguish between low flow due to bladder outlet obstruction and that due to a poorly contractile bladder. Some

Figure 4.4
Uroflowmetry.
(a) A normal flow rate.
(b) In prostatic obstruction.

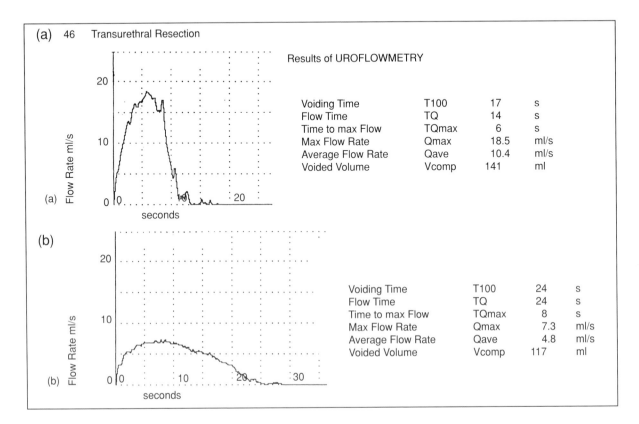

studies suggest that men with poor outcomes are more likely to have had higher flows pre-operatively compared with those with good outcomes[32-34], whereas other studies report equivalent improvements in symptoms whether or not pre-operative flow rate is high or low[27,35]. In the more recent Veterans Administration trial of TURP versus watchful waiting, Bruskewitz *et al*[28] found that flow rate could not predict the likelihood of a good symptomatic outcome after TURP.

So, whether one measures flow rate or not prior to TURP will probably depend very much on whether one is working in North America (in which case you may well not) or Europe (in which case guidelines recommend that you should).

Pressure-flow studies

Pressure-flow studies are probably better at predicting symptomatic outcome after TURP than are residual urine volume and flow rate. However, most patients without obstruction have a good outcome and the time and cost of performing pressure-flow studies routinely is perceived by most urologists as not worth the effort. A Gallup Organization poll of urologists carried out in the USA in 1995 perhaps provides the most telling statement about what practising urologists regard as important pre-operative 'urodynamic' measurements[36]. Of this random sample of 514 urologists, 53% routinely measured urine flow rates when evaluating men with symptoms of BPH, 71% routinely estimated residual urine volume and only 11% routinely used pressure-flow studies. This must tell us something about the perception urologists have of the ability of these tests to help them in day to day decision making in men presenting with urinary symptoms thought to be due to BPH.

Renal ultrasonography

Koch has shown that renal ultrasound is only useful if serum creatinine is elevated above the normal range. The percentage of patients having upper tract dilatation on ultrasound according to their serum creatinine level was: creatinine <115 μmol/l, 0.8%; creatinine 115–130 μmol/l, 9%; and creatinine >130 μmol/l, 33%[37]. As a consequence Koch and colleagues recommended upper tract imaging only if the creatinine level was >130 μmol/l, if the residual urine volume was >150 ml with a serum creatinine between 115 and 130 μmol/l or in patients presenting with urinary retention.

In terms of diagnostic tests in patients with LUTS who we are considering for TURP we culture the urine and measure serum creatinine. We obtain a frequency volume chart where nocturia is a prominent symptom. We do not routinely measure urine flow rate or post-void residual urine volume, nor do we routinely perform renal ultrasonography in patients with a serum creatinine below 130 μmol/l.

Recurrent acute urinary retention

A focused history and examination combined with selected tests along the lines of those discussed above for a man presenting with symptoms should be carried out in any patient presenting with urinary retention.

Retention may be precipitated by a variety of factors in the absence of a significant degree of prostatic obstruction, and when the precipitating factor has resolved or been removed, the patient may enjoy many years of normal voiding without requiring a TURP. The classic example would be postoperative urinary retention. This can be managed by a short period with a catheter and is often followed by successful voiding once the patient is more mobile, postoperative pain has settled down and the effects of anaesthetic and other drugs have washed out of his system.

Remember to exclude the rare but important causes of retention other than simple prostatic obstruction. Be particularly wary of the man with a history of constipation and of back pain which keeps him awake at night, especially if this has become severe in the weeks before the episode of retention. A neurological cause for retention should be excluded in such cases.

Many urologists will try to avoid proceeding straight to TURP after just one episode of retention, instead recommending a trial of catheter removal, with or without an alpha-blocker, in the hope that the patient will void spontaneously and avoid the need for operation. A trial without catheter is clearly not appropriate in cases where there is back pressure on the kidneys, so-called high pressure retention (see below). About a quarter of men with acute retention will void successfully after a trial without catheter[38–40]. Of those who pass urine successfully after an initial episode of retention, about 50% will go back into retention within a week, 60% within a month and 70% after a year. This means that after 1 year, only about 1 in 10 men originally presenting with urinary retention will not have gone back into retention. Recurrent retention is more likely in those with a flow rate <5 ml/s or average voided volumes of <150 ml. An alpha-blocker started 24 hours before a trial of catheter removal increases the chances of voiding successfully (30% taking placebo voiding successfully, and 50% taking an alpha-blocker[41]). However, whether continued use of an alpha-blocker after an episode of acute retention reduces the risk of a further episode of retention[42] is not yet known.

Comparable studies with prostate-shrinking treatments such as finasteride have not been done in patients who have already had an episode of retention. However, patients in retention from malignant prostatic obstruction may void successfully after a few weeks of an indwelling catheter and an LHRH agonist such Zoladex with cyproterone acetate 'cover'[43]. Hampson reported that in men presenting with acute retention with associated prostate cancer diagnosed on needle biopsy (retention volume <800 ml), 30% voided successfully within 1 month of starting treatment, another 30% voided within 2 months of starting treatment and another 20% voided at 3 months. Conversely, only 40% of those with larger retention volumes voided successfully after treatment with hormone therapy. Thus, a substantial proportion of men with malignant retention can avoid the need for TURP by treatment with hormone therapy, and for the elderly, frail man this may be an appealing option.

It is our pratice to recommend a trial of catheter removal in all men presenting with acute retention, as long as there is no evidence of back pressure on the kidneys. We give patients with retention and malignant prostates the option of treatment with an LHRH agonist followed by catheter removal 2–3 months after commencement of treatment.

High pressure chronic retention
Mitchell[16] defined high pressure chronic retention of urine as maintenance of voiding, with a bladder volume of >800 ml and an intravesical pressure above 30 cm H_2O, often accompanied by hydronephrosis[44]. Over time this leads to renal failure. When the patient is suddenly unable to pass urine, so-called acute-on-chronic high pressure retention of urine has occurred.

A man with high pressure retention who continues to void spontaneously may be unaware that there is anything wrong. He will often have no sensation of incomplete emptying and his bladder seems to be insensitive to the gross distension. Often the first presenting symptom is that of bedwetting. This is such an unpleasant and disruptive symptom that it will cause most people to visit their doctor. In such cases inspection of the abdomen will show gross distension of the bladder, which may be confirmed by palpation and percussion of the tense bladder. On catheterization a large volume of urine is drained from the bladder (often in the order of 1–2 L and sometimes much greater). The serum creatinine will be elevated and an ultrasound will show hydronephrosis with a grossly distended bladder if the scan is done before relief of retention. These patients may develop a profound diuresis following drainage of the bladder and a small percentage show a postural drop in blood pressure. It is wise to admit such patients for a short period of observation, until the diuresis has settled. A few will require intravenous fluid replacement if they experience a symptomatic fall in blood pressure when standing.

The treatment choices for high pressure chronic retention, whether the patient is able to void spontaneously or has gone into retention, are either a TURP or a long-term catheter[45]. A trial without catheter is clearly not appropriate in cases where there is back pressure on the kidneys. Very rarely a patient who wants to avoid a TURP and does not want an indwelling catheter will be able to empty their bladder by intermittent self-catheterization, but such cases are exceptional.

Recurrent haematuria due to benign prostatic enlargement

An enlarged, vascular prostate may cause recurrent episodes of frank haematuria, sometimes resulting in clot retention or anaemia. Clearly other causes of haematuria such as bladder or renal cancer should be excluded. In terms of treatment there is some evidence that finasteride may be helpful. Kearney and colleagues[46] reported that 41 of 53 (77%) patients given finasteride for recurrent haematuria due to BPH experienced no further bleeding and similar results have been reported by others[47,48]. However, the effectiveness of finasteride compared with placebo has not been tested. We try to avoid TURP in patients whose main symptom is haematuria due to BPH, preferring instead to treat such cases with a 5-alpha reductase inhibitor.

Bladder stone

The presence of a bladder stone (Fig. 4.5) is a classic indication for TURP. In an autopsy study of over 1600 men and women, Grosse found that bladder stones were eight times more frequent in men with histological evidence of BPH (3.4% vs 0.4%). This implies that bladder stones are caused by bladder outlet obstruction due to BPH[49].

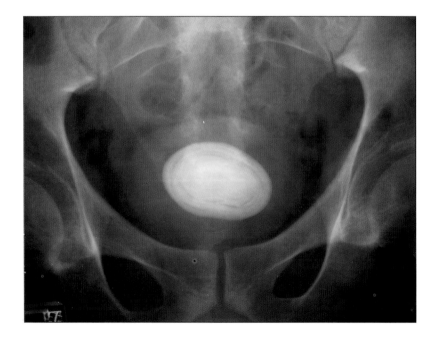

Figure 4.5
A bladder stone.

Preparation for TURP in the weeks before surgery

Stopping antiplatelet drugs and non-steroidal anti-inflammatory drugs (NSAIDs)

It is our current practice to stop antiplatelet drugs, including NSAIDs, 10 days prior to surgery.

The risk of postoperative bleeding in patients taking these drugs should be balanced against the risks of stopping antiplatelet therapy. There are no hard and fast rules. In a recent editorial review in the *British Journal of Urology* Mak and Amoroso stated that 'consideration should be given to withholding these agents before elective surgery', but no specific advice was given beyond this[50].

In a series of 125 TURPs, Thurston and Briant[51] reported that 50% of patients on aspirin (seven of 14) required more than 2 units of blood post-TURP compared with 30% in those not on aspirin. While this is not a great difference, those on aspirin who did require blood received on average 10 units each, suggesting that the postoperative bleeding in those on aspirin could be very heavy indeed. This was not a prospective study randomizing one group to aspirin and the other to placebo, so other differences between the aspirin and non-aspirin groups (such as greater age in the aspirin group) could explain the higher transfusion rate in the former. Wierod *et al*[52] found that patients undergoing TURP while on aspirin or NSAIDs received significantly more units of blood transfused than those not on these drugs: 11% of those on aspirin or NSAIDs required 2 or more units of blood compared with 5% of those not on these drugs.

The majority of studies support stopping these agents several days before elective surgery (10 days before for aspirin and 7 days before for the newer agents such as clopidrogel).

Anaesthetists are concerned about the possibility of causing epidural haematomas in patients undergoing regional anaesthesia such as epidurals while on antiplatelet drugs and NSAIDs. The combination of an antiplatelet agent with an NSAID seems to be worse than either agent alone[53]. This is another reason for stopping these drugs prior to TURP.

Haemoglobin, creatinine, typing and saving serum

It goes without saying that the haemoglobin level should be checked before any operation where there is the potential for blood loss. Serum creatinine should also be checked to determine whether there is impairment of renal function. Serum should be grouped and saved, as blood transfusion is required in a significant percentage of men. In the National Prostatectomy Audit approximately 8% of patients undergoing TURP for retention and 3% of those undergoing TURP for symptoms required >2 units of blood.

Immediate pre-op preparation for TURP

Antibiotics

It is our current practice to give antibiotic prophylaxis for all patients undergoing TURP. Our choice of antibiotic is based on urine culture results done some weeks before surgery (a mid-stream specimen in those not in retention and a catheter specimen in those who presented with urinary retention). If an organism is grown which is sensitive to a specific antibiotic, we start treatment with this antibiotic 48 hours before operation and continue these for a total of 10 days (which for the majority of patients with an organism cultured before surgery means a short course of antibiotics continued after discharge). If the urine is sterile, we still give antibiotic prophylaxis in the form of oral nitrofurantoin 1 hour before the patient is called to the operating theatre, with a dose of intravenous gentamicin (1.5 mg/kg of weight) at induction of anaesthesia. When the catheter is removed a few days after surgery, again we administer a prophylactic dose of 100 mg of oral nitrofurantoin, again 1 hour before the catheter is removed. This policy is based on advice from our microbiology department, which routinely audits the organisms grown on urine culture, and appropriate antibiotic sensitivities.

Giving every patient antibiotics raises the chance of breeding multi-resistant organisms and also runs the risk of antibiotic-associated complications such as allergic reactions and anaphylaxis. However, in practice if the prophylactic antibiotics are restricted to either a single dose or a 24-hour course, antibiotic resistance will either not occur or will be of no consequence. The risk of antibiotic resistance and of allergic reactions must be balanced by the risk of postoperative urinary tract infection and septicaemia.

Positive blood cultures and the risk of septicaemia seem to be reduced by routine prophylaxis[54]. A large and well designed randomized placebo-controlled study of over 750 men showed that in men with *sterile* urine prior to TURP, septicaemia occurred in 1.5% of patients receiving no antibiotic prophylaxis, but did not occur in those receiving a single dose or a short course of intravenous ceftazidime[55]. It could be argued that routine antibiotic prophylaxis is expensive, but the cost of avoiding the need to treat septicaemia – which often requires a period in the Intensive Care Unit – will more than offset the costs of a policy of routine prophylaxis. This study also showed that the postoperative UTI rate was substantially lower for those who received antibiotic prophylaxis. Again, this is likely to offset the costs of a policy of routine prophylaxis.

The optimum antibiotic prophylaxis prior to TURP has not been established. It is wise to seek the advice of your local microbiology department with regard to the local bacterial flora and patterns of antibiotic resistance, and to base your policy on their advice.

Antibiotics in patients with heart murmurs and artificial heart valves

The *British National Formulary*, a joint publication of the British Medical Association and the Royal Pharmaceutical Society of Great Britain[56] is widely used in the UK as a reference for indications for drug treatments. For patients with heart murmurs and those with prosthetic heart valves it recommends that 1 g of i.v. amoxycillin with 120 mg of gentamicin should be given at induction of anaesthesia, with an additional dose of oral amoxycillin 500 mg 6 hours later (substituting vancomycin 1 g for those who are allergic to penicillin).

Antibiotic prophylaxis for patients with joint replacements

The American Academy of Orthopaedic Surgeons (AAOS) and the American Urological Association (AUA) have issued joint advice on antibiotic prophylaxis in such patients[57]. Their advice is that antibiotic prophylaxis is not indicated for urological patients who have pins, plates or screws, nor for most patients with total joint replacements. They did, however, recommend that antibiotics be given to all patients undergoing urological procedures, including TURP within 2 years of a prosthetic joint replacement, for those who are immunocompromised (e.g. rheumatoid patients, those with systemic lupus erythematosus, drug-induced immunosuppression including steroids), and for those with co-morbidities including a history of previous joint infection, haemophilia, HIV infection, diabetes and malignancy.

The antibiotic regime that has been recommended is a single dose of a quinolone, such as 500 mg of ciprofloxacin, 1–2 hours pre-operatively, plus ampicillin 2 g i.v. and gentamicin 1.5 mg/kg 30–60 minutes pre-operatively (substituting vancomycin 1 g i.v. for patients who are allergic to penicillin). It is obviously sensible to culture the patient's urine pre-operatively and use alternative drugs if a specific organism is grown.

However, in the UK a Working Party of the British Society for Antimicrobial Chemotherapy[56] has stated that 'patients with prosthetic joint implants (including total hip replacements) do not require antibiotic prophylaxis … The Working Party considers that it is unacceptable to expose patients to the adverse effects of antibiotics when there is no evidence that such prophylaxis is of any benefit'. This advice is based on the rationale that joint infections are caused by skin organisms that get onto the prosthesis at the time of the operation and that the role of bacteraemia as a cause of seeding, outside the immediate postoperative period, has never been established.

Our policy is to use the same antibiotic prophylaxis as for patients without joint prostheses. Clearly those surgeons who work in the USA are likely to follow the advice of the AUA.

Prophylaxis against deep venous thrombosis and pulmonary embolism

As with many surgical procedures, TURP is associated with a risk of venous thromboembolism, in the form of deep venous thrombosis (DVT) or more seriously pulmonary embolus (PE). There is good evidence that patients undergoing TURP are in a hypercoagulable state[58]. In contemporary studies of complications following TURP (those published since 1990), between 0.1 and 0.2% of patients experience a pulmonary embolus[59] (see Chapter 11).

All patients undergoing TURP in our department are fitted with above-knee TED stockings (thromboembolism stockings) and these are worn until discharge. In addition, we routinely use intermittent pneumatic compression boots (Fig. 4.6) during the operation and until the patient starts to mobilize after the operation (usually the morning after surgery). We encourage early postoperative mobilization.

The American College of Chest Physicians (ACCP) Guidelines on prevention of venous thromboembolism are generally regarded to be the standard of care for DVT and pulmonary embolus prevention[60]. They are based on an extensive review of the literature relating to the prevention of venous thromboembolism. The quality of the evidence establishing the optimal DVT prophylaxis for urologic surgery is not as good as that for orthopaedic surgery and for this reason the ACCP guidelines state that for urological patients 'the optimal approach to thromboprophylaxis is not known'. This uncertainty presumably accounts for the variable approach to DVT and pulmonary embolus prophylaxis shown in a recent survey of British urologists; 80% of urologists responded to the survey. Three-quarters routinely used prophylaxis in men undergoing TURP and a quarter did not[61]. Of those who employed prophylaxis, 80% used mechanical methods, and 20% used heparin, either alone or with anti-thromboembolic stockings.

Figure 4.6
Above-knee TED stockings (thromboembolism stockings) (a) and intermittent pneumatic compression boots (b) used to reduce the risk of deep venous thrombosis.

(a)

(b)

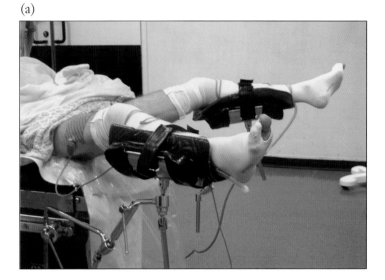

The options for prophylaxis include early postoperative mobilization, TED stockings, subcutaneous heparin (low dose unfractionated heparin or one of the newer low molecular weight heparins) or intermittent pneumatic compression boots. TED stockings provide graduated, static compression of the calves, thereby reducing venous stasis, and are known to reduce the risk of thrombosis and embolism after surgery[62]. Heparin, a sulphated glycosaminoglycan, is a naturally occurring anti-coagulant in human tissue, which inhibits thrombin (factor Xa) and other intrinsic pathway coagulation factors. In unfractionated preparations the heparin molecules are polymerized with molecular weights ranging from 5000 to 30 000 daltons. Low molecular weight heparin is depolymerized so the molecular weight is in the order of 4000–5000 daltons. Intermittent pneumatic compression boots which are placed around the calves are intermittently inflated and deflated, thereby increasing the flow of blood in the veins of the calf. This has been shown to reduce the risk of thrombosis after urological surgery[63].

The American Guidelines on DVT and pulmonary embolus prevention and also the British Thromboembolic Risk Factors (THRIFT) Consensus Group[64] categorize the risk of development of venous thromboembolism from low to moderate to high risk. Low risk patients are defined by both groups as those aged under the age of 40 who are undergoing minor surgery, defined as surgery lasting <30 minutes, and with no additional risk factors. No specific measures to prevent DVT are required in such patients other than early mobilization. Clearly, patients undergoing TURP are not low risk, according to this definition. Increasing age and duration of surgery increase the risk of thrombosis and pulmonary embolism. High risk patients include those undergoing non-major surgery (defined by THRIFT as that lasting >30 minutes) who are aged >60. Most patients undergoing TURP are likely to be aged >60 years and will therefore fall into a higher risk group.

The ACCP recommends that such patients should receive either low dose unfractionated heparin 8-hourly or once-daily low molecular weight heparin or should be fitted with intermittent pneumatic compression boots. Combining one or other of these measures with above-knee TED stockings worn throughout the duration of the patient's hospital stay would seem a sensible way of reducing the risk of DVT and pulmonary embolus after TURP. The only contraindications to TED stockings are peripheral vascular disease and peripheral neuropathy. Patients may have additional risk factors such as a history of previous DVT or pulmonary embolism, and in this situation the recommendations are to use a combination of preventative measures, such as heparin together with intermittent pneumatic compression boots.

What is the risk of bleeding when heparin is used as DVT prophylaxis in patients undergoing TURP? The studies that have addressed this question have involved small numbers of patients, are inadequately powered from a statistical perspective and poorly designed, and moreover the results are contradictory. Wilson and colleagues[65] showed no difference in blood loss in 30 patients randomized to receive 5000 units of unfractionated heparin 2 hours before surgery when compared with 30 patients who received no heparin. A third of patients in each group received a blood transfusion. In a double-blind prospective study comparing heparin against normal saline, Bejjani et al[66] found no difference in the risk of pulmonary embolus or postoperative blood loss, but the study comprised just 34 patients. Conversely, Sleight[67] reported that low dose subcutaneous heparin significantly increased blood loss during and after TURP. In this non-randomized, non-blinded study comparing blood loss in 50 control patients followed by 48 patients who received heparin, 38 units of blood were required in the heparin group and 7 in the control group, for comparable resected volumes.

It is difficult to draw conclusions from these studies. Some surgeons favour use of subcutaneous heparin and do not perceive an increased risk of peri-operative bleeding with its use. Others do not use it, presumably because of a perceived fear of haemorrhage. Practice in situations where there are no specific guidelines is often based upon personal experiences. The surgeon who has experienced the death of a patient from pulmonary embolus is probably more likely to use heparin, whereas the surgeon who has experienced problems with heavy postoperative bleeding in a patient on heparin will probably use an alternative form of prophylaxis, such as anti-thromboembolic stockings or intermittent pneumatic compression boots. It is our current practice *not* to use heparin as thrombosis prophylaxis.

If you do use subcutaneous heparin as DVT prophylaxis, it is important to be aware of the potential risk of a spinal haematoma that can occur with spinal anaesthesia. Although rare, this complication can be devastating, leading to permanent paralysis. It occurs more frequently with low molecular weight heparin than with low dose unfractionated heparin. For those who use low molecular weight heparin, the American guidelines[60] state that insertion of a spinal needle should be delayed until the anticoagulant effect of low molecular weight heparin is minimal, which is approximately 12 hours after administration of subcutaneous low molecular weight heparin. It should also not be given for 2 hours after the spinal needle has been inserted. These guidelines also apply to low dose unfractionated heparin. Thus, if using heparin there is a 14-hour window (12 hours before and 2 hours after) around insertion of the spinal needle when it should not be given. Clearly communication with your anaesthetist is important to avoid such problems.

How should one manage those patients who are already on warfarin therapy because of a recent DVT, atrial fibrillation or because they have an artificial heart valve? The options are to keep them on warfarin while you do the TURP, or to stop the warfarin with or without anticoagulant cover with heparin.

One study suggests that transurethral resection may safely be performed despite warfarin treatment[68]. Four of the 14 patients in this latter study required transfusion of 2–4 units of blood and fresh frozen plasma was given in three. Only one case of clot retention was reported and no other serious complications occurred. Again, however, the numbers in this study were low and many surgeons will feel uncomfortable performing TURP in a fully anticoagulated patient. The decision has to be based on the individual patient's problems. Certainly withdrawing anticoagulant therapy can be associated with thromboembolic complications that threaten life or limb.

Stopping warfarin clearly exposes the patient to an increased risk of thromboembolism. In addition, there is some evidence that stopping warfarin can cause a rebound increase in clotting factors, leading to a hypercoagulable state[69], so compounding that which already exists in the patient undergoing TURP[58]. It has been estimated that a patient on warfarin for atrial fibrillation has a risk of stroke during the 4–6 days for which their International Normalized Ratio (INR) is subtherapeutic of up to 0.3%[70]. For a patient on warfarin because of venous thromboembolism, the risk of a recurrent DVT while off warfarin is approximately 40% within a month of the first DVT and approximately 10% at 3 months. For such patients it is best to postpone surgery for 3 months. For patients on warfarin because of a prosthetic heart valve, the risk of a stroke when warfarin is stopped is up to about 0.4% per day during which the INR is subtherapeutic[70].

For those who are not happy to perform TURP on a fully warfarinized patient, the ACCP Consensus Conference on Antithrombotic Therapy gives advice on management of oral anticoagulation around the time of surgical procedures[71,72]. For patients with a low risk of thromboembolism (e.g. DVT >3 months ago or atrial fibrillation with no prior history of stroke), warfarin should be stopped approximately 4 days before surgery, to allow the INR to return to a near-normal level, and prophylaxis such as subcutaneous unfractionated heparin (e.g. 5000 u every 8–12 hours) or low molecular weight heparin should be administered only at the time of surgery (the last dose of heparin being given 12 hours before surgery). It takes approximately 4 days for the INR to return to ≤1.5 in most patients, at which level surgery is safe[73]. For patients with an intermediate risk of thromboembolism (e.g. DVT between 1–3 months ago, those with artificial aortic valves) warfarin should be stopped approximately 4 days before surgery, to allow the INR to return to a near-normal level, and low dose subcutaneous unfractionated heparin (5000 u every 8–12 hours) or low molecular weight heparin should be started 2 days before surgery. For patients with a high risk of thromboembolism (e.g. DVT within the last month; those with mechanical mitral heart valves or old model – ball and cage – valves; atrial fibrillation with a history of stroke), stop warfarin approximately 4 days before surgery, allow the INR to return to a near-normal level and start unfractionated heparin as an intravenous infusion in hospital as the INR falls. The APTT (activated partial thromboplastin time) should be kept at approximately 2.5. The intravenous heparin is stopped about 3–4 hours before surgery so that the anticoagulant effect has worn off at the time of surgery and it is restarted as soon as possible after surgery, the precise timing depending on the colour of the urine in the irrigant fluid.

Shaving

There is no need to shave the skin before transurethral prostatectomy.

Anaesthesia

Many techniques of anaesthesia are suitable for transurethral surgery. No particular technique is uniquely suited to endoscopic work. Deliberate hypotension is preferred by some surgeons but in our experience it is not the level of the blood pressure which is critical so much as the absence of venous congestion.

Spinal anaesthesia is used by many anaesthetists as a routine. There are certain advantages to the patient being awake during the procedure. Although TUR syndrome is uncommon, one of the earliest indications that this is occurring can come from the awake patient reporting visual disturbance such as flashing lights. This early warning can allow the surgeon to end the procedure rapidly.

Position on the table

Special tables adapted for endoscopic surgery have the advantage that they can be raised or lowered by the surgeon. In many institutions, however, one must make do with the ordinary operating table, using

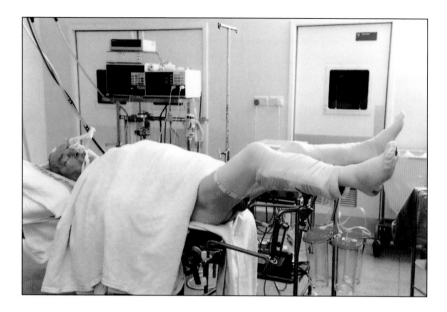

Figure 4.7
Adjustable Lloyd-Davies supports.

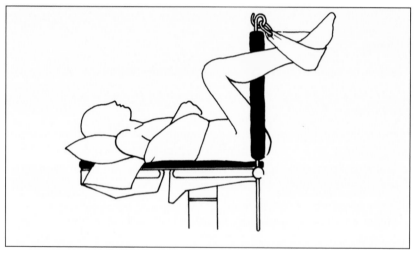

The wrong position for endoscopic surgery.

appropriate supports for the legs. Many different types of support are available (Fig. 4.7), and the important thing is that the legs are kept in the correct position with the thighs making an angle of no more than 45° with the plane of the table (Fig. 4.8). To have the legs in this almost flat position puts less strain on the heart[74]. The so-called lithotomy position, as used in operations on the anus, produces an awkward angulation of the prostate as well as sometimes causing backache afterwards.

Before applying the surgical drapes, the surgeon should take a few seconds to check that the patient is not in contact with any metal such as the drip stand or metal on the operating table, that pressure points are protected, and that the patient has above-knee TED stockings on (and

Figure 4.8
Mitchell slings, which allow the legs to be almost horizontal.

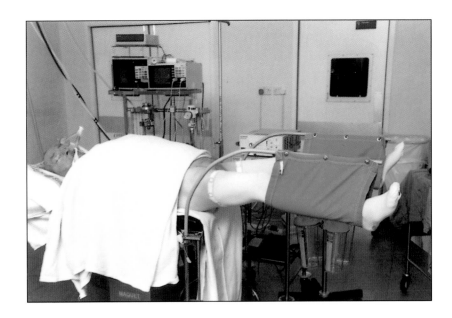

Flowtron intermittent pneumatic compression boots if these are to be used). Ensure that the patient is positioned at the end of the table so that the resectoscope can be moved freely. If the patient is positioned too far from the end of the table it will be difficult to swing the resectoscope downwards when access to the prostate in the 10 to 2 o'clock position is required (Fig. 4.9).

Diathermy pad

The earth pad is placed on the thigh, if necessary shaving a very hairy thigh. The appropriate safety devices should be checked to ensure that adequate contact has been made.

Skin cleansing

The skin of the genitalia and scrotum should be cleaned with a non-alcoholic antiseptic agent: iodine is avoided in view of the risk of causing a severe allergic reaction on the skin of the scrotum. The cleansing solution is applied with swabs held in forceps in the usual way. It is necessary to retract the prepuce and clean behind it.

Drapes

The legs are enclosed in roomy leggings or special disposable TUR drapes which are provided with a finger-cot to allow rectal examination during the procedure (Fig. 4.10). The camera is covered in a camera sleeve (Fig. 4.11) or a camera which can be sterilized between cases is used.

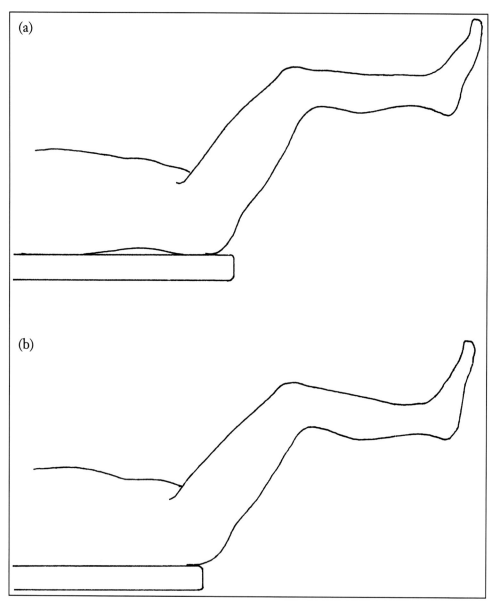

(a)

(b)

Figure 4.9
(a) Positioning the patient too far up the table can make it difficult to swing the resectoscope downwards when access to the 10 to 2 o'clock position is required. (b) The correct position of the patient relative to the end of the operating table.

Preparation of the urethra

The urethra must be properly lubricated before introducing any instrument, and here the surgeon should follow the example of the engineer who always fills a cylinder with oil before inserting a piston into it. We use water-soluble gel containing dilute chlorhexidine: thereafter all the instruments are well 'buttered' with gel before being inserted. This is repeated whenever one feels the instrument dragging on the urethra.

Figure 4.10
All-in-one drape for transurethral resection.

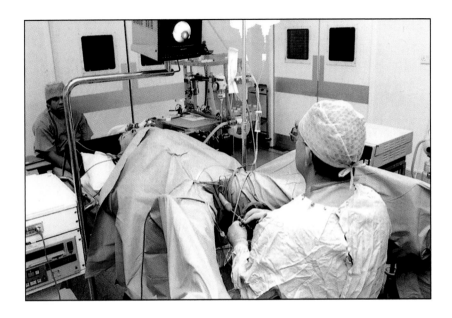

Figure 4.11
The camera is covered in a camera sleeve.

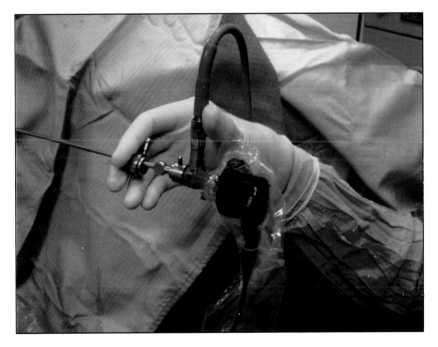

Urethroscopy

After lubricating the urethra it is examined from end to end using the 0° or 30° telescope advanced under direct vision. This reveals a surprising number of soft annular strictures in the normal bulbar urethra. Once within the prostatic urethra care is taken to estimate the size of the gland and the distance from verumontanum to sphincter and to bladder neck. The sphincter is identified carefully.

Cystoscopy

The interior of the bladder is inspected with a 30° or 70° telescope. Special search is made for small tumours, especially those that may lie hidden behind the bump of the middle lobe, calculi that might need to be crushed and evacuated, and diverticula which must all be carefully examined to rule out stone or cancer.

Urethrotomy

Once the decision has been taken to go ahead with transurethral resection the 24 Ch sheath is introduced. If the urethra is at all tight, avoid the temptation to force the resectoscope sheath into a urethra that is too small to accept it. It takes just a few minutes to pass an Otis or similar urethrotome, and incise the urethra at 12 o'clock along its last 4 or 5 cm (Fig. 4.12). The urethrotome is passed with its blades closed, right into the bladder. Withdraw it past the external sphincter, open the blades to 30 Ch in the mid-bulb, advance the knife and withdraw the instrument. If the urethra is examined after 6 weeks or so all that is left of the incision is a fine white line (Fig. 4.13).

Bailey and Shearer[75] performed a prospective study on 210 consecutive patients undergoing TURP, randomizing them either to full-length pre-

Figure 4.12
(a) Otis urethrotome. Courtesy of KeyMed.
(b) Clean incision of urethra.
(c) Large calibre sheath goes in easily.
(d) Heals without narrowing.

(a)

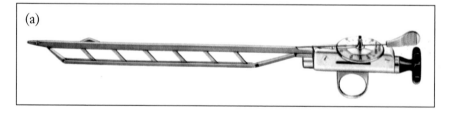

(b)   (c)   (d)

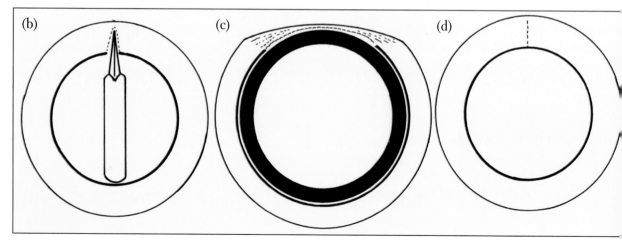

Figure 4.13
After a few weeks the site of urethrotomy is seen as a thin white scar, without any stricture.

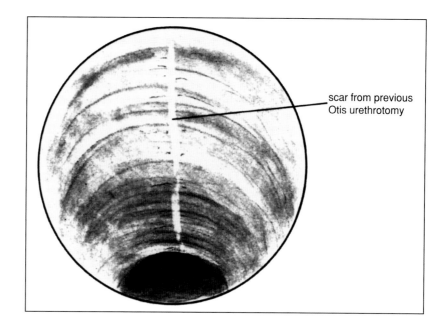

scar from previous
Otis urethrotomy

TURP internal urethrotomy (with the urethrotome set to 30 Ch) or to pre-operative urethral dilatation (to 30 Ch), according to the day of the week on which surgery was performed. Strictures were diagnosed on the basis of symptoms suggestive of a stricture (it was not deemed ethical to perform routine postoperative urethroscopy). Two patients in the urethrotomy group (2%) and 9 in the dilatation group (10%) developed strictures. Those in the dilatation group were at the external meatus, in the navicular fossa, at the peno-scrotal junction or in the membranous urethra.

And finally...

Once the resectoscope is in position within the prostatic urethra, make yourself comfortable. Position the irrigation tubing, the light lead and the camera so that they will not become tangled in a great knot as you swing the instrument clockwise and anticlockwise through 360°. Some surgeons like to lock the camera in position, while others prefer to let it hang loosely in the 6 o'clock position. It does not matter, as long as you know where you are in relation to the verumontanum. Position the foot pedals in the most comfortable position. Some surgeons like both the diathermy and cutting current pedals on one foot, others prefer one on the left and the other on the right foot. Position the height of the patient and of your stool so that your hand and arm are comfortable. Use a stool with wheels so that you can adjust your position relative to the patient with ease. Check that you can move the resectoscope freely from side to side and up and down, without hitting the patient's legs or the operating table. If you are not happy with the position you or the patient are in, change it until you are happy. Now you can begin.

References

1. Adshead J, Sinclair A, Williams G. *Procedure Specific Consent Forms for Urological Surgery*. British Association of Urological Surgeons, London, 2003.
2. Reynard JM, Yang Q, Donovan JL *et al*. The ICS-'BPH' study: uroflowmetry, lower urinary tract symptoms and bladder outlet obstruction. *Br J Urol* 1998;82:619–23.
3. Barry MJ, Fowler FJ Jr, O'Leary MP *et al*. The American Urological Association symptom index for benign prostatic hyperplasia. *J Urol* 1992;148:1549–57.
4. Lepor H, Machi G. Comparison of AUA symptom index in unselected males and females between fifty-five and seventy-nine years of age. *Urology* 1993;42:36–41.
5. Abrams P. New words for old – lower urinary tract symptoms for 'prostatism'. *BMJ* 1994;308:929–30.
6. Roehrborn CG, Bartsch G, Kirby R *et al*. Guidelines for the diagnosis and treatment of benign prostatic hyperplasia: a comparative international overview. *Urology* 2001;58:642–50.
7. Irani J, Brown CT, van der Meulen J, Emberton M. A review of guidelines on benign prostatic hyperplasia and lower urinary tract symptoms: are all guidelines the same? *Br J Urol Int* 2003;92:937–42.
8. AUA Guidelines. http://hstat.nlm.nih.gov/ftrs/arahcpr
9. EAU Guidelines. http://www.uroweb.org/files/uploaded_files/bph.pdf
10. WHO (International Consensus Committee) Guidelines. http://www.who.int/ina-ngo/ngo/ngo048.htm
11. Australian Guidelines. http://www.health.gov.au/nhmrc/publications/pdf/cp42.pdf
12. German Guidelines. http://dgu.springer.de/leit/pdf/3_99.pdf
13. Singapore Guidelines. http://www.urology-singapore.org.html/guidelines_bph.htm
14. Malaysian Guidelines. http://www.mohtrg.gov.my/guidelines/bph98.pdf
15. UK Guidelines. http://www.rcseng.ac.uk/publications/
16. Mitchell JP. Management of chronic urinary retention. *BMJ* 1984;289:515–16.
17. National Institute for Clinical Excellence Guidance. Urinary tract outflow symptoms (prostatism) in men – Referral practice guidelines. October 2000. www.nice.org.uk
18. EAU Guidelines (2001) for diagnosis of BPH. *Eur Urol* 2001;40:256–63.
19. Neal DE. The National Prostatectomy Audit. *Br J Urol* 1997;79(Suppl 2):69–75.
20. McConnell JD, Barry MJ, Bruskewitz RC *et al*. *Benign Prostatic Hyperplasia: Diagnosis and Treatment. Clinical Practice Guideline*. Agency for Health Care Policy and Research, Public Health Service, US Department of Health and Human Sciences, Rockville, MD; publication no. 94-0582, 1994.
21. Denis L, Griffiths K, Khoury S, *et al* (Health Publication Ltd). *Fourth International Consultation on Benign Prostatic Hyperplasia (BPH), Paris 1997*. Plymbridge Distributors, Plymouth, UK, 1998; pp. 669–83.
22. Wasson JH, Reda DJ, Bruskewitz RC *et al*. A comparison of transurethral surgery with watchful waiting for moderate symptom of benign prostatic hyperplasia. The Veterans Administration Cooperative Study Group on Transurethral Resection of the Prostate. *N Engl J Med* 1995;332:75–9.
23. Bates TS, Sugiono M, James ED *et al*. Is the conservative management of chronic retention in men ever justified? *Br J Urol Int* 2003;92:581–3.
24. Birch NC, Hurst G, Doyle PT. Serial residual urine volumes in men with prostatic hypertrophy. *Br J Urol* 1988;62:571–5.
25. Bruskewitz RC, Iversen P, Madsen PO. Value of post-void residual urine determination in evaluation of prostatism. *Urology* 1982;20:602–4.
26. Dunsmuir WD, Feneley M, Corry DA *et al*. The day-to-day variation (test-retest reliability) of residual urine measurement. *Br J Urol* 1996;77:192–3.

27. Neal DE, Ramsden PD, Sharples L *et al*. Outcome of elective prostatectomy. *BMJ* 1989;299:762–7.
28. Bruskewitz RC, Reda DJ, Wasson JH *et al*. Testing to predict outcome after transurethral resection of the prostate. *J Urol* 1997;157:1304–8.
29. Riehmann M, Goetzmann B, Langer E *et al*. Risk factor for bacteriuria in men. *Urology* 1994;43:617–20.
30. Hampson SJ, Noble JG, Rickards D, Milroy EG. Does residual urine predispose to urinary tract infection. *Br J Urol* 1992;70:506–8.
31. Reynard JM, Peters TJ, Lim C, Abrams P. The value of multiple free-flow studies in men with lower urinary tract symptoms. *Br J Urol* 1996;77:813–18.
32. Abrams PH. Prostatism and prostatectomy: the value of urine flow rate measurement in the pre-operative assessment for operation. *J Urol* 1977;117:70–1.
33. Abrams PH, Griffiths DJ. The assessment of prostatic obstruction from urodynamic measurements and residual urine. *Br J Urol* 1979;51:129.
34. Jensen KM-E, Bruskewitz RC, Iversen P, Madsen PO. Spontaneous uroflowmetry in prostatism. *Urology* 1984;24:403–9.
35. Dorflinger T, Bruskewitz RC, Jensen KM-E *et al*. Predictive value of low maximum flow rate in benign prostatic hyperplasia. *Urology* 1986;27:569–73.
36. Gee WF, Holtgrewe HL, Albertsen PC *et al*. Practice trends in the diagnosis and management of benign prostatic hyperplasia in the United States. *J Urol* 1995;154:205–6.
37. Koch WF, Ezz el Din KE, De Wildt MJ *et al*. The outcome of renal ultrasound in the assessment of 556 consecutive patients with benign prostatic hyperplasia. *J Urol* 1996;155:186–9.
38. Murray K, Massey A, Feneley RC. Acute urinary retention – a urodynamic assessment. *Br J Urol* 1984;56:468–73.
39. Hastie KJ, Dickinson AJ, Ahmad R, Moisey CU. Acute retention of urine: is trial without catheter justified? *J R Coll Surg Edinb* 1990;35:225–7.
40. Djavan B, Madersbacher S, Klingler C, Marberger M. Urodynamic assessment of patients with acute urinary retention: is treatment failure after prostatectomy predictable. *J Urol* 1997;158:1829–33.
41. McNeill SA, Daruwala PD, Mitchell IDC *et al*. Sustained-release alfuzosin and trial without catheter after acute urinary retention. *Br J Urol Int* 1999;84:622–7.
42. McNeill SA. Does acute urinary retention respond to alpha-blockers alone? *Eur Urol* 2001;9(Suppl 6):7–12.
43. Hampson S, Davies JA, Morris SB *et al*. The use of LH-RH analogues in patients with retention and carcinoma of the prostate. *J Urol* 1993;149:428A.
44. Abrams P, Dunn M, George N. Urodynamic findings in chronic retention of urine and their relevance to results of surgery. *BMJ* 1978;2:1258–60.
45. George NJR, O'Reilly PH, Barnard RJ, Blacklock NJ. High pressure chronic retention. *BMJ* 1983;286:1780–3.
46. Kearney MC, Bingham JB, Bergland R *et al*. Clinical predictors in the use of finasteride for control of gross hematuria due to benign prostatic hyperplasia. *J Urol* 2002;167:2489–91.
47. Carlin BI, Bodner DR, Spirnak JP, Resnick MI. Role of finasteride in the treatment of recurrent hematuria secondary to benign prostatic hyperplasia. *Prostate* 1997;15:180–2.
48. Miller MI, Puchner PJ. Effects of finasteride on hematuria associated with benign prostatic hyperplasia: long-term follow-up. *Urology* 1998;51:237–40.
49. Grosse H. Frequency, localization and associated disorders in urinary calculi. Analysis of 1671 autopsies in urolithiasis. *Z Urol Nephrol* 1990;83:469–74.
50. Mak S, Amoroso P. Stop those antiplatelet drugs before surgery. *Br J Urol* 2003;91:593–4.
51. Thurston AV, Briant SL. Aspirin and post-prostatectomy haemorrhage. *Br J Urol* 1993;71:574–6.
52. Wierod FS, Frandsen NJ, Jacobsen JD *et al*. Risk of haemorrhage from transurethral prostatectomy in acetylsalylic acid and NSAID-treated patients. *Scand J Urol Nephrol* 1998;32:120–2.

53. Benzon HT, Wong HY, Siddiqui T, Ondra S. Caution in performing epidural injections in patients on several antiplatelet drugs. *Anesthesiology* 1999;91:1558–9.
54. Hall JC, Christiansen KJ, England P *et al*. Antibiotic prophylaxis for patients undergoing transurethral resection of the prostate. *Urology* 1996;47:852.
55. Hargreave TB, Botto B, Rikken GHJM *et al*. European Collaborative Study of Antibiotic Prophylaxis for Transurethral Resection of the Prostate. *Eur Urol* 1993;23:437–43.
56. British National Formulary. British Medical Association and the Royal Pharmaceutical Society of Great Britain (September 2003), ISBN 0-85369-556-3.
57. The American Academy of Orthopaedic Surgeons (AAOS) and the American Urological Association (AUA) – Advisory statement. *J Urol* 2003;169:1796.
58. Bell CR, Murdock PJ, Pasi KJ, Morgan RJ. Thrombotic risk factors associated with transurethral prostatectomy. *Br J Urol Int* 1999;83:984–9.
59. Donat R, Mancey-Jones B. Incidence of thromboembolism after transurethral resection of the prostate (TURP). *Scand J Urol Nephrol* 2002;36:119–23.
60. Geerts WH, Heit JA, Clagett PG *et al*. Prevention of venous thromboembolism. *Chest* 2001;119:132S–175S.
61. Golash A, Collins PW, Kynaston HG, Jenkins BJ. Venous thromboembolic prophylaxis for transurethral prostatectomy: practice among British urologists. *J R Soc Med* 2002;95:130–1.
62. Clagett GP, Reisch JS. Prevention of venous thromboembolism in general surgical patients. Results of meta-analysis. *Ann Surg* 1988;208:227–40.
63. Soderdahl DW, Henderson SR, Hansberry KL. A comparison of intermittent pneumatic compression of the calf and whole leg in preventing deep venous thrombosis in urological surgery. *J Urol* 1997;157:1774–6.
64. Lowe GDO, Greer IA, Cooke TG *et al*. Risk of and prophylaxis for venous thromboembolism in hospital patients. Thromboembolic Risk Factors (THRIFT) Consensus Group. *BMJ* 1992;305:567–74.
65. Wilson RG, Smith D, Paton G, Gollock JM, Bremner DN. Prophylactic subcutaneous heparin does not increase operative blood loss in transurethral resection of the prostate. *Br J Urol* 1988;62:246.
66. Bejjani BB, Chen DCP, Nolan NG, Edson M. Minidose heparin in transurethral prostatectomy. *Urology* 1983;22:251–4.
67. Sleight MW. The effect of prophylactic subcutaneous heparin on blood loss during and after transurethral prostatectomy. *Br J Urol* 1982;54:164–5.
68. Parr NJ, Lohn CS, Desmond AD. Transurethral resection of the prostate without withdrawal of Warfarin therapy. *Br J Urol* 1989;64:623–5.
69. Genewein U, Haeberli A, Straub PW. Rebound after cessation of oral anticoagulation therapy: the biochemical evidence. *Br J Haematol* 1996;92:479–85.
70. Spandorfer JM. The management of anticoagulation before and after procedures. *Med Clin North Am* 2001;85:1109–16.
71. Ansell J, Hirsh J, Dalen J *et al*. Managing oral anticoagulant therapy. Sixth ACCP Consensus Conference on Antithombotic Therapy. *Chest* 2001;119:22S–38S.
72. Meyer JP, Gillatt DA, Lush R, Persad R. Managing the warfarinized urological patient. *Br J Urol Int* 2003;92:351–4.
73. Kearon C, Hirsh J. Management of anticoagulation before and after elective surgery. *N Engl J Med* 1997;336:1506–11.
74. Kedar S, Gaitini L, Vaida S *et al*. The influence of patient positioning on the hemodynamic changes in TURP patients with severe coronary disease. *Eur Urol* 1995;27:23.
75. Bailey MJ, Shearer RJ. The role of internal urethrotomy in the prevention of urethral stricture following transurethral resection of the prostate. *Br J Urol* 1979;51:28–31.

Chapter 5

The basic skills of transurethral resection

Just as in general surgery it is necessary to learn to make a clean incision with the knife, to tie a secure knot, to handle tissue with delicacy and to secure haemostasis with the minimum of trauma and tissue necrosis, so in transurethral surgery there are certain basic steps which the beginner has to master. Many of them can be learned on models and appreciated by watching a more experienced surgeon at work. Others can only be learned solo.

Cutting a chip

Cutting chips from prostate or bladder tumours can and must be practised before the beginner tries to resect in a live patient. A number of surgical 'workshops' provide such experience, and use models which have been developed to feel as close to the 'real thing' as is possible. The loop of the resectoscope cuts like a knife through butter without any effort: but it requires a little time to do its work. The cutting is carried out by a halo of sparks between the diathermy electrode and the tissues (see page 21). The cutting takes place without contact, but it takes a little time for the sparks to do their work. No force is ever required. The rate at which you work is limited by the rate of disruption of the tissues.

The shape of the chip is like a canoe (Fig. 5.1). It is as wide and deep as the loop, and its length is determined by the travel of the loop plus

Figure 5.1
The TUR chip is shaped like a canoe; it should be as deep and broad as the loop, and as long as the travel of the loop in and out of the sheath plus the distance you move the sheath.

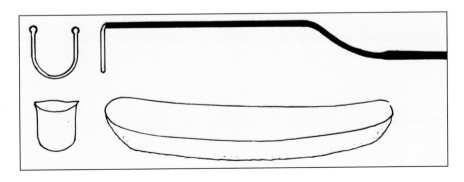

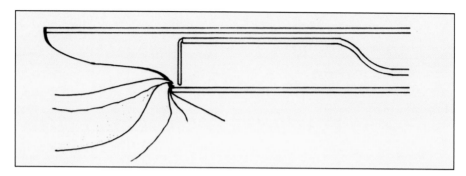

Figure 5.2
The usual method of cutting the chip off against the edge of the sheath.

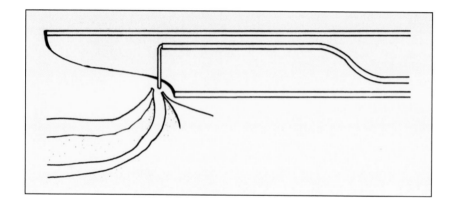

Figure 5.3
Cutting the chip off before the loop enters the sheath prevents any possible damage to the telescope.

the extra length gained by moving the sheath in and out. There are two methods of cutting off the chip. The usual method is to sever the chip against the edge of the resectoscope sheath and for this reason many of the old masters such as Barnes insisted on a loop which entered 1 or 2 mm inside the sheath[1] (Fig. 5.2). The second technique, advocated by Nesbit, was to bring the loop out completely before entering the sheath[2] (Figs 5.3 and 5.4).

If the loop goes too far inside the sheath sparks may damage the lens of the telescope and cause expensive damage, and for this reason some instrument makers design the loop so that it will not go inside the sheath. In practice, most urologists use the Barnes method, and will bend the loop: this is perfectly safe so long as there is still a gap between loop and lens (Fig. 5.5).

In time the edge of the sheath always gets more or less burnt away and when this is corrected by bending the loop the result can be disastrous,

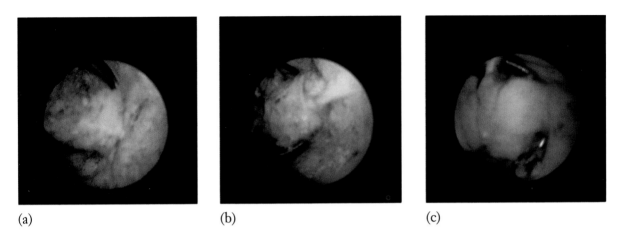

(a) (b) (c)

Figure 5.4
Cutting a chip: (a) the loop is sunk into its full depth, (b) drawn towards you and (c) cut off before the loop enters the sheath.

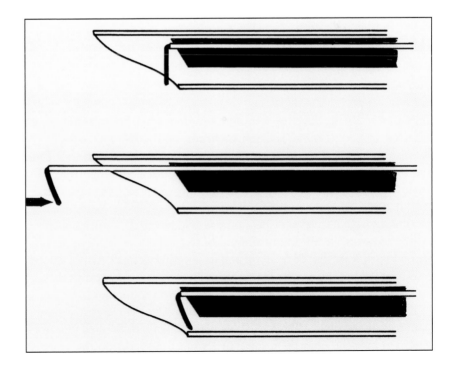

Figure 5.5
It is safe to bend the loop to allow it to enter the tip of the sheath so long as there is a gap between loop and telescope.

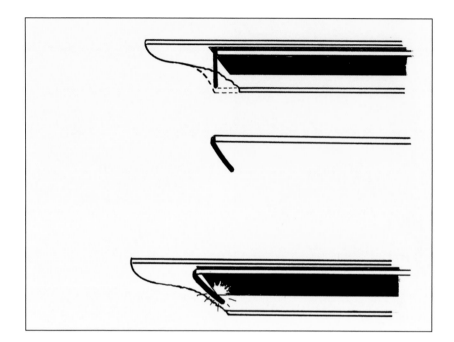

Figure 5.6
If the end of the sheath has been burnt away, and you continue to bend the loop, you risk damage to the telescope from the diathermy spark.

with a spark arcing across the lens, thereby fracturing it (Fig. 5.6). The first rule, then, when starting to put the resectoscope together at the beginning of the operation, is to check the end of the sheath and the position of the loop. Send for an undamaged sheath even if this causes delay in the operation. A spare resectoscope sheath is a great deal cheaper than a new telescope.

Rhythm

It is important to develop a smooth rhythm when performing transurethral surgery (Fig. 5.7). Begin by lifting up the handpiece to let the loop sink in as you start the stroke, and end by depressing it to lift out the loop. In a bladder tumour the action is similar although one must take care not to sink the loop too deeply into the wall of the bladder.

When resecting the bulk of the lateral lobes of the prostate, once the landmarks have been established, time is saved by making sure that every stroke removes the maximum amount of tissue, i.e. the depth of the chip should be at least that of the loop and its length as long as that of the lateral lobe even if this means moving the sheath outwards, always making sure that you know the exact situation of the verumontanum.

If the electrode does not spark cleanly it will not cut, but will coagulate or char the tissue (Fig. 5.8). This is most likely to occur if you press the loop into the prostate instead of letting the sparks do the work. A crust of carbonized tissue may cover the loop. Clean it and start again.

Figure 5.7
Cutting a chip: (a) lift the resectoscope to allow the loop to sink in, (b) keep it level as you cut the chip and (c) depress the sheath to cut off the chip.

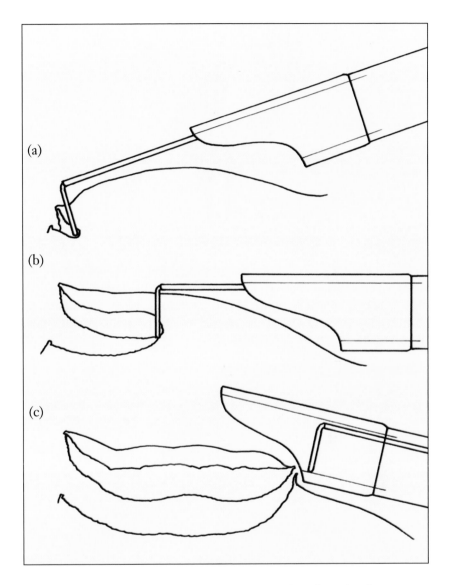

If the loop does not cut at all, do not respond by asking for the current to be increased. Instead, carry out the following checks:

1. Make sure that the loop is sitting firmly in its holder. A 'click' can be felt and heard as the loop fits into the holder.
2. Check that the loop is not broken.
3. Check that the diathermy plate is securely attached to the thigh.
4. Check that the diathermy lead is attached to the machine.
5. Check that the wire within the diathermy lead has not worked loose at either end.
6. Check the irrigating fluid: a common mistake is for the theatre team to hang a bag of saline instead of glycine.

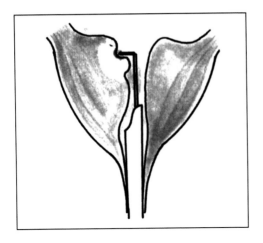

Figure 5.8
If the loop does not strike sparks it will cause deep local coagulation.

If all these items have been checked and the loop still does not cut, you must change the diathermy machine. You cannot resect with a loop which merely chars: it drags in the tissues, makes it difficult to cut cleanly, and worse, risks producing a deep burn in the underlying tissues which may damage the sphincter.

Figure 5.9
If the loop does not cut, check these causes of failure before asking for the current to be increased.

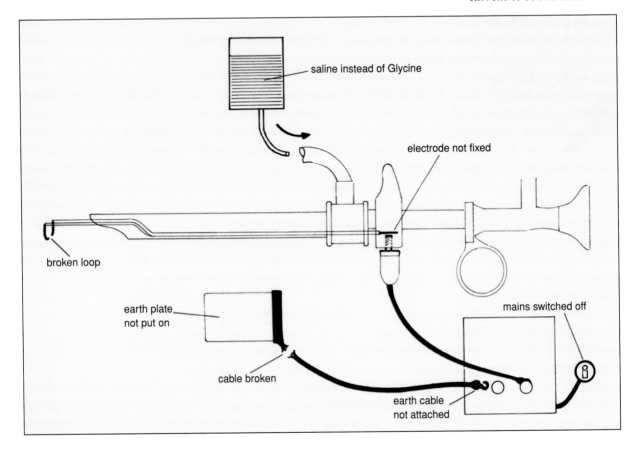

Haemostasis

Most of the light oozing which occurs during a resection comes from small veins which are cut as you resect the adenoma. This type of bleeding is minimized by using a continuous flow Iglesias irrigating system, but it should be stopped as you go along in order to keep a clear view. Any arterial bleeder should be controlled as soon as you see it by touching it with the loop and applying the coagulating current for a moment (Fig. 5.10). There is the typical noise of the coagulating circuit but there should be no charring or burning, only cessation of bleeding and a little whitening of the tissue.

Figure 5.10
Typical endoscopic appearances of sealing a small artery.

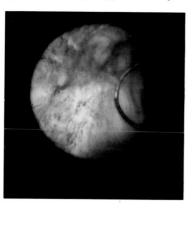 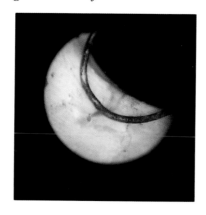 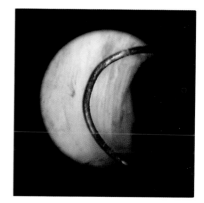

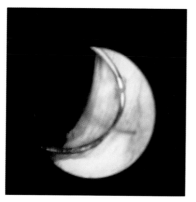 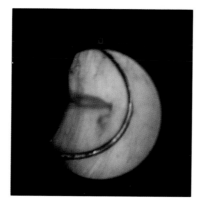

When an artery is larger or thickened by atheroma it may be more difficult to close it off merely by touching its mouth. A useful trick is to compress the tissue to one side or other of the orifice of the artery (Fig. 5.11) so as to squeeze its walls together and allow the coagulating current to seal them.

Occasionally you will be misled by 'bounce' bleeding, when a fierce jet of blood rebounds off the opposite wall of the prostatic fossa: the appearance is easily recognized once it has been seen before (Fig. 5.12). The wily operator soon learns to turn his attention to the contralateral wall of the prostatic fossa to seek the true source of bleeding.

Another common source of confusion is the artery which is shooting out straight at the telescope. All you can see is a uniform red haze. The trick is to advance the resectoscope beyond the bleeder, angulate it to compress the vessel, and then slowly withdraw the sheath until the opening of the artery is betrayed by the emergence of a puff of blood (Fig. 5.13).

Coagulating just upstream of the artery will seal it off (Fig. 5.14). When you encounter large veins, multiple vessels set close together, or several atheromatous arteries which do not seal with the loop, change the loop for the roly-ball electrode (Fig. 5.15) and apply this sparingly

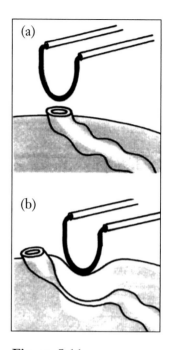

Figure 5.11
(a) A larger vessel may not be controlled by coagulating its mouth; the trick is (b) to squeeze the walls together by applying the loop just to one side to seal them with the coagulating current.

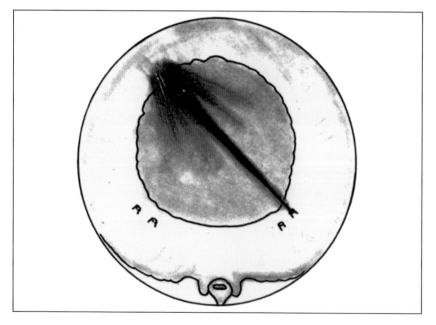

Figure 5.12
Bounce bleeding.

Figure 5.13
When an artery points straight at you all you can see is a red blur. The trick is to advance the sheath, tilt it to squeeze the vessel, and coagulate just upstream.

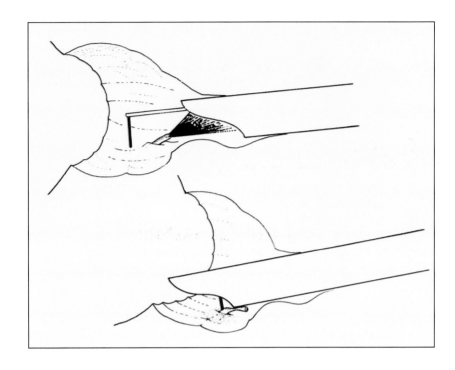

Figure 5.14 (left)
An artery bleeding straight at you. The loop will coagulate it just upstream.

Figure 5.15 (right)
Coagulation with the loop.

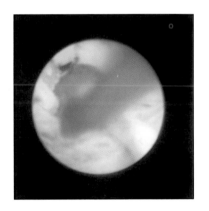
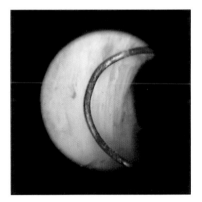

to the source of the haemorrhage. Take care not to overdo the coagulation with the roly-ball: it produces heat at a depth which is proportional to the square of its diameter and invites late secondary haemorrhage.

Prophylactic coagulation

Sometimes it is obvious from the moment you pass the cystoscope that the resection is likely to be bloody. You can save yourself trouble by making a prophylactic attempt to control the main arteries before you

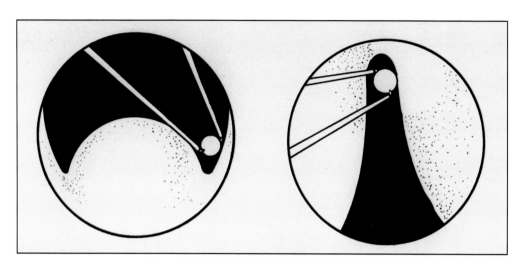

Figure 5.16
Prophylactic coagulation of the main prostatic arteries at 2, 5, 7 and 10 o'clock.

start to resect. Using the roly-ball coagulate the prostate at 2, 5, 7 and 10 o'clock (Fig. 5.16) where the main arteries enter the gland. This simple measure minimizes subsequent bleeding, and may be repeated later on during the resection should bleeding recur.

Veins

Veins are more difficult to detect than arteries, especially if the pressure of the irrigating fluid is equal to, or greater than, the pressure in the veins of the pelvis. For this reason you may see no venous bleeding at all during the resection, but as soon as the handpiece is removed there is a copious flow of blood.

Having sealed off all the arteries, the trick in finding the little veins is to slow down the inflow of irrigating fluid by adjusting the tap on the resectoscope until you can hardly see the tissue: little clouds of blood betray the position of the veins, which should be coagulated. It is worth taking time to go over the entire inner surface of the capsule at the end of the operation to seal them all. Time spent on this manoeuvre is time well spent.

Even so, there are some patients in whom, despite prolonged and patient haemostasis, there is still a copious ooze of venous blood. Here tamponade is effective. A catheter is passed on a curved introducer to make sure it does not catch under the bladder neck. Sterile water (40 ml) is injected into the balloon while it is well inside the bladder, and then the catheter is firmly drawn down so that the balloon compresses the

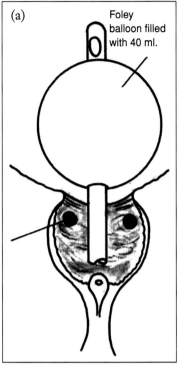

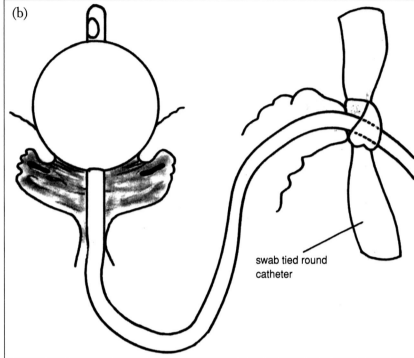

Figure 5.17
The Foley balloon is filled with 40 ml of sterile water (a) and pulled down to compress the veins at the bladder neck (b): traction is maintained by a gauze swab tied round the catheter and pulled back onto the glans penis.

neck of the bladder where most of the offending veins are situated (Fig. 5.17). Pull the catheter down, and maintain traction for 8–10 minutes, passing the time by discussing politics or football with your anaesthetist. Before doing so, ask the nurse not to clear the equipment away, but to keep it sterile in case you need to re-insert the resectoscope to achieve better haemostasis. It is far easier and faster to sort the bleeding out now while the patient is on the operating table, anaesthetized, and the equipment is still available, than to bring him back from recovery and start all over again.

Often the bleeding will have been controlled by this period of traction. If not, never hesitate to reinsert the resectoscope to double-check that you have not missed a bleeding vessel. Briskly bleeding arteries just inside the bladder neck at roughly the 12 o'clock position can easily be missed, so look here in particular.

Once you are happy that there are no more bleeding vessels to control, reinsert the catheter and maintain traction by means of the Salvaris swab: two gauze swabs are tied moderately tightly around the catheter and pushed up against the glans penis. These swabs should be removed after 20–30 minutes lest a pressure sore be formed on the glans.

Evacuation of the chips

Whenever one breaks the rhythm of resection to remove chips, time is wasted so keep the number of evacuations to the minimum, i.e. when the chips begin to fall back into the empty prostatic fossa and get in the way of the loop.

Of all instruments for removing clot and chips from the bladder, the evacuator designed by Milo Ellik[3] is the most simple and effective (Fig. 5.18a). Make sure that two of them are always filled and ready. Make sure also that you have mastered the knack of filling them and getting rid of all the air. The purpose of the bulb is to allow the irrigating fluid to go in and out of the bladder, to swirl it around and allow the chips and clot to float out of the bladder and fall down into the chamber. It must be used gently: if used roughly it is possible to rupture the bladder (particularly in old ladies with thin bladders who have undergone bladder tumour resection). The irrigation inflow valve can be left open as a sort of 'safety valve' to take some of the pressure off the bladder each time the Ellik is squeezed. Some surgeons prefer a wide nozzle hand syringe (called by some a Toomey syringe) to the Ellik: readers should try for themselves. Disposable, one-use only sterile Elliks are used in many hospitals nowadays, partly because of concerns about adequacy of sterilization of the components of the old multi-use Elliks (Fig. 5.18b). The receptacle for the prostate chips or bladder tumour can

(a)

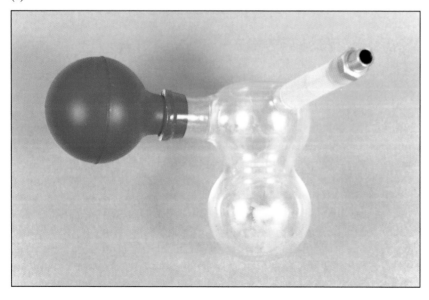

Figure 5.18
(a) Ellik's evacuator.

Figure 5.18 (*continued*)
(b) Disposable, one-use only sterile Ellik evacuator.
(c) The chips of resected tissue can be sent for pathological examination in the container of the Ellik.

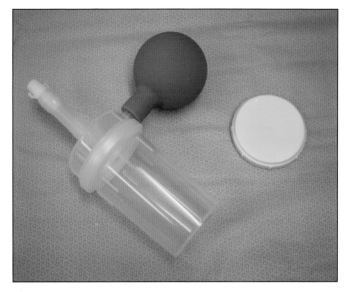

(b)

(c)

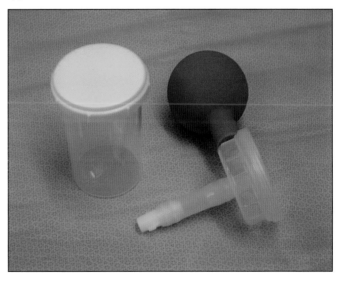

be filled with formalin after the operation is over and sent directly to the pathologist as the specimen pot. The disposable Elliks have the added advantage of a flap valve which stops evacuated tissue from flying back into the bladder, and they do not break when you drop them on the floor.

Keeping a clear view

Nothing is more important in resecting prostate or bladder tumour than being able to see what you are doing. There are many causes for a dim or obscured view, and some of them are worth mentioning for the beginner.

1. Bubbles on the lens may be caused by hydrolysis of the water by the electric sparks and cannot be avoided, but a more tiresome (and avoidable) source of bubbles can be traced to faulty connections of the tube and bag of irrigating fluid. The continuous flow resectoscopes minimize both types of bubble, but do not entirely avoid them (Fig. 5.19). When bubbles form, stop the flow of irrigant for a second

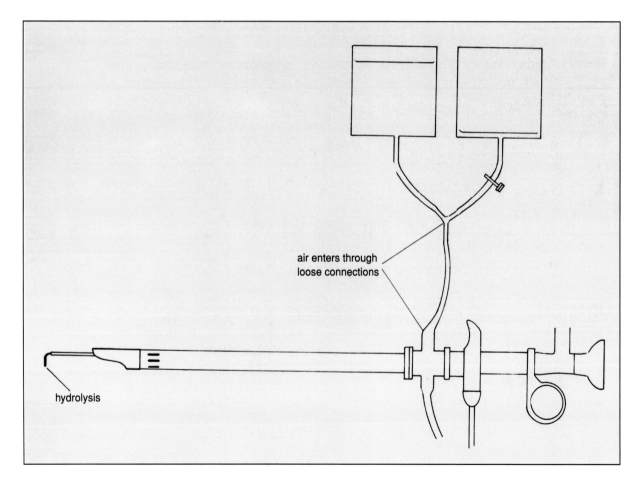

Figure 5.19
Causes of bubbles in the field of vision.

and allow water to run out. If the bubbles persist, tap the telescope smartly in and out a few times.

2. A particularly irritating habit of the novice is to finger the eyepiece with a glove moistened with saline or lubricating gel. Others, given their first chance to look down the telescope, huff and puff on the eyepiece. These lenses are made of soft optical glass and should only be cleaned with soft lint rather than cotton gauze which might scratch them. The best prevention is vigilance on the part of the surgeon and the application of the general rule that the eyepiece is regarded as surgically 'dirty'. Water may also not have been wiped off the lens of the telescope or the camera before the camera is attached to the telescope. Check that they are both dry before connecting them.

3. In conventional irrigating systems the most common cause for want of clear vision is obstruction of the water inflow (Fig. 5.19), usually because an inattentive nurse has let the bag run out. This happens on a boringly regular basis, so keep an eye on the bag from time to time and warn the nurse that you need more fluid well in advance. Sometimes the inflow becomes kinked or twisted. In continuous flow systems there may be imbalance between the negative pressure in the suction and the rate of inflow of the irrigating fluid. For this reason inflow and outflow taps must be under the control of the surgeon.

4. Whatever system of irrigation is used the inflow will stop when the bladder is so full that it can take no more. Since this means that the pressure inside the bladder has risen, this is a state of affairs that should never be allowed to occur. This situation can occur with con-tinuous irrigation, although it is much less likely to do so. If it does, the balance between inflow and outflow is wrong and must be adjusted. Most surgeons develop a sixth sense when the bladder is nearly full and when it is time to empty it out, and most resectoscopes begin to leak before this critical moment has been reached.

5. From time to time a chip of prostate or bladder tumour will be stuck to the lens or jammed between loop and sheath. In either case it is necessary to remove the handpiece. The lens should be cleaned using the jet of irrigating fluid or a piece of sterile lint. Blood that has been allowed to coagulate on the lens is a different matter. Use a broken wooden orange stick such as used for microbiological cultures: the wood does not scratch the optical glass.

6. If the telescope has gone misty, there is nothing you can do about it. Send for a spare and get on with the operation. The telescope will probably have to be returned to the manufacturer to get rid of water vapour.

References

1. Barnes RW. *Endoscopic Prostatic Surgery*. London: Kimpton, 1943.
2. Nesbit RM. *Transurethral Prostatectomy*. Springfield: Thomas, 1943.
3. Ellik M. A modification of the evacuator. *J Urol* 1937;38:327.

Chapter 6

Transurethral resection technique for benign prostatic enlargement

Figure 6.1

The tissue removed during an enucleative open prostatectomy (a) is the same as that removed by TUR (b). In both, the inner zone adenoma is removed from the 'surgical capsule' of compressed outer zone.

Although several different techniques of transurethral resection have been described, their aim is essentially the same, to remove all the adenomatous tissue from the inner zone, leaving the compressed outer zone intact: the so-called 'surgical capsule'. The tissue which is removed during transurethral resection is therefore in theory identical with the tissue removed by an enucleative open operation[1,2] (Fig. 6.1). The various techniques of transurethral resection differ only in the order in which the bulk of tissue is removed. Two plans are described here: neither is in the least bit original and no particular preference is claimed for either.

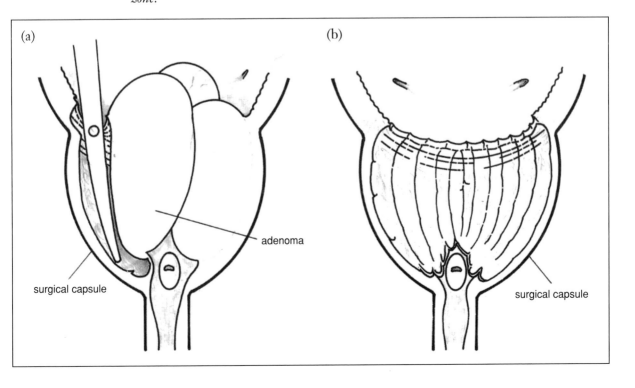

(a)　　　　　　　　　　　　　(b)

adenoma

surgical capsule

surgical capsule

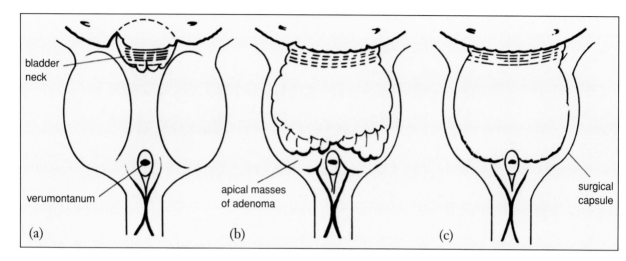

bladder neck

verumontanum

(a)

apical masses of adenoma

(b)

(c)

surgical capsule

Figure 6.2
The three stages of transurethral prostatectomy: (a) the landmarks are located, (b) most of the adenoma is removed, (c) the apical tissue is trimmed from either side of the verumontanum.

The important thing is that you should have a plan and stick to it, or else you will certainly get lost. Try each of these methods and choose the one which suits you best.

In both methods there are three stages (Fig. 6.2):

1. Establishing the landmarks.
2. Removing the main bulk of tissue.
3. Tidying up.

In each method the resection begins with a preliminary urethroscopy and cystoscopy, careful lubrication of the urethra, and an internal urethrotomy if there is the slightest tightness of the resectoscope sheath (see page 70).

1. Establishing the landmarks

The landmarks in transurethral resection are the same whether you remove much tissue or only a little: the distal limit to the resection is the verumontanum, which stands like a lighthouse just proximal to that special region of the prostatic urethra which contains the supramembranous intrinsic component of the external sphincter (Fig. 6.3). This is a ring of elastic tissue, striated and unstriated muscle, quite distinct from and above the levator ani[3]. It is the essential part of the continence mechanism and must not be damaged.

Make sure that you have seen the sphincter: bring the resectoscope out beyond it, cut off the water flow and see it contract like the anus in its characteristic way (Fig. 6.4). As you do this you will note an even more important feature: as the sheath of the resectoscope passes out

Figure 6.3

The three components of the sphincter mechanism of the bladder, bladder neck, intramural external sphincter (just distal to the verumontanum) and levator ani.

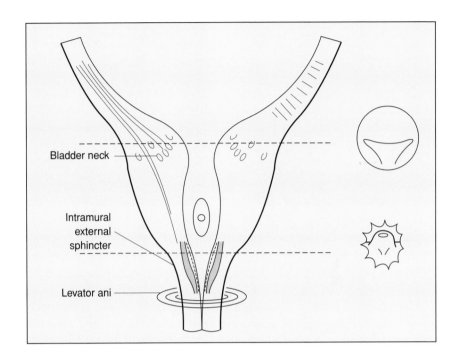

Figure 6.4

(a) Diagram of the external sphincter, just downstream of the verumontanum and (b) endoscopic photograph taken from just downstream of the sphincter.

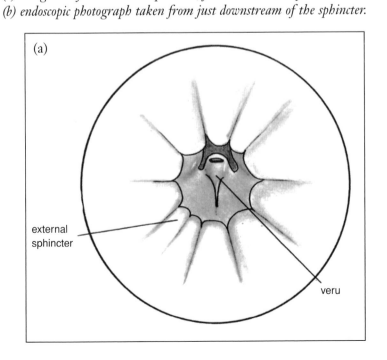

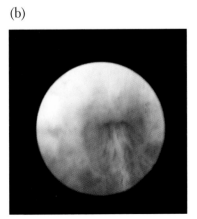

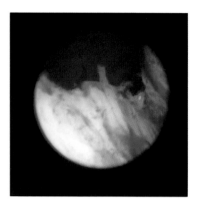 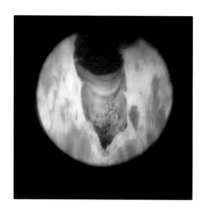

Figure 6.5
In a patient with a very small middle lobe the first cut reveals the transverse smooth muscle fibres of the bladder neck.

beyond the sphincter it instantly becomes more loose. Recognizing this sensation is of great importance: it is as important as for the blind man to know what it feels like to step off the pavement onto the road. It is an instant warning that you are too far down the urethra for safety.

The proximal limit to the resection is the ring of muscle at the neck of the bladder. Having identified the verumontanum and the external sphincter, the next step is to find the ring of muscle at the bladder neck in the posterior middle line. The purpose of defining this proximal limit is to prevent you from inadvertently encroaching on the trigone and ureteric orifices. In some patients there is virtually no adenoma in the region of the middle lobe and the first loopful of tissue reveals muscle fibres immediately under the urothelium (Fig. 6.5). In others it is necessary to resect a considerable volume of adenoma before the bladder neck is exposed (Fig. 6.6). Once these fibres have been laid bare, they are left alone for the time being, even though it may be necessary to return to the bladder neck and trim more of it away at the end of the resection.

When the adenoma is very big the anatomy is distorted, and the lumps of adenoma in the apex of each lateral lobe extend well down below the verumontanum, distorting the supramembranous intrinsic component of the external sphincter (Fig. 6.7). When the time comes to resect this apical tissue great care is taken to lift it up with a finger in the rectum so that the loop does not cut the corner and injure the sphincter. It is equally important to refrain from coagulating in this region for fear of injuring the sphincter.

Having found the muscle fibres of the bladder neck, you now complete the removal of the middle lobe from the bladder neck down to just above the verumontanum (Fig. 6.8). You should now be able to see verumontanum and bladder neck in the same field of view and easily reorientate yourself if you get lost (Fig. 6.9).

The value of the verumontanum as a landmark is recognized by all experienced resectionists. In the old days of open prostatectomy it was not

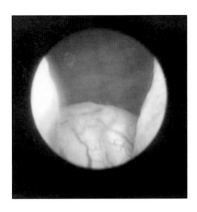

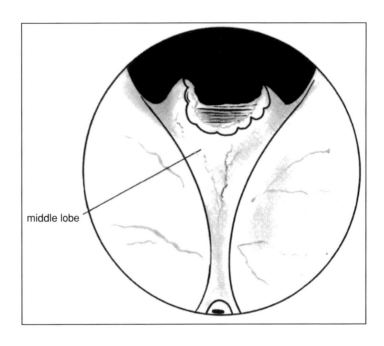

middle lobe

Figure 6.6
When there is a larger middle lobe more tissue must be removed before the bladder neck is exposed.

uncommon to see the verumontanum in the specimen, and the patients were not always incontinent because the intrinsic component of the external sphincter remained behind. But the verumontanum lies just upstream of the supramembranous sphincter and wantonly to remove it is not only to vandalize a useful landmark which never causes obstruction to the flow of urine, but also to guarantee the end of any chance of ejaculation.

Figure 6.7
In the small prostate: (a) the verumontanum is well upstream of the sphincter, but in a big bulky prostate (b) the lateral lobe adenomas bulge down past the verumontanum and distort the sphincter.

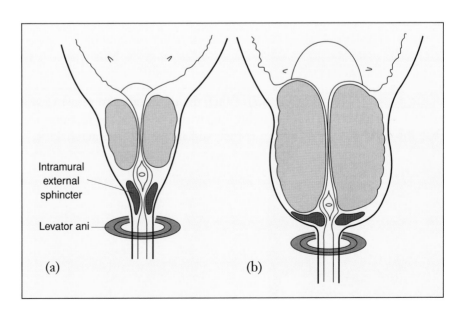

Intramural external sphincter

Levator ani

(a)   (b)

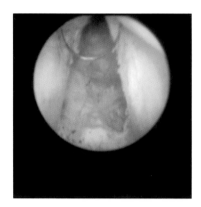

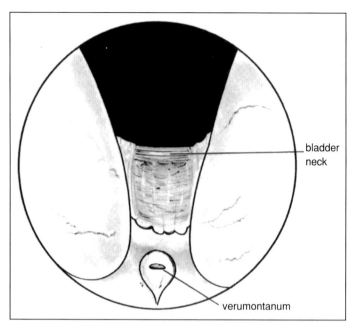

Figure 6.8
All the middle lobe tissue should be removed from the bladder neck down to just upstream of the verumontanum.

In the course of defining the bladder neck fibres it is not uncommon to create a small perforation under the edge of the trigone: there is a tell-tale appearance as if of a spider's web, and sometimes a distinct black hole in the connective tissue under the neck of the bladder (Fig. 6.10). By themselves these are not important, but they do mean you must take care not to pass the beak of the resectoscope under the trigone.

Once the middle lobe has been neatly cleaned out, take time to coagulate Badenoch's large arteries at 5 and 7 o'clock if these have not been completely controlled (Fig. 6.11).

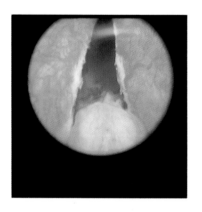

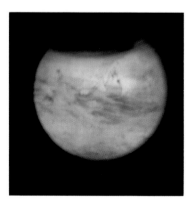

Figure 6.9 (left)
All the middle lobe is resected. You can see clearly from the middle lobe to the bladder neck.

Figure 6.10 (right)
Correctly resected middle lobe: there is a cobweb appearance under the bladder neck.

Figure 6.11
After resecting all the middle lobe, make sure that Badenoch's arteries at 5 and 7 o'clock have been controlled.

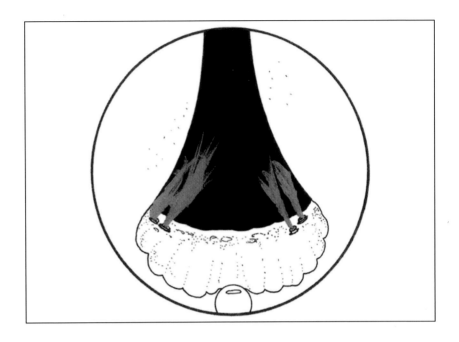

2. Removing the main bulk of tissue

Keeping the landmarks in mind, the next stage of the operation is to remove the main bulk of adenoma.

1. First method

In the first method to be described, you rotate the resectoscope to bring the anterior commissure into view at 12 o'clock (Fig. 6.12). The object is now to liberate one of the lateral lobes from the capsule. Begin by taking one or two careful chips at 1 o'clock until the bladder neck fibres and the capsule are disclosed, remembering that the prostate is very thin anteriorly (Fig. 6.13). Continue to deepen the trench until the lateral

Figure 6.12 (left)
The anterior commissure.

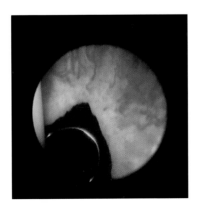
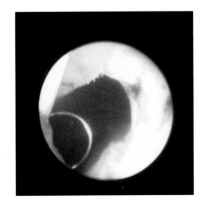

Figure 6.13 (right)
After the first one or two chips the capsule is exposed at 1 o'clock.

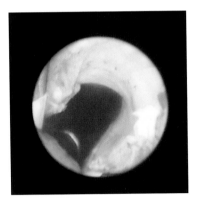

Figure 6.14
The trench is deepened and the left lateral lobe falls backwards.

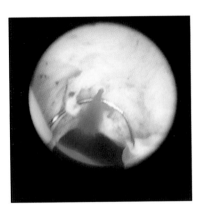

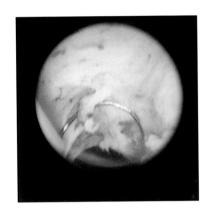

Figure 6.15
The 2 o'clock arteries of Flocks need to be carefully controlled.

lobe falls backwards into the defect left by removal of the middle lobe (Fig. 6.14). In doing this you may come across the little arteries of Flocks at 2 o'clock, which should be carefully coagulated[4] (Fig. 6.15).

The next step is to remove the lump of lateral lobe which has fallen inwards and away from the capsule. Removing this part is usually relatively bloodless, because the main arteries have already been controlled at 2 and 5 o'clock. Trim the top of the lateral lobe away in a series of even cuts, keeping the surface flat (Fig. 6.16). Do not make the mistake of hollowing out the lateral lobe or you will find that a thin shell of tissue will flop down and conceal the verumontanum (Figs 6.17 and 6.18).

Make sure that each stroke of the resectoscope loop cuts its chip off completely: do not make the mistake of leaving a chip attached at its distal end like a pine cone (Fig. 6.19).

At this stage you can leave the most distal nubbin of apical tissue just near the verumontanum. Go over the whole of the inner surface of the prostatic 'capsule' from which you have removed the lateral lobe and make sure that all the bleeding has been stopped.

Figure 6.16
Trim the top of the lateral lobe evenly, keeping its surface flat.

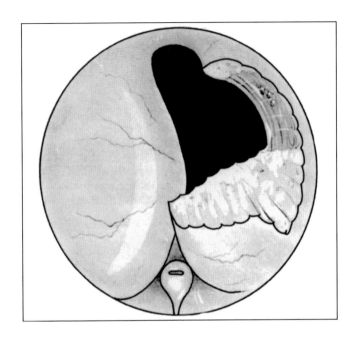

Figure 6.17
Avoid the mistake of hollowing out the lateral lobe and leaving a thin shell on the medial side.

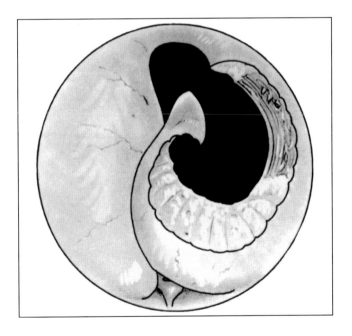

Check the position of the verumontanum and bladder neck, and then turn your attention to the other side. You will find that the anterior commissure seems to have moved and your original 2 o'clock trench now seems to be at 12 o'clock. Make a second trench (Fig. 6.20), detach

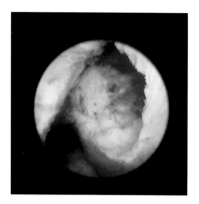

Figure 6.18
Left lateral lobe hollowed out: the medial edge needs to be trimmed flat before it flops down and covers up the verumontanum.

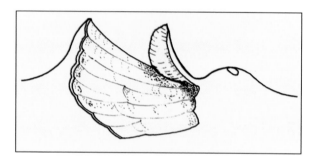

Figure 6.19
Make sure that every chip is detached. Do not make a pine cone of your resection.

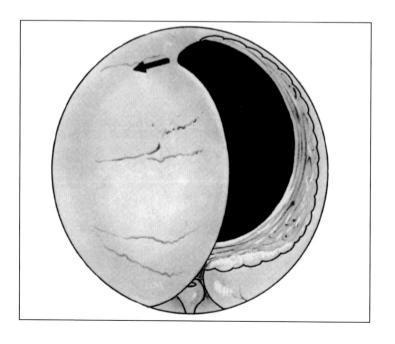

Figure 6.20
Beginning the second lateral trench. Note that the anterior commissure seems to have moved over to the right.

Figure 6.21
Beginning the resection of the right lateral lobe.

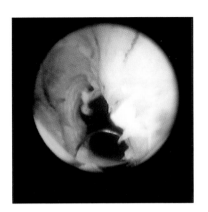 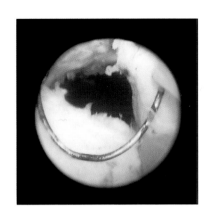

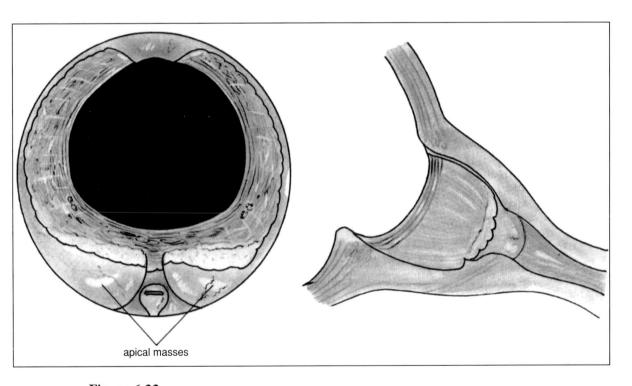

apical masses

Figure 6.22
Both lateral lobes are now removed, leaving only a little nubbin of apical tissue on either side of the verumontanum.

the other lateral lobe, cut it away quickly and cleanly (Fig. 6.21), leaving only the nubbin of apical tissue adjacent to the verumontanum (Fig. 6.22). Go over the exposed 'capsule' and control the bleeding.

2. Second method

Many surgeons find it more comfortable to remove the bulk of the lateral lobes in one circular sequence (Fig. 6.23). After removing the middle lobe (as above) you start by taking one lateral lobe from the bottom upwards, across the commissure between the lateral lobes, and then down the other lateral lobe to the starting point (Figs 6.24 and 6.25). It is important to start each chip at the level of the bladder neck and continue the cut down to the downstream limit of the adenoma, at the level of the verumontanum, in order to maintain a clear plan of progress. Long chips are achieved by moving the sheath in the urethra (Fig. 6.26). As you deepen the cut under the lateral lobe so the length of cut must be shortened to follow the barrel shape of the 'capsule' (Fig. 6.27).

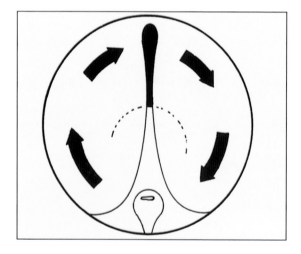

Figure 6.23
Richard Notley plan of resection: after removing the middle lobe, the operator starts at 7 o'clock and works all round the clock.

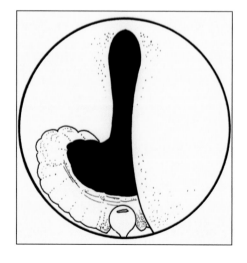

Figure 6.24
Beginning to resect the right lateral lobe, from 7 to 9 o'clock.

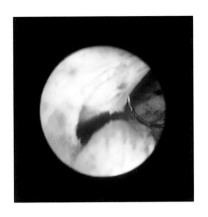
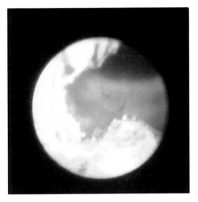
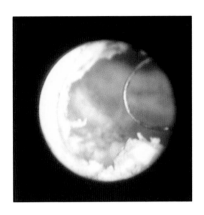

Figure 6.25
The right lobe is progressively resected from 7 to 9 o'clock.

Figure 6.26
Long chips are made by adding movement of the sheath (b) to the movement of the loop (a).

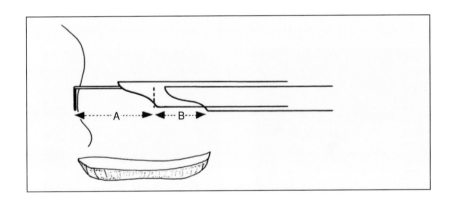

Figure 6.27
Resecting the right lateral lobe.

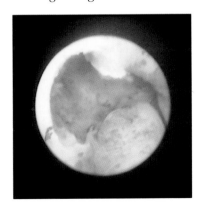
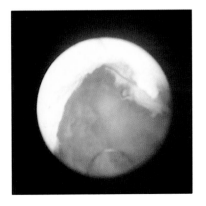
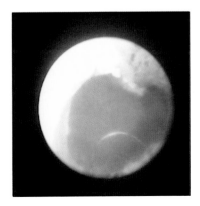

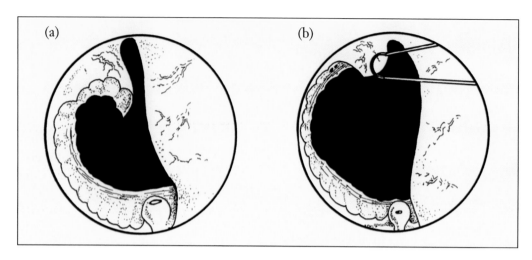

Figure 6.28

(a) Take care not to hollow out the lateral lobe.

(b) Near the commissure, where the adenoma is very thin, direct the loop laterally, not upwards.

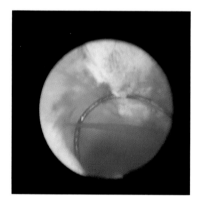 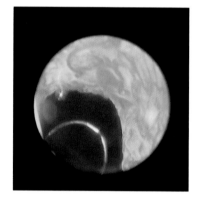 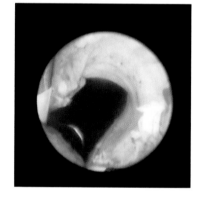

Figure 6.29
Flock's 10 o'clock artery will need to be coagulated.

Figure 6.30
Continuing the resection across the anterior midline to the left.

Figure 6.31
Continuing to resect the left lateral lobe, which has now fallen back.

As your resection approaches the anterior commissure a mass of tissue will be seen hanging down. Remember again that the prostate is very thin here: do not hollow it out (Fig. 6.28) but trim it away with the loop pointing laterally rather than upwards. The 10 o'clock arteries of Flocks will be found here and must be carefully coagulated (Fig. 6.29).

The resection can then be carried across the midline at 12 o'clock, bearing in mind that there is not much depth of adenoma in this part of the gland (Fig. 6.30). Continue the clockwise resection until the rest of the lateral lobe is removed (Fig. 6.31), sparing only the tissue adjacent to the verumontanum.

3. Tidying up

In the third stage the apical tissue that has been left behind is removed very carefully. The danger here is that the sphincter may be damaged, and you do not start this part of the resection until you have completely controlled the bleeding and have a really clear view. Repeatedly check the position of the verumontanum and sphincter. Take only very short chips. It often helps to insert one finger in the rectum to lift up the verumontanum and offer the apical tissue to the loop rather than digging with the loop to scoop it out (Fig. 6.32). The finger in the rectum provides a very precise sensation of the amount of tissue remaining and of the nearness of the loop. Bleeding is seldom severe in the region of the apex and one should be very sparing in the use of the coagulating current.

After emptying the bladder, withdraw the sheath beyond the sphincter, and then gradually advance it: this will show where you have left adenoma behind. The usual places are just on either side of the verumontanum, and up at 2 and 10 o'clock. These are all carefully trimmed

Figure 6.32
A finger in the rectum lifts the apical tissue up to the resectoscope loop.

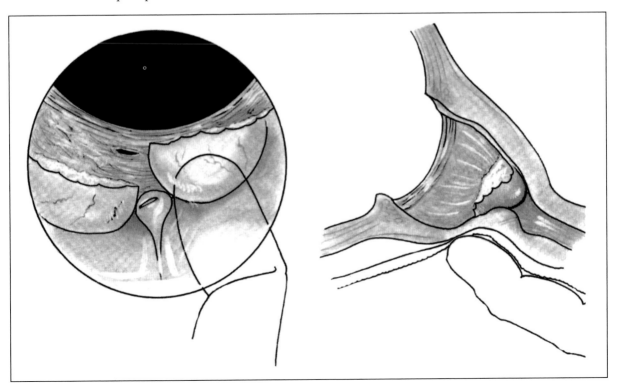

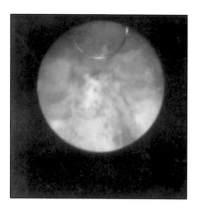

Figure 6.33
Trim the apical tissue with great care to preserve the verumontanum.

away (Fig 6.33). In removing the tissue adjacent to the verumontanum err on the side of caution. A gram or two of adenoma in this situation does not cause outflow obstruction, and a damaged sphincter can never be restored.

Resection of the larger prostate >50 g

Thanks to the instruments of today there is virtually no limit to the size of prostate that can be resected transurethrally so long as the surgeon can keep clearly orientated and maintain concentration and patience. It is unwise to attempt to resect a bulky gland when the resectoscope sheath does not slip easily over a huge mound of middle lobe, or when there is so much oedema and bleeding from the margin of the prostate that it is impossible to keep one's bearings. Such cases are uncommon, and it is interesting to see how seldom experienced resectionists need to perform an open prostatectomy. Be guided by your own common sense and judgement. Never be deceived by pride or by a sense of letting down your patient by embarking on a transurethral resection when you are not comfortable and confident: far better to do a clean, safe, open enucleative prostatectomy. On the other hand, if you can see clearly enough to keep your bearings, it is hardly more difficult to remove 100 g than 40 g, since the steps of the operation are the same even though they take a little longer.

Stage 1

With a really bulky prostate there is much to be said for a preliminary coagulation of the main prostatic arteries at 10, 2, 5 and 7 o'clock using the roly-ball before taking out any tissue (Fig. 6.34).

In the first stage the middle lobe is often very bulky and bulges up and over the trigone (Fig. 6.35). It must be resected evenly along its top so

Figure 6.34
Prophylactic coagulation at 10, 2, 5 and 7 o'clock before starting to resect.

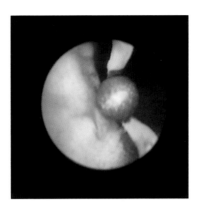

Figure 6.35
The middle lobe can be very large.

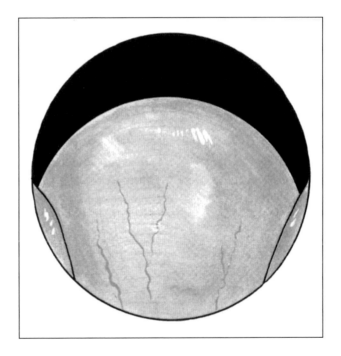

that the mound is kept level and flat, otherwise it is easy to cleave it into two halves by a single deep channel in the middle which leaves you bewildered and confused by what now seem to be two lateral lobes (Fig. 6.36). In removing the larger middle lobes the large 5 and 7 o'clock arteries will be exposed on either side and thoroughly coagulated (Fig. 6.37). It is wise to remove the whole of the middle lobe right down to within a few millimetres of the verumontanum. There is a tiresome tendency for a clot to sit just proximal to the verumontanum, making it difficult to see clearly. A finger in the rectum makes it easier to check on the position of the verumontanum and complete the resection of the middle lobe (Fig. 6.38).

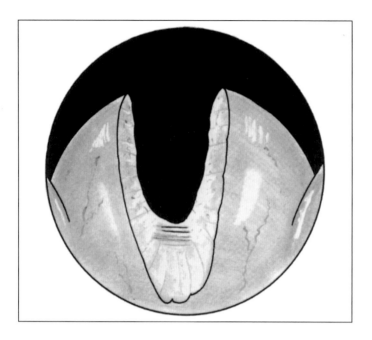

Figure 6.36
If you do not resect the middle lobe evenly you end up with a deep trench and 'two' middle lobes, which can be very confusing.

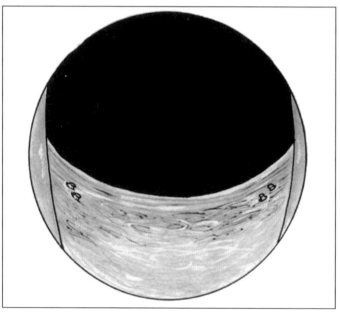

Figure 6.37
After resecting all the middle lobe, make sure that the 5 and 7 o'clock arteries are completely controlled.

As always, make sure of the haemostasis before going on to the next stage of the resection.

Stage 2

With large glands it is better to attempt to remove the whole of one lateral lobe than nibble away at both. If you prefer the first method, start

Figure 6.38
A finger in the rectum makes it easier to check on the position of the verumontanum.

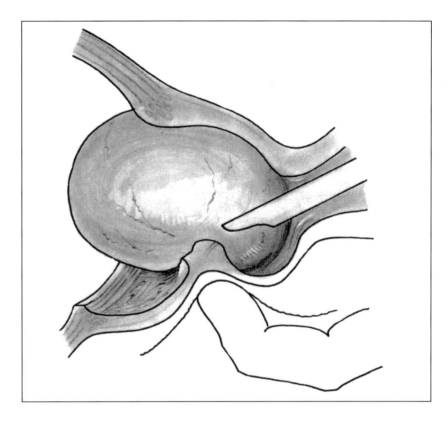

Figure 6.39
Start the trench near the anterior commissure.

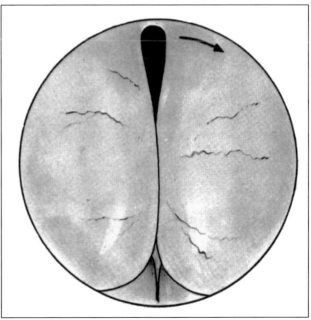

the trench near the anterior commissure (Fig. 6.39), where the adenoma is always very thin, seal off Flocks' arteries, allow the lateral lobe to fall down, and then cut it away with long even strokes, making sure you do not hollow it out (Fig. 6.40). A finger in the rectum will help to offer the adenoma to the loop rather than you having to dig into the barrel-shaped cavity of the capsule (Fig. 6.41).

If you take big long chips and move the sheath as well as the loop, you are less likely to create cliffs of unresected tissue half way down the prostatic urethra which may cause you to lose your bearings, but of course, you must not let the loop go past the verumontanum at this stage.

Once the first lateral lobe has been removed, saving only the apical tissue (Fig. 6.42), go over the inside of the barrel carefully to stop all the bleeding; if necessary using the roly-ball. If you put off getting haemostasis at this stage you will find that when you return everything is confused by tenacious clot which conceals the origin of the bleeding. If there has been a considerable loss of blood, it is sensible to consider stopping the operation when one lateral lobe has been removed. The patient will often be able to pass urine perfectly well.

If all is well, go ahead and remove the other lateral lobe in the same way (Figs 6.43 and 6.44). It is of no importance which lobe you resect first but it is wise to get into the habit of doing things in the same order, a rule which is especially valuable when you are teaching others.

The third stage in removal of a very large prostate is more difficult because the apical tissue often extends some way distal to the verumontanum (Fig. 6.45) where there is often a definite edge, 'Nesbit's white line', marking the distal limit of the adenoma[5]. The problem is to know

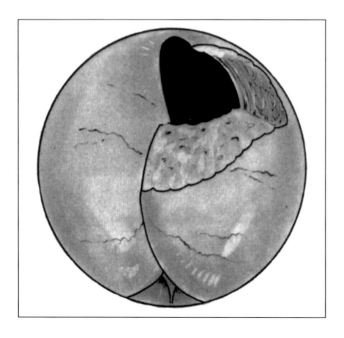

Figure 6.40
Trim the lateral lobe evenly and avoid hollowing it out.

Figure 6.41
A finger in the rectum helps to push the adenoma medially towards the loop.

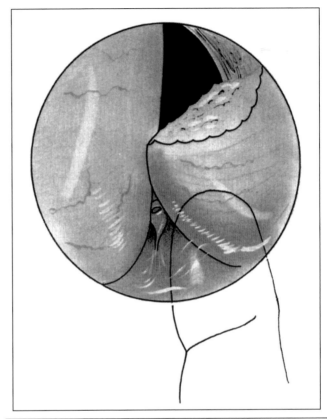

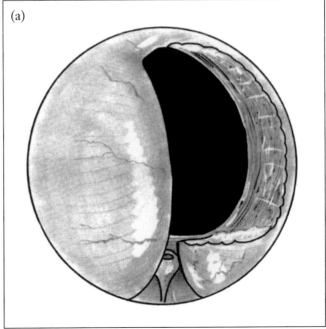

(a)

Figure 6.42
(a) Endoscopic and (b) lateral view after nearly all the left lateral lobe has been removed leaving only a small apical mass level with the verumontanum.

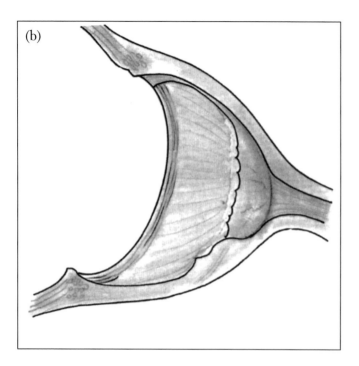

(b)

Figure 6.42 (*continued*)

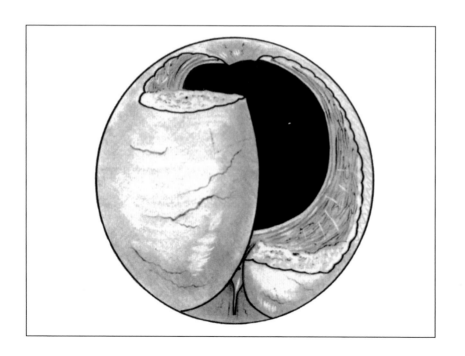

Figure 6.43
Removal of the right lateral lobe.

Figure 6.44
Both lateral lobes removed: apical tissue remains level with verumontanum.

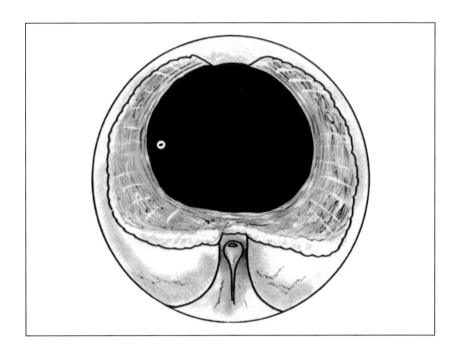

(a)

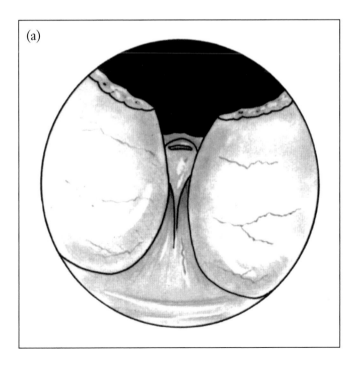

Figure 6.45
(a) Endoscopic and (b) lateral view of a large prostate showing how the apices of the lateral lobe can extend downstream of the verumontanum.

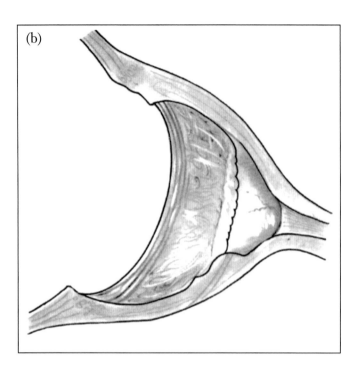

(b)

Figure 6.45 (*continued*)

how much of this has to be removed if all the obstruction is to be relieved, without risking damage to the sphincter.

With a finger in the rectum to lift up the apical tissue, and taking very short bites with the loop, the bulk of the adenoma is trimmed away. A back-cut from just above Nesbit's white line helps to define the distal limit of resection (Fig. 6.46).

Once the lateral lobes have been removed and the apices trimmed up, withdraw the resectoscope again distal to the sphincter and slowly advance it to identify any remaining tissue at 2 and 10 o'clock (Figs 6.47 and 6.48).

Finally, make a careful bimanual examination after emptying out the bladder. Usually all that is felt is a ridge of tissue on either side of the midline, exactly the same as after an enucleative prostatectomy (Fig. 6.49).

Perforations

Page[6] showed that the tissue remaining in the outer zone after removing the adenoma from the 'capsule' was composed of a compressed adenoma, which was in fact thinner than the loop of the resectoscope. There was no such thing as a true anatomical capsule, or at best only a paper-thin layer of connective tissue which was continuous with that

Figure 6.46
(a) A finger in the rectum lifts up the apex, well clear of the verumontanum. (b) Short back-cuts with the loop define the lower edge of the apex.

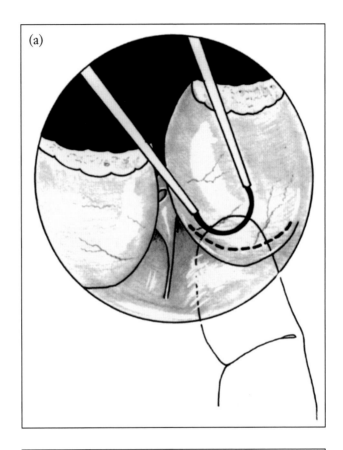

(a)

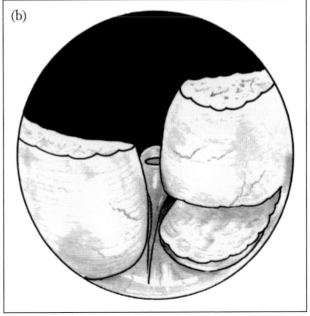

(b)

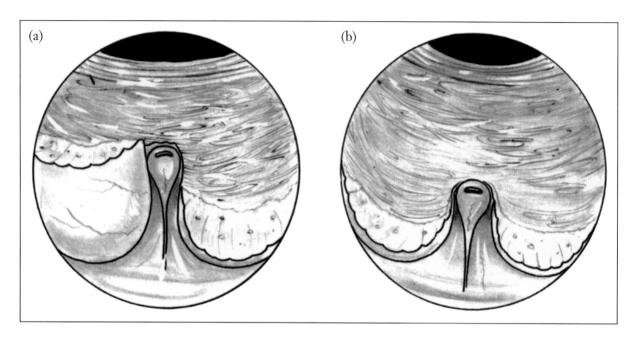

Figure 6.47
(a) First one and then (b) the other apices are cleared, leaving an intact verumontanum.

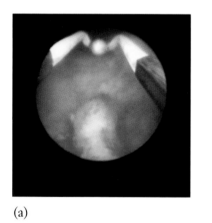
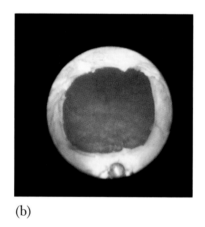

(a)   (b)

Figure 6.48
(a) The resection is complete: the verumontanum is intact, and (b) the cavity of the prostate has been clearly hollowed out.

which surrounded the vessels in the periprostatic fat. What we recognize as 'capsule' is in fact nearly a perforation. It is small wonder then that at the end of a resection it is usual to see little patches of fat (Fig. 6.50), and sometimes the dark hole which is actually the lumen of a vein (Fig. 6.51). These little perforations are not dangerous and there is no need to drain the retropubic space even though there is always some extravasation of the irrigating fluid into it.

Figure 6.49
Bimanual palpation will reveal any lumps of prostate that have been left behind.

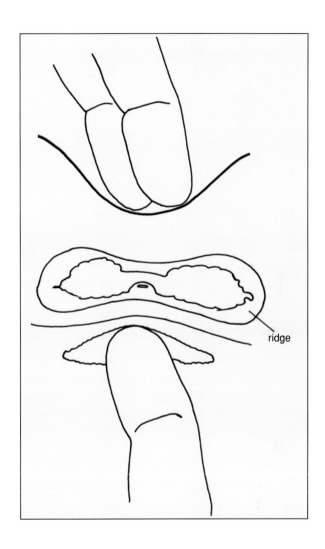

ridge

Figure 6.50
Capsule exposed, and a perforation showing fat globules.

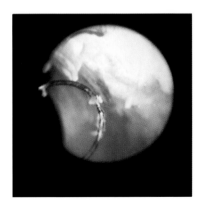
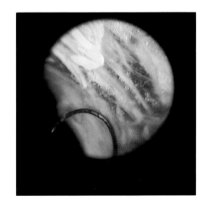

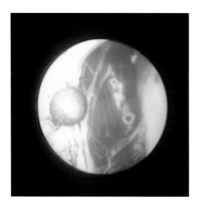

Figure 6.51
*Deep perforation, probably
the lumen of a vein.*

The same deep cut which has revealed fat may have damaged a large vein, which is not controlled by coagulation. In such an event the resection should be completed as quickly as possible and the bleeding controlled with tamponade (see page 85).

Perforations under the trigone

During the first stage of transurethral resection, as the bladder neck is being exposed under the middle lobe, it is very common to see small perforations which give the tell-tale appearance of a spider's web. By themselves these are not important, but there is a risk that the beak of the resectoscope may be driven inadvertently under the trigone, between the bladder muscle and the fascia of Denonvilliers. If this happens it produces a startling sight down the resectoscope (Fig. 6.52) but

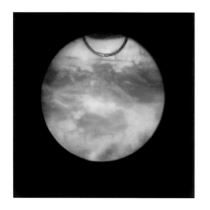 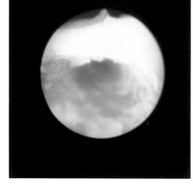 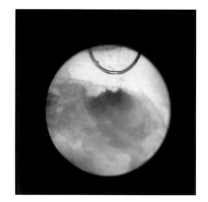

Figure 6.52
Perforation under the bladder neck.

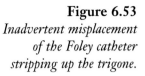

Figure 6.53
Inadvertent misplacement of the Foley catheter stripping up the trigone.

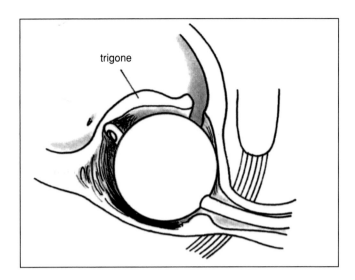

trigone

is not particularly dangerous: the danger is if the catheter is placed in this space and the balloon is inflated there (Fig. 6.53) – hence the precaution of passing the catheter on an introducer.

Catheters and drainage

Whatever the size of the gland the operation is concluded by putting in a suitable catheter and arranging through and through irrigation (Fig. 6.54). It is not necessary to use a catheter larger than 22Ch, but some surgeons prefer one made of PVC to latex. The irrigation is continued until the existing bag of glycine is finished, and then continued with saline. If the bleeding is more than a very faint pink the balloon should be filled with 40 ml and traction maintained (see page 85).

At this stage do not be in a hurry: have no hesitation in withdrawing the catheter and reinserting the resectoscope if haemostasis is not perfect. A few minutes of extra care at this stage may save hours of misery later on. If the patient has an endotracheal tube, wait for this to be removed, and wait for postoperative coughing and straining to have stopped before allowing the patient to go to the recovery room.

In the recovery room the team should all know how important it is to keep the irrigation flowing and how necessary it is to summon the surgical team if the catheter is blocked. It is easy to irrigate or change the catheter in the recovery room and, when in doubt, the patient can be returned to the theatre for a second look.

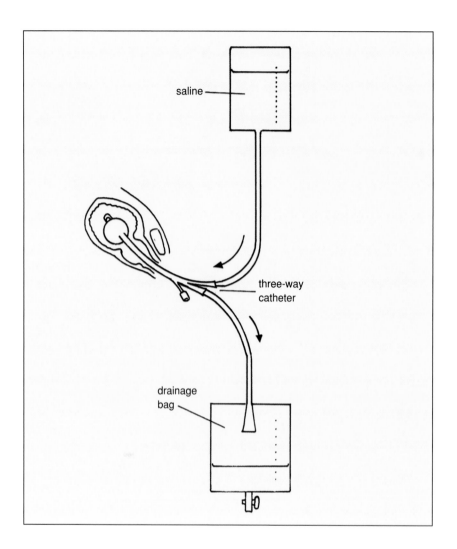

saline

three-way
catheter

drainage
bag

Figure 6.54
*Routine three-way
irrigation system.*

The mildly hypotensive patient should be allowed to recover his normal blood pressure naturally, not by aggressive fluid replacement. Particular care must be taken with the bradycardiac hypotensive patient, a common enough situation after halothane anaesthesia. It may be better to correct the bradycardia with atropine rather than attempt to restore the blood pressure by fluids. A confused patient complaining of pain should be allowed to recover his senses, when rational discussion of the discomfort can often allay his unhappiness without the automatic recourse to morphine which may prolong the period of postoperative recovery. The patient should only be allowed to return to the ward when the irrigation is running freely, is no darker than *vin rosé* and the patient is fully conscious.

Bladder neck dyssynergia

Younger patients may have outflow obstruction that seems to be caused by a failure of the α-adrenergic smooth muscle of the bladder neck to relax in synchrony with the contraction of the detrusor[7]. The predominant symptom is frequency, and urodynamics will show an abnormally high detrusor pressure and a poor flow-rate. A therapeutic trial of α-blockers such as prazosin is given, and if the patient is relieved of symptoms, but dislikes the side effects of the drug, the option can be put to him of incision of the bladder neck. It is important that he fully understands the risk of retrograde ejaculation and the possibility of being rendered infertile.

After the usual urethroscopy and cystoscopy, an incision is made with a Collings' knife through the ring of bladder neck muscle. Classically the incisions were made at 5 and 7 o'clock but the proximity of the neurovascular bundles to the penis suggests that incisions at 2, 10 or 6 o'clock may be preferable[8] (Fig. 6.55).

The small fibrous prostate

A different type of narrowing of the bladder neck is seen in patients with severe outflow obstruction but hardly any prostate to feel on rectal examination. They do not respond to α-blockers, and on resection the tissue is white and gristly and usually shows fibrous tissue on histological examination. Occasionally a more active granulation tissue is found in the specimen, in which case the patient should be carefully followed because recurrent stenosis of the bladder neck is then very likely. Mere

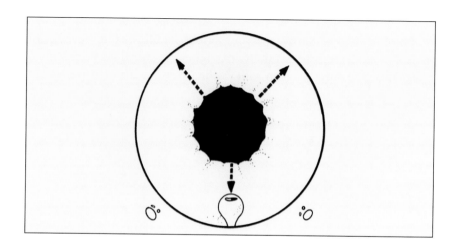

Figure 6.55
Bladder neck incisions which avoid the neurovascular bundles to the penis.

incision does not result in an open bladder neck and it is better to perform a circumferential resection, leaving only a strip of mucosa in the region of the anterior commissure (Fig. 6.56).

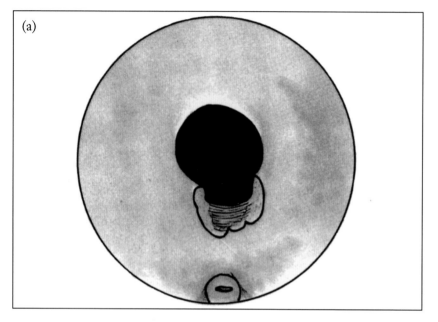

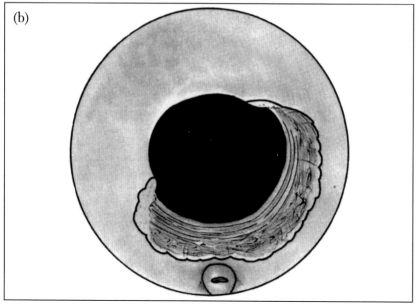

Figure 6.56
Transurethral resection of a small fibrous prostate.
(a) First cuts.
(b) Left half resected.

References

1. Green JSA, Bose P, Thomas DP *et al*. How complete is a transurethral resection of the prostate? *Br J Urol* 1996;77:398.
2. Blandy JP, Fowler CG. Prostate: structure and function. In *Urology*, 2nd edn. Oxford: Blackwell Science, 1996;363–74.
3. Gosling JA, Dixon JS, Humpherson RR. *Functional Anatomy of the Urinary Tract*. London: Gower, 1982.
4. Flocks RH. The arterial distribution within the prostate gland: its role in transurethral prostatic resection. *J Urol* 1937;37:524.
5. Nesbit RM. *Transurethral Prostatectomy*. Springfield, IL: Thomas, 1943.
6. Page BH. The pathological anatomy of digital enucleation for benign prostatic hyperplasia and its application to endoscopic resection. *Br J Urol* 1980;52:111.
7. Caine M. Reflections on alpha blockade therapy for benign prostatic hyperplasia. *Br J Urol* 1995;75:265.
8. Donker PJ, Droes JTPM, van Ulden BM. Anatomy of the musculature and innervation of the bladder and the urethra. In: Williams DI, Chisholm GD (eds) *Scientific Foundations of Urology*, Vol. 2. London: Heinemann, 1976:32.

Chapter 7

Transurethral resection of bladder tumours

The reasons for transurethral resection of a bladder tumour (TURBT) are to:

1. Provide accurate information with regard to bladder tumour grade and local stage.
2. Treat superficial bladder tumours, TURBT being the mainstay of treatment for the majority of such tumours (supplemented by intravesical chemotherapy and immunotherapy).
3. Palliate symptoms, such as bleeding, in invasive cancers where cystectomy or radiotherapy are not appropriate.
4. Debulk large tumours prior to radiotherapy.

In a small percentage of patients, transurethral resection of muscle invasive bladder tumours can be curative, as suggested by the absence of any residual tumour in the bladders of a number of patients who undergo cystectomy for muscle invasive disease diagnosed on an initial TURBT[1]. However, most patients with a diagnosis of a muscle invasive tumour will usually proceed to cystectomy (or radiotherapy), and thus it is only with the benefit of hindsight that it becomes apparent that the TURBT cured the cancer.

Preparations for TURBT

These are much the same as for TURP. TURBT is usually a shorter procedure than TURP and above-knee TED stockings (thromboembolism stockings) may be all that is necessary for DVT prophylaxis (provided that it is anticipated that the procedure will not last too long). However, if there are additional risk factors for venous thromboembolism then additional prophylaxis such as intermittent pneumatic calf compression may be necessary.

There have been no placebo-controlled randomized studies of antibiotic propylaxis for TURBT. We routinely culture the urine beforehand and use a similar antibiotic regime to that used for TURP.

Again, as for TURP some surgeons will prefer to stop drugs that might predispose to bleeding, such as aspirin and non-steroidal anti-inflammatory agents. Heavy bleeding after TURBT is uncommon, but checking the patient's blood group and saving some serum prior to TURBT is a sensible precaution.

If you anticipate that the resection is likely to be short, then consider using water rather than glycine. In theory this may cause lysis of freely floating tumour cells, so helping to prevent implantation of tumour cells in raw areas of resected bladder. For longer resections, glycine should be used to reduce the risk of intravascular haemolysis and possible TUR syndrome.

Formal resection versus fulguration of bladder tumours

Before deciding whether to resect a bladder tumour or to 'coagulate' it with a Bugbee electrode or the roly-ball, one should have a clear idea of the objectives of removal of the bladder tumour. If the tumour is to be removed for accurate staging and grading to decide the need for adjuvant treatment such as cystectomy or radiotherapy then a formal resection is required. Similarly, some tumours may be too large for roly-ball coagulation and therefore formal resection will be the only way in which the tumour can be removed to stop it from bleeding. If however, further aggressive surgical treatment is not contemplated, for example because the patient is very elderly and frail or has significant medical problems, and if it can be destroyed easily with the roly-ball or Bugbee electrode, then one will be more inclined to 'coagulate' the tumour using one or other of these electrodes. There is little point in resecting a tumour aggressively, thereby exposing the patient to the risk of uncontrollable bleeding or bladder perforation, if accurate staging information is not required and if the tumour can be confidently removed by coagulation alone. The bladders of little old ladies can be particularly thin and not infrequently discretion (in the form of roly-ball diathermy coagulation) is the better part of valour. Rather than coagulating the tumour it is easier to use the roly-ball with the cutting current, as the tissue so treated is vaporized rather than coagulated. Coagulated tissue tends to stick to the electrode, which has to be cleaned frequently as a consequence.

Small tumours

When the tumour is very small it can be pinched off together with its base and a layer of bladder muscle with the sharp 'cold' cup forceps. The base is then touched with the diathermy to stop any bleeding. An

Figure 7.1
Insulated biopsy forceps.

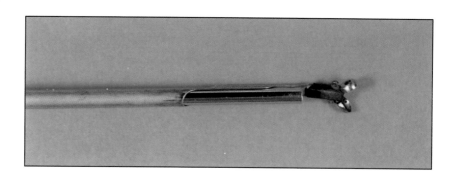

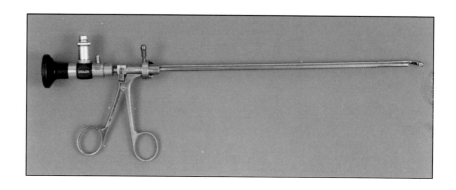

Figure 7.2
Very small tumours are easily coagulated with the Bugbee electrode.

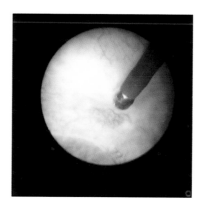 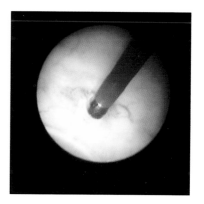

insulated biopsy forceps is available which can do both things without changing instruments (Fig. 7.1). When there are multiple superficial tumours a few of them are removed in this way and the remainder are coagulated with the roly-ball or Bugbee electrode (Fig. 7.2).

Biopsy

After removing the obvious tumour, many surgeons routinely take small mucosal biopsies from apparently normal bladder (Fig. 7.3). The cup forceps are thrust at once into formalin to give histology free from the artefact caused by picking the biopsy off a gauze swab with a needle.

Mossy patches

Flat pink patches without obvious exfoliative tumour should be biopsied and then coagulated with the roly-ball electrode. When there is an extensive area of this superficial tumour the process can be speeded up by using the cutting current.

The average pedunculated tumour

The majority of superficial tumours are from 1 to 3 cm in diameter on a well-defined stalk. One or two large vessels can be seen entering the stalk from the adjacent mucosa. These may be coagulated with the roly-ball prior to formal resection. These tumours are too large to be removed with the cup biopsy forceps, but a single cut of the diathermy loop can often lift them off the bladder with a generous divot of muscle (Fig. 7.4), and the base is then thoroughly coagulated (Fig. 7.5). If you have not obtained a generous sample of the base of the tumour and the

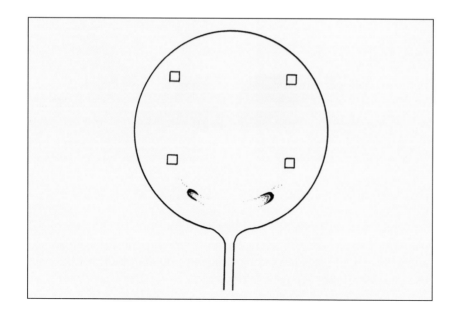

Figure 7.3
Random biopsies taken from the four quadrants of the bladder.

Figure 7.4
Resection of a small papillary tumour, base and all.

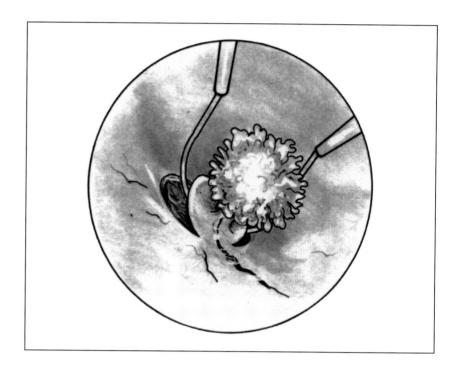

Figure 7.5
The roly-ball is used to coagulate the base.

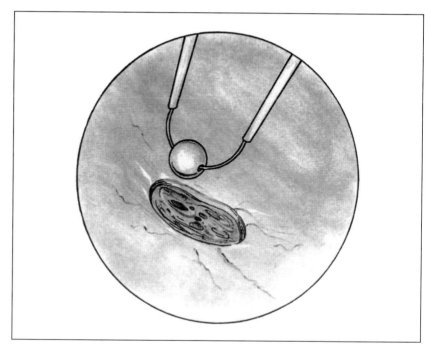

adjacent bladder wall, the cold cup forceps or the loop of the resecto-scope can be used to take an additional biopsy from the base of the stalk. This specimen can be sent in a separately labelled pot to indicate that this represents the part of the tumour that was immediately adjacent to the bladder wall. The cold cup forceps may allow better preservation of the tumour architecture, which makes subsequent histological examination of the tumour easier.

Larger papillary tumours 4–6 cm diameter

The first difficulty when resecting the larger papillary tumours with the conventional irrigating system is that the tumour seems to move away from the telescope as the bladder fills up, and you find yourself trying to hit a moving target. As soon as you start to resect the bleeding makes the vision even worse. This difficulty is very largely overcome by using the Iglesias-type continuous flow resectoscope. If the inflow and outflow are correctly adjusted the tumour stays put and can be resected according to a methodical plan.

The second difficulty is that even though the stalk of the tumour may be quite narrow, the bush flops over and hides it, and until the big blood vessels in the stalk have been coagulated, resection of the bush is followed by more or less furious bleeding.

Do not attack the bush of the tumour as if you were trimming a hedge. Direct your attack at the stalk. It will probably be necessary to start by resecting the fronds of the bush which hide the stalk from you (Figs 7.6

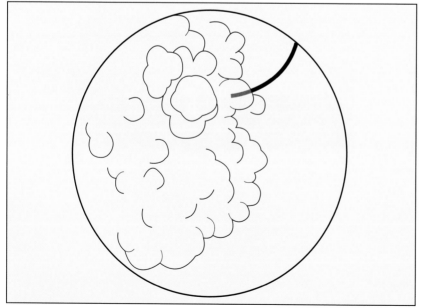

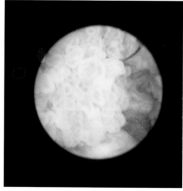

Figure 7.6
The first aim is to expose the stalk by resecting the overhanging bush.

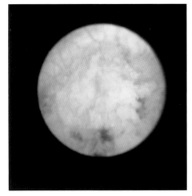

Figure 7.7
Overlying bush resected to reveal the stalk.

and 7.7). As soon as you see the edge of the stalk, apply the roly-ball electrode to the stalk to coagulate it, and render the rest of the resection relatively bloodless (Fig. 7.8).

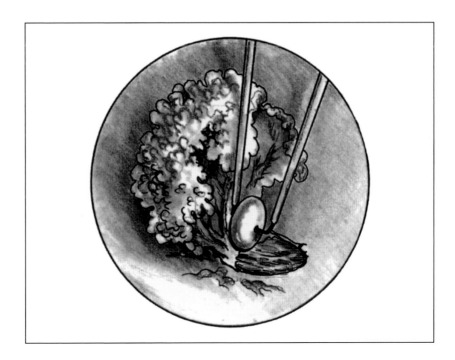

Figure 7.8
Once the stalk has been found, use the roly-ball to coagulate the main vessels.

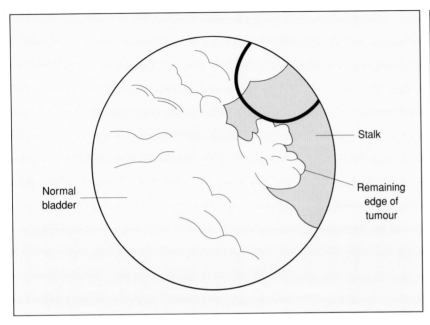

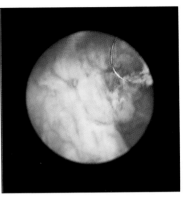

Figure 7.9
Trimming remaining tumour from the edge of the stalk.

Then, having found the edge of the stalk, work round it, continuing to resect more and more of the overlying tumour until it has all been removed. Towards the end of the process you will find it easier to work from healthy bladder towards the stalk (Fig. 7.9). Finally, send pieces from the muscle in the base of the stalk for separate section to help the histopathologist establish how deeply it has invaded (Fig. 7.10). Make

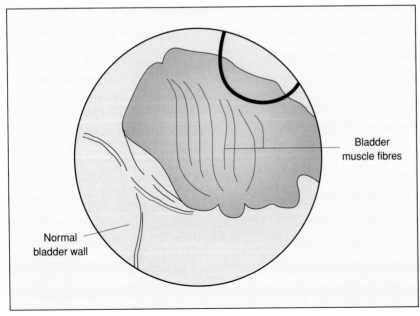

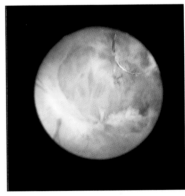

Figure 7.10
A separate biopsy, taken from the stalk, is sent to detect muscle invasion.

Figure 7.11
The base is coagulated with the roly-ball to achieve complete haemostasis.

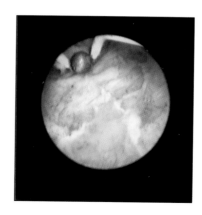

sure that the tissues from the bush and the stalk are sent in separate specimen pots to the laboratory, labelled 'bush' and 'stalk' respectively. Finally, go over the base of the stalk thoroughly with the roly-ball electrode to effect haemostasis and coagulate the layer of bladder muscle deep to your resection (Fig. 7.11). Haemostasis must be complete, for unlike the prostate there is no way of effecting tamponade in the bladder.

After resection is complete, empty the bladder and perform a careful bimanual examination: induration in the wall of the bladder remaining after resection suggests invasion of muscle, and puts the tumour stage into T3.

Once haemostasis is complete, set up continuous irrigation as for a routine prostatectomy (see page 153).

Second-look TURBT

In some circumstances a second TURBT is carried out some weeks after the first resection. This is done where the preliminary pathology report suggests a high grade, non-invasive tumour or an intermediate grade tumour that is equivocally into muscle. The rationale for the second-look TURBT is to establish whether there really is no muscle invasion. In such cases, be particularly careful when taking further biopsies from the original tumour site, as the bladder wall here may be very thin and therefore prone to perforation. A cold cup biopsy may be safer than a formal loop resection where the bladder appears especially thin.

Very large papillary tumours

Very rarely one encounters a group of giant papillomas that daunt even the most experienced resectionist. It is true that with the continuous irrigating cystoscope it is usually possible to resect them in the way described above, but occasionally the bleeding is so furious that it is impossible to see where to start.

There are two options here. Resect as many of the tumours that you can see, as long as you are able to maintain a clear field of view, and then come back on another day to finish the job, rather than risk perforating the bladder. Alternatively, consider using prolonged high pressure cysto-distension – Helmstein's technique. This is very rarely used nowadays, and the majority of younger urologists will probably never have seen, let alone used it. Nonetheless we have retained a description of the technique for the rare cases where it may still be required[2,3]. The technique requires a very long period of continuous epidural anaesthesia because it relies on compression of the tumour by the balloon to produce ischaemic necrosis.

Under continuous epidural anaesthesia, which will produce a measure of hypotension, a large balloon is placed in the bladder tied to a catheter. Specially made and tested balloons are available for the purpose, but in the beginning Helmstein and others used ordinary toy balloons. The pressure inside the balloon is monitored continuously, as it is distended with glycine and the pressure is kept up for 6 hours (Fig. 7.12).

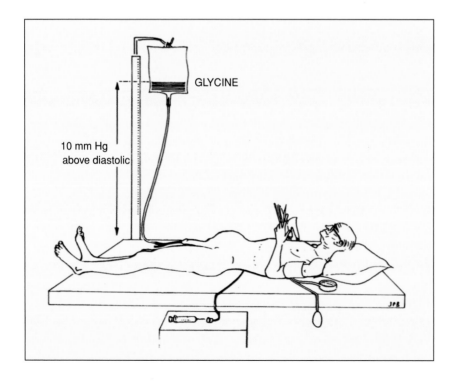

Figure 7.12
Helmstein's distension method.

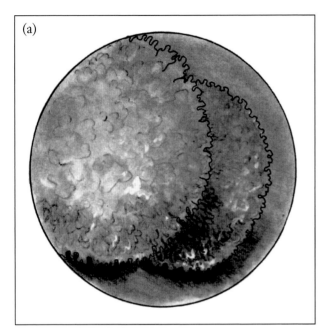

(a)

Figure 7.13
Three weeks after the Helmstein treatment, the bulky tumours (a) have sloughed away leaving only stumps (b) which are then resected.

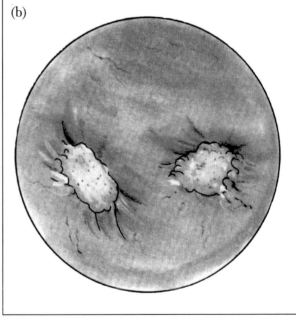

(b)

After the balloon is let down the ischaemic tissue of the tumour sloughs and an irrigating catheter may be necessary for the next few days until all the necrotic debris has come away. The bladder is re-examined after 3 weeks, by which time only the stumps of the previous tumours will be found. These are resected for staging in the usual way (Fig. 7.13).

Invasive solid tumours

When there is histological evidence of invasion of muscle the distinction between pT2 and pT3 is made according to the finding of induration on bimanual palpation after resection of the tumour is complete. Thus, after resection of a T2 tumour no mass or induration will remain, but after resection of a T3 cancer a mass or induration will still be palpable.

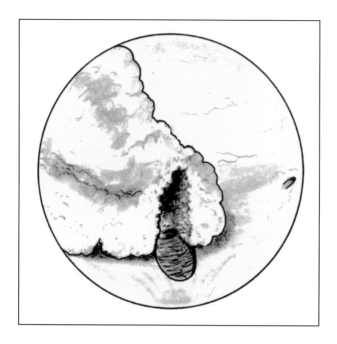

Figure 7.14
Large solid tumour: a deep biopsy which must include muscle, is taken from its edge for staging purposes.

The purpose of TURBT for solid tumours, where the patient is a candidate for aggressive adjuvant treatment such as radiotherapy or cystectomy, is to provide accurate grading and local staging information. It is not necessary to resect all the exophytic tumour, particularly if cystectomy is planned, as the purpose of the cystectomy (obviously) is to remove all residual cancer. For patients where radiotherapy is contemplated many surgeons feel that TURBT controls bleeding and provides symptomatic relief from frequency and strangury, and many radiotherapists prefer that the bulk of the intravesical tumour should be removed, leaving less to be destroyed by irradiation. To get evidence of tumour grade and stage, a good deep biopsy that reaches well into bladder muscle is required (Fig. 7.14).

Resecting tumours in inaccessible places

Tumours on the anterior wall and in the dome can sometimes be very difficult to reach. In this situation, decompress the bladder somewhat. This, combined with your free hand applying suprapubic pressure may bring the tumour within reach of the loop of the resectoscope. It is sometimes easier to use the roly-ball to treat such tumours, as this can be controlled more safely than the loop of the resectoscope. Sometimes inclining the table so that the patient is in the head-down position may make the resection a little easier, particularly where there is a large 'overhang' of lower abdomen. If these tricks fail, then ask for the long resectoscope.

Tumours in diverticula can present a problem. The bladder wall in the depths of a diverticulum is thin, and it is safer to use the cold cup biopsy forceps to remove tumours here, with roly-ball diathermy for coagulation.

Resecting tumours in the region of a ureteric orifice

From time to time a tumour is located right at the ureteric orifice and the surgeon's concern may be that resection or diathermy in this location could damage the ureter with subsequent scar formation and stricturing. None of the authors have ever seen this complication over many years of cumulative experience. The usual outcome is a gaping ureteric orifice ('golf-hole' ureteric orifice).

Management of this theoretical problem is based on anecdote. The use of pure cutting current will reduce the likelihood of scarring occurring, but clearly coagulating current may be required to stop bleeding. You can simply resect the tumour, leave the resected ureteric orifice alone and hope for the best. Alternatively, an insulated guidewire can be positioned in the ureter before the resection is done, so that you can subsequently place a JJ stent easily. This can be left in place for a couple of weeks and then removed. A follow-up intravenous urogram (IVU) will establish whether there is any significant hold-up to the flow of contrast through the ureter. However, as already stated, in practise we have not seen this problem and therefore leaving a JJ stent in place is probably unnecessary.

Occasionally the tumour completely obscures the ureteric orifice and in this situation one has no choice other than to resect it and then try to find the lumen of the ureter to allow placement of a JJ stent. Sometimes the lumen instantly becomes apparent; at other times it cannot be found. Again, a follow-up IVU will determine whether the ureteric orifice is obstructed, in which case a nephrostomy with antegrade balloon dilatation and stenting can be used to deal with the stricture. Again, it is our cumulative experience that ureteric obstruction is very rare and therefore such precautions are probably unnecessary.

Adjuvant chemotherapy for superficial tumours

Every patient who has been treated for a bladder tumour will be carefully followed up by regular check cystoscopy, nowadays using the flexible cystoscope. There is considerable evidence that prophylactic adjuvant immunotherapy with Bacillus Calmette-Guérin (BCG) or chemotherapy with mitomycin will diminish the number of recurrences, and when multiple tumours are seen, when they recur very frequently and in large numbers or where there is associated carcinoma *in situ*, these agents should be used[4,5].

Perforation

The bladder wall is often perforated during transurethral resection of a tumour and it is not uncommon to see the glistening globules of fat in the site of the stalk (Fig 7.15). As with the prostate, this is very seldom of any consequence provided that all the bleeding has been controlled. Extravasation of irrigating fluid is minimized by using a continuous irrigating resectoscope. The bladder should be drained.

The exception is when there is a tumour on the dome of the bladder and a deep resection of an invasive tumour has resulted in a perforation into the peritoneal cavity. This is very rare. It calls for laparotomy, not only to close the hole in the bladder and control bleeding, but also to make sure that any thermal injury to adjacent bowel is correctly over-sewn or resected (see Chapter 11).

There have been reports of spread of cancer cells into the peritoneal cavity following bladder perforation[6].

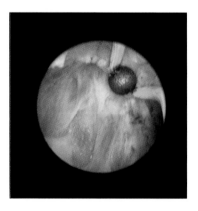

Figure 7.15
Perforation through the wall of the bladder into fat.

References

1. Herr HW. Transurethral resection in regionally advanced bladder cancer. *Urol Clin North Am* 1992;9:695–700.
2. Helmstein K. Treatment of bladder carcinoma by a hydrostatic pressure technique. *Br J Urol* 1972;44:434.
3. England HR, Rigby C, Shepheard BGF, Tresidder GC, Blandy JP. Evaluation of Helmstein's distension method for carcinoma of the bladder. *Br J Urol* 1973;45:593.
4. Tolley DA, Parmar MK, Grigor KM *et al*. The effect of intravesical mitomycin C on recurrence of newly diagnosed superficial bladder cancer: a further report with 7 years of follow-up. *J Urol* 1996;155:1233–8.
5. Lamm DL, Crawford ED, Blumenstein B *et al*. Maintenance BCG immunotherapy for recurrent Ta, T1 and Tis transitional cell carcinoma of the bladder: a randomized prospective Southwest Oncology Group Study. *J Urol* 2000;163:1124–9.
6. Myldo JH, Weinstein R, Shah S *et al*. Long term consequences from bladder perforation and/or violation in the presence of transitional cell carcinoma: results of a small series and a review of the literature. *J Urol* 1999;161:1128–32.

Chapter 8

Carcinoma and other disorders of the prostate and bladder

Carcinoma of the prostate

Since cancer usually arises in the peripheral zone of the prostate, when a small nodule is felt on rectal examination it is better to get tissue for histology by means of a transrectal biopsy, a procedure which today is most accurately performed under transrectal ultrasound control[1,2]. The later management of the small prostatic nodule is still a matter for debate which is beyond the scope of this monograph, and unfortunately is of little relevance to the large number of men who present at a stage when their cancer is not confined to the prostate, but is causing severe symptoms from outflow obstruction.

For these men transurethral resection of the prostate is but one incident in the management of their cancer, but at least to start with it is the one that is most necessary in order to relieve symptoms. The investigations and preparation are identical to those that apply to benign enlargement, and the urethroscopy and cystoscopy are the same standard preliminary.

One difficulty is often encountered with prostatic cancer, where a carcinoma has made the entire prostate and prostatic urethra rigid, as if made of concrete, and it is difficult to pass the resectoscope. Direct visualization of the urethra with a visual obturator can help negotiate a way through the prostate and into the bladder. If this fails, a helpful trick is to pass a filiform bougie, perhaps with a dog-leg bend at its tip (Fig. 8.1), to negotiate a tortuous pathway into the bladder. Once the filiform bougie is in place, an angled Timberlake obturator is fitted into the resectoscope sheath (Fig. 8.2), and the whole gently passed, following the filiform into the bladder. Once in the bladder, the tissue around the internal meatus is then resected, and at once the resectoscope sheath becomes mobile and the rest of the resection is straightforward.

If the angled Timberlake obturator is not available, the same procedure can be followed by passing the resectoscope sheath over a flexible Phillips follower which screws onto the filiform (Fig. 8.3).

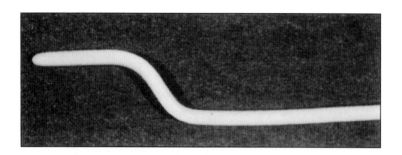

Figure 8.1
A dog-leg bend on the end of a filiform bougie assists in getting it past a tortuous carcinoma of the prostate.

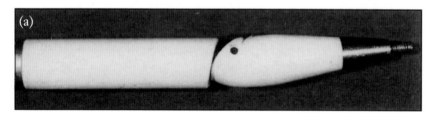

Figure 8.2
(a) An angled Timberlake obturator can be (b) screwed on to a filiform.

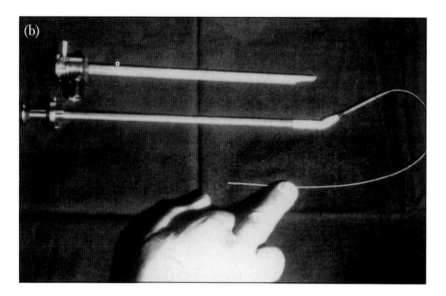

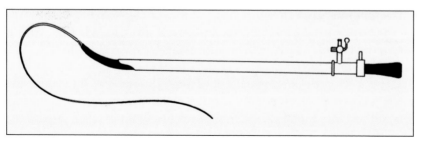

Figure 8.3
Alternative method of passing a resectoscope sheath through a hard, narrow prostate cancer using a flexible Phillips follower attached to the filiform.

In many cancers the landmarks may be difficult to find. Often the verumontanum is displaced or distorted by tumour, and sometimes the external sphincter is infiltrated by growth which makes it lumpy and

Figure 8.4

The external sphincter and verumontanum are often distorted by carcinoma of the prostate.

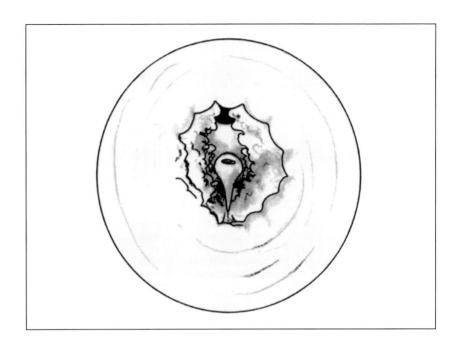

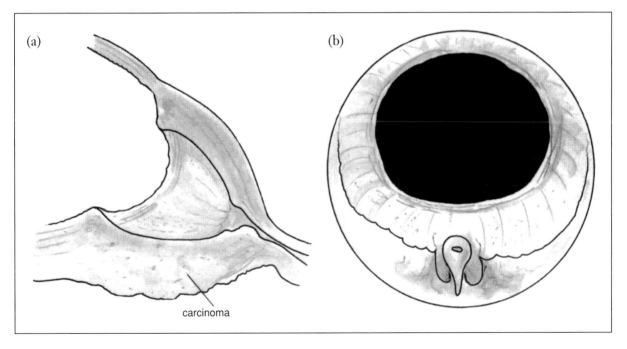

(a)

(b)

carcinoma

Figure 8.5

In cancer the intention is only to carve a funnel-shaped cone from the bladder neck to the verumontanum.

rigid (Fig. 8.4). Since the cancer usually arises in the peripheral and caudal outer zone of the prostate and invades the capsule early on, you must not expect to find the usual difference in appearance between the 'bread' of the adenoma and the fibrous lacework of the 'capsule'. Instead the object of the operation is to carve an adequate funnel through the tumour from verumontanum to bladder neck (Fig. 8.5), through which the patient can pass urine. There is no point in attempting to do more. You should be extra careful when resecting in the region of the verumontanum and sphincter in the hope of preserving continence.

In resecting prostatic cancers it is particularly helpful to work with one finger in the rectum, which will give a three-dimensional concept of the position of the resectoscope and the loop, even when the cancer has made the whole field stiff and unfamiliar.

As a rule, bleeding is less profuse in cancer of the prostate, but one precaution should not be forgotten in men who present with widespread metastases, namely the possible presence of prostatic fibrinolysins which may prevent normal coagulation. Be wary of this, especially in the patient who gives a story of spontaneous bleeding and bruising.

It has been suggested on many occasions that transurethral resection might allow cancer cells to enter the circulation and so encourage dissemination of metastases. The evidence is disturbing, but inconclusive[3,4]. When the requirement is to confirm a diagnosis and establish the grade of the tumour, needle biopsies guided by transrectal ultrasound are more useful.

Calculi in the prostate

Small multiple calculi are so common as to be a normal component of the prostate[5] and they usually lie in the plane between inner and outer zones (Fig. 8.6), so that when they are reached in the course of

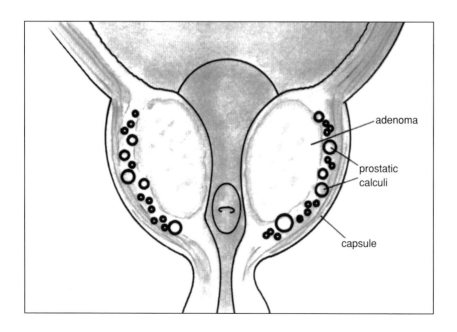

adenoma

prostatic
calculi

capsule

Figure 8.6
Small calculi are often found in the plane between the inner and outer zones of the prostate.

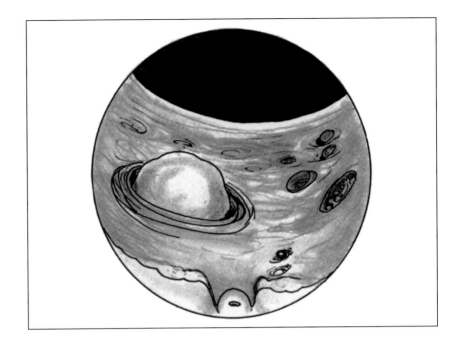

transurethral resection of a benign gland it is a good indication that the 'capsule' has been reached and you have gone far enough. Sometimes the stones are so large that the loop of the resectoscope is broken when trying to dislodge them (Fig. 8.7).

Less common are the very large stones which protrude into the lumen of the prostatic urethra and sometimes extend up into the bladder. They are always half-covered by a layer of prostatic tissue (Fig. 8.8). This has

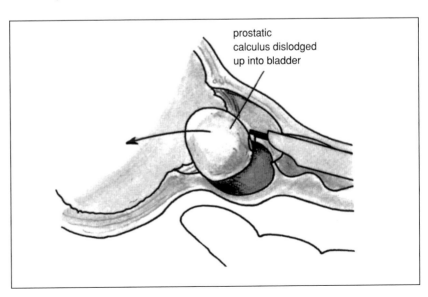

prostatic
calculus dislodged
up into bladder

Figure 8.8
After uncapping the adenoma over a big prostatic stone it is pushed upwards into the bladder where it can be crushed and evacuated.

to be resected before it is possible to push the stone up into the bladder, where it can be crushed and evacuated in the usual way[6].

Abscess of the prostate

Nowadays it is rare to see an abscess of the prostate, but it should always be suspected when a patient has fever, painful or difficult urination, and a very tender prostate on rectal examination[7]. Usually the prostate is more swollen on one side than the other. Sometimes the abscess bursts as soon as it is touched by the resectoscope; more often it is necessary to sink the loop of the resectoscope into the abscess, when pus pours out and the distended prostate collapses like a pricked balloon (Fig. 8.9).

Chronic prostatitis

This is a diagnosis to be made with the utmost caution, and requires bacteriological confirmation by Stamey's method[8], and perhaps histological confirmation by biopsy under transrectal ultrasound control. Occasionally it is accompanied by outflow obstruction, which in these cases must be proven by urodynamic measurements. Transurethral resection is likely to leave behind continuing infection in the residual outer zone tissue and relapse of symptoms is very likely to occur.

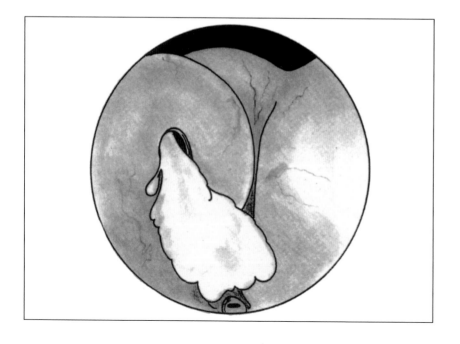

Figure 8.9
Opening an abscess of the prostate with the loop.

For the patient who complains of pain in the prostate and has no evidence of microbiological infection or the histological stigmata of inflammation, transurethral resection is contraindicated: it will almost certainly make the patient worse[9].

External sphincterotomy

In males with neuropathic lesions of the bladder an increase in the detrusor pressure may threaten the upper tracts; an incision of the bladder neck is often performed in the hope of allowing the bladder to empty at a lower pressure[10]. In some cases, however, the external sphincter remains closed, and the dangerous increase in detrusor pressure persists. In such patients a deliberate incision of the external sphincter may be necessary so that the bladder will become incontinent, and the patient voids without any increase in pressure into a condom urinal.

The classical site for the incision into the external sphincter was at 5, 6 or 7 o'clock, but to avoid injury to the neurovascular bundles of the penis the sphincterotomy incision should be made at 12 o'clock (Fig. 8.10).

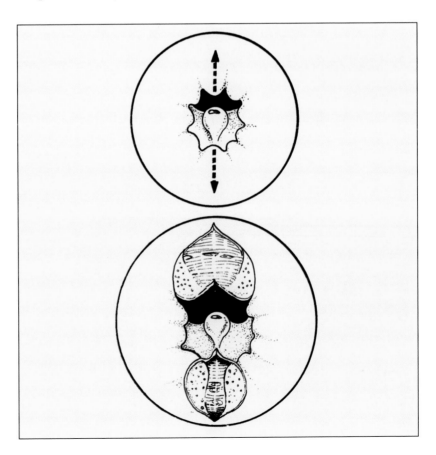

Figure 8.10
Sphincterotomy. Midline incisions avoid the neurovascular bundles to the penis.

Bladder calculi

Small stones are often found behind enlarged prostates. There are few calculi which cannot be crushed and evacuated. A number of instruments are now available for crushing bladder calculi including the optical lithotrite (Fig. 8.11), stone-crushing forceps (Fig. 8.12) and Mauermayer's stone punch (Fig. 8.13).

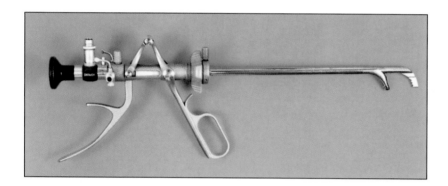

Figure 8.11
Storz optical lithotrite.

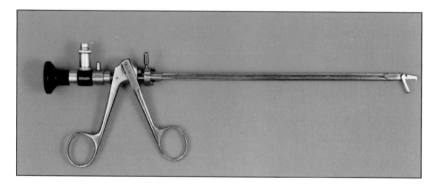

Figure 8.12
Storz stone-crushing forceps.

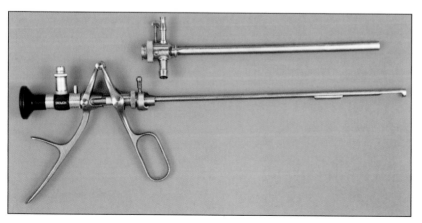

Figure 8.13
Mauermayer's stone punch.

Figure 8.14
Crushing a small calculus with Mauermayer's stone punch.

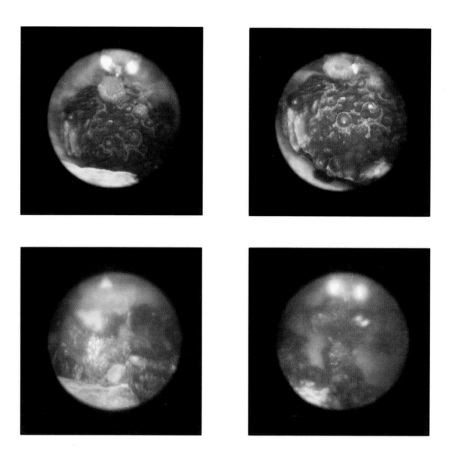

These optical instruments are ideal for small calculi, and allow the stone to be broken up under vision and evacuated with an Ellik evacuator (Fig. 8.14). Larger stones can be fragmented by a combination of electrohydraulic lithotripsy and the Mauermayer stone punch. Very large stones will require open cystolithotomy.

However, the classical blind lithotrite (Fig. 8.15), remains the most effective and rapid instrument for all but the smallest stones and it is a

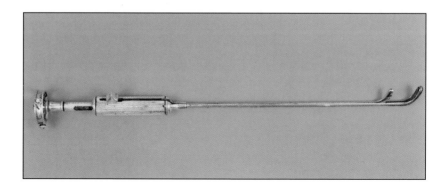

Figure 8.15
Freyer's classical lithotrite.

pity that its use is a skill which is dying out, despised by a generation of urologists reared on electrohydraulic or ultrasonic lithotriptors[11].

When there has been a large stone that has been present for a long time it is prudent to take a mucosal biopsy of any suspicious area in view of the occasional complication of squamous cell cancer[12].

When the patient has a bulky middle lobe it can be difficult to see the stone. It is then more convenient to resect most of the middle lobe, then crush and evacuate the stone, and complete the transurethral resection in the usual way.

Diverticula of the bladder

Small saccules are commonly present in association with prostatic obstruction and can be disregarded (Fig. 8.16). Larger diverticula must always be fully examined by passing the cystoscope inside them to rule out cancer or a stone; be particularly suspicious of a diverticulum whose opening is oedematous or inflamed. If you cannot see inside clearly, make sure that the diverticulum is innocent by means of a CT scan. When it harbours a stone or a tumour, or when there is continuing infection, the diverticulum should be removed, but since the prostate is often quite a small one, it is easier to perform the prostatectomy transurethrally and then go on to do the diverticulectomy in the usual way[13].

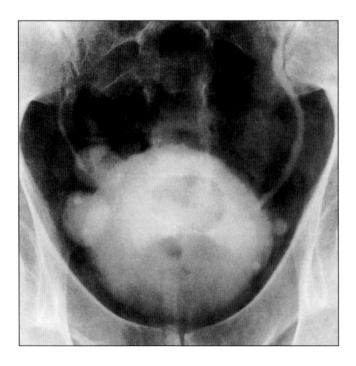

Figure 8.16
Multiple small diverticula are often found with a trabeculated bladder.

Urethral strictures and transurethral resection

Strictures may be found in patients who need transurethral resection of a bladder tumour. To allow the passage of the resectoscope it is necessary to dilate them or perform an optical urethrotomy. The optical urethrotome (Fig. 8.17) may be passed over a guidewire or a ureteric catheter if the way through the stricture cannot be seen clearly (Fig. 8.18). The incision is made at 12 o'clock right through the fibrous stricture into healthy tissue (Fig. 8.19). Urethrotomy by itself does not

Figure 8.17
Sachse optical urethrotome (Storz).

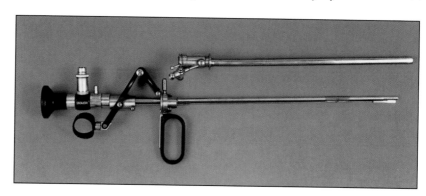

Figure 8.18
A guidewire or ureteric catheter may be passed through the stricture if the way through is not clear.

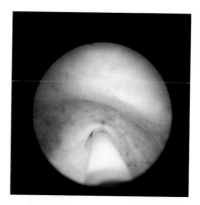

Figure 8.19
Internal optical urethrotomy using a ureteric catheter as guide.

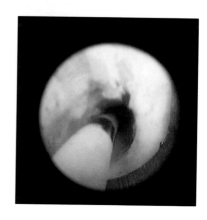

produce a long-lasting cure, indeed its results are virtually indistinguishable from traditional dilatation[14], and so every patient must be followed up with intermittent dilatation or self-catheterization. When there is a bladder tumour to be resected prudence suggests that dilatation may be preferable in view of the possible implantation of cancer cells into the raw area in the urethra, although such cases must be exceedingly rare.

References

1. Weaver RP, Noble MJ, Weigel JW. Correlation of ultrasound guided and digitally directed biopsies of palpable prostatic abnormalities. *J Urol* 1991;145:516.
2. Stamey TA. Making the most out of six systematic sextant biopsies. *Urology* 1995;45:2.
3. Meacham RB, Scardino PT, Hoffman GS *et al*. The risk of distant metastases after transurethral resection of the prostate versus needle biopsy in patients with localized prostate cancer. *J Urol* 1989;142:320.
4. Duncan W, Catton CN, Warde P *et al*. The influence of transurethral resection of prostate on prognosis of patients with adenocarcinoma of the prostate treated by radical radiotherapy. *Radiother Oncol* 1994;31:41.
5. Hassler O. Calcifications in the prostate gland and adjacent tissues: a combined biophysical and histological study. *Path Microbiol* 1968;31:97.
6. Emmet JL. Transurethral removal of large prostatic calculi. *Proc Staff Meet Mayo Clin* 1941;16:289.
7. Trapnell J, Roberts JBM. Prostatic abscess. *Br J Surg* 1970;57:565.
8. Meares EM, Stamey TA. Bacteriological localization patterns in bacterial prostatitis and urethritis. *Invest Urol* 1968;5:492.
9. Blandy JP, Fowler CG. Prostate – inflammation. In: *Urology*, 2nd edn. Oxford: Blackwell Science, 1996:375–9.
10. Reynard JM, Vass J, Sullivan M, Mamas M. Sphincterotomy and the treatment of detrusor-sphincter dyssynergia: current status, future prospects. *Spinal Cord* 2003;41:1–11.
11. Swift-Joly J. *Stone and Calculous Disease of the Urinary Organs*. London: Heinemann, 1929.
12. Tannenbaum SI, Carson CC, Tatum A, Paulson DF. Squamous carcinoma of the urinary bladder. *Urology* 1983;22:597.
13. Blandy JP. *Operative Urology*, 2nd edn. Oxford: Blackwell Science, 1986: 123–5.
14. Steenkamp JW, Heyns CF, de Kock MLS. Dilatation versus internal urethrotomy as out-patient treatment for male urethral stricture – a prospective, randomized clinical trial. *Br J Urol* 1996;77(Suppl 2):11.

Chapter 9

Routine postoperative care after transurethral resection

In the recovery room

From the operating table the patient goes to the recovery room where, in addition to monitoring the usual vital signs, the airway and the intravenous drip (if there is one), the nursing team pay particular attention to the three-way catheter and its irrigating system (Fig. 9.1).

Figure 9.1
Recovery room: vital signs are monitored; the three-way irrigating system is kept running briskly, and nursing staff keep an eye on the suprapubic region. The penile swab used for tamponade is removed before the patient returns to the ward.

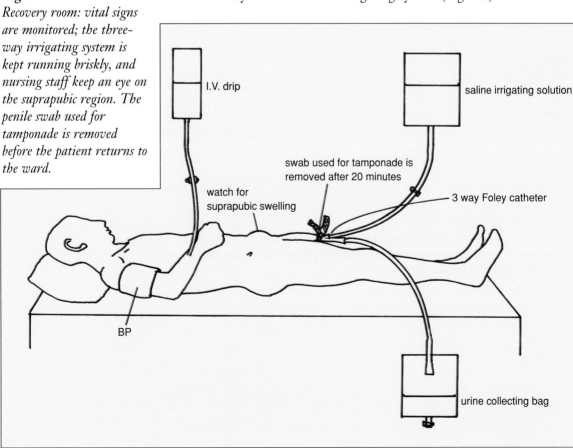

I.V. drip

saline irrigating solution

swab used for tamponade is
removed after 20 minutes

watch for
suprapubic swelling

3 way Foley catheter

BP

urine collecting bag

It is a sensible idea to get to know your recovery room staff. Spend a few moments telling them what operation you have done, and what problems you anticipate. Try to become actively involved in teaching the young recovery nurse about how you like the patient to be managed in the recovery room. Listen to the opinions of the nurses and avoid dismissing their suggestions in what may appear to be an arrogant fashion. It is a good idea to pass through the recovery room from time to time to check that all is well with the patients you have operated on. You might identify problems at an early stage when they are easier to correct and at the very least you will gain a reputation as a surgeon who takes an active interest in the postoperative care of your patients.

A few surgeons prefer to use a two-way catheter, and rely on the patient's own urine to keep the bladder irrigated. If necessary, intravenous fluids and a diuretic are given to encourage an adequate output of urine. The authors mistrust this system, fearing that it courts the risk of dilutional hyponatraemia, particularly in a patient with an inappropriate secretion of antidiuretic hormone, but it has some advocates.

Some surgeons prefer to leave the catheter to drain freely, only irrigating it with a hand syringe if the flow is blocked. The disadvantage of this method is the risk of introducing infection whenever the bladder is irrigated with a syringe[1].

In the usual technique with the three-way catheter the purpose of the irrigation is to dilute the blood so that a clot will not form to block the catheter. The rate of inflow of the saline is adjusted from time to time to keep the outflow a pale pink *vin rosé* colour, and as a rule the rate of inflow can be cut down after about 20 minutes.

Blocked catheter

1. The bag may be too full and its valve squeezed shut (Fig. 9.2). For this reason the drainage bags should be emptied long before they are full. Get into the habit of emptying the bag just before the patient leaves the operating theatre and of reviewing the patient in the recovery room from time to time to check that the catheter bag is not being neglected and allowed to overfill.
2. A small clot may have obstructed the catheter.
3. A chip of prostate may have stuck in the eye of the catheter.

In both these latter cases the first thing is to apply a bladder syringe to the end of the catheter and give it a good suck: this will often start the flow. If not, some of the irrigant should be drawn up in the syringe until it is about half-full, and about 20 ml injected before smartly aspirating again with the object of clearing the eye of the catheter.

Figure 9.2
If the valved drainage bag is allowed to get too full, the valve is closed and drainage ceases.

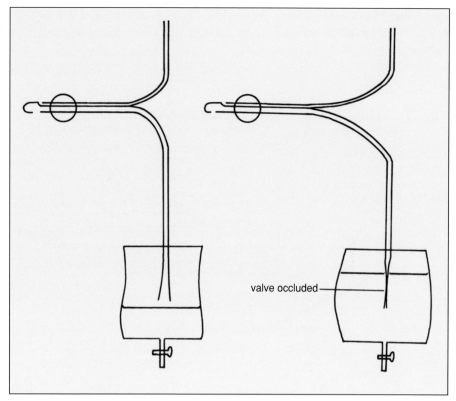

valve occluded

If neither of these tricks works, the catheter must be changed. It is no good persisting in vain attempts to syringe a catheter which is blocked: it will result in overdistension of the bladder, which adds to the patient's distress and restlessness.

Let down the balloon of the catheter and withdraw it. The offending chip of prostate may declare itself stuck in the eyeholes in the end of the catheter. Place a curved introducer in a new catheter and take care not to catch the bladder neck as you introduce it. More or less clear urine usually runs out at once, and when the bladder is empty irrigation can be started again.

If the bladder has been allowed to become full of clot then the patient should be returned to the theatre without delay. This is one of the chief advantages of having the recovery room close to the operating theatre: a message from the recovery room nurse will bring one of the surgical team within seconds, who can check the situation and make the decision to return the patient or not without delay. Experienced nursing staff usually know when it is time to return the patient and the young surgeon does well to take heed of their advice. It is far better to err on the side of caution than waste valuable time, while the patient may be continuing to bleed, fiddling with a bladder syringe and a hopelessly blocked catheter.

Clot evacuation

Once re-anaesthetized the patient is repositioned, cleaned and draped as for a transurethral resection. The catheter is removed and the resectoscope passed again. Often this will allow a clot or chip to emerge and the problem is solved, but it is always wise to look into the bladder and irrigate out any clots that may be there with the Ellik evacuator (Fig. 9.3). When the bladder has been emptied, check the cavity of the prostate for any source of bleeding. It is rare that you will find any: the bleeding (as with the tonsil bed) has usually stopped when the clot has been evacuated. Rarely you may find a little tag of prostate which seems to be keeping a small vein open: resect it and coagulate the vein.

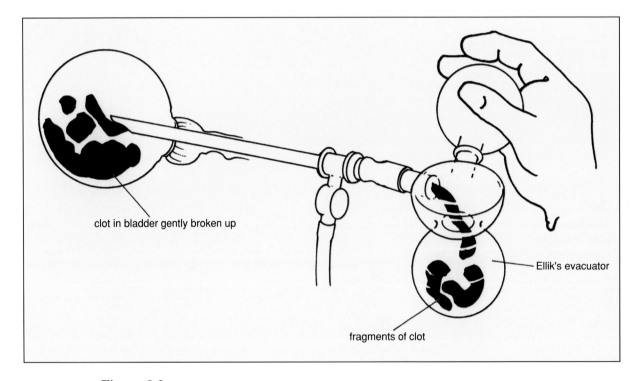

clot in bladder gently broken up

Ellik's evacuator

fragments of clot

Figure 9.3
Clot retention. The resectoscope sheath is passed and the Ellik evacuator is used to break up the clot and suck it out.

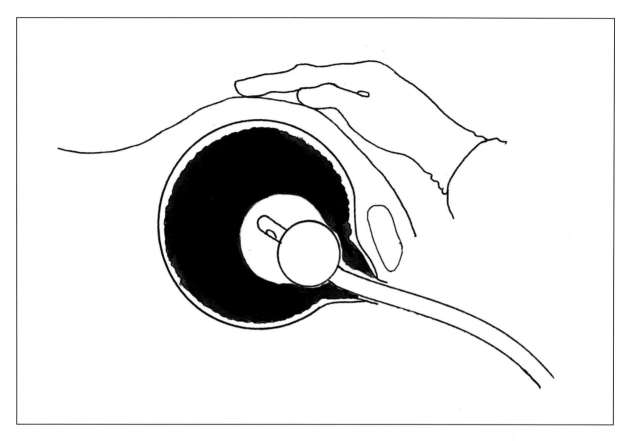

Figure 9.4
The end of the irrigating catheter has become surrounded by clot, preventing effective irrigation of the bladder.

Very occasionally there may appear to be normal flow of urine into and out of the bladder, the urine may be only lightly blood-stained, but the patient may complain that their bladder feels full. Examination reveals a tensely distended bladder which is dull to percussion. The distended bladder suggests that the catheter is blocked, but this does not fit with the apparently normal flow of irrigant through the drainage system. What may have happened is that the patient's bladder has filled up with clot as a consequence of persistent bleeding from the prostate, and the end of the catheter has become surrounded by clot (Fig. 9.4). Irrigant simply passes out from the irrigation channel at the tip of the catheter and then directly back out of the bladder again through the outflow channel of the catheter. Attempts at evacuation of the thick clot through the catheter using a bladder syringe will not work. The only way to deal with this is to take the patient back to theatre, evacuate the clot from the bladder and find and control the source of the persistent bleeding. The clue to diagnosing this uncommon event is simple clinical examination of the patient's abdomen.

Major reactionary haemorrhage

Mercifully very rare, major reactionary haemorrhage may take place without warning. If there is time, and the general condition of the patient permits, the bladder should be emptied with the Ellik and the source of bleeding coagulated, if possible, or controlled by traction on the Foley catheter. Exceptionally, the bleeding is impossible to control by these means, and it is necessary to open the patient and pack the prostate bed.

The retropubic space is opened through a Pfannenstiel incision. The bladder is retracted as for a Millin's prostatectomy and the capsule is incised transversely[2]. All clot is evacuated and the prostatic bed is firmly packed with gauze. Allow plenty of time for loss of blood to be restored, and then remove the pack, try to identify the source of bleeding, and suture the offending vessel. If the bleeding continues, pack it with two vaginal packs. The second pack should be tied to the first. Close the wound with a large suprapubic tube in the bladder, leaving the end of the second pack protruding through the wound. Book theatre for 24 hours later, so that you can remove the packs under general anaesthetic, with a full prostatectomy set ready and waiting in case you encounter continued bleeding. Withdraw the pack gently. Usually the bleeding will have stopped, but if it has not, you will be in the best position to control it.

Fortunately this emergency is rare, but there are few urologists of experience who have not had to pack the prostate once or twice. The important thing is not to procrastinate when the patient is losing blood rapidly: it is better to have to explain an unexpected Pfannenstiel incision to a living patient than to his widow.

Sedation

Transurethral resection is seldom painful unless the wall of the bladder or the trigone has been resected, or a large middle lobe has had to be removed. Then the patient may have a fierce desire to pass urine and the bladder may be thrown into involuntary detrusor spasms which nothing will control, and urine may escape alongside the catheter.

A sacral or caudal epidural anaesthetic minimizes this kind of post-operative discomfort and will last for several hours. Pethidine or morphine will relieve pain but do not prevent detrusor spasm, and they may lull the recovery staff into a sense of false security so that they may not realize that the pain and leakage are in fact due to a blocked catheter. Because transurethral resection is not usually a painful procedure, it is wise not to prescribe postoperative analgesic drugs as a routine in order to avoid this hazard. If the patient is in pain, find out why, before prescribing analgesia. Most commonly the patient who is apparently in pain will settle down as he regains full consciousness and can understand that there is a catheter in his penis.

Return to the ward

As soon as the patient has recovered consciousness and the irrigating system has settled down to an even flow, then the patient may go back to the ward. During the journey it is important that the irrigation is not inadvertently shut off, and as soon as the patient arrives on the ward the irrigating system should be checked to make sure that the fluid is running and that the bag has not become overfilled (Fig. 9.5). Thereafter the patient's vital signs are checked at intervals of 15, and later 30, minutes.

Figure 9.5
Return to the ward. Inflow and outflow must be measured. Ward staff should check that the penile swab has been removed. As the colour of the outflow becomes less blood-stained the rate of inflow is cut down.

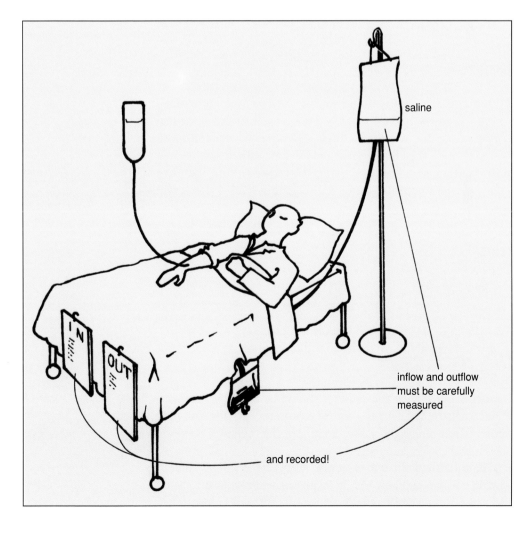

When the patient comes round he may well be hungry and thirsty and there is no reason why he should not be allowed to drink so long as he is not nauseated. Within 4–6 hours most patients are fully alert, may take a light meal and may start to drink as they please. If blood loss needs to be made up then the intravenous cannula should be retained until all the blood has been given. If the bleeding has stopped and the patient is taking fluids well there is no need to keep the drip up.

Recording the irrigating fluid

The volume of fluid run into the bladder and the urine collected should be continuously recorded and totted up every hour to make sure that there is no large discrepancy that might suggest that the bladder is becoming overdistended, or that there is an excessive loss of fluid into the veins (see page 116).

Ambulation

Early mobilization is a good way of preventing the development of deep venous thrombosis and patients should be encouraged to sit out of bed as soon as possible – the evening of their operation or the following morning – or as soon as the effects of the epidural anaesthetic have worn off. The next day they should be encouraged to walk around the ward carrying their catheter and the drip for the irrigating fluid if this is still needed (Fig. 9.6).

Irrigation

When the effluent is clear, or contains only a little staining of altered brownish blood, the irrigation may be discontinued – usually after about 12 hours.

Removing the catheter

Common sense dictates when the catheter should be removed. Sundays and public holidays are bad days to remove a catheter, and for the same reason it is better to remove the catheter early in the morning than late at night.

When a patient has had chronic retention with a huge floppy bladder year in and year out, it is unlikely that his detrusor will regain the ability to expel the urine for several days. Most patients, however, pass water within a few hours of removing the catheter.

Figure 9.6
First postoperative day. The patient may walk around, carrying his irrigating drip and urine bag.

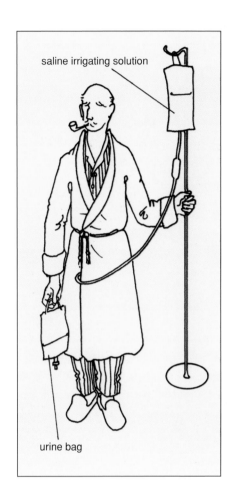

If the catheter is taken out within 6–12 hours of the resection, as one may be tempted to do when the bleeding has been exceptionally well controlled, urine may escape from capsular perforations and give rise to stinging and pain on urination. For this reason it is usual to remove the catheter after about 48 hours. Warn the patient that removing the catheter is a little uncomfortable and ensure that it is taken out slowly and gently. The very apprehensive patient deserves a little sedation beforehand.

Failure to void after removing the catheter

There are three reasons for this:

1. The most common reason is that the patient finds it so uncomfortable to start to void that the process is inhibited. He shuts his external

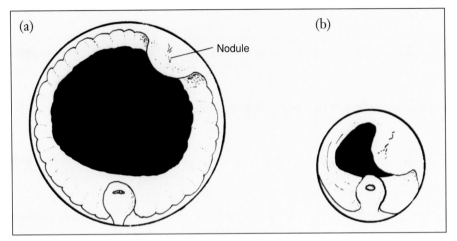

Figure 9.7
If a small nodule of tissue has been left behind after removing a large prostate, leaving a large cavity, it is very easy to overlook it at the time (a), but it becomes all too obvious when the prostatic cavity has contracted (b).

sphincter tightly and even when the bladder is painfully distended, cannot void.

2. The patient has detrusor failure from chronic retention.
3. Insufficient tissue may have been removed, usually at 2 or 10 o'clock, for when the prostatic capsule shrinks down a tiny lump becomes relatively large compared with the lumen of the prostatic urethra (Fig. 9.7).

When a patient cannot pass urine within an hour or two of removing the catheter one should not wait for the bladder to become painfully distended, but replace the catheter as soon as the patient has any discomfort, or whenever the bladder can be felt. Be aware of the pitfall of the patient with a big floppy detrusor who may be passing small amounts of urine but is quietly building up a huge residual.

Allow 3 or 4 days of rest, and then remove the catheter a second time and see if the patient can void. The man with the first, most common, type of failure to void will now do so without difficulty.

The patient with significant obstruction due to residual prostatic tissue should be returned to the theatre and the offending tissue resected: it is usually only a few grams.

The patient with detrusor failure poses a more serious problem. There is seldom any pain, but he soon returns to the state of chronic retention with overflow in which he arrived in hospital. In nearly every case the detrusor function returns after about 4 weeks of catheter drainage. He should be allowed to go home with an indwelling catheter on free drainage (Fig. 9.8). On no account should the patient be provided with a spigot or tap, or there will be a serious risk of accumulation of infected urine in the bladder with resulting septicaemia.

Figure 9.8

If failure to resume voiding is due to atony of the detrusor, a period of continuous catheter drainage is necessary. The patient may go home wearing a silicone rubber catheter connected to a leg drainage bag. Never permit a spigot to be used.

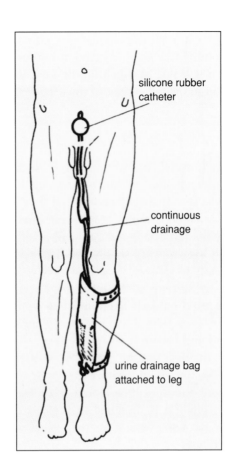

After about a month, the patient is re-admitted to hospital overnight for the catheter to be removed, under antibiotic cover. The patient is carefully monitored to make sure that residual urine does not gradually accumulate: the best method is to check this with an ultrasound scan. Cholinergic drugs are often recommended for this type of detrusor failure but they do not work in practice when the problem has been long-standing.

The frequency with which failure to void occurs is discussed further in Chapter 12.

Deliberate sphincterotomy

Some very old demented men with chronic retention have a detrusor which is irrevocably damaged and never recovers the strength to empty the bladder. A permanent indwelling catheter may not be tolerated, and may prevent them from being cared for in sheltered accommodation for the elderly. In such a patient it may be a kindness to perform an external sphincterotomy (see page 147) and fit him with a penile sheath, but such a decision will not be taken lightly and only in consultation with the geriatrician in overall charge of the care of the patient.

Going home

Most men can leave hospital after transurethral resection of the prostate or even a large bladder tumour within 4–5 days of the operation, but it is important to make sure that they understand that the raw area inside them will not be healed up completely for some time. They should rest quietly. Many patients (especially doctors, and practically all surgeons) think they can rush back to work simply because they have felt no pain. Nothing is more likely to give rise to secondary haemorrhage. Tell them they must take it easy. In reply to the inevitable question, 'What do you mean, Doctor?', a good guide is anything they would normally do in their carpet slippers (Fig. 9.9). They may potter around the house, go next door for a chat and have friends round to see them, but they must not play golf, walk the dog, dig the garden or mow the lawn. Surgeons must not operate. No one should drive a car.

This carpet-slipper convalescence should go on for 2 weeks after the patient has left hospital. It is designed to prevent the physical effort which might increase the pressure in the pelvic veins and provoke secondary haemorrhage.

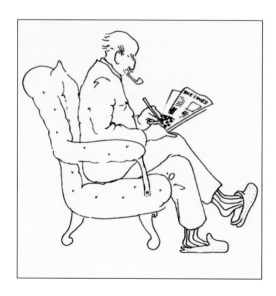

Figure 9.9
'Carpet-slipper' convalescence is enjoined for 2 weeks after leaving hospital.

After this time the patient should gradually return to normal life, increasing his activities day by day, go for walks, play a few holes of golf and go shopping. The rate of his progress will usually be regulated by the patient's frequency and urgency, which take a little while to subside. Ideally this second period is one of getting back into training for a normal life, and if your patient can afford it, he should go away for a holiday in the sun before returning to work, or the equally strenuous life of modern-day retirement. The holiday should be postponed until 3 or 4 weeks after the operation, this being the risk period for secondary haemorrhage.

It is not uncommon for a patient to experience some haematuria a few weeks after TURP. His urine may have completely cleared of blood for a couple of weeks, and then he may experience a sudden episode of seemingly heavy haematuria, with some residual bleeding for a few days afterwards. This usually resolves spontaneously, and unless accompanied by symptoms of urethral burning or scalding on urination, is not a sign of urinary infection. Passing blood in the urine is always alarming and understandably the patient may think that something is wrong. If you warn the patient before he is discharged that this may happen, then it is far easier to reassure him that all is well, and that the bleeding will in all probability settle down without the need for any active treatment.

Fluid intake

During the period of carpet-slipper convalescence your patient should drink freely – about 3 l a day – so that the overconcentrated urine does not sting when he voids, and debris is washed away from the healing prostatic fossa. It matters not a jot what he drinks and there is no medical reason why he should not take a little alcohol if he wants to: one never encourages a patient to get drunk, but there is no physiological or pharmacological reason why he should be denied this little solace in time of trouble. After the first 2 weeks he may drink as much or as little fluid as he pleases.

Diet

There are no restrictions on what a man may or may not eat after transurethral surgery. Constipation is to be avoided since the passage of a stiff motion may provoke straining and start secondary haemorrhage. Plenty of bran and vegetables is sufficient for most men, and a bulk laxative for those inclined to be constipated will keep postoperative bowel actions soft and comfortable.

Antibiotics

If prophylactic antibiotics have been given because the patient had been catheterized, or there was known urinary infection, there is no consensus as to how long they should be continued. It is probably wise to keep up the antibiotic cover until the catheter is removed, and for 24 hours thereafter. Where there is a special risk of systemic infection, e.g. in patients with implanted foreign bodies or mitral valve disease, a more prolonged course may be advisable and should be planned with the help of the patient's cardiologist and your microbiologist (see Chapter 4).

References

1. Symes JM, Hardy DG, Sutherns K, Blandy JP. Factors reducing the rate of infection after transurethral surgery. *Br J Urol* 1972;44:582.
2. Blandy JP. *Operative Urology*, 2nd edn. Oxford: Blackwell Science, 1986:168–76.

Chapter 10

Complications occurring during transurethral resection

Bleeding

Because bleeding is the chief cause of difficulty and danger in any form of prostatectomy, surgeons have been trying to discover how to limit blood loss for more than a century. In the UK National Prostatectomy Audit[1] bleeding severe enough to require the operation to be stopped occurred in 20 of 4226 TURPs (0.7%) and in 20 (0.4%) packing of the prostate was required to stop the bleeding. In the postoperative period return to the operating theatre to control major bleeding was reported in 0.6% of cases.

The way to obtain haemostasis during the operation has been described (see page 181–3) and is usually sufficient to permit a clean resection for which no blood replacement is needed. Nevertheless from time to time haemorrhage can be copious, unexpected and daunting. However skilled the resector, it is always necessary to be prepared, to know the patient's haemoglobin and to have his blood grouped and serum saved in the laboratory. In very large prostates and very large bladder tumours where considerable blood loss is to be expected it is safer to have 2 units of blood standing by.

Adjuvant methods of limiting blood loss

Claims have been made that cooling the tissues with ice-cold irrigating fluid may reduce blood loss, but were based on resection of very small amounts of tissue. In theory, one would expect the natural clotting mechanisms to work best at normal temperature, and in practice the technique led to a sometimes alarming fall in core temperature[2–6]. Hypotensive anaesthesia was used extensively for retropubic prostatectomy some 30 years ago and is revived from time to time for transurethral surgery, but the benefit in terms of limiting blood loss must be offset by the risk of cerebrovascular accident and coronary thrombosis, both hazards of any surgical procedure in this age group.

Many other agents have been tried with the object of limiting blood loss, including oestrogens, injecting the prostate with vasoconstrictors, carbazochrome salicylate, kutapressin, oestrogens and aprotinin, all without significant benefit[7–11]. Cyclokapron and its precursor ε-amino-caproic acid were in vogue for a time, and then given up when it was found that they caused intraglomerular thrombosis[12,13]. They might have limited postoperative blood loss, but had no effect on bleeding during the operation. Dicynene, said to reduce capillary fragility, had no advantage when bleeding was serious[14].

More important than any of these adjuvant agents is a good technique of haemostasis at the time of operation, and the use of a simple method of measuring blood loss in the operating theatre, e.g. a colorimeter to estimate the haemoglobin in the bucket[15].

Extraperitoneal perforation during TURP

This complication was discussed earlier (see page 116). It occurred in 0.25% of cases in the National Prostatectomy Audit[1]. The capsular per-foration in itself is not a problem. The danger is from fluid absorption when a large volume of fluid has been allowed to escape into the circulation (Fig. 10.1a). Occasionally fluid introduced with the Ellik evacuator does not suck back, or a change in the character of the respi-ration and a coldness and swelling of the suprapubic tissues may suggest that there has been a massive loss of fluid. This is why it is so helpful to get a mental image of the appearance of the patient's lower abdomen before starting a TURP – it allows one to establish whether the distension has occurred since the operation started or whether it simply represents years of over-indulgence at the dinner table!

As in most times in surgery when things go wrong they get worse if you dither and delay. Stop the resection. If there is significant abdomi-nal distension make the decision to proceed with open drainage of the retropubic space. Have things made ready as soon as possible. Make a Pfannenstiel incision. Expose the bladder, open it between stay sutures and evacuate the clot. Complete the prostatectomy (if it is not already complete) by enucleating the remaining adenoma with the finger[16]. Get exact haemostasis by sutures, and if you can see the hole in the capsule, close it with a stitch. Only when all the bleeding is controlled should you close the wound with a suprapubic and urethral catheter and a drain to the retropubic space.

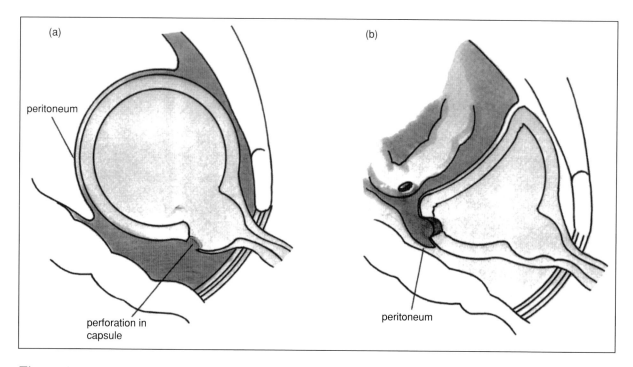

Figure 10.1

(a) Extraperitoneal perforation; fluid extravasates around the prostate and the base of the bladder.

(b) Intraperitoneal perforation; the main danger is of inadvertent injury to the bowel.

Extraperitoneal and intraperitoneal perforation during resection of a bladder tumour

Small perforations into the perivesical tissues are not uncommon when resecting small tumours of the bladder and so long as you have secured good haemostasis and all the irrigating fluid is being recovered, no additional steps are required except that perhaps one should leave the catheter in for 4 rather than 2 days.

Trainees are sometimes uncertain whether a perforation is extraperitoneal or intraperitoneal. Establishing this can sometimes be difficult, because both can cause marked distension of the lower abdomen – an intraperitoneal perforation by allowing escape of irrigating solution directly into the abdominal cavity and an extraperitoneal perforation by expanding the retroperitoneal space, with fluid then diffusing directly into the peritoneal cavity. The fact that a suspected intraperitoneal perforation was actually extraperitoneal becomes apparent only at laparotomy when no hole can be found in the bladder!

When there is no abdominal distension, the volume of extravasated fluid is likely to be low and if the perforation is small it is reasonable to manage the case conservatively. Achieve haemostasis, pass a catheter and send the patient to the recovery room. Make frequent visits to see the patient. If the patient remains well, you may continue conservative management. If things are not right – worsening abdominal pain and distension – then proceed to laparotomy. In most cases everything will settle down and the hole in the bladder will heal spontaneously if a catheter is left *in situ* for 10 days or so. The patient can go home in a couple of days and will have been spared the morbidity and longer hospital stay that is required after laparotomy.

However, in cases where there is marked abdominal distension, whether the perforation is extraperitoneal or intraperitoneal is in many senses academic – the important thing is to explore the abdomen, principally to drain the large amount of fluid which can compromise respiration in an elderly patient by splinting the diaphragm, but also to check that loops of bowel adjacent to the site of perforation have not been injured at the same time. Failing to make the diagnosis of an intraperitoneal diagnosis, particularly if bowel has been injured, is a worse situation to be in than performing a laparotomy for a suspected intraperitoneal perforation, but then finding that the perforation was 'only' extraperitoneal.

The diagnosis of an intraperitoneal perforation is obvious if you can actually see loops of bowel (Fig. 10.1b). The tell-tale sign of the Ellik evacuator not sucking back can occur with both intraperitoneal and extraperitoneal perforation and this therefore tells you that something is wrong, rather than what is wrong.

When there is marked abdominal distension, or where it is obvious that the perforation has been made right through into the peritoneum (Fig. 10.1b) or, as is often the case, the perforation is obscured and accompanied by haemorrhage, then it is necessary to explore the abdomen.

The bladder is again approached through a Pfannenstiel incision or lower abdominal incision, opened between stay sutures, the clot is evacuated, the bleeding controlled and the hole sewn up (Fig. 10.2). Then the peritoneum should be opened, which is easily done whether the incision is a Pfannenstiel or lower abdominal one. This allows you to see if there is any blood-stained fluid inside. Adjacent loops of small and large bowel should be pulled out and searched for diathermy damage. A hole in the small bowel is closed in its transverse axis (Fig. 10.3). A hole in the colon should be protected with a temporary loop-colostomy.

Perforation into the rectum

Although this is much dreaded, it is rare. In the National Prostatectomy Audit[1] it was reported in 0.25% of 4226 TURPs. Rectal perforation is so uncommon that management is decided on a case by case basis. Most

Figure 10.2
As soon as the bladder is opened the perforation is obvious.

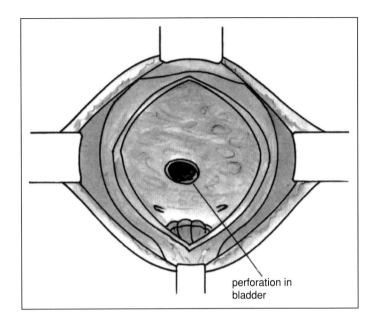

perforation in bladder

Figure 10.3
A small burn in the small bowel is oversewn in its transverse axis.

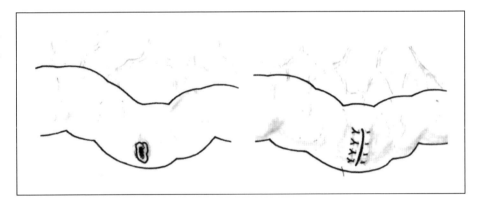

urologists nowadays will not perform colostomies on a regular basis, and from the perspective of avoiding possible later litigation, it is a sensible idea to involve a colorectal surgeon in subsequent management decisions and indeed with performing the colostomy if this is deemed to be necessary. If the perforation is large, many would recommend a defunctioning colostomy with a catheter left in situ for about 3 weeks. This may be a urethral or suprapubic catheter, but the latter may be more comfortable. If the perforation is small, then an indwelling catheter for a few weeks may be all that is necessary. However, bear in mind that the injury will have been caused by the diathermy, rather than by a sharp knife, and as a consequence the edges of the perforated bowel will have been devitalized and therefore may not heal. If in doubt, err on the side of performing a colostomy.

If a defunctioning colostomy and a suprapubic cystostomy is used, after about 6 weeks most of these fistulae will have healed, and in the rare case that persists the fistula can be closed through a perineal approach or by one of Parks' operations using a sleeve of rectal wall[17,18].

Broken sheath

In days when sheaths were generally made of plastic they sometimes broke across, leaving the tip in the urethra. Even today the tip of a steel sheath may come away. Occasionally one can see the edge of the detached portion with a cystoscope and draw it out with biopsy forceps (Fig. 10.4). An alternative trick is to pass a Foley catheter through the lumen of the detached portion, leave it for 10–14 days, and when the catheter is removed the piece of sheath will usually come away (Fig. 10.5).

Broken loop

A fragment of inert wire broken off in the course of a transurethral resection can do no possible harm unless in the fullness of time it migrates into the bladder and acts as a nucleus for a stone to form. By all means look for it and remove it with a biopsy forceps if you find it, but otherwise, complete the resection with another loop. An X-ray in the

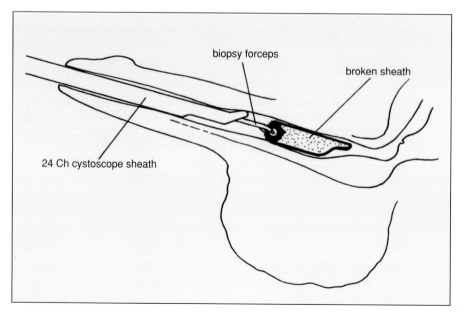

biopsy forceps

broken sheath

24 Ch cystoscope sheath

Figure 10.4
A broken-off tip of a resectoscope may be recovered with a biopsy forceps.

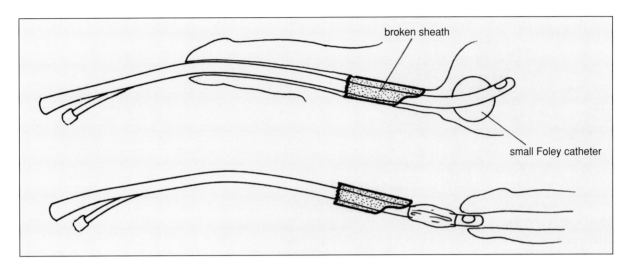

Figure 10.5
If a small Foley catheter can be passed through the broken fragment of resectoscope sheath, it is left for about 10 days; when it is removed, the sheath comes with it.

Figure 10.6
Plain X-ray showing resectoscope loop in the prostate. It caused no trouble and was left alone.

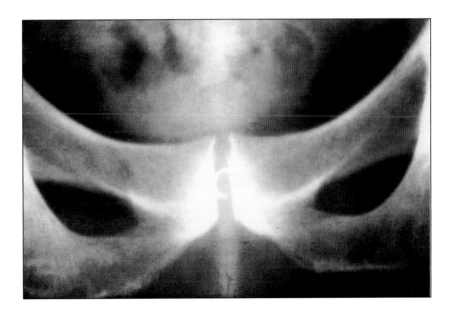

postoperative period will reveal the loop (Fig. 10.6), but if the patient is comfortable there is no need to hunt for it. What you tell the patient is of course for you to decide in the interests of the peace of mind of your patient rather than what you fear his lawyers might say, but you will probably find that it simplifies things to tell him, explaining that there are many old soldiers who still carry with them bullets and shrapnel fragments from past wars, and many surgeons routinely use metal clips for haemostasis. A man may well feel aggrieved and insulted if he finds out later and you had not told him.

Explosions

The mixture of hydrogen and oxygen formed by hydrolysis of water by diathermy sparks, along with air introduced in the irrigating fluid, collects into a bubble at the vault of the bladder. This is sometimes an explosive mixture, so if you are resecting tumour from the vault, push down on the suprapubic region to indent the vault and displace the bubble away from the loop. The authors have never seen this terrible complication but the accounts of it in the literature make grim reading[19].

Obturator jump

If a bladder tumour is situated on the lateral wall of the bladder, resection may be complicated by brisk spasms of the adductors of the ipsilateral leg – the obturator jump. This occurs when low frequency harmonic currents generated by the diathermy stimulate the obturator nerve. Apart from giving you a box on the ears, this surprising event may cause you to perforate the wall of the bladder with the cutting loop. There is no certain way to avoid this phenomenon, but steps can be taken to reduce the likelihood of it taking place.

First, be aware of the possibility whenever you are resecting tumours near the ureteric orifice. It is particularly easy to stimulate the obturator nerve just above and lateral to the ureteric orifice. If you see a tumour in this location, and it is small and the purpose of treating the tumour is for local control only, then use the roly-ball to coagulate the tumour, rather than trying to formally resect it. If the patient is not a candidate for radical treatment of a muscle invasive bladder tumour, there is little point in exposing them to the potential risk of bladder perforation from an aggressive resection causing an obturator kick.

However, if it is important to determine the precise stage of the tumour because you need to decide whether radical treatment such as cystectomy or radiotherapy will be required, then you will have to perform formal resection of the tumour. Even if you do not need precise staging information, the tumour may simply be too large for adequate local control by roly-ball vaporization. In these situations, turn down the current until it is barely cutting. The obturator nerve may no longer be stimulated by the lower current. Get two assistants to stand one on either side of the patient, and to grasp the patient's thighs and lower abdomen firmly, underneath the sterile drapes. This can help to stabilize the pelvis, preventing it from rocking to one side or other if the obturator nerve is stimulated. Next, ask your anaesthetist to intubate the patient and paralyse his muscles. Curare-related agents work by blocking depolarization of the neuromuscular end plates, but this blockade can be overcome by supramaximal nerve stimulation. Paralysis with agents such as suxamethonium, which depolarize the end plates and prevent repolarization, overcomes the problem, but their action is short-lived, and repeated administration may lead to other problems so that anaesthetists are understandably not enthusiastic to use repeated doses. Finally, just as you are about to start resecting, be prepared to quickly withdraw the resectoscope into the prostatic urethra so that if an obturator kick does occur, the end of the resectoscope will not go shooting through the bladder.

The obturator nerve may be anaesthetized locally by injecting local anaesthetic directly into the nerve (Fig. 10.7). Using a long spinal needle aim for the obturator foramen, entering the needle halfway between the mid-inguinal point and the pubic tubercle, aiming downwards and medially, aspirating and injecting alternately until the bony medial edge

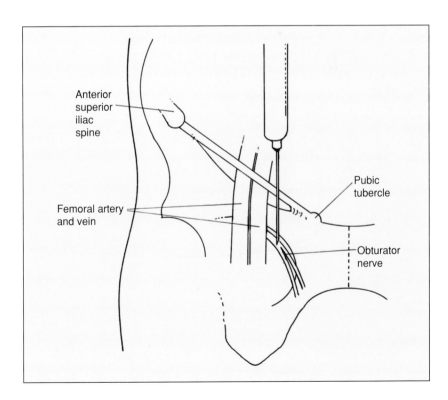

Figure 10.7
Injection of local anaesthetic into the obturator nerve.

of the obturator foramen is encountered. If the femoral vein is inadvertently entered, press on the puncture for 5 minutes.

Erection

Penile erection can develop insidiously and the operator must constantly be on the lookout for it, as it is exceedingly dangerous. It is the authors' experience that erection is most common in patients who are too lightly anaesthetized, often by an inexperienced anaesthetist. In the National Prostatectomy Audit[1] an erection caused the operation to be stopped in 0.2% of cases.

The first sign that anything is going wrong may be that the resectoscope seems to be unduly tight in the urethra, or that the view has become obscured by new bleeding. Feel the penis; early engorgement is quite obvious. Stop now, before it is too late.

The erection can be reversed with an injection directly into the corpus cavernosum of 200 micrograms of phenylephrine diluted in normal saline[20]. This can be repeated. If the erection fails to subside immediately then you should seriously consider terminating the operation. It is better to come back another day rather than lose one's way and risk damaging the sphincter.

Failure to recognize that an erection is taking place and failure to reverse it may result in the resectoscope being forced out of the urethra, with the result that the operator may easily mistake the external sphincter for prostate, and resect it. The result is irreversible incontinence (Fig. 10.8).

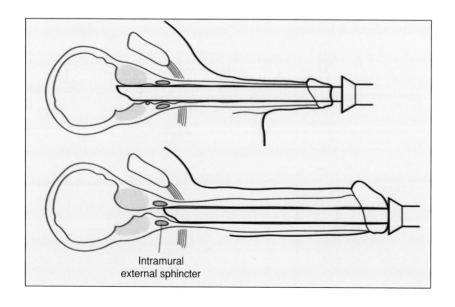

Intramural
external sphincter

Figure 10.8

During an erection the short flaccid penis becomes elongated, forcing the resectoscope out. It is easy to mistake external sphincter for prostate, especially when bleeding confuses your view.

The 1 hour rule and transurethral resection

An interesting myth has been handed down from one generation of resectors to the next, without any basis in measurement or experiment, namely that resection must be completed within 60 minutes or disaster will befall. The myth probably took its origin in the early days of transurethral resection when the surgeon often gave his own spinal anaesthetic, and patients began to recover sensation after about an hour.

Clearly, the longer the operation goes on, the more time there is for blood to be lost and irrigating fluid to enter the veins, and if the resection takes more than 1 hour, it usually means that the gland is very large (when there is more likely to be more of both) or the resector has been unduly slow in removing what gland there is. Time alone is no more relevant to endoscopic than to any other kind of surgery, and if you can make a better job of the operation by taking 61 minutes it is illogical to call a halt at 59.

While the 1 hour rule is certainly great nonsense there is never any excuse for dawdling. This is nothing new in surgery; operating time is not wasted by taking care and trouble over the steps of any operation, but in indecision – fiddling about and wondering what to do next. It is a commonplace in surgery that master craftsmen neither hurry nor watch the clock, but they never waste a movement. So it should be in transurethral resection. Keep your landmarks ever in view; know where you are and what you are cutting. Cut with a confident rhythm and stop the bleeding as you go. Transurethral resection is no work for the picker and scratcher.

The TUR syndrome

Early in the history of transurethral resection it was recognized that if distilled water was allowed to run into the circulation it would lead to haemolysis, haemoglobinuria and possibly even renal failure[21-24] (Fig. 10.9). Accordingly a number of non-ionizing solutions were introduced which would be more or less isotonic and fail to cause haemolysis, e.g. 2.5% glucose, Cytal (a proprietary mixture of sorbitol and mannitol) and 1.5% glycine.

Although these solutions avoided the risk of haemolysis, they did not avoid the dangers that arose from intravenous infusion of a large volume of water into the blood. This dilutes the normal electrolytes, especially sodium, leading to a lowering of the membrane potential on the cell wall (the latter is necessary for nerve conduction and muscle contraction). This is soon followed by an increase in intracellular water, resulting in cell oedema (Fig. 10.10). A normal patient can cope with a surprisingly

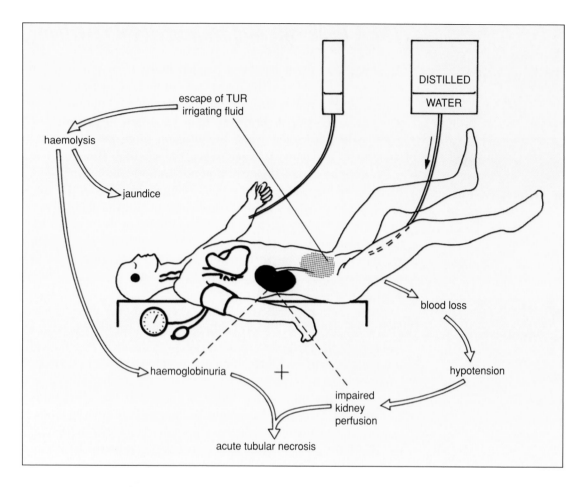

Figure 10.9
*The hazards of using
distilled water as the
irrigating medium.*

large volume of water added to his bloodstream in this way, responding with a prompt diuresis that gets rid of the surplus water. But not all transurethral resection patients are normal; many are already on the brink of heart failure, and in as many as 25% there is an inappropriate secretion of pituitary antidiuretic hormone[25]. An additional factor, hitherto unnoticed, may be the effect of endotoxins due to bacteraemia during the resection[26].

Diagnosis – symptoms, signs and tests

In the National Prostatectomy Audit[1] the TUR syndrome occurred in 0.5% of cases. It is characterized by a number of symptoms and signs which may be present in variable degree depending on the severity of the condition. These include confusion, nausea, vomiting, hypertension, bradycardia and visual disturbances.

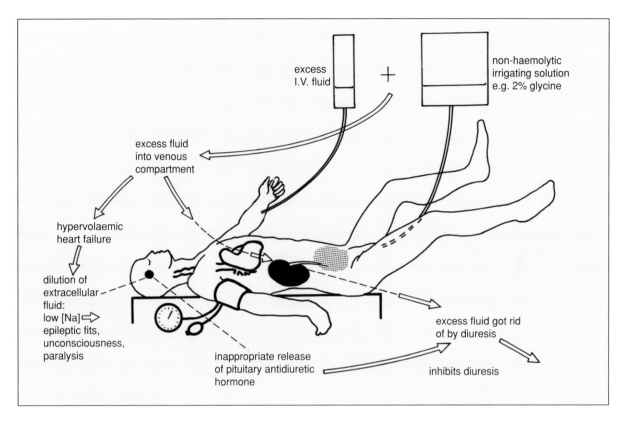

Figure 10.10

The dilutional syndrome.

The diagnosis of the TUR syndrome calls for a high degree of awareness on the part of the urological team. It may be ushered in with restlessness and hypertension, and rapidly proceed to what appears to be a grand mal seizure. If the patient is under spinal anaesthesia and is therefore awake during the procedure, they may report visual disturbances such as flashing lights. This can be a very helpful warning that significant amounts of glycine (and therefore fluid) are being absorbed and that corrective measures should be started. One of the authors was once explaining this feature of TUR syndrome to a junior anaesthetic colleague when the patient suddenly complained of flashing lights. The operation was quickly brought to a conclusion and the patient responded rapidly to intravenous frusemide and fluid restriction, without going on to develop the more serious manifestations of advanced TUR syndrome.

Pathophysiology

The TUR syndrome is characterized by biochemical, haemodynamic and neurological disturbances. Dilutional hyponatraemia is the most important – and serious – factor leading to the symptoms and signs. The serum sodium usually has to fall to below 125 mmol/l before the patient becomes unwell. The hypertension is due to fluid overload. Visual disturbances may be due to the fact that glycine is a neurotransmitter in the retina.

Predicting and preventing development of the TUR syndrome and definitive treatment

Prevention is better than cure. Try to avoid the development of the TUR syndrome by limiting resection time, avoiding aggressive resection near the capsule and by reducing the height of the irrigant solution. Madsen and Naber[27] demonstrated that increasing the height of the irrigation fluid from 60 to 70 cm above the patient increased fluid absorption by a factor of two.

If the resection has been long and bloody, assume that the patient is going to develop the TUR syndrome and take corrective measures before the patient starts developing symptoms. Send a sample of blood for sodium measurement, and give 20–40 mg of intravenous frusemide to start off-loading the excess fluid that has been absorbed. If the serum sodium comes back as being normal, you will have done little harm by giving the frusemide, but if it comes back at <125 mmol/l, you will have started treatment already and thereby may have prevented the development of severe TUR syndrome.

It is possible to measure the quantity of fluid escaping into the patient if a special weighing machine is added to the ordinary operating table[28]. Nowadays it is also possible to monitor the concentration of sodium in the blood with a sodium-sensing electrode[29], or more easily, by adding a little alcohol to the irrigating fluid and constantly monitoring the expired air with a breathalyser[30]. This allows one to estimate the volume of excess fluid that has been absorbed.

Many techniques have been used to avoid the TUR syndrome. A suprapubic cannula and the continuous irrigating cystoscope of Iglesias are commonly used[31]. In practice the TUR syndrome is rarely seen in most modern departments, partly because of these precautions, and perhaps because of sparing use of intravenous fluids[32,33] and careful measurement of the volumes of fluid that are irrigated in and out of the bladder.

In a patient who is not too ill, and is having a good diuresis, it is safe to wait and let him get better. Intravenous frusemide can be given to hasten the excretion of the excess water that has been absorbed.

References

1. Neal DE. The National Prostatectomy Audit. *Br J Urol* 1997;79(Suppl 2):69–75.
2. Madsen PO, Kaveggia L, Atassi SA. The effect of oestrogens (premarin) and regional hypothermia on blood loss during transurethral prostatectomy. *J Urol* 1964;92:314.
3. Madsen PO, Bohlman DC, Madsen RE. Local hypothermia during transurethral surgery. *Anesth Analg* 1965;44:734.
4. Robson CT, Sales JL. Effect of local hypothermia on blood loss during transurethral resection of the prostate. *J Urol* 1966;95:393.
5. Serrao A, Mallik MK, Jones PA, Hendry WF, Wickham JEA. Hypothermic prostatic resection. *Br J Urol* 1976;48:685.
6. Walton JK, Rawstron RE. The effect of local hypothermia on blood loss during transurethral resection of the prostate. *Br J Urol* 1981;53:258.
7. Creevy CD. Aids to hemostasis during transurethral prostatic resection. *J Urol* 1965;93:80.
8. Madsen PO, Straugh AE, Barquin OP, Malek GH. The lack of hemostatic effect of polyestradiolphosphate and carbazochrome salicylate in transurethral prostatectomy. *J Urol* 1968;99:786.
9. Weisenthal CL, Meade RC, Owenby J, Irwin RI. An investigation of kutapressin as a hemostatic agent in transurethral surgery of the prostate. *J Urol* 1961;86:346.
10. Pearson BS. The effects of Trasylol and aminocaproic acid in post prostatectomy haemorrhage. *Br J Urol* 1969;41:602.
11. Lawrence ACK, Ward-McQuaid JN, Holdom GL. Effect of EACA on blood loss after retropubic prostatectomy. *Br J Urol* 1966;38:308.
12. Madsen PO, Strauch AE. The effect of aminocaproic acid on bleeding following transurethral prostatectomy. *J Urol* 1996;96:255.
13. Vinnicombe J, Shuttleworth KED. Aminocaproic acid in the control of haemorrhage after prostatectomy. *Lancet* 1966;1:230.
14. Symes JM, Offen DN, Lyttle JA, Blandy JP, Chaput de Saintonge DM. The effect of Dicynene on blood loss during and after transurethral resection of the prostate. *Br J Urol* 1975;47:203.
15. Wilson RG, Smith D, Paton G, Gollock JM, Bremner DN. Prophylactic subcutaneous heparin does not increase operative blood loss during and after transurethral resection of the prostate. *Br J Urol* 1988;62:246.
16. Blandy JP. *Operative Urology*, 2nd edn. Oxford: Blackwell Science, 1986:400–3.
17. Tiptaft RC, Motson RW, Costello AJ, Paris AMI, Blandy JP. Fistulae involving rectum and urethra: the place of Parks' operations. *Br J Urol* 1983;55:711.
18. Blandy JP. *Operative Urology*, 2nd edn. Oxford: Blackwell Science, 1986:357–9.
19. Hansen RE, Iversen P. Bladder explosions during uninterrupted transurethral resection of the prostate. *Scand J Urol Nephrol* 1979;13:211.
20. Montague DK, Jarow J, Broderick GA, *et al.* American Urological Association guidelines on the management of priapism. *J Urol* 2003;170:1318–24.
21. Creevy CD. Hemolytic reactions during transurethral prostatic resection. *J Urol* 1947;58:125.
22. Bunge RG, Barker AP. Hemolysis during transurethral prostatic resection. *J Urol* 1948;60:122.
23. Creevy CD, Reiser MP. The importance of hemolysis in transurethral prostatic resection: severe and fatal reactions associated with the use of distilled water. *J Urol* 1963;89:900.
24. Beirne GJ, Madsen PO, Burns RO. Serum electrolyte and osmolarity changes following transurethral resection of the prostate. *J Urol* 1954;93:83.
25. Rao PN. Fluid absorption during urological endoscopy. *Br J Urol* 1987;60:93.

26. Sohn MH, Vogt C, Heinen G, Erkens M, Nordmeyer N, Jakse G. Fluid absorption and circulating endotoxins during transurethral resection of the prostate. *Br J Urol* 1993;72:605.
27. Madsen PO, Naber KG. The importance of the pressure in the prostatic fossa and absorption of irrigating fluid during transurethral resection of the prostate. *J Urol* 1973;109:446–52.
28. Coppinger SW, Lewis CA, Milroy EJG. A method of measuring fluid balance during transurethral resection of the prostate. *Br J Urol* 1995;76:66.
29. Watkins-Pitchford JM, Payne SR, Rennie CD, Riddle PR. Hyponatraemia during transurethral resection: its practical prevention. *Br J Urol* 1984;56:676.
30. Hahn RG. Ethanol monitoring of extravascular absorption of irrigating fluid. *Br J Urol* 1993;72:766.
31. Iglesias JJ, Stams UK. How to prevent the TUR syndrome. *Urologe* 1975;14:287
32. Gale DW, Notley RG. TURP without TURP syndrome. *Br J Urol* 1985;57:708.
33. Goel CM, Badenoch DF, Fowler CG, Blandy JP, Tiptaft RC. Transurethral resection syndrome: a prospective study. *Eur Urol* 1992;21:15.

Chapter 11

Complications after transurethral resection

Three large, contemporary audits provide useful information on outcomes and complications after TURP. These are the UK National Prostatectomy Audit[1-3], Mebust's Cooperative Study from North America[4] and the Northern Region Audit[5].

The National Prostatectomy Audit[1-3] was a prospective audit conducted on operations performed in four health regions of the UK over a 6-month period in 1992. The majority of patients in this study underwent TURP (4624 patients representing 86% of all patients in the study), TURP combined with bladder neck incision (4.6% of patients), or bladder neck incision alone (5.7% of patients). Only 1.6% of patients underwent open prostatectomy. Thus, the National Prostatectomy Audit essentially represents the outcome from TURP. Mebust *et al*[4] retrospectively evaluated outcome following TURP at 13 participating institutions in the USA with a total of 3885 patients. In the Northern Audit[5], data were collected prospectively from 12 sites in one UK health region, on 1400 prostatectomies. TURP was the form of prostatectomy performed in 98% of cases. Complications reported by these studies, with additional information provided by other studies, are documented below.

Death

In 1989 Roos and co-workers[6] reported that the death rate within 90 days of TURP was significantly higher than after open prostatectomy. This sent shockwaves through the urological community. The 90-day mortality after TURP amongst the 37 000 Danish men in this study who formed the most recent group of patients operated on – between 1977 and 1985 – was 2.5%. For open prostatectomy in the Danish patients 90-day mortality was 2.7%, but for the other centres mortality after open prostatectomy was lower when compared with TURP. For the entire group of patients in the Roos study, the relative risk of death 90 days after TURP compared with open prostatectomy was 1.45.

Roos and co-authors admitted that it was not possible to 'rule out potential confounding effects of unmeasured characteristics of patients' and it is likely that the higher mortality after TURP was due to a greater degree of co-morbidity in those patients undergoing TURP when compared with those undergoing open prostatectomy. When one thinks about it, a patient with significant co-morbidity is more likely to be offered a TURP rather than an open prostatectomy so that those undergoing TURP may be less fit than those undergoing open prostatectomy. This view is supported by data from Western Australia[7]. In this large population-based cohort study of mortality after TURP and open prostatectomy, after adjusting for co-morbidity the relative mortality of TURP over open prostatectomy was 1.2 (CI 0.99–1.23). In a study of almost 66 000 TURPs performed in Scotland between 1968 and 1989, Hargreave et al[8] found that the relative risk of death after TURP compared with open prostatectomy was 1.1. There had been suggestions that the fluid balance changes occurring as a consequence of using irrigation fluid during the process of TURP could in some way lead to an increased 'strain' on the heart of frail patients, but interestingly no difference in the risk of dying from ischaemic heart disease (including myocardial infarction) was found between the TURP and open prostatectomy groups in the Australian study.

In the contemporary series of TURPs, the National Prostatectomy Audit[3] reported a hospital mortality rate (death before discharge) of 0.8% for patients undergoing TURP for urinary retention and 0.2% for those with symptoms alone. Overall mortality in the Northern Region Audit was 0.9% at 30 days[5]. For elective admissions this was 0.5% and 2.4% for emergency admissions. In Mebust's series 0.23% of patients died within 30 days of surgery[4].

Infective complications

Septicaemia

Different incidences of *bacteraemia* are reported after transurethral resection, ranging from as low as 1.6% to 58%, more commonly when the urine is infected before operation[9–11]. Disturbingly, as many as 55% of men were found to have positive blood cultures even though their preoperative urine had been sterile[12], while if bacterial endotoxins were measured the proportion rose even higher[13]. Fortunately only a small proportion of men in whom bacteria or endotoxins are found go on to develop septicaemic shock, which is relatively rare and always unexpected.

In the National Prostatectomy Audit septicaemia occurred in 1.9% of men undergoing TURP for retention and 1.3% of those with symptoms

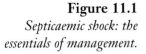

Figure 11.1

Septicaemic shock: the essentials of management.

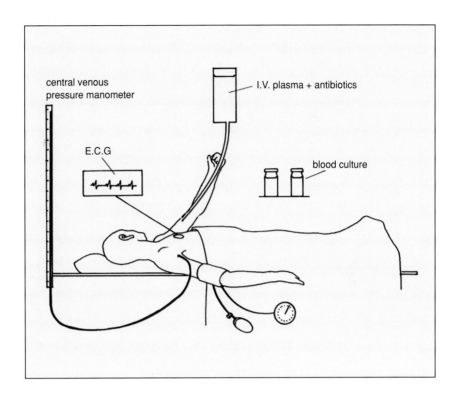

alone. The Northern Region Audit reported a sepsis rate of 8% (varying between 0 and 17% depending on the hospital). Although in Mebust's series of 3885 TURPs the septicaemia rate was not given, of the 9 post-operative deaths, 5 were due to sepsis (presumably with urine as the source) leading to multi-organ failure. In the European Collaborative Study of Antibiotic Prophylaxis for TURP (see Chapter 4), postoperative septicaemia occurred in 1.5% of patients with sterile urine prior to surgery, where no antibiotic prophylaxis had been given at the time of surgery[14].

Septicaemic shock is most likely to occur on the day of operation, or when the catheter is removed. A high fever and rigors, sometimes with flushing of the skin, precedes haemodynamic instability with hypotension. As soon as the diagnosis is suspected (on the basis of a fever), urine and blood should be cultured and empirical intravenous antibiotic treatment started, with generous infusion of intravenous fluids (Fig. 11.1). An early, aggressive approach can prevent the development of hypotension and subsequent multi-organ failure. There should be a low threshold for requesting care in a high dependency unit or intensive care unit. Fortunately death from septicaemic shock after transurethral resection is now rare, although it is still dangerous in men over 80[15,16]. Treating culture-positive urine with several days of antibiotics prior to TURP and antibiotic prophylaxis in all patients (even those with culture-negative urine) probably reduces the rate of septicaemia. Even in patients with sterile urine before TURP, septicaemia can still occur, and a policy of giving prophylactic antibiotics to all patients before TURP may reduce this risk[14].

Urinary infection

The reported incidence of urinary infection after transurethral resection varies from 6 to 100%. In the National Prostatectomy Audit proven UTI occurred either before or after discharge in 13% of patients undergoing prostatectomy for retention and 4.6% of those undergoing prostatectomy for symptoms alone. Comparable figures in Mebust's series were 4.3% and 1.5%.

Much can be done to reduce infection by strict attention to aseptic drill when changing the catheter bag and when irrigating the bladder. If organisms enter the closed system it becomes a culture and they are rapidly carried up into the bladder on the interface of bubbles[17]. Experience and quality control in the management of the catheter is one major reason for bringing urological patients together in one ward area. Even so, the incidence of urinary infection inexorably rises when any catheter has been in the bladder for more than 5 days, by which time a continuous biofilm of bacteria has come to coat the catheter from external meatus to bladder.

Fortunately the clinical effects of this bacterial colonization of the bladder are seldom of any consequence. Upper tract infection, as judged by rigors, a high temperature, or pain in the loin, is rare. Bacteraemia (as pointed out above) is even more rare. As a rule, within a few days of removing the catheter, the infected system has cleansed itself and infection which persists for more than 6 weeks after transurethral resection is so unusual that it makes one suspect persistent residual urine or a diverticulum.

Routine antibiotic prophylaxis in patients with sterile urine prior to TURP has been shown to substantially reduce the chance of postoperative symptomatic UTI[14].

Epididymitis

Once the bane of open prostatectomy, epididymitis is so rarely seen in hospital after TURP that the old practice of routine prophylactic vasectomy has long been given up. In the 1970s prophylactic vasectomy was being performed in up to 95% of prostatectomy patients[18], but by the

1980s this had fallen to 10%[4] and nowadays it is simply no longer part of routine practice.

However, epididymitis is still reported, albeit rarely. In the National Prostatectomy Study it occurred in 5% of men, whether undergoing TURP for retention or symptoms alone[2,3]. When epididymitis does occur it may give rise to systemic illness out of proportion to the local signs, and require intensive antibiotic treatment. If unchecked, epididymitis may proceed to suppuration and even loss of a testicle.

Urethritis

The catheter always provokes some discharge of mucus around the catheter. The normal secretions of the urethra accumulate at the external meatus to form a crust which should be cleansed regularly to remove a potential source of infection. In some patients there is an unusually severe reaction to the catheter, and this may be followed by a stricture, probably from chemical or allergic irritation[19]. In some cases this may represent a latex allergy, and clearly latex-containing catheters should be avoided in individuals with a history of latex allergy.

Osteomyelitis

One very rare infective complication of transurethral resection is vertebral osteomyelitis, which is presumably a late aftermath of bacteraemia, although patients who develop this have seldom had any noteworthy postoperative symptoms (Fig. 11.2). The infection begins in the intervertebral disk, and typically the patient complains of backache which comes on several weeks or months after the operation, is difficult to localize and steadily gets worse. There are almost no physical signs, and it is only when the characteristic erosion of the vertebral body is eventually demonstrated by computerized tomography or magnetic resonance imaging that the diagnosis is made. Intensive treatment with antibiotics usually cures the condition quickly. The difficulty is to make the diagnosis.

Deep venous thrombosis and pulmonary embolism

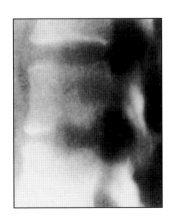

Figure 11.2
X-ray showing osteomyelitis of vertebra.

Deep venous thrombosis (DVT) has been reported in between 4 and 10% of patients after TURP[20], although contemporary series suggest that the rate is somewhat lower, only 0.2% of patients in the National Prostatectomy Audit[2] being diagnosed with a DVT after TURP. In this same audit pulmonary embolus was reported in 0.1% of men. From other reports of outcome after TURP, published since 1990, 0.1–0.5% of men develop a pulmonary embolus after TURP[21].

Pulmonary embolism was diagnosed in 11 out of the 166 cases of death within 30 days of TURP analysed by the National Confidential Enquiry into Perioperative Deaths in 1993/1994, although the true proportion might well have been somewhat higher[22].

DVT and pulmonary embolus prophylaxis is discussed in Chapter 4.

Cerebrovascular accident

From time to time an elderly man with a cardiac history or a previous small stroke comes into hospital, undergoes a transurethral resection, does well, and returns rejoicing to his family. A few weeks later he dies with a sudden stroke and the urologist blames himself, feeling that perhaps if no operation had been done the patient might have survived. In the National Prostatectomy Audit[2] stroke occurred in 0.3% of men after TURP. There is an increased risk of postoperative stroke if the patient has had a history of cerebral or myocardial infarction within the last 3 months.

Failure to void after postoperative catheter removal

It is depressing when a patient fails to void following catheter removal a few days after TURP. Inevitably the patient thinks that something has gone wrong and the surgeon, particularly the trainee, is concerned that not enough obstructing tissue has been removed. In fact this is rarely the case; although failure to void is a common occurrence after TURP, a second 'trial of catheter removal' a few weeks later is usually successful.

Mebust et al[4] reported failure to void in 6.5% of men and in the National Prostatectomy Audit[3] 9% of those with acute retention and 2.3% in those who had a TURP for symptoms alone failed to void on catheter removal after the operation. In the latter study, a permanent catheter was required in 1% and 0.1% of men respectively.

Reynard and Shearer[23] reviewed a series of 381 consecutive TURPs performed by four experienced surgeons over an 18-month period. Failure to void did not occur after TURP done for symptoms alone, but it was suprisingly frequent after TURP done for retention. Most significantly it could be predicted from the retention volume – the volume of urine drained at the initial presentation. Acute retention was defined as painful inability to void with a catheter volume of <800 ml of urine, chronic retention as maintenance of voiding with a residual urine volume of >500 ml (average residual volume in this group was 1400 ml, and ranged from 500 to 3000 ml) and acute-on-chronic retention as painful inability to void with a catheter volume of >800 ml of urine (average retention volume in this group was 1300 ml, and ranged from 900 to 5000 ml). Using these definitions, failure to void after TURP was reported in 10%, 38% and 44%, respectively. Only 1% of patients ultimately failed to void at repeat catheter removal 6 weeks later (thus requiring a long-term catheter), all having presented with chronic retention.

Why should the patient not void after the initial catheter removal, even though an adequate volume of tissue has been removed? This presumably relates to a degree of swelling of the residual prostatic tissue, possibly combined with postoperative urethral pain which inhibits normal voiding and in some cases with the added problem of a poorly contractile bladder[24]. Given a few additional weeks of catheterization after TURP, the oedema has settled down, the resection margin has shrunk a little and the patient has recovered from the effects of surgery. Successful voiding is the norm. There is some evidence that detrusor pressure increases over the course of several months in patients who initially fail to void after TURP, but ultimately regain the ability to void spontaneously[24].

As with so many surgical operations, it is much better to warn the patient in advance that problems can be encountered postoperatively and that failure to void might occur. The patient can be reassured that there is a 99% chance that they will ultimately be free of a catheter.

Secondary haemorrhage

Bleeding in the early postoperative phase has been dealt with on page 81–3. Very commonly there is a small secondary bleed about the 10th postoperative day which the patient should be warned about. In the National Prostatectomy Study it caused difficulty in passing urine in 10% of patients[2].

What is far less common is for haemorrhage to occur months or years later. Often there is some new cause for it, e.g. cancer of the bladder or kidney, and all cases require a complete urological investigation (such as urine culture and cytology, flexible cystoscopy and renal ultrasonography). But in a number of men all that can be found is some regrowth of the prostatic adenoma and, after a biopsy to rule out cancer of the prostate, nothing else needs to be done. However, within this group is a small number who continue to bleed. The options for such patients include a prolonged course of 5-alpha reductase inhibitors (see Chapter 4) or a further TURP.

Urethral stricture

The true incidence of stricture after transurethral surgery is probably rather higher than is admitted in most series, and it depends on how the diagnosis is made. If the patient has no symptoms he is unlikely to have his flow rate measured, let alone his urethra investigated by urethrogram, urethroscopy or urethral ultrasound. The usual problem is a narrowing just inside the external meatus, presenting about 8 weeks after the operation with the symptom of spraying on micturition. It is easily treated by regular dilatation using a short straight sound. The patient can be taught to pass a Lofric® catheter of appropriate calibre on himself. The annual toll of these strictures is diminishing, thanks probably to the increasing use of narrow resectoscope sheaths and the use of prophylactic internal urethrotomy[25].

Other sites for postoperative stricture are at the penoscrotal junction, the bulb and the external sphincter (Fig. 11 .3). Occasionally optical urethrotomy is required, but usually these strictures are easily managed by dilatation supplemented by regular self-catheterization.

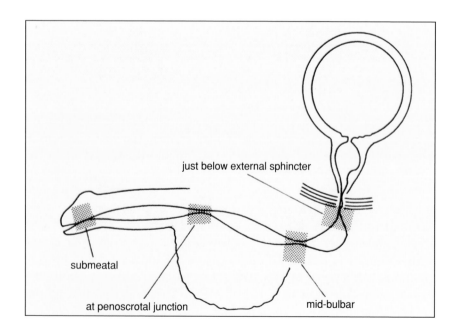

just below external sphincter

submeatal

at penoscrotal junction

mid-bulbar

Figure 11.3
Main sites of post transurethral resection strictures.

Bladder neck stenosis

Formerly common after open prostatectomy this is rare after transurethral surgery. At an interval of some months after transurethral resection the patient comes back with a return of symptoms and is found to have a tight membrane at the level of the bladder neck (Fig. 11.4). It is easily put right with a urethrotome or a bee-sting electrode (Fig. 11.5), but it does tend to recur, perhaps because (as histology often shows) there is evidence of granuloma in the tissue. Bladder neck stenosis is not prevented by incision of the bladder neck[26].

Vesico-ureteric junction stricture and ureteric reflux

The ureteric orifice, where the ureter drains in the bladder, is close to the bladder neck. Very rarely it is possible for the loop of the resectoscope to cut across the lower end of the ureter at this point during a TURP, particularly if there is a large middle lobe such that the loop of the resectoscope has to be advanced well into the bladder to allow this lobe to be resected. In theory this may lead either to vesicoureteric reflux or to obstruction of the kidney, although none of the authors have ever encountered this complication over many years of practice. Reflux of urine occurs because the flap valve mechanism of the ureteric orifice is disrupted. Obstruction occurs as a consequence of contraction of scar

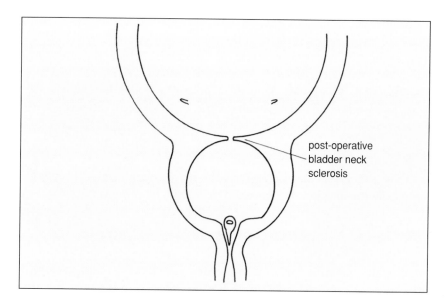

post-operative
bladder neck
sclerosis

Figure 11.4
Bladder neck stenosis
following prostatectomy.

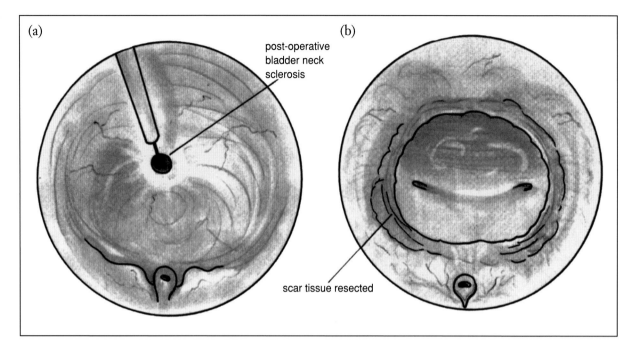

(a)

(b)

post-operative
bladder neck
sclerosis

scar tissue resected

Figure 11.5
Bladder neck stenosis.
(a) The hole in the
diaphragm is incised with
the bee-sting electrode or
Collings knife and then
(b) the scar tissue is cut
away all round.

tissue around the healing ureteric orifice and this process constricts the lumen of the ureter. This problem can be avoided by making a mental note at the start of resection of the location of the ureteric orifices. At the end of the resection some surgeons find it comforting to look at the ureteric orifices just to check that they have not been damaged.

Where a bladder tumour overlies the ureteric orifice, it is impossible to remove the tumour without deliberately cutting across the ureteric orifice. Leaving a JJ stent in the ureter for a few weeks after the TURBT may reduce the risk of contraction of the ureteric orifice. If possible, try to place a guidewire (preferably insulated) into the ureter before starting the resection. This can make it easier to pass a JJ stent after the resection, because the lumen of the ureter may be lost once the tumour has been resected. Placing a JJ stent in the ureter before the resection runs the risk of cutting through the stent, and the proximal part of the stent may then be very difficult to retrieve.

If the ureter does become scarred, the stricture can be managed endoscopically (by incision or dilatation) or (rarely) by reimplantation.

The need to repeat transurethral resection

One of the old criticisms of transurethral resection was that it was less thorough than surgical enucleation, and this was certainly true in the days when instrumentation was so poor. Today it is probably less common, but it was disturbing to find that about 12% of transurethral resections were revision procedures[5]. The Roos study[6] found a re-operation rate after TURP of approximately 12% versus 4.5% after open prostatectomy. Of course the prostate will continue to grow and this will account for a proportion of such patients who need to undergo repeat TURP.

Incontinence

Far from causing incontinence, TUR often cures the incontinence that is present in a quarter of patients before operation. Nevertheless, one in 10 men remain incontinent afterwards and the operation seems to cause incontinence in as many as 6%[2]; nothing is a greater disaster for an otherwise fit patient. In a proportion of cases the cause is poor selection of the patient, whose symptoms were really due to detrusor instability from some other cause. In such patients transurethral resection may change a picture of severe frequency into one of disabling incontinence.

The incidence of incontinence after TURP falls with time. This is probably due to spontaneous resolution of bladder overactivity (detrusor instability) in a substantial proportion of patients.

Technical error at the time of operation can also cause incontinence. In such a patient endoscopy will show a tell-tale defect in the external sphincter, usually at 10 or 2 o'clock, and perusal of the notes may yield the story that during the operation the patient developed an erection, the surgeon lost his way, and the sphincter was cut in mistake for adenoma.

The investigation of post TUR incontinence requires urodynamic investigations to determine the state of the detrusor, and endoscopy to reveal the sphincter. The treatment is often unsatisfactory. The choice is between wearing incontinence pads or an incontinence appliance such as a condom sheath, injection of urethral bulking agents such as marcoplastique in the bladder neck and/or membranous urethra or an artificial implanted sphincter. In days gone by a Cunningham clip was sometimes applied to the penis, but ischaemic necrosis could develop at the site where the clip was worn. The artificial urinary sphincter usually provides a satisfactory degree of continence, but this is at the price of a further operation which carries certain risks. The greatest worry is infection of the implanted sphincter, which almost always requires complete removal of the device and weeks of nursing care of the wound, often in hospital. The urethral cuff of the artificial sphincter applies a constant pressure to the urethra and as a consequence the underlying urethra may atrophy so that the cuff no longer fits snugly around it, and the incontinence recurs. A more extreme effect of this pressure on the urethra is that of urethral erosion, which leads to recurrent incontinence and ultimately device infection. Being a mechanical device, sooner or later the artificial sphincter will simply break down and require replacement[27].

Sexual dysfunction after transurethral resection

In all, 40% of men in the National Prostatectomy Audit were unhappy with their postoperative sexual function[28].

There are three separate elements to sexual dissatisfaction after transurethral surgery. The first is retrograde ejaculation, about which urologists have been aware of for many years, and must routinely warn all their patients as it occurs in about two out of three men[28]. It is probably caused by the removal of the bladder neck, which normally closes during ejaculation, and is necessarily removed along with the obstructing adenoma.

The second component is erectile impotence. For many years this was given little thought, but some 70% of men are still sexually active in their 70s, and of these 10–30% will be rendered impotent afterwards[2,29–31]. Erectile function can improve after TURP. Indeed, 20% of men in the UK National Prostatectomy Audit reported an improvement in erectile function after TURP[28].

There is a third component, namely the lack of the sensation of orgasm. This may relate to a deficiency in contraction of muscular tissue in the prostate and seminal vesicles. In the National Prostatectomy Audit 52% of men described absent or altered sensation of orgasm.

Dunsmuir and Emberton[30] found a strong association between the presence of retrograde ejaculation and sensation of impaired orgasm: 60% of men with retrograde ejaculation reported impaired orgasm, compared with only 16% of men who retained antegrade ejaculation after TURP. The occurrence of retrograde ejaculation after TURP implies that a more extensive resection has taken place than in men where no retrograde ejaculation occurs. It is conceivable that a more extensive resection, particularly if capsular perforation occurs, could damage the cavernous nerves and arteries which are located in the periprostatic tissues.

For the surgeon the crucial thing is that these matters are discussed with the patient before the operation, particularly when there is no life-threatening complication such as ureteric obstruction or severe infection, and especially in the younger patient who may not have completed his family. It was disturbing to find in one large audit that a note had been made to the effect that these matters had been discussed with the patient at the time of getting consent in <30% of records[32]. At the very least patients are likely to be upset if they are not warned about the possibility that significant sexual dysfunction can occur following TURP. In a proportion this will lead to anger and the possibility of litigation[28].

References

1. Emberton M, Neal DE, Black N *et al*. The National Prostatectomy Audit: the clinical management of patients during hospital admission. *Br J Urol* 1995;75:301–16.
2. Neal DE. The National Prostatectomy Audit. *Br J Urol* 1997;79(Suppl 2):69–75.
3. Pickard R, Emberton M, Neal DE. The management of men with acute urinary retention. *Br J Urol* 1998;81:712–20.
4. Mebust WK, Holtgrewe HL, Cockett ATK *et al*. Transurethral prostatectomy: immediate and postoperative complications. A cooperative study of 13 participating institutions evaluating 3885 patients. *J Urol* 1989;141:243–7.
5. Thorpe AC, Cleary R, Coles J *et al*. Deaths and complications following prostatectomy in 1400 men in the Northern Region of England. *Br J Urol* 1994;74:559–65.
6. Roos NP, Wennberg J, Malenka DJ *et al*. Mortality and reoperation after open and transurethral resection of the prostate for benign prostatic hyperplasia. *N Engl J Med* 1989;320;1120–4.
7. Holman CD, Wisniewski ZS, Semmens JB *et al*. Mortality and prostate cancer risk in 19,598 men after surgery for benign prostatic hyperplasia. *Br J Urol Int* 1999;84:37–42.
8. Hargreave TB, Heynes CF, Kendrick SW *et al*. Mortality after transurethral and open prostatectomy in Scotland. *Br J Urol* 1996;77:547–53.
9. Kiely EA, McCormack T, Cafferkey MT, Faliner FR, Butler MR. Study of appropriate antibiotic therapy in transurethral prostatectomy. *Br J Urol* 1989;64:61.
10. Hall JC, Christiansen KJ, England P *et al*. Antibiotic prophylaxis for patients undergoing transurethral resection of the prostate. *Urology* 1996;47:852.
11. Ibrahim AIA, Bilal NE, Shetty SD, Patil KP, Gomaa H. The source of organisms in the post-prostatectomy bacteremia of patients with pre-operative sterile urine. *Br J Urol* 1993;72:770.
12. Robinson MRG, Arudpragasam ST, Sahgal SM *et al*. Bacteraemia resulting from prostatic surgery: the source of bacteria. *Br J Urol* 1982;37:551.
13. Sohn MH, Vogt C, Heinen G *et al*. Fluid absorption and circulating endotoxins during transurethral resection of the prostate. *Br J Urol* 1993;72:605.
14. Hargreave TB, Botto B, Rikken GHJM *et al*. European Collaborative Study of Antibiotic Prophylaxis for Transurethral Resection of the Prostate. *Eur Urol* 1993;23:437–43.
15. Phair JP. Approach to bacteremia (Gram positive/negative and septic shock). In: Kelley WN (ed.) *Textbook of Internal Medicine*. Philadelphia: Lippincott, 1989: 1796–800.
16. Edwards JD. Management of septic shock. *BMJ* 1993;306:1661.
17. Ramsay JWA, Garnham AJ, Mulhall AB *et al*. Biofilms, bacteria and bladder catheters. *Br J Urol* 1989;64:395.
18. Melchior J, Valk WL, Foret JD, Mebust WK. Transurethral prostatectomy: computerized analysis of 2223 consecutive cases. *J Urol* 1974;112:634–42.
19. Blandy JP. Urethral stricture. *Postgrad Med J* 1980;56:383.
20. Brenner DW, Fogle MA, Schellhammer PF. Venous thromboembolism. *J Urol* 1989;142:1403–11.
21. Donat R, Mancey-Jones B. Incidence of thromboembolism after transurethral resection of the prostate (TURP). *Scand J Urol Nephrol* 2002;36:119–23.

22. Lunn JN, Devlin HB, Hoile RW. The Report of the National Confidential Enquiry into Perioperative Deaths 1993/1994. London: NCEPOD, 1996.

23. Reynard JM, Shearer RJ. Failure to void after transurethral resection of the prostate and mode of presentation. *Urology* 1999;53:336–9.

24. Djavan R, Madersbacher S, Klingler C *et al*. Urodynamic assessment of patients with acute urinary retention: is treatment failure after prostatectomy predictable? *J Urol* 1997;158:1829–33.

25. Edwards LI, Lock R, Powell C, Jones P. Post-catheterization urethral strictures: a clinical and experimental study. *Br J Urol* 1983;55:53.

26. Woodhouse E, Barnes R, Hadley H, Rothman C. Fibrous contracture of bladder neck. *Urology* 1979;13:393.

27. Gundian JC, Barrett DM, Parulkar BG. Mayo Clinic experience with the AS800 artificial urinary sphincter for urinary incontinence after transurethral resection of prostate or open prostatectomy. *Urology* 1993;41:318.

28. Dunsmuir WD, Emberton M. Surgery, drugs and the male orgasm. *BMJ* 1997;314:319.

29. Hanbury DC, Sethia KK. Erectile function following transurethral prostatectomy. *Br J Urol* 1995;75:12.

30. Dunsmuir WD, Emberton M. There is significant sexual dysfunction following TURP. *Br J Urol* 1996;77:39 (161) abstract.

31. Samdal F, Vada K, Lundmo P. Sexual function after transurethral prostatectomy. *Scand J Urol Nephrol* 1993;27:27.

32. Thorpe AC, Cleary R, Coles J *et al*. Written consent about sexual function in men undergoing transurethral prostatectomy. *Br J Urol* 1994;74:479.

Chapter 12

The role of alternatives to transurethral resection

Guidelines

As discussed in Chapter 4, to decide the most appropriate treatment for patients presenting with lower urinary tract symptoms thought to be due to BPH, the urologist should be aware of so-called clinical practice guidelines (CPGs) which summarize the available options. Guidelines started to appear in the early 1990s as an attempt to standardize treatment. This was a consequence of reports which showed wide variations in TURP rates both within and between countries. The fact that the treatment you received depended not so much on what condition you had, but more on where you lived, suggested that there was no consensus on the indications for TURP. Therefore, in an attemp to define more precisely the indications for treating BPH symptoms, clinical practice guidelines were established.

A number of clinical practice guidelines have been published and they have recently been reviewed[1,2], (see also Chapter 4 page 44). Precisely which guidelines you use will depend to a considerable degree on which country you are working in. In essence there are few differences between them, in terms of their treatment recommendations (although their recommendations for diagnostic tests to complement the diagnosis of 'BPH' vary considerably – see Chapter 4). All recommend documenting the severity of the patient's symptoms using the IPSS, the International Prostate Symptom Score. This provides a baseline against which the effects of treatment can be measured. The IPSS also measures the 'bother' caused by the patient's symptoms – the degree to which the patient's symptoms trouble him. A man may have a high symptom score, but may not be bothered by his symptoms. Clearly, one would tend towards recommending watchful waiting in such an individual, rather than active treatment.

Using guidelines in your practice is not obligatory, but with the ever-present threat of litigation you need to be able to defend a decision not to use them. They thus provide a certain amount of protection from litigation, quite apart from helping day to day management decisions.

Why do men seek treatment for their symptoms?

There are several reasons. Firstly the symptoms may be bothersome. Secondly, there may be the fear that the symptoms are a warning that acute urinary retention will develop. Thirdly, the patient may be concerned that their symptoms indicate that they have prostate cancer. It is important to establish what the patient wants from his consultation with you. Once reassured that the likelihood of urinary retention and prostate cancer is low, he may not want treatment for symptoms which on the surface may appear quite bad and may be quite happy to adopt a policy of watchful waiting.

Watchful waiting

The first option that should be discussed with the patient is watchful waiting. Numerous studies have shown that in a substantial proportion of men symptoms do not progress, even for those with severe symptoms.

In a study now regarded as a classic, Ball *et al*[3] followed 107 men with watchful waiting over a 5-year period. In none was there an absolute indication for surgery. Half of the patients were obstructed on urodynamic testing. A third of the patients got better, just under half stayed the same, a quarter got worse (of whom eight underwent TURP) and only 2% went into retention. This study had been preceded by another which suggested that urinary symptoms improved in approximately 30% of men in the placebo arm of a BPH drug study[4].

Data from the placebo arm of the PLESS study (Proscar long-term efficacy and safety study) in which 1500 men with moderate to severe symptoms were randomized to placebo, showed that the average symptom score had fallen by 1 point at 4 years of follow-up[5]. Clearly symptoms got worse in some men, but better in others. The Wasson study of watchful waiting versus TURP has shown that for the man with moderate symptoms who chooses watchful waiting, the risk of progression to retention, worsening symptoms or need for TURP is relatively low[6]. Of those men on watchful waiting 40% noticed an improvement in their symptoms, 30% got worse and TURP was required in about a quarter. In the five centres study[7], 500 men referred by their family doctors for consideration for TURP were managed non-operatively after viewing an educational programme. Over the following 4-year period a proportion of the men chose drug treatment or surgery. For men with mild, moderate or severe symptoms, 10%, 24% and 39%, respectively, had undergone surgery at the end of 4 years. For the same symptom categories, 63%,

45% and 33% were still not receiving any treatment at the end of 4 years. Almost a quarter of men who initially presented with severe symptoms noted an improvement in their symptoms, to mild or moderate.

On the basis of these studies we can say that symptoms, even if severe, do not necessarily get worse even over fairly long periods of time. This forms the foundation of watchful waiting as an option for many patients, even if the symptoms at baseline are severe.

Drug treatment

Where a patient has bothersome symptoms and wants active treatment, a 5-alpha reductase inhibitor or an alpha-blocker will usually be the first line of treatment.

Alpha-blockers

The alpha-blockers act on the so-called 'dynamic' component of prostatic obstruction, which is thought to be mediated by alpha-adrenergic-dependent smooth muscle contraction in the stroma of the prostate.

Relative to the improvement in symptoms after TURP, that seen with the alpha-blockers is modest. The average improvement in symptom score after TURP is about 85%[8]. While clearly some of this may represent a placebo response, this improvement is considerably better than that seen with the alpha-blockers which result in a 10–30% improvement in symptom score relative to placebo[9]. In real terms, the average improvement in symptom score is about 4–5 points over and above an improvement with placebo of 2–3 points. This improvement in symptom score must be considered in the context of the smallest perceptible change in symptom score that a man can detect, which is 3 points. It is therefore difficult to describe the symptomatic effect of alpha-blockers as anything other than modest.

Furthermore, not all patients respond to an alpha-blocker. If one defines 'response' as a >25% improvement in symptoms relative to placebo (a fairly modest definition of improvement), most studies describe response rates of 30–40%[10]. The mean probability for improvement in symptom score after TURP is in the order of 80%, i.e. 8 out of 10 men will notice an improvement in their symptoms after TURP[8,11].

A substantial proportion of men will also stop taking their medication as time goes by, either because of side effects or because of a perceived lack of effectiveness. The side effects of alpha-blockers include asthenia (weakness – 5%), dizziness (6%), headache (2%), postural hypotension (1%) and retrograde ejaculation (8%)[10]. Overall approximately 15–30% of men report some constellation of side effects.

5-Alpha reductase inhibitors

Generally speaking, 5-alpha reductase inhibitors are used for the larger prostate. They inhibit the conversion of testosterone to dihydrotestosterone, the more active androgen in the prostate. This causes shrinkage of the prostatic epithelium and therefore a reduction in prostate volume. This takes some months to occur, so urinary symptoms will not improve initially.

A number of large studies have reported on the effectiveness of these drugs. These include the SCARP (Scandinavian BPH Study Group)[12], PROSPECT[13] (Proscar safety plus efficacy Canadian 2-year study) and PROWESS studies[14] and more recently the PLESS study[5] (Proscar long-term efficacy and safety study). All these studies show symptom improvement over placebo in the order of 2–3 points on the IPSS and improvements in flow rate in the order of 1–2 ml/s. The PLESS data also show a small reduction in the risk of urinary retention (see below).

The side effects of the 5-alpha reductase inhibitors are generally speaking fairly mild and principally centre around sexual problems such as loss of libido in 5%, impotence in 5% and reduced volume of ejaculate in a few percent. This low side effect profile is reflected in the relatively low drop-out rate in the PLESS study, two-thirds of men assigned to finasteride remaining on the drug at 4 years of follow-up and 50% of those on finasteride in the SCARP study remaining on the drug at 6 years.

Anticholinergics

For a man with frequency, urgency and urge incontinence – symptoms suggestive of an overactive bladder – one can consider an anticholinergic such as oxybutynin or tolterodine. There is concern that these drugs could precipitate urinary retention in men with bladder outlet obstruction, but in fact the risk of this occurring is probably very low[15].

Combination therapy

An alternative to a single drug is to use a combination of an alpha-blocker and a 5-alpha reductase inhibitor. In the MTOPS (Medical Therapy of Prostatic Symptoms) study[16] this combination prevented progression of BPH, progression being defined as a worsening of symptom score by 4 or more, or the development of complications such as UTI or acute urinary retention.

In the Veterans Affairs combination therapy study[17] 1200 men were randomized to placebo, finasteride, terozosin or a combination of terazosin and finasteride. At 1 year of follow-up, finasteride had reduced the symptom score by an average of 3 points relative to placebo, whereas terazosin alone or in combination with finasteride had reduced the symptom score by an average of 6 points.

The PREDICT (Prospective European Doxazosin and Combination Therapy) study[18] randomized over 1000 men to placebo, finasteride, doxazosin or a combination of finasteride and doxazosin. The differences in symptom score (International Prostate Symptom Score) at baseline and at 1 year of follow-up were –5.7 and –6.6 for placebo and finasteride, and –8.3 and –8.5 for doxazosin and combination therapy. In another study over 1000 men were randomized to alfuzosin, finasteride or a combination. At 6 months the improvement in the IPSS was not significantly different in the alfuzosin versus the combination group[19].

Thus, most studies except for the MTOPS suggest that combination therapy is no more useful than an alpha-blocker alone. Enthusiasm for dual therapy has been dampened somewhat by the Prostate Cancer Prevention Trial[20]. In this study of over 18 000 men who were randomized to receive finasteride or placebo over a 7-year period, those in the finasteride group had a lower prevalence of prostate cancer detected on prostate biopsy. However, higher grade tumours, which are biologically more aggressive than low grade cancers were more common in the finasteride group. The jury is out on whether finasteride causes higher grade cancers or not.

Phytotherapy

An alternative drug treatment for BPH symptoms, and one which is widely used in Europe and increasingly in North America, is phytotherapy: 50% of all medications consumed for BPH symptoms are phytotherapeutic ones[21]. These attractively named agents include the African plum (*Pygeum africanum*), purple cone flower (*Echinacea purpurea*), South African star grass (*Hipoxis rooperi*) and saw palmetto berry (*Seronoa repens, Permixon*).

Saw palmetto contains an anti-inflammatory, antiproliferative, oestrogenic drug with 5-alpha reductase inhibitory activity, derived from the American dwarf palm. It has been compared with finasteride in a large double-blind, randomized trial, and equivalent (40%) reductions in symptom score were found with both agents over a 6-month period[22]. A meta-analysis of 18 randomized controlled trials of almost 3000 men suggests that *Seronoa repens* produces similar improvements in symptoms and flow rates to those produced by finasteride[23].

South African star grass (*Hipoxis rooperi*), which is marketed as Harzol, contains beta-sitosterol, which may induce apoptosis in prostate stromal cells, by causing elevated levels of TGF-beta$_1$ (transforming growth factor). In a 6-month randomized, double-blind, placebo-controlled study involving 200 men, the IPSS improved by 2 points with placebo and by 7 points with beta-sitosterol[24].

For other agents, such as *Urtica dioica* (stinging nettle) and the African plum the studies that set out to establish their effectiveness involved small numbers of patients, placebo groups were seldom included and follow-up was short. Many lack sufficient statistical power to prove conclusively that the various agents work[25].

Practice in 'real life'

So, in practice, what does the average urologist do for a man with symptoms of BPH? In a recent survey of American urologists who were specifically questioned about their management of BPH symptoms[26], for mild symptoms (AUA score 0–7) 77% recommended watchful waiting, 21% alpha-blockers and 1% finasteride.

For the moderately symptomatic man (AUA score 8–19) alpha-blockers were recommended by 88%, finasteride by 1% and TURP by 1% of urologists for prostate estimated to be <40 ml in volume. For the moderately symptomatic man with a prostate larger than 40 ml, alpha-blockers were recommended by 69%, finasteride by 10% and TURP by 9% of urologists.

For the severely symptomatic patient, alpha-blockers were recommended 58% of the time for smaller prostates and 45% of the time for larger prostates. TURP was recommended for 31% of severely symptomatic patients with prostates <40 ml in volume and for 38% with prostates >40 ml. Thus, watchful waiting is being used by a large proportion of urologists, particularly for patients with mild symptoms, and many are using drug treatments even for the severely symptomatic man. It seems sensible to at least give the patient the option of avoiding surgery. It is always a relief that this was done when a complication develops after surgery.

'Am I likely to develop retention of urine?'

Many patients are understandably concerned that their urinary symptoms may be a harbinger for the development of acute urinary retention. This may influence their decision to seek help for symptoms which they may perceive as indicating a risk of subsequent retention and it may affect the type of treatment they choose.

In a community-based study from North America, Jacobsen *et al*[27] prospectively followed a cohort of over 2000 men for a period of 4 years to identify risk factors for acute urinary retention. Pre-study symptom scores and flow rates were obtained for the whole group, and in a subsample transrectal ultrasonography was used to determine prostate volume. The presence of lower urinary tract symptoms, a low maximum flow rate, and enlarged prostate and old age were asociated with an increased risk of urinary retention. In those aged 40–49 years with mild symptoms (AUA symptom score ≤7), approximately 3 men in every 1000 experienced an episode of retention each year, compared with 9 men in every 1000 in those aged 70–79 years. For those with moderate or severe symptoms, 3 of every 1000 men aged 40–49 years went into retention every year, and for those aged 70–79 years, 34 of every 1000 men experienced urinary retention each year. These data are reassuring, as they suggest that even for the elderly man with moderate to severe symptoms, the chance of an episode of urinary retention is only 3 in 100 per year.

Adjusting for age and flow rate, those with an AUA symptom score of ≥8 had a 2.3-fold increased risk of going into urinary retention when compared with those with an AUA score of ≤7. Those men with a peak flow rate of <12 ml/s had a 4-fold increased risk of urinary retention when compared with those with a flow rate of >12 ml/s. Prostate volume >30 ml was associated with a 3-fold increased risk of urinary retention compared with those with prostate volumes <30 ml.

The PLESS data[5] have been widely publicized as showing a substantial reduction in the risk of urinary retention. In this 4-year follow-up study, 42 of 1471 men on finasteride went into urinary retention (3%), while 99 of 1404 on placebo experienced an episode of retention (7%). This represents an impressive 43% *relative* reduction in risk in those taking finasteride. However, the *absolute* risk reduction over a 4-year period is a less impressive 4%. And of course, it is the absolute reduction in risk that patients are interested in. So, finasteride does reduce the risk of retention, but it is reducing the risk of an event which is actually quite rare, as suggested by the fact that 93% of men on placebo in this study did not experience retention over a 4-year period. Put another way, to prevent 1 episode of retention, 25 men would have to continue treatment with finasteride for 4 years.

Surgical alternatives to TURP

TURP or other surgical alternatives are used where complications of BPH have developed (such as urinary retention), where medical treatment has not worked or where the effects of such treatment have worn off. The search for alternative surgical treatments essentially started with the Roos paper, which reported a seemingly higher mortality and re-operation rate after TURP when compared with open prostatectomy[28]. The search was on for less invasive treatments, with lower morbidity and mortality, but with similar efficacy.

There are two broad categories of alternative surgical techniques – the minimally invasive and the invasive. All are essentially heat treatments, delivered at variable temperature and power and producing variable degrees of coagulative necrosis of the prostate or vaporization of prostatic tissue. The emphasis, particularly for the more invasive options such as TUVP (transurethral electrovaporization) and laser prostatectomy, has been directed towards trying to reduce blood loss while maintaining effective relief of symptoms.

Minimally invasive surgical alternatives to TURP

These include transurethral radio-frequency needle ablation of the prostate (TUNA), transurethral microwave thermotherapy (TUMT) and high intensity focused ultrasound (HIFU).

Transurethral radio-frequency needle ablation of the prostate – TUNA

Low level radio-frequency is transmitted to the prostate via a transurethral needle delivery system, the needles which transmit the energy being deployed in the prostatic urethra once the instrument has been advanced into the prostatic urethra. The procedure is done under local anaesthetic, with or without intravenous sedation. The resultant heat causes localized necrosis of the prostate.

In a randomized trial comparing TUNA with TURP, Bruskewitz et al[29] reported a low complication rate after TUNA with a substantial reduction in symptom score (13 points) at 1 year of follow-up compared with a similar reduction in symptom score after TURP (15 points). Flow rate after TURP had increased by 12 ml/s at 1 year, compared with a 6 ml/s increase after TUNA. Roehrborn et al[30] reported similar results. It seems that, on average, the improvement in flow rate at 12 months post-treatment is in the order of 6 ml/s and the improvement in symptom score averages about 13 points[31]. Side effects include bleeding in about one-third of patients, urinary tract infection in 10% and urethral stricture in about 2%. No adverse effects on sexual function have been reported.

TUNA has recently been endorsed as a minimally invasive treatment option for symptoms associated with prostatic enlargement by the UK National Institute for Clinical Excellence (NICE)[32], although concerns were expressed relating to the long-term effectiveness of the treatment, a concern similarly expressed in EAU Guidelines[33]. Only time will tell whether TUNA falls out of favour as a treatment which simply delays the need for TURP, but Gee's survey of practice among North American urologists suggests that very few are offering this treatment – only 3% of urologists were performing TUNA in 1997[26].

Transurethral microwave thermotherapy – TUMT

Microwave energy can be delivered to the prostate via an intraurethral catheter, with a cooling system to prevent damage to the adjacent urethra. The microwave energy produces heating of the prostate, leading to coagulative necrosis. Subsequent shrinkage of the prostate relieves obstruction. There is also evidence that TUMT causes thermal damage to adrenergic neurons and this heat-induced blockade of the adrenergic pathway may account for at least some of the reported symptomatic improvement[34].

Many published reports of outcomes after TUMT are open studies, where all patients have received treatment and where there is no control group. In trials comparing TUMT with sham 'treatments' (where the intraurethral microwave catheter is inserted, but the machine is not turned on), improvements in symptom scores in the order of 10 points on the IPSS have been reported, in as many as three-quarters of men[35–40]. Symptomatic improvement appears to be greater when using microwave systems that deliver higher energy to the prostate. One study, however, found an equivalent improvement in symptom score in treated patients and in those undergoing sham treatment with the machine turned off[41]. This suggests that the improvements in symptoms score, at least in this study, represented a placebo effect. In those studies where symptoms improve, the maximal improvement is usually apparent within 3–6 months of treatment and the improvement seems to be durable, at least over a 3-year period[42].

D'Ancona et al[43] compared TUMT with TURP in 52 patients. Symptoms improved in 56% after TUMT compared with 74% after TURP. TURP relieved obstruction in 90% of the TURP patients and 70% of the TUMT patients. Sexual side effects after TUMT, such as impotence and retrograde ejaculation, were less frequent than after TURP. The period of catheterization after TUMT is longer than with TURP (in this study averaging 4 days after TURP and 12 days after TUMT) and urinary infection and irritative urinary symptoms are more common after TUMT.

TUMT is really an intermediate treatment between drugs and more invasive methods. It has the obvious advantage that it can be performed under local anaesthetic, although where higher energy systems are used intravenous sedation may be required. It may have less of an effect on sexual function than TURP, but post-treatment catheterization is longer, on average, than that after TURP. It is a less effective treatment for improving bladder outflow obstruction than TURP. On the basis of these effects, EAU Guidelines[33] state that TUMT 'should be reserved for patients who prefer to avoid surgery or who no longer respond favourably to medication'.

High intensity focused ultrasound – HIFU

A focused ultrasound beam can be used to induce a rise in temperature in the prostate, or indeed in any other tissue to which it is applied. For HIFU treatment of the prostate a transrectal probe is used. A general anaesthetic or heavy intravenous sedation is required during the treatment. Preliminary data suggested a reduction in symptom score in the order of 12 points[44,45]. There are no data comparing HIFU against other surgical treatments for BPH and it should therefore, as EAU Guidelines state, be regarded as an investigational therapy.

Invasive surgical alternatives to TURP

These include laser prostatectomy and TUVP.

TUVP

TUVP uses a combination of vaporization and dessication of prostatic tissue. A number of electrode configurations have been designed to maximize the efficiency of vaporization. TUVP has been compared against TURP in a number of well designed, randomized, single-blinded studies.

Over the short term (up to about 1 year of follow-up) TUVP seems to be as effective as TURP for symptom control and relief of bladder outlet obstruction[46]. In this same study operating time and in-patient hospital stay were equivalent, although more patients required blood transfusion after TURP compared with TUVP (9 versus 2). Over a 5-year period symptomatic relief after TUVP is maintained and re-operation rates are equivalent to TURP[47].

Thus, TUVP seems to be very nearly equivalent to TURP in terms of symptom relief, relief of obstruction, complications and re-operation rate. It has the potential disadvantage over TURP of not allowing histological examination of tissue which is removed, so prostate cancers cannot be detected. Recently, NICE in the UK has endorsed its use as a surgical treatment option for prostatic symptoms[48].

Laser prostatectomy

Several different techniques of 'laser prostatectomy' evolved during the 1990s using laser energy to coagulate, vaporize or resect the prostate. The precise effect – coagulation or vaporization – depends on the laser type, the time for which it is applied and the total laser energy that is delivered to the prostate. A single laser system may produce a combination of coagulation and vaporization, with one effect predominating. A number of different laser delivery systems have been used for laser treatment of the prostate.

Transurethral ultrasound-guided laser-induced prostatectomy – TULIP
TULIP was performed using a probe consisting of a Nd:YAG laser adjacent to an ultrasound transducer, with a balloon designed to keep the laser at a defined distance from the prostate. This probe was swept backwards and forwards from the bladder neck to the verumontanum under ultrasound guidance. No comparative studies of TULIP versus TURP have been reported, although data from the TULIP National Human Cooperative Study Group[49] suggested improvement in symptom scores in the order of 70% at 6 months of follow-up. However, less modest improvements with longer follow-up suggest that the effects are not durable[50]. TULIP is no longer used and this may partly be because urologists were not comfortable with a technique that did not allow direct visualization of the tissue being treated.

Other laser delivery systems were developed using either an end-firing laser fibre applied directly onto the surface of the prostate ('contact' laser), a side-firing delivery system (so-called visual laser ablation of the prostate, VLAP) or a laser fibre introduced directly into the prostate, the so-called interstitial laser system. All these systems allowed direct visualization of the prostatic urethra during treatment.

Visual laser ablation of the prostate – VLAP
The side-firing system used either a mirror to reflect or a prism to refract the laser energy at various angles (usually 90°) from a laser fibre located in the prostatic urethra onto the surface of the prostate. Some vaporization of the surface of the prostate occured, but the principal tissue effect was one of coagulation. The coagulated tissue underwent necrosis and then sloughs over the course of several weeks.

Two well designed studies, both with a 12-month follow-up, have compared outcomes in patients randomized to VLAP or TURP. Cowles *et al*[51] reported a reduction in the AUA symptom score of 13 after TURP and 9 after VLAP, with an increase in flow rate of 7 ml/s after TURP and 5 ml/s after VLAP. Anson *et al*[52] found very similar improvements in

AUA symptom score, of 13 and 10 after TURP and VLAP respectively, and improvements in flow rate of 12 ml/s and 6 ml/s, respectively. Longer-term results are difficult to assess. In those studies that have reported on long-term outcome, many patients have been lost to follow-up[53]. Of those patients who were available for follow-up (only a third of the total originally treated), 16% of the TURP patients and 38% of the VLAP patients had required further surgical treatment.

The results have to be weighed against the advantages of VLAP. No blood transfusions were required after VLAP; indeed, it can be performed safely on patients on full anticoagulation. Nor did TUR syndrome occur, as normal saline is used as the irrigant during the procedure. Retrograde ejaculation occurred in approximately 30% of men. Postoperative urinary retention developed in 30%.

Contact laser prostatectomy

Contact laser prostatectomy produces a greater degree of vaporization than VLAP, allowing the immediate removal of tissue. This has the potential advantage of reducing the likelihood of postoperative retention, which is a problem with VLAP. A variety of specialized laser fibre tips were developed, made of sapphire, configured into a variety of shapes. Like VLAP, contact laser prostatectomy uses normal saline as the irrigation solution, so that TUR syndrome does not occur.

Contact laser prostatectomy was compared with TURP in the Oxford Laser Prostate Trial. Patients were randomized to TURP or laser prostatectomy. At 3 months of follow-up the improvement in AUA symptom score was 12 in the TURP group and 7 in the laser group[54]. By 1 and 3 years of follow-up, the improvement in symptom score was 12 following TURP and 11 after laser prostatectomy. Re-operation (principally TURP) was required in 9% of the TURP group and 18% of the laser group at 3 years of follow-up[55].

The mean duration of catheterization was 1 day after laser prostatectomy and 2 days after TURP, but the re-catheterization rate was higher in the laser group, 28% of laser patients failing to void after the postoperative catheter was removed compared with 12% in the TURP group. Thus, the hoped-for reduction in postoperative retention was not realized.

Interstitial laser prostatectomy – ILP

ILP is performed by transurethral placement of a laser fibre directly into the prostate. This produces a zone of coagulative necrosis some distance from the prostatic urethra, thereby avoiding damage to the prostatic urethra and eliminating postoperative voiding problems such as urinary retention. Open studies where all subjects were treated by ILP have shown improvements in symptom scores of between 30 and 90%. In a randomized study comparing ILP with TURP, AUA symptom score improved by 18 points after TURP and by 12 points after ILP, at 3 months of follow-up[56]. Postoperative urinary retention does not appear to have been a problem following ILP, but whether these short-term improvements in symptoms have been sustained is not known.

Holmium laser prostatectomy

The wavelength of the holmium:YAG laser is such that the energy of this form of laser is strongly absorbed by water within prostatic tissue. At the energy levels delivered it produces vaporization at the tip of the laser fibre. Its depth of penetration is <0.5 mm and thus it can be used to produce precise incisions in tissue. It has the added advantage of all laser techniques that it can be used with normal saline, and so TUR syndrome does not occur during holmium laser prostatectomy. When the beam is 'de-focused', it provides excellent haemostasis.

The holmium laser can be used for contact vaporization (holmium-only laser ablation of the prostate, HoLAP), for resection (holmium laser resection of the prostate, HoLRP[57]) or for enucleation of the prostate (holmium laser enucleation of the prostate, HoLEP). These different techniques developed in progression. Initially the holmium laser was used for contact vaporization, but this was time-consuming and only suitable for small prostates. With increasing experience advocates of the technique appreciated that the holmium laser could incise tissue and in this way chips of prostate could be formally resected, which could then be evacuated from the bladder in the usual way. In a large, randomized study comparing HoLRP with TURP, symptomatic and urodynamic outcomes at 2 years were similar, with a lower transfusion rate and shorter hospital stay after HoLRP[58].

Holmium laser resection led to the development of holmium laser enucleation (HoLEP) of the prostate. In this technique the lobes of the prostate are dissected off the capsule of the prostate and then pushed back into the bladder. A transurethral tissue morcellator is introduced into the bladder and used to slice the freed lobes into pieces that can then be removed. As with HoLRP, HoLEP has been compared with TURP in well designed, randomized studies. Improvement in symptom scores and flow rates are equivalent, and although the operation time with HoLEP is longer, catheter times and in-hospital stays are less with HoLEP[59–62].

So why does not everyone use HoLEP rather than TURP? This is partly because the laser units are costly, but these capital costs can be off-set to a degree by using the laser for other procedures such as treatment of ureteric and renal calculi. One should, however, bear in mind that the more costly a piece of equipment, the more costly the repairs. Many hospitals will only be able to afford one laser unit and thus when the laser breaks down, as will occasionally happen, you will have to wait for the laser to be repaired and this may take some time.

Evidence suggests that approximately 20–30 procedures need to be done under supervision before results similar to those of a more experienced surgeon are achieved[63]. For the surgeon who has completed his training, or for those in training jobs that do not offer experience in HoLEP or HoLRP, it is clearly difficult to gain the necessary experience to be able to operate safely on one's own. There are only a limited number of centres, principally in New Zealand and North America, where these techniques of prostatectomy are practised regularly, and so opportunities for training are limited.

Summary

A substantial proportion of men who opt for no active treatment of their symptoms – watchful waiting – will experience no worsening of their symptoms, even over several years. A patient, once reassured that his symptoms may not get worse, that he does not have prostate cancer and that he is unlikely to develop acute urinary retention, may well decide not to have any active treatment. Drug treatments for BPH produce only modest improvements in symptom scores when compared with placebo, and in the case of alpha-blockers a significant proportion of men stop taking their medication over the course of time because of side effects. The efficacy of combination therapy with both an alpha blocker and finasteride appears to be no better than that with alpha-blockers alone. Phytotherapy seems to produce improvements in symptoms equivalent to those with finasteride.

Minimally invasive treatments such as TUNA and TUMT produce symptom improvements that are intermediate between drug treatments and TURP, and at least in the case of TUMT these effects seem to be durable over a 3-year period. The morbidity after both TUNA and TUMT is less than that associated with TURP. The more invasive procedures of TUVP and holmium laser prostatectomy produce results which are equivalent to TURP. Longer-term results are needed to allow the precise role of these alternative surgical techniques in BPH treatment to be defined.

Thus, there is a wide range of potential treatment options for men presenting with BPH symptoms. In general terms, clinical practice guidelines recommend surgical treatment over medical therapy where complications such as renal impairment or recurrent acute retention have developed, or where medical therapy has failed to control severe symptoms. In uncomplicated cases, these guidelines state the importance of patient preference in deciding which treatment to have.

In terms of the precise technique used to treat the prostate in those patients who opt for surgical treatment, unless there are clear benefits of one technique over another, the majority of surgeons will tend to use the technique that they feel provides the best results in their hands.

References

1. Roehrborn CG, Bartsch G, Kirby R *et al*. Guidelines for the diagnosis and treatment of benign prostatic hyperplasia: a comparative international overview. *Urology* 2001;58:642–50.
2. Irani J, Brown CT, van der Meulen J, Emberton M. A review of guidelines on benign prostatic hyperplasia and lower urinary tract symptoms: are all guidelines the same? *Br J Urol Int* 2003;92:937–42.
3. Ball AJ, Feneley RC, Abrams PH. Natural history of untreated "prostatism". *Br J Urol* 1981;53:613–16.
4. Theodorides P, Bourke JB, Griffin JP *et al*. Clinical trial of gestronol hexanoate (SH582) in benign prostatic hypertrophy. *Proc R Soc Med* 1972;65:130–1.
5. McConnell JD, Bruskewitz R, Walsh PC *et al*. The effect of finasteride on the risk of acute urinary retention and the need for surgical treatment among men with benign prostatic hyperplasia (PLESS). *N Engl J Med* 1998;338:557–63.
6. Wasson JH, Reda DJ, Bruskewitz RC *et al*. A comparison of transurethral surgery with watchful waiting for moderate symptoms of benign prostatic hyperplasia. The Veterans Affairs Cooperative Study Group on Transurethral Resection of the Prostate. *N Engl J Med* 1995;332:75–9.
7. Barry MJ, Fowler FJJ, Bin L *et al*. The natural history of patients with benign prostatic hyperplasia as diagnosed by North American urologists. *J Urol* 1997;157:10–14.
8. McConnell JD, Barry MD, Bruskewitz RC *et al*. The BPH Guideline Panel. *Benign Prostatic Hyperplasia: Diagnosis and Treatment. Clinical Practice Guideline*. Agency for Health Care Policy and Research, Public Health Service, US Department of Health and Human Sciences, Rockville, MD; publication no. 94-0582, 1994.
9. Boyle P, Robertson C, Manski R *et al*. Meta-analysis of randomized trials of terazosin in the treatment of benign prostatic hyperplasia. *Urology* 2001;58:717–22.
10. Lowe F. Alpha-1-adrenoceptor blockade in the treatment of benign prostatic hyperplasia. *Prostate Cancer Prostatic Dis* 1999;2:110–19.
11. Neal DE. The National Prostatectomy Audit. *Br J Urol* 1997;79(Suppl 2):69–75.
12. Andersen JT, Ekman P, Wolf H *et al*. Can finasteride reverse the progress of benign prostatic hyperplasia? A two-year placebo-controlled study. The Scandinavian BPH Study Group. *Urology* 1995;46:631–7.
13. Nickel J, Fradet Y, Boake RC *et al*. Efficacy and safety of finasteride therapy for benign prostatic hyperplasia: results of a 2-year randomised controlled trial (the PROSPECT study). PROscar Safety Plus Efficacy Canadian Two Year Study. *Can Med Assoc J* 1996;155:1251–9.
14. Marberger MJ. Long-term effects of finasteride in patients with benign prostatic hyperplasia: a double-blind, placebo-controlled, multicenter study. PROWESS Study Group. *Urology* 1998;51:677–86.
15. Reynard J. Does anticholinergic medication have a role for men with lower urinary tract symptoms/benign prostatic hyperplasia either alone or in combination with other agents? *Curr Opin Urol* 2004;14:13–16.
16. McConnell JD, Roehrborn CG, Bautista OM *et al*. The long-term effect of doxazosin, finasteride, and combination therapy on the clinical progression of benign prostatic hyperplasia. *N Engl J Med* 2003;349:2387–98.

17. Lepor H, Williford WO, Barry MJ *et al*. The efficacy of terazosin, finasteride, or both in benign prostatic hypertrophy. *N Engl J Med* 1996;335:533–9.
18. Kirby RS, Roerborn C, Boyle P *et al*. Efficacy and tolerability of doxazosin and finasteride, alone or in combination, in treatment of symptomatic benign prostatic hyperplasia: the Prospective European Doxazosin and Combination Therapy (PREDICT) trial. *Urology* 2003;61:119–26.
19. Debruyne FM, Jardin A, Colloi D *et al*. Sustained-release alfuzosin, finasteride and the combination of both in the treatment of benign prostatic hyperplasia. *Eur Urol* 1998;34:169–75.
20. Thompson IM, Goodman PJ, Tangen CM *et al*. The influence of finasteride on the development of prostate cancer. *N Engl J Med* 2003;349:215–24.
21. Chapple C. BPH disease management. Introduction and concluding remarks. *Eur Urol* 1999;36(Suppl):1–6.
22. Carraro JC, Raynaud JP, Koch G *et al*. Comparison of phytotherapy (Permixon) with finasteride in the treatment of benign prostatic hyperplasia: a randomized international study of 1089 patients. *Prostate* 1996;29:231–40.
23. Wilt JW, Ishani A, Stark G *et al*. Saw palmetto extracts for treatment of benign prostatic hyperplasia: a systematic review. *JAMA* 1998;280:1604–8.
24. Berges RR, Windeler J, Trampisch H *et al*. Randomized, placebo-controlled, double-blind clinical trial of beta-sitosterol in patients with benign prostatic hyperplasia. *Lancet* 1995;345:1529–32.
25. Lowe FC, Fagelman E. Phytotherapy in the treatment of benign prostatic hyperplasia: an update. *Urology* 1999;53:671–8.
26. Gee WF, Holtgrewe HL, Blute M *et al*. 1997 American Urological Association Gallup Survey: changes in diagnosis and management of prostate cancer and benign prostatic hyperplasia and other practice trends from 1994 to 1997. *J Urol* 1998;160:1804–7.
27. Jacobsen SJ, Jacobson DJ, Girman CJ *et al*. Natural history of prostatism: risk factors for acute urinary retention. *J Urol* 1997;158:481–7.
28. Roos NP, Wennberg J, Malenka DJ *et al*. Mortality and reoperation after open and transurethral resection of the prostate for benign prostatic hyperplasia. *N Engl J Med* 1989;320:1120–4.
29. Bruskewitz R, Issa M, Roehrborn CG *et al*. A prospective, randomised, 1 year clinical trial comparing transurethral needle ablation (TUNA) to transurethral resection of the prostate for the treatment of symptomatic benign prostatic hyperplasia. *J Urol* 1998;159:1588–94.
30. Roehrborn CG, Issa MM, Bruskewitz R *et al*. Transurethral needle ablation (TUNA) for benign prostatic hyperplasia: 12-month results of a prospective multicenter study. *Urology* 1998;51:415–21.
31. Fitzpatrick JM, Mebust WK. Minimally invasive and endoscopic management of benign prostatic hyperplasia. In: Walsh PC, Retik AB, Vaughan ED, Wein AJ (eds) *Campbell's Urology*, 8th edn. Saunders, Philadelphia, PA, 2002.
32. National Institute for Clinical Excellence. Transurethral Radiofrequency Needle Ablation of the Prostate, National Institute for Clinical Excellence Interventional Procedure Guidance. London: NICE, 2003.
33. De la Rosette J, Alivizatos G, Madersbacher S *et al*. EAU Guidelines. Benign prostatic hyperplasia. *Eur Urol* 2001;40:256–63.
34. Bdesha AS, Schachter M, Sever P *et al*. Radioligand-binding analysis of human prostatic alpha-1 adrenoreceptor density following transurethral microwave therapy. *Br J Urol* 1996;78:886–92.
35. de la Rosette JJMCH, de Wildt MJAM, Alivizatos G *et al*. Transurethral microwave thermotherapy (TUMT) in benign prostatic hyperplasia: placebo versus TUMT. *Urology* 1994;44:58–63.
36. Blute ML, Patterson DE, Segura JW *et al*. Transurethral microwave thermotherapy v sham treatment: double-blind randomized study. *J Endourol* 1996;10:565–73.

37. de Wildt MJAM, Hubregtse M, Ogden C *et al*. A 12 month study of the placebo effect in transurethral microwave thermotherapy. *Br J Urol* 1996;77:221–7.
38. Larson TR, Blute ML, Bruskewitz RC *et al*. A high-efficiency microwave thermo-ablation system for the treatment of benign prostatic hyperplasia: results of a randomized, sham controlled, prospective, double-blind, multicenter clinical trial. *Urology* 1998;51:731–42.
39. Roehrborn CG, Preminger G, Newhall P *et al*. Microwave thermotherapy for benign prostatic hyperplasia with the Dormier Urowave: results of a randomized, double blind, multicenter, sham-controlled study. *Urology* 1998;51:19–28.
40. Djavan B, Ghawidel K, Basharkhah A *et al*. Pre-treatment prostate-specific antigen as an outcome predictor of targeted transurethral microwave thermotherapy. *Urology* 2000;55:51–7.
41. Nawrocki JD, Bell TJ, Lawrence WT *et al*. A randomized controlled trial of transurethral microwave therapy. *Br J Urol* 1997;79:389–93.
42. Ramsey EW, Miller PD, Parsons K. Transurethral microwave thermotherapy in the treatment of benign prostatic hyperplasia: results obtained with the Urologix T3 device. *World J Urol* 1998;16:96–101.
43. D'Ancona FCH, Francisca EAE, Witjes WPJ *et al*. Transurethral resection of the prostate vs high-energy thermotherapy of the prostate in patients with benign prostatic hyperplasia: long-term results. *Br J Urol* 1998;81:259–64.
44. Sullivan LD, McLoughlin MG, Goldenberg LG *et al*. Early experience with high-intensity focused ultrasound for the treatment of benign prostatic hyperplasia. *Br J Urol* 1997;79:172–6.
45. Madersbacher S, Kratzik C, Susani M, Marberger M. Tissue ablation in benign prostatic hyperplasia with high intensity focused ultrasound. *J Urol* 1994;152:1956–61.
46. McAllister WJ, Karim O, Plail RO *et al*. Transurethral electrovaporization of the prostate: is it any better than conventional transurethral resection of the prostate? *Br J Urol Int* 2003;91:211–14.
47. Hammadeh MY, Madaan S, Hines J, Philp T. Transurethral electrovaporization of the prostate after 5 years: is it effective and durable. *Br J Urol Int* 2000;86:648–51.
48. National Institute for Clinical Excellence. *Interventional Procedure Guidance 14*. London: NICE, 2003.
49. McCullough DL, Roth RA, Babayan RK *et al*. Transurethral ultrasound-guided laser-induced prostatectomy: National Human Cooperative Study results. *J Urol* 1993;150:1607–11.
50. Chatzopoulos C, Lorge FJ, Opsomer RJ *et al*. Transurethral ultrasound-guided laser-induced prostatectomy: a critical evaluation. *J Endourol* 1996;10:463–76.
51. Cowles RS, Kabalin JN, Childs S *et al*. A prospective randomised comparison of transurethral resection to visual laser ablation of the prostate for the treatment of benign prostatic hyperplasia. *Urology* 1995;46:155–8.
52. Anson K, Nawrocki J, Buckley J *et al*. A multicenter randomised prospective study of endoscopic laser ablation versus transurethral resection of the prostate. *Urology* 1995;43:305–10.
53. McAllister WJ, Absalom MJ, Mir K *et al*. Does endoscopic laser ablation of the prostate stand the test of time? Five year results from a multicentre randomised controlled trial of endoscopic laser ablation against transurethral resection of the prostate. *Br J Urol Int* 2000;85:437–9.
54. Keoghane S, Cranston DW, Lawrence KC *et al*. The Oxford Laser Prostate Trial: a double-blind randomised controlled trial of contact vaporisation of the prostate against transurethral resection: preliminary results. *Br J Urol* 1996;77:382–5.
55. Keoghane S, Lawrence K, Gray A *et al*. A double-blind randomised controlled trial and economic evaluation of transurethral resection vs contact laser vaporisation for benign prostatic enlargement. *Br J Urol Int* 2000;85:74–8.
56. Whitfield N. A randomized prospective multicenter study evaluating the efficacy of interstitial laser coagulation. *J Urol* 1996;155:318A.

57. Gilling PJ, Cass CB, Cresswell MD *et al*. Holmium laser resection of the prostate: preliminary results of a new method for the treatment of benign prostatic hyperplasia. *Urology* 1996;47:48–51.
58. Gilling PJ, Kennett KM, Fraundorfer MR *et al*. Holmium laser resection of the prostate (HoLRP) versus transurethral resection of the prostate (TURP): results of a randomised trial with 2 years follow-up. *J Endourol* 2000;14:757–60.
59. Gilling PJ, Kennett KM, Westenberg AM *et al*. Holmium laser enucleation of the prostate (HoLEP) is superior to TURP for the relief of bladder outflow obstruction (BOO): a randomised trial with 2 year follow-up. *J Urol* 2003;169:1465.
60. Gilling PJ, Kennett KM, Fraundorfer MR. Holmium laser enucleation of the prostate for glands larger than 100 g – an endourologic alternative to open prostatectomy. *J Endourol* 2000;14:529–31.
61. Moody JA, Lingeman JE. Holmium laser enucleation for prostate adenoma greater than 100 gm: comparison to open prostatectomy. *J Urol* 2001;165:459–62.
62. Kuntz RM, Lehrich K. Transurethral holmium laser enucleation versus transvesical open enucleation for prostate adenoma greater than 100 g: a randomized prospective trial of 120 patients. *J Urol* 2002;168:1465–9.
63. El-Hakim A, Elhilali MM. Laser enucleation of the prostate can be taught: the first learning experience. *Br J Urol Int* 2002;90:863–9.

Chapter 13

Medico-legal aspects of transurethral resection

It is an unfortunate fact of surgical life that the risk of being involved in litigation has increased enormously during the latter part of the twentieth century and into the twenty-first century, to the extent that today few surgeons get through their professional lifetime without being sued at least once. Transurethral resection seems to cause rather less litigation than many other procedures, but has its own areas of risk, which need to be considered.

Litigation after any operation more often than not arises because something unexpected occurs. The patient believes, or the relatives believe, that something has gone wrong. They then interpret this as having been due to an error by the surgeon, and go on to make the assumption that such an error on his part must have involved negligence. Litigation follows.

Any surgeon may make a mistake from time to time, but only a very few are incompetent. However, every surgeon owes the patient a duty of care. If that duty of care is breached then the Court may adjudge that breach to be negligent. A breach of duty may be founded upon a positive act or acts of 'commission' by the surgeon (i.e. carelessly doing something which he/she ought not to have done), but it may equally be founded on an act or acts of 'omission' (i.e. carelessly failing to do something which he/she ought to have done). Lawyers refer to the surgeon's negligent breach of his duty of care as his 'liability'. Any harm, damage and consequential financial loss suffered by the patient as a result of (or – in legal jargon – 'causation by') a negligent breach of care is the basis upon which the Court assesses compensation: such compensation is known as 'damages'. The amount (or 'quantum') of an award of damages will depend upon the extent of the harm, damage and consequential financial loss which is proved in any given case. Sometimes, an award will not involve compensation for financial loss and will be confined to damages for so-called 'pain and suffering' (for example, where a patient is not in employment and/or where the harm suffered by him is relatively minor and has no permanent effects). Where, on the other hand, the harm suffered results in a permanent and serious disability which restricts (or even prevents) the patient from carrying on with his pre-operation employment, then obviously the award of damages will be very much larger.

The judgement as to whether an act or omission is negligent is a subtle one. It has to be related to a bedrock of basic standards of knowledge below which one cannot go. It also must be related to standards of experience; so an act or omission which causes a problem may not be found by a Court to be negligent if performed (or not performed) by a junior trainee, but would be so found if done (or not done) by a consultant of many years' standing. The point in time when the supposedly negligent act or omission took place will also be significant – a complication that was acceptable 5 years ago may no longer be so, due to changes in techniques, preventative measures or understanding. The judgement of what is negligent may vary as practices vary, surgery being an imprecise art. It is a defence to a civil action in negligence if it can be shown that, in relation to a particular act or omission, a body of surgeons would have done (or not done) the same even if others disagree. This is the so-called *Bolam* defence. Latterly this defence has been qualified so that an act/omission is defensible only so long as there is a logical basis for the act or omission (the *Bolitho* modification of the *Bolam* defence).

But litigation may start when there has been no negligence. Probably 50% of allegations have no basis in fact, so why should they be made? A few arise from malice, or the perception that there is money to be made, and some arise from the distorted perception by a diseased mind of what has happened. Sometimes there is arrogance on the part of the surgeon, who may feel that the patient has no right or need to be given explanations – in years gone by this was a commonplace attitude, but is happily rare today. There may be a simple lack of courtesy on the part of the surgeon – polite surgeons do not often get sued without reason. However, most unfounded allegations of negligence arise from a simple failure to communicate between patient and surgeon. This can on the one hand arise as a result of a failure by the surgeon to explain clearly and, on the other, by a failure of the patient to understand what is being said. Most commonly the loss of proper communication is a failure by the surgeon to judge his or her patient's ability to understand the situation. It is sometimes hard to realize just how ignorant a person may be about the workings of his or her body, let alone understand how the surgeon intends to modify it. That ignorance has little to do with social or educational status – a High Court judge may have less understanding of anatomy or physiology than a filing clerk. So the surgeon must put as much thought, skill and care into the explanation of the treatment as has been put into the diagnosis and investigation of the condition about to be treated.

Failure of communication is not, of course, restricted to the pre-operative period. Good communication is essential after the operation, even if nothing untoward occurs. If complications do occur, if something went wrong during the operation or if something unexpected occurred, good communication becomes even more important, as this is when the idea of litigation may germinate. A clear explanation that is understood by the patient and the relatives, if necessary accompanied by an apology (which is not an admission of liability), will go a very long way towards preventing that germ of suspicion growing into subsequent litigation. It is the regular experience of many lawyers that the first real explanation ever understood by the patient was that given in the litigation expert witness's report.

Clearly it is necessary to ensure that the standard of history taking, physical examination and investigation before an operation are appropriate. Similarly it is essential to ensure that the operation is done carefully and accurately and that aftercare is appropriate. It is absolutely vital to document all this activity accurately and legibly in a set of records written at the time, so that, if necessary, you can prove what you did and why. This takes time, particularly because it must be done for every single case, but it is time well spent. Remember, if you haven't documented what you said, it could be argued that you never said it!

With today's atmosphere of potential litigation it is easy to fall into a defensive attitude and to over-investigate patients. However, the sensible surgeon can avoid litigation, or mitigate litigation, by appropriate care in these areas without going to extremes – there is no need to resort to doing magnetic resonance or CT scanning in men with bladder outflow obstruction, for example. Such elaborate investigations need only be done if circumstances indicate that it is necessary. As noted in Chapter 4, the most rigourously constructed BPH guidelines are actually those that recommend the least number of routine investigations, so more is not necessarily better.

It is necessary to warn patients of certain outcomes of your proposed operation, or the possible complications that may arise. In the past these have been selected on the basis of their frequency of incidence, their severity or their unpleasantness. For example, it is necessary to warn men that they will have troublesome urinary frequency with pain on uri-nation, urgency and possible urge incontinence when the catheter is first removed after TURP. Although these symptoms are not a sign of a significant problem, they are unpleasant and universal, so you must tell your patient that they will occur. Deep vein thrombosis and pulmonary embolism, on the other hand, are rare complications after TUR and in the past did not warrant a warning. Although the possible outcome was grave, the risk was small. However, the medico-legal climate has changed and it is now necessary to warn of this complication because some complications carry such far-reaching consequences that they merit explanation even if the risk is so small. All urological surgeons will be familiar with the necessity to warn of the possible spontaneous late return of fertility after vasectomy – the incidence is tiny, but its effect is not. The possible significance of such a small risk was brought into the medico-legal arena many years ago when a neurosurgeon was sued successfully by a patient who developed a rare but well-documented complication after an operation (*Sidaway*). This significance has been underlined recently by an Australian High Court decision in 1992 that an ophthalmic surgeon was guilty of negligence for not warning of the tiny risk (1 in 40 000) of losing vision in the normal eye after surgery to the contralateral eye[1] (*Rogers v. Whittaker*). So the *Bolam* test – the defence that a group of reasonably competent doctors would have done the same – may no longer be the impregnable defence that it has been in the past, as the Courts may move away from it towards a Rogers and Whittaker 'reasonable patient' test in cases involving consent.

The difficulty that the surgeon now has to face will be in deciding what a reasonable patient would wish to know. On whose advice or on what evidence will the Court make a decision about what a reasonable patient would want to know? Using the *Bolam* test, expert witnesses provide evidence to the court and, using this information, the Court makes a decision. If the test becomes the *Rogers v. Whittaker* test, the court will have to make its own assessment of whether a risk was a material one or not. There may be additional problems in adopting the *Rogers v. Whittaker* approach to what a patient thinks is appropriate, as the perception of information provided or not provided may change with events. Once a patient knows more about a risk or complication – usually when they have just experienced it – they are likely to think that information about this risk should have been given prior to the procedure. For the doctor, all of this presents the dilemma of uncertainty and there is a risk that surgeons may respond by overloading patients with information.

Complications may occur after any operation. In a perfect world it should be possible to quantify the risk of any particular complication, but many episodes go unpublished in the literature, so that any survey of operative outcomes is necessarily incomplete and the true incidence of a complication may be significantly greater than is actually recognized. Documented complications in themselves are not reasonable grounds for litigation, unless there is clear evidence that the appropriate skill has not been used, or the necessary precautions were omitted. It is easy to assume that because a particular complication of a certain operation is a recognized complication its occurrence cannot be regarded as arising from negligence. However, if it can be demonstrated that the complication occurred because the surgeon failed to take a specific precaution that had been identified beforehand as appropriate to eliminate or lessen the incidence of that complication the Court may find the surgeon negligent. For example, septicaemia is a recognized complication of TURP and antibiotic prophylaxis can reduce the risk of this occurring. Failure to give antibiotic prophylaxis to an at-risk patient undergoing TURP who subsequently develops septicaemia could be construed as negligence.

Things change. Whether for better or worse may be a matter of opinion, but sometimes a surgeon has failed to notice a change going on in attitudes or practices affecting aspects of his or her work. A complication arising after an operation that hitherto he or she had thought was a recognized and acceptable risk of the particular procedure may have become an unacceptable one. This may arise as a result of any one of a number of reasons, commonly because of a better understanding of the causes of the problem, and therefore its prevention, but also because of progress in specific treatment for the problem or its cause. Constant attention to the current medical literature, continuing medical education (CME) and participation in departmental death and complication meetings with appropriate departmental audit should be a guard against such failures to keep up to date.

So, if the surgeon sets out to investigate a patient using appropriate and established tests, establishes a diagnosis according to orthodox contemporary knowledge, gives appropriate advice, writes that sequence of events clearly in the records and finally makes sure that the patient really understands what is proposed, he or she should be immune from suit. Or that is the theory!

Like any other operation transurethral resection is open to the possibility of litigation. How may this be coped with? There are a number of general principles and a number of specific areas of risk.

It goes without saying that clear communication is essential at all times. Use simple words. Speak in the vernacular rather than using technical terms – talk of peeing, not micturition, balls, not testicles – to ensure understanding. Use simple images. Ensure that the message is being received – is his deaf-aid working? Are your words being understood by a patient whose first language is not the same as your own? Repeat the explanation if in doubt, changing the words and images if necessary. Clear, simple diagrams are useful tools in the promotion of understanding. Perhaps you can keep a diagram of the bladder and prostate before and after transurethral resection on the desk, which you can show to the patient during the consultation. You may draw such diagrams in the patient's notes. This is not only a good way of explaining the reasons why a procedure is needed and the possible risks, but also serves as a permanent record of the efforts you made to explain the nature of the procedure. When you have finished your explanation of the plan of treatment it is a sensible idea to ask the patient what it is he thinks you are going to do. Do not just ask if has understood what you have said, get him to tell you what he has understood you to have said. If he cannot explain it to you, you have not made it clear to him.

The most senior member of the operating team should provide the explanation, preferably the operating surgeon. The individual providing the explanation should then obtain the patient's signed consent for the operation planned and should countersign the declaration to say that the procedure has been explained. It has become common practice for this to be done at the end of the final pre-operative consultation, rather than leaving it until admission to the ward. In the UK all hospitals have recently adopted a standardized form for this purpose. More recently still the British Association of Urological Surgeons (BAUS) Procedure Specific Consent Forms have been produced in an attempt to stan-dardize the process of consent for urological surgery. The process of obtaining consent has become fairly tedious and time-consuming. Unfortunately it is the only way you can guard yourself against vexatious litigation, so it is actually time well spent. Pre-operative explanation and consent is <u>not</u> for the admitting house surgeon, the ward nursing staff, the anaesthetist or a passing medical student.

Pre-admission clinics are now widespread in the UK, where patients are screened and examined by junior staff at a suitable interval before the admission for the planned operation. While the notes from these clinics need to be recorded with care, these clinics – generally speaking – are not appropriate places for the main explanation of the proposed surgery to be given, or consent obtained, as the doctors seeing the patients are usually junior members of the surgical team. However, if a consultant is able to be present at the pre-admission clinic, then consent may be taken at this time if it was not obtained at the clinic when the decision to operate was made. There is much to be said for obtaining consent some days or weeks before the operation. This provides a cooling off period, allowing the patient time for contemplation, giving him the opportunity to ask questions that did not originally spring to mind and giving him time to change his mind.

Many urological surgeons provide an explanatory pamphlet or leaflet that sets out the information they wish to transmit to the patient about transurethral resection. If you decide to use such an explanatory pam-phlet, how do you set about creating it? First of all it needs to be couched in simple language. Then it may be divided conveniently into several sections, arranged in a logical sequence to present the informa-tion you wish to impart. A good place to start is with an explanation of what the prostate is and what it does, followed by a very brief explana-tion of the mechanics of the proposed operation.

Next the document should set out what the patient needs to know and do <u>before coming into hospital</u>, especially if he is to be admitted on the day of the proposed surgery. This section should include such matters as whether or not to take their regular medication (e.g. stopping their regular aspirin a week prior to admission), having a bath or shower before admission, going without food and drink, pre-operative bowel action, etc. It is wise to give some suggestions as to what arrangements need to be made at home, before admission, in preparation for return there after the operation, especially if it is your practice to send the patient home within a day or so of surgery. This is particularly important for an elderly man who lives alone or who has a frail or disabled spouse.

Then the leaflet should describe what the patient may expect <u>on admission to the ward</u>. This should include a brief outline of what the nursing staff will do and that there will be a visit from the surgeon and anaesthetist, who will explain their plans and provide an opportunity for any further questions to be asked by the patient. Most hospitals provide general information to all patients concerning the planned admission, so the TUR pamphlet does not need to go into exhaustive detail if the situation has been described clearly already – find out what your hospital provides so that you do not duplicate information unnecessarily.

The pamphlet should then describe what will happen immediately <u>after the operation</u>, which will depend upon your local practices. This section should contain information about the urethral catheter, what a catheter is and does, why it will not fall out, that it is connected to a urine bag and whether or not it will be connected to a bladder washout. It is wise to provide a warning that the patient's first waking sensation after transurethral resection is usually a fierce desire to urinate but that the catheter is taking care of that problem. Make sure, by a clear explanation, that the presence of blood in the catheter urine is to be expected and is not an indication that all is not well. Mention the use of postoperative painkillers and how to get them if necessary. Explain what happens when the catheter is removed, when it is likely to be removed and what will happen when it has been removed – urinary frequency, dysuria, urgency, temporary leaks, etc.

The final section should include a brief outline about what is likely to happen <u>after going home</u>. This should include the plan for postoperative review in the urology clinic as well as what to do if things do not seem right. Advice about the timing of resumption of physical activities (including sexual intercourse) is essential. Tell your patient when he may reasonably expect to be able to drive his car and when it is sensible to go back to work, bearing in mind the nature of your patient's work – an office worker can probably expect to go back to full work earlier than a labourer. The possibility of unexpected secondary haemorrhage, both minor and major, and what to do about it should be included in this section.

This may sound a daunting catalogue, but it can usually be condensed into a few sides of A5 paper with a little thought. The advantage of such a leaflet is that the patient can take it home and refer to the various points when a doubt arises, or when he cannot remember what you told him. It is also useful reading for the patient's spouse! Its final function is to be available as a rebuttal to the tales of his well-meaning friends who take such innocent pleasure in telling him grisly tales of what happened to their grandfather or uncle when they had a prostate operation, often many years before!

Possible complications may be included in this pamphlet if you wish. There is a risk that providing too much information may simply mean than none of it gets read by the patient. However, if your pamphlet does contain an explanation of possible complications no one can claim subsequently that they were not given the information.

Make sure that the staff of the ward into which your patient is to be admitted all know exactly what operation is proposed, what explanation has been given and what warnings have been provided. Ensure that your particular habits are clearly understood by the nursing staff, perhaps you aim to remove the catheter after transurethral resection after 24 hours regardless of circumstances, whereas your colleague removes it when he is happy that there is no more haematuria. There is nothing worse than a patient receiving contradictory information. Many hospitals use a set of individual ward protocols to ensure that all the necessary points are covered for each operation.

With regard to risks and complications, how much information should you provide? The amount and nature of the information that patients receive can be daunting for the surgeon and frightening for the patient. However, do not forget that it is your duty as a surgeon to give adequate information to the patient concerning the benefits and risks of a procedure, unpleasant though that information may be. No one likes to talk about serious complications, but you should not shy away from discussing these issues with the excuse that you are trying to 'protect' the patient. There are a number of complications associated with TURP that must be discussed with each man advised to undergo transurethral resection. The BAUS Procedure Specific Consent Forms do not require that you mention every single complication that can occur after TURP. While it is quite obviously impossible to mention all possible complications, erring on the side of giving more information rather than less is a safe practice to adopt, bearing mind the case-law mentioned above. Litigation is far more likely to occur if you have *not* warned a patient of a particular complication than if you have warned him that it could occur. Patients often want more information than we think they do and one should be careful to avoid the assumption that they don't want to hear about particular risks. The BAUS Procedure Specific Forms do provide a basis upon which consent can be obtained.

It is perfectly possible to talk gently about any serious risks without frightening the patient, but it will depend on you having already established a friendly relationship and perhaps by emphasizing the likelihood that a serious complication is <u>not</u> going to happen. For instance a risk of a 1 in 200 chance of death can be put the other way round – that 199 out of 200 men leave hospital fit and well, which sounds like better odds!

Occasionally you will meet a patient who specifically expresses a desire <u>not</u> to know about any unpleasant or serious risks. A way around this is to suggest to the patient that he is actually putting you in a difficult position and that it is unacceptable to perform a procedure that does carry significant risks without being able to explain in advance what these risks are. An alternative is to talk to a close relative or friend about the risks, with the patient's consent. In any case, making sure the relatives are au fait with the ins and outs of the proposed operation is a good principle to follow when obtaining consent for any procedure. It is to be borne in mind that, if a very serious complication does occur, it will often be a close relative with whom you will be communicating afterwards.

It is worth bearing in mind that in the light of the Bristol paediatric heart scandal[2] there is a move towards surgeons being required to warn patients of their individual outcomes and complications, rather than relying on national or international figures. Audit of your own outcomes will allow you to modify the discussion with regard to the complications discussed in the next few paragraphs.

There are a number of specific points that must be discussed with each man being advised to undergo transurethral resection. The patient must understand that there are various complications that may occur, the reasons for them if they do occur and their management. He must also know that certain things are an inevitable sequel of the procedure and <u>will</u> happen. The BAUS Procedure Specific Consent Forms recommend that all men should be aware of the alternatives to TURP such as observation, drug treatments, catheters or open prostatectomy. All men need to know that after a TURP there will be blood in the urine after the operation, with a warning that very occasionally this is severe and may need blood transfusion and rarely return to the operating theatre. Absorption of irrigating fluid leading to confusion and heart failure (the TUR syndrome) should be mentioned as a rare possibility. The BAUS Procedure Specific Consent Forms recommend that the patient should be warned that very rarely perforation of the bladder can occur, even during TURP, and that this may require a longer period of catheter drainage than normal, or even a formal open operation for its repair.

What should we tell men about to have a TURP?

- With regard to the postoperative period, it is essential that everyone knows that they will have frequency, burning and urgency of micturition for a while after the catheter has been removed and that this may take a matter of weeks to subside, but is part of the natural healing process. In this context the risk that detrusor instability associated with the existing bladder outflow obstruction may not subside postoperatively must be mentioned, which can lead to a degree of urge incontinence.
- It is sensible to warn that some men cannot urinate when the catheter is removed postoperatively so that it needs to be replaced temporarily. The risk of this occurring after a TURP for symptoms alone is very low, but if the TURP is being done in a man with retention of urine the risk of not being able to void goes up to around 1 in 5–10. The greater the retention volume the higher the risk, so it may be difficult to get men with long-standing chronic retention voiding spontaneously.
- The risk of severe bleeding mentioned above can be set out, making clear that it is very unlikely to happen.
- The inevitability of minor bleeding occurring after the patient has gone home must be mentioned and the warning given that the occasional man will have a brisk and alarmingly red bleed a couple of weeks after the operation. Give the reassurance that it will stop spontaneously and the advice to drink generously to help wash it away. It is not necessary to mention the possibility of clot retention as that is very unusual and a warning may cause unnecessary anxiety.
- The remote possibility of TUR syndrome should be included.
- It is wise to mention the small risk of postoperative bladder infection.
- The patient should be told that a pathologist will examine the tissue that is removed at TURP and that in a proportion of cases a prostate cancer will inadvertently be found and this may require further investigation and treatment.

The longer-term outcomes, complications and risks then need to be dealt with.

- If the operation is being done for symptoms alone, the patient should be made aware that a proportion of men may not experience any improvement in their symptoms. This may occur in the order of 20% of cases. Some symptoms, such as nocturia and urgency are less likely to improve than are hesitancy and poor flow.

- It is essential to warn <u>all</u> men about to have a transurethral resection of the prostate or bladder neck, or a bladder neck incision, that they are more likely than not to have retrograde ejaculation of semen postoperatively and that this will be a permanent situation. This occurs after approximately 20% of bladder neck incisions and at least 75% of TURPs. It is absolutely essential to discuss this with younger men, particularly because of the desire to retain fertility in this age group. Many older men accept retrograde ejaculation as no more than a curious occurrence, but some find it intolerable not to have been warned of the likelihood. This warning must be documented in the clinical record, as should all potential risks and complications.
- It is necessary to warn that there is a risk of erectile dysfunction postoperatively. Make a note that you have told the patient that there is a chance that he may permanently lose the ability to get an erection. This is a rather long-winded way of saying impotence, but not all men understand what impotence is. For a condition where the implications both for the patient and for the doctor can be profound, it is important to make it as clear as possible what you mean. Statistics available are almost certainly incomplete, but it does seem that somewhere around 5–10% of men undergoing transurethral surgery for bladder outflow obstruction will suffer erectile dysfunction postoperatively and that this figure will tend to increase with the passage of years and with the 'quality' of erections prior to surgery. Most men who are actually capable of penetrative sexual intercourse before transurethral resection of the prostate or bladder neck, or bladder neck incision, will continue to be able to enjoy worthwhile sexual intercourse afterwards, although usually without ejaculation. Not all men are completely honest about their sexual prowess, or their sexual activity may have ceased to be a matter of great concern, but it is necessary to warn all men that there is a small risk of losing the ability to get a worthwhile erection. Never assume that it is not likely to be a cause for concern because the patient in question is over ninety! This warning should also be documented in the clinical record.
- Mention should be made of the possibility that the sensation of orgasm may be lost or altered after TURP. In the National Prostatectomy Audit this occurred in 52% of men.
- The risk of urinary incontinence needs to be mentioned, if only to emphasize that it is a small risk in the region of 3% unless there are predisposing pre-operative causes.
- Similarly the small risk of urethral stricture after endoscopic surgery must be mentioned, again if only to underline its low incidence.
- Finally the chance of needing a repeat operation for a late return of symptoms must be quantified – about 10–20% after 10 years.

For TURBT, the BAUS Procedure Specific Consent Forms give useful guidance. You should warn your patient of a number of points.

- The patient should be made aware that radiotherapy or cystectomy may become necessary after the findings of the TURBT are known.
- There will be a need for a catheter after the operation, almost certainly with bladder irrigation.
- There will be urinary burning and frequency when the catheter is removed.
- There is a risk of postoperative bleeding, occasionally requiring clot evacuation, both immediately after the operation and then secondarily after they have gone home.
- The small risk of perforation of the bladder requiring prolonged catheter drainage or even open surgical repair should be explained.
- The patient should be told that additional treatment such as intravesical chemotherapy might be necessary.
- It must be made clear that you cannot guarantee that complete removal of the cancer with cure of the disease can be achieved by this operation alone. Make it clear that recurrence may occur, so that follow-up is necessary.

Litigation based upon these risks can usually be avoided if it is possible to demonstrate clearly that they have been aired with the patient pre-operatively. If a pamphlet is used it is necessary to record in the clinical notes that the patient has been given one. Clear contemporaneous notes of the warnings given are the best way of proving that you have discussed the risks pre-operatively. This is time-consuming, but so is trying to defend a case because your documentation does not provide adequate support for what you said or what you think you said to the patient!

Having said all that, there is a risk that you will get involved in litigation when strange and rare complications arise, but these should be entirely defensible. The occurrence of what is a recognized complication of an operation is defensible if a clear warning has been provided (and can be <u>demonstrated</u> to have been provided) and the necessary precautions against its occurrence had been taken. Some complications of certain operations are all too well recognized, but are not defensible against an allegation of negligence if there are reasonable and established methods of avoiding them which the surgeon has not followed.

References

1. Rogers v. Whittaker (1992) 67 ALJR 47.
2. Horton R. How should doctors respond to the GMC's judgements on Bristol? *Lancet* 1998;351:1900–1.

Index

Note: page numbers in *italics* refer to figures